Emerging Materials and Technologies for Bone Repair and Regeneration

This book covers advancements in the field of bone repair and regeneration. It introduces bone development, repair, and regeneration and details different biomaterials and technologies involved in the fabrication and characterization of bone-related scaffolds and implants. The book explores nanotechnological intervention and folklore phytomedicines and their prospects in regenerating bone including major bone related disease conditions, infection, and their tackling via tissue engineering strategies.

FEATURES:

- Covers polymer materials and technologies for bone repair and regeneration based on tissue engineering
- Defines the interdisciplinary mechanism of bone tissue repair ranging from the fields of material science, nanotechnology, and phytomedicine includes basic sciences, scaffolds, and bone infection
- Examines fabrication and characterization methods for the bone repair materials
- Reviews fundamentals of interlinked mechanisms of bone development, repair, and regeneration.

This book is aimed at graduate students and researchers in biomedical and tissue engineering and biomaterial sciences.

Emerging Materials and Technologies

Series Editor: Boris I. Kharissov

The *Emerging Materials and Technologies* series is devoted to highlighting publications centered on emerging advanced materials and novel technologies. Attention is paid to those newly discovered or applied materials with potential to solve pressing societal problems and improve quality of life, corresponding to environmental protection, medicine, communications, energy, transportation, advanced manufacturing, and related areas.

The series takes into account that, under present strong demands for energy, material, and cost savings, as well as heavy contamination problems and worldwide pandemic conditions, the area of emerging materials and related scalable technologies is a highly interdisciplinary field, with the need for researchers, professionals, and academics across the spectrum of engineering and technological disciplines. The main objective of this book series is to attract more attention to these materials and technologies and invite conversation among the international R&D community.

Emerging Materials and Technologies for Bone Repair and Regeneration
Edited by Ashok Kumar, Sneha Singh, and Prerna Singh

Mechanics of Auxetic Materials and Structures
Farzad Ebrahimi

Nanomaterials for Sustainable Hydrogen Production and Storage
Edited by Jude A. Okolie, Emmanuel I. Epelle, Alivia Mukherjee, and Alaa El Din Mahmoud

Calcium-Based Materials
Processing, Characterization, and Applications
Edited by S.S. Nanda, Jitendra Pal Singh, Sanjeev Gautam, and Dong Kee Yi

Advanced Synthesis and Medical Applications of Calcium Phosphates
Edited by S.S. Nanda, Jitendra Pal Singh, Sanjeev Gautam, and Dong Kee Yi

Non-Metallic Technical Textiles
Materials and Technologies
Mukesh Kumar Sinha and Ritu Pandey

Smart Micro- and Nanomaterials for Drug Delivery: Two-Volume Set
Edited by Ajit Behera, Arpan Kumar Nayak, Ranjan K. Mohapatra, and Ali Ahmed Rabaan

Smart Micro- and Nanomaterials for Drug Delivery: Volume One
Edited by Ajit Behera, Arpan Kumar Nayak, Ranjan K. Mohapatra, and Ali Ahmed Rabaan

Smart Micro- and Nanomaterials for Pharmaceutical Applications
Edited by Ajit Behera, Arpan Kumar Nayak, Ranjan K. Mohapatra, and Ali Ahmed Rabaan

Friction Stir-Spot Welding
Metallurgical, Mechanical and Tribological Properties
Edited by Jeyaprakash Natarajan and K. Anton Savio Lewise

For more information about this series, please visit: www.routledge.com/Emerging-Materials-and-Technologies/book-series/CRCEMT

Emerging Materials and Technologies for Bone Repair and Regeneration

Edited by Ashok Kumar, Sneha Singh, and Prerna Singh

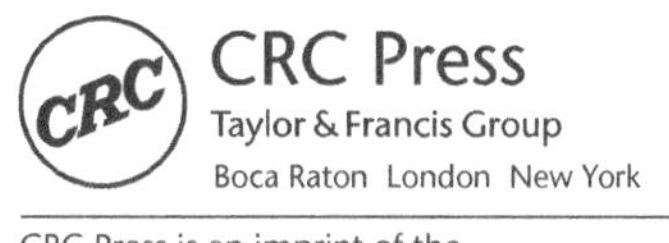

CRC Press is an imprint of the
Taylor & Francis Group, an **informa** business

Designed cover image: Cover image presents the 3D micro-CT picture acquired using CTVox that shows the T10 vertebrae of a guinea pig, where a defect area of 2 mm was filled with bioactive ceramic material for bone regeneration (Editor's unpublished work).

First edition published 2025
by CRC Press
2385 NW Executive Center Drive, Suite 320, Boca Raton FL 33431

and by CRC Press
4 Park Square, Milton Park, Abingdon, Oxon, OX14 4RN

CRC Press is an imprint of Taylor & Francis Group, LLC

Library of Congress Cataloging-in-Publication Data
Names: Kumar, Ashok, 1963– editor. | Singh, Sneha, editor. | Singh, Prerna, Ph.D. editor.
Title: Emerging materials and technologies for bone repair and regeneration / edited by Ashok Kumar, Sneha Singh, and Prerna Singh.
Other titles: Emerging materials and technologies.
Description: First edition. | Boca Raton, FL : CRC Press, 2024. | Series: Emerging materials and technologies | Includes bibliographical references and index.
Subjects: MESH: Bone Regeneration | Tissue Engineering—methods | Biocompatible Materials—therapeutic use | Nanotechnology—methods | Bone Diseases—therapy
Classification: LCC R857.T55 (print) | LCC R857.T55 (ebook) | NLM WE 202 | DDC 610.28—dc23/eng/20240506
LC record available at https://lccn.loc.gov/2024002936
LC ebook record available at https://lccn.loc.gov/2024002937

ISBN: 978-1-032-30927-9 (hbk)
ISBN: 978-1-032-30932-3 (pbk)
ISBN: 978-1-003-30731-0 (ebk)

DOI: 10.1201/9781003307310

Typeset in Times
by Apex CoVantage, LLC

Support Material URL: www.routledge.com/9781032309279

Dedicated to our
Mentor, Parents, & Family

Contents

II Application of Nanotechnology and Phytomedicines for Bone Repair and Regeneration

About the Editors

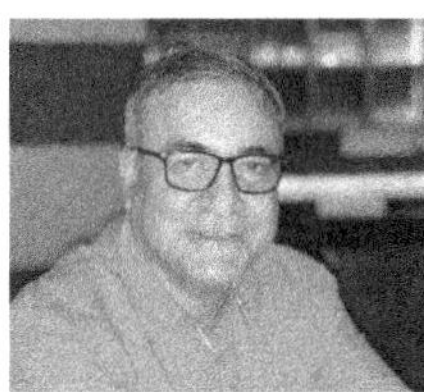

Prof. Ashok Kumar is a chair professor of bioengineering at the Department of Biological Sciences and Bioengineering, Indian Institute of Technology (IIT), Kanpur, India. He received his Ph.D. in Biotechnology from IIT Roorkee. He conducted his postdoctoral research at Nagoya University, Japan, and Lund University, Sweden. He has published more than 230 research papers, edited five books, has many patents granted/filed, and has transferred technologies to industry. His areas of research interest include biomaterials, tissue engineering, regenerative medicine, bioprocess engineering, and environmental biotechnology. Prof. Kumar has been conducting active national and international research collaborations and has been recognized with various awards and appreciations for his outstanding research contributions. He has been conferred the honorary doctorate, D.Sc. Technology by Aalto University, Finland.

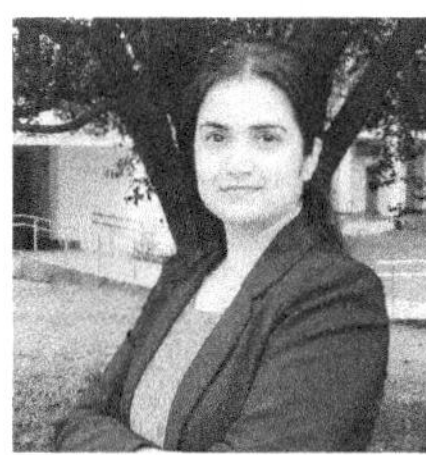

Dr. Sneha Singh is an assistant professor in the Department of Bioengineering and Biotechnology at Birla Institute of Technology, Mesra, Ranchi, India (BIT Mesra). She received her Ph.D. in the domain of nanobiotechnology from BIT. She has published many peer-reviewed research papers, book chapters, edited books, and patents to her credit. Her research interests span nanobiotechnology, biomaterials and tissue engineering, phytomedicines, antimicrobials and regenerative medicine specializing in nanomaterials, phytobioactives, and smart biomaterials for biomedical applications while conducting active research collaborations with eminent institutions nationally and internationally.

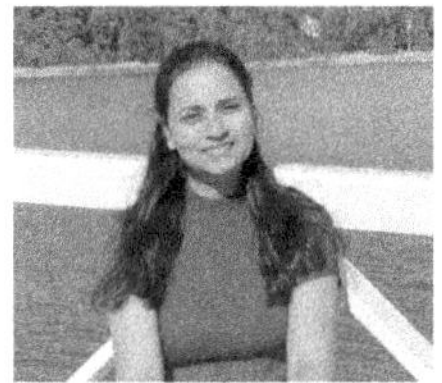

Dr. Prerna Singh is a postdoctoral fellow in the Department of Biological Sciences and Bioengineering, IIT Kanpur, India. She received her Ph.D. in biotechnology from Banaras Hindu University, India, in 2017. Her research areas include biomaterials, tissue engineering, regenerative medicine, stem cell research, and phytomedicine. She has significant peer-reviewed research articles, granted patent, book chapters and edited issues in journals among her scientific accomplishments. She is presently working in the area of biocompatible scaffolds for bone and soft tissue engineering. She has been involved in international and national collaborative research work with Aalto University, Finland; IIT Delhi; SKUAST, Kashmir; BIT Mesra, and BHU.

About the Editors

[illegible] ... Technology from Aalto University, Finland.

Dr. Sneha Singh is [illegible] ... [illegible] ... nationally and internationally.

[illegible]

Contributors

Vamsi Krishna Balla
Bioceramics & Coating Division
CSIR-Central Glass & Ceramic Research Institute
Kolkata, West Bengal, India

Kaushita Banerjee
Department of Biomedical Sciences
School of Bioscience and Technology
Vellore Institute of Technology
Vellore, Tamil Nadu, India

Bikramjit Basu
Centre of Excellence for Dental and Orthopedic Applications and Centre for Biosystems Science and Engineering, Materials Research Centre
Indian Institute of Science
Bangalore, Karnataka, India

Diana Arredondo Bernal
ITESM
Monterrey, N.L, 64700, Mexico

Nimet Bölgen
Chemical Engineering Department, Engineering Faculty
Mersin University 33110
Mersin, Türkiye

Kanta Chakraborty
School of Medical Science and Technology
Indian Institute of Technology
Kharagpur, India

Sergio Omar Martinez Chapa
ITESM
Monterrey, N.L, 64700, Mexico

Kaushik Chatterjee
Department of Materials Engineering
Indian Institute of Science
Bangalore, Karnataka, India

Naibedya Chattopadhyay
Division of Endocrinology
CSIR-Central Drug Research Institute
Centre for Research in Anabolic Skeletal Targets in Health and Illness
Lucknow, U.P., India

Gaurav Chauhan
ITESM
Monterrey, N.L, 64700, Mexico

Vianni Chopra
Chemical Biology Unit,
Institute of Nano Science and Technology
Mohali, Punjab, India

Samir Das
School of Medical Science and Technology
Indian Institute of Technology
Kharagpur, India

Sayan Das
School of Medical Science and Technology
Indian Institute of Technology
Kharagpur, India

Rahul Deka
Department of Bioengineering and Biotechnology
Birla Institute of Technology, Mesra
Ranchi, Jharkhand, India

Didem Demir
Department of Chemistry and Chemical Process Technologies
Mersin Tarsus Organized Industrial Zone Technical Sciences Vocational School
Tarsus University 33100
Tarsus, Mersin, Türkiye

Raghavendra Dhanenawar
Department of Biotechnology
National Institute of Pharmaceutical Education and Research
Ahmedabad, Gandhinagar, Gujarat, India

Santanu Dhara
School of Medical Science and Technology
Indian Institute of Technology
Kharagpur, India

Sabrina Ehnert
Siegfried-Weller Institute for Trauma Research, BG Trauma Center
University of Tuebingen
Schnarrenbergstrasse 95
72070 Tuebingen, Baden-Württemberg, Germany

Deepa Ghosh
Chemical Biology Unit
Institute of Nano Science and Technology
Mohali, Punjab, India

Rupita Ghosh
Department of Biological Sciences and Bioengineering
Centre for Environmental Science and Engineering
Indian Institute of Technology Kanpur
Kanpur, U.P., India

N. H. Gowtham
Centre of excellence for Dental and orthopedic applications, Materials Research Centre
Indian Institute of Science
Bangalore, Karnataka, India

Archita Gupta
Department of Bioengineering and Biotechnology
Birla Institute of Technology, Mesra
Ranchi, Jharkhand, India

Sneha Gupta
Department of Biological Sciences and Bioengineering
Indian Institute of Technology Kanpur
Kanpur, U.P., India

Tanjot Kaur
Department of Biotechnology, Bhupat & Jyoti Mehta School of Biosciences
Indian Institute of Technology Madras
Chennai, Tamil Nadu, India

Chandra Khatua
Centre for Nanotechnology
Indian Institute of Technology Roorkee
Roorkee, Uttarakhand, India

Ashok Kumar
Department of Biological Sciences and Bioengineering, Centre for Environmental Science and Engineering, Center for Nanosciences, The Mehta Family Centre for Engineering in Medicine, Center of Excellence for Orthopedics and Prosthetics, Gangwal School of Medical Sciences and Technology
Indian Institute of Technology Kanpur
Kanpur, U.P., India

Kanishka Kunal
Department of Bioengineering and Biotechnology
Birla Institute of Technology, Mesra
Ranchi, Jharkhand, India

Biswanath Kundu
Bioceramics & Coating Division
CSIR-Central Glass & Ceramic Research Institute
Kolkata, West Bengal, India

Debrupa Lahiri
Centre for Nanotechnology
Department of Metallurgical and Materials Engineering
Indian Institute of Technology Roorkee
Roorkee, Uttarakhand, India

Harishkumar Madhyastha
Department of Cardiovascular Physiology, Faculty of Medicine
University of Miyazaki
Miyazaki, Japan

Radha Madhyastha
Department of Cardiovascular Physiology, Faculty of Medicine
University of Miyazaki
Miyazaki, Japan

Arkodip Mandal
Department of Materials Engineering
Indian Institute of Science
Bangalore, Karnataka, India

Masugi Maruyama
Department of Cardiovascular Physiology, Faculty of Medicine
University of Miyazaki
Miyazaki, Japan

Shreya Mehrotra
Department of Biological Sciences and Bioengineering
Centre for Environmental Science and Engineering
Indian Institute of Technology Kanpur
Kanpur, U.P., India

Sanjay Kumar Mehta
Department of Bioengineering and Biotechnology
Birla Institute of Technology, Mesra
Ranchi, Jharkhand, India

Mitali Mishra
Centre of Excellence for Indian Knowledge Systems
School of Medical Science and Technology
Indian Institute of Technology
Kharagpur, West Bengal, India

Erick Orozco Morato
Department of Skeletal Biology and Regeneration
University of Connecticut Health Center
Farmington, Connecticut 06030

Eshita Mukherjee
Centre for Nanotechnology
Indian Institute of Technology Roorkee
Roorkee, Uttarakhand, India

Lakshmi S. Nair
Department of Skeletal Biology and Regeneration
University of Connecticut Health Center
Farmington, Connecticut 06030

Yuichi Nakajima
Department of Cardiovascular Physiology, Faculty of Medicine
University of Miyazaki
Miyazaki, Japan

Sandhya Natesan
Department of Biotechnology
Bhupat & Jyoti Mehta School of Biosciences
Indian Institute of Technology Madras
Chennai, Tamil Nadu, India

Aman Nikhil
Department of Biological Sciences and Bioengineering
Indian Institute of Technology Kanpur
Kanpur, U.P., India

Andreas K Nüssler
Siegfried-Weller Institute for Trauma Research
BG Trauma Center
University of Tuebingen
Schnarrenbergstrasse 95
72070 Tuebingen, Baden-Württemberg, Germany

Ashiq Hussain Pandit
Department of Biological Sciences and Bioengineering
Centre for Environmental Science and Engineering
Indian Institute of Technology Kanpur
Kanpur, U.P., India

Konica Porwal
Division of Endocrinology
CSIR-Central Drug Research Institute
Centre for Research in Anabolic Skeletal Targets in Health and Illness
Lucknow, U.P., India

Irfan Qayoom
Department of Biological Sciences and Bioengineering
Indian Institute of Technology Kanpur
Kanpur, U.P., India

Deepak Bushan Raina
Department of Clinical Science Lund, Orthopedics
Lund University
Lund, Scania, Sweden

Baisakhee Saha
School of Medical Science and Technology
Indian Institute of Technology
Kharagpur, India

Erdem Aras Sezgin
Department of Orthopedics and Traumatology
Aksaray University Faculty of Medicine
Aksaray, 68200, Türkiye

Shazia Shaikh
Department of Biological Sciences and Bioengineering
Centre for Environmental Science and Engineering
Indian Institute of Technology Kanpur
Kanpur, U.P., India

Vidushi Sharma
Centre of Excellence for Dental and Orthopedic Applications
Materials Research Centre
Indian Institute of Science
Bangalore, Karnataka, India

Mayank Singh
Department of Biotechnology
Bhupat & Jyoti Mehta School of Biosciences
Indian Institute of Technology Madras
Chennai, Tamil Nadu, India

Prerna Singh
Department of Biological Sciences and Bioengineering
Indian Centre for Environmental Science and Engineering
Indian Institute of Technology Kanpur
Kanpur, U.P., India

Sneha Singh
Department of Bioengineering and Biotechnology
Birla Institute of Technology, Mesra
Ranchi, Jharkhand, India

Akshay Srivastava
Department of Medical Devices
National Institute of Pharmaceutical Education and Research
Ahmedabad, Gandhinagar, Gujarat, India

Ekta Srivastava
Department of Biological Sciences and Bioengineering
Indian Institute of Technology Kanpur
Kanpur, U.P., India

D.C. Sundaresh
Sri Sathya Sai Institute of Higher Medical Sciences
Sri Sathya Sai General Hospital, EPIP Area
Whitefield, Bangalore, Karnataka, India

Greeshma Thrivikraman
Department of Biotechnology
Bhupat & Jyoti Mehta School of Biosciences
Indian Institute of Technology Madras
Chennai, Tamil Nadu, India

Ashok Vaseashta
International Clean Water Institute
Manassas, Virginia
Institute of Biomedical Engineering and Nanotechnologies
Riga Technical University
Riga, Latvia

Nozomi Watanabe
Department of Cardiovascular Physiology, Faculty of Medicine
University of Miyazaki
Miyazaki, Japan

Akash Yadav
Department of Biotechnology
National Institute of Pharmaceutical Education and Research
Ahmedabad, Gandhinagar, Gujarat, India

Foreword

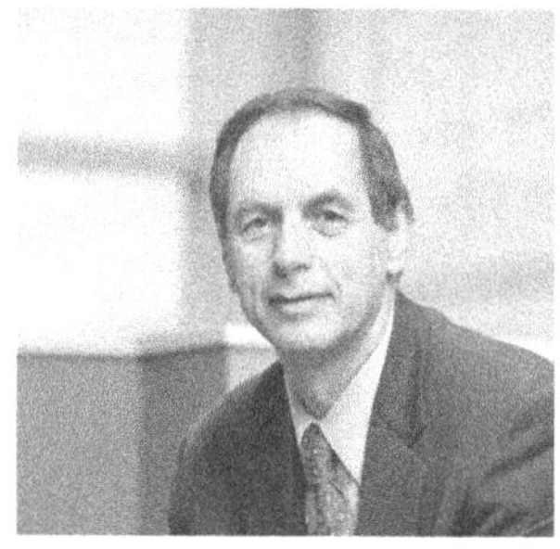

Recently, many bone-promoting materials have been studied worldwide; there has been a huge shift toward bioactive, resorbable, multifunctional biomaterials for bone tissue engineering applications. Recently an upsurge toward amalgamation of nanotechnology and tissue engineering has empowered the field with potentially upgraded functional nanobiomaterials. Owing to the unique physicochemical properties of nanomaterials, their use in bone scaffolds has been a timely and important research topic. Further, to impart functionality and bioactivity, the use of natural compounds and/or bioactive cues of natural origin has been recognized as a promising strategy to overcome the side effects of synthetic osteogenic molecules.

Emerging Materials and Technologies for Bone Repair and Regeneration highlights the current advances in the field of bone repair and regeneration along with the classical and well-established practices. Details on new domains such as 3D printing and emerging materials provide the reader with a deeper, cutting-edge comprehension of the field. Novel areas and materials are elaborately discussed with respect to technology, development and clinical evaluation. Furthermore, this book explores the fundamental features of different materials involved in bone healing ranging from their synthesis, characterization and effect on repair mechanisms.

The book introduces bone development, repair and regeneration emphasizing the correlation of the processes while further encompassing details about different biomaterials and technologies involved in fabricating and characterizing bone-related scaffolds and implants. The book also highlights the realm of nanotechnological intervention and folklore phytomedicines and their prospects in regenerating bone. The book finally discusses the major bone-related disease conditions, infection and their tackling via tissue engineering strategies while also elaborating on the theragnostic advancement in this field and its applications.

This book completely spans the journey from the inherent bone repair/regeneration process to the development of advanced biomaterials, ethnomedicine and cutting-edge strategies for bone diseases and defects. The significance and impact of a book is often related to the expertise of the senior editor. It is exciting that this book was edited by globally recognized experts and a team that has vast experience in bone regeneration. This is clearly reflected in the uniquely comprehensive and updated coverage of highly relevant topics. The book is highly recommended—for anyone from scientists who wish to enter into this exciting field all the way to established experts.

Joachim Kohn, Ph.D.

Joachim Kohn, PhD, FBSE
President, International Union of Societies for Biomaterials Science and Engineering
Distinguished Professor Emeritus, Rutgers University, New Jersey, USA
June 28, 2023

Preface

Bone tissues generally have self-healing capability and repair through regeneration. This unique fracture healing is well coordinated through the extracellular matrix, differentiating cells, and biogenic cues. The interplay between these elements significantly affects orthopedic procedures. The biomaterials and nanomaterials mimic the microarchitectural arrangement and extracellular matrix surrounding the osseous tissues, although phytomedicines and the sustained release of synthetic as well as natural bioactive cues are also crucial during bone regeneration. In short, understanding the current research and advancements with regard to material development and the technologies involved thereof is highly desired.

The contributors to this book explore different materials and technologies involved in bone repair and regeneration with particular emphasis on their fabrication, characterization, and role in orthopedics. The book will provide an interdisciplinary view of currently available biomaterials, nanomaterials, and phytomedicines in terms of their bone regeneration potential. Essential parts involved during the complete process of bone regeneration are accompanied by ranges of biomaterials for the surfaces of regenerated tissues. A complete understanding of the biomaterial precursors and different fabrication procedures is critical in the clinical acceptance of orthopedic substitutes.

Nanomaterials are highly encouraged due to the microarchitectural similarity arrangement to that of osseous tissues. Natural treatment options have traditionally been the first choice since ancient times. Therefore, an in-depth understanding of the available phytomedicines for repairing fractured bones is also highly desired.

Emerging Materials and Technologies for Bone Repair and Regeneration contains three broad sections: The first section includes the introduction and a synthesis and characterization of biomaterials, while the second part deals with the application of nanotechnology and phytomedicines for bone repair and regeneration. The third section encompasses advancing and applying tissue engineering toward orthopedic concerns. Each section comprises different chapters pertaining to both basic and advanced understanding of these concepts.

The chapters are contributed by renowned researchers, professors, and scientists from different parts of the globe working in interdisciplinary research areas. The book will provide a comprehensive illustration of the available and most-researched materials and technologies involved in bone repair. The first part, comprising Chapters 1–7, will introduce bone development, repair, and regeneration, emphasizing the correlation of the processes while encompassing details about different biomaterials and advanced technologies involved in the fabrication and characterization of bone-related scaffolds and implants.

Section I begins with a comprehensive discussion about the cellular mechanism and crosstalk among the cells involved in maintaining bone homeostasis for efficient bone repair and regeneration. The section progresses to the requirements of various biomaterials in bone tissue engineering and their relevance in different clinical settings. The section subsequently provides a detailed overview of emerging materials, design and advanced fabrication strategies, and characterization in analyzing bone substitutes for their successful application.

The second section of the book, comprising Chapters 8–11, highlights nanotechnological interventions, folklore phytomedicines, and their prospects in regenerating bone. The section discusses the advances in nanoscale materials that have brought revolutionary improvement in material development for therapeutic and bone-regenerative applications ranging from the sustained delivery of biogenic cues to providing nanotopographic architecture.

Section II focuses on various nanotherapeutics and nutra-nanoceuticals and their interactions in bone biology to maintain healthy bone. The section unravels the emerging avenue of nano-scaffolds, their fabrication, and their efficacy during bone diseases. The section also elaborately discusses different groups of phytobioactives, their structural identification in modulating bone metabolism, and the effects of the constituents on repairing bone tissues evidenced through different in vitro and in vivo models. The section also highlights the promising local delivery strategies beneficial in enhancing the bioavailability of the osteogenic phytobioactives. This will not only help to understand the complex mechanism involved behind their effects but will also help in designing future treatment strategies for bone repair.

The third section, covering Chapters 12–19, deals with applications and advancements in tissue engineering strategies for various bone diseases, infections, diagnosis, and therapy. The section discusses cellular and molecular events during skeletal homeostasis and other pathophysiological situations giving rise to various bone diseases. The section also highlights different in vitro and in vivo bone models and clinical applications of biomaterials, providing crucial insights into new technologies developed for bone disease.

Chapters in this section are dedicated to highlighting new advanced materials like ultra-high-molecular-weight polyethylene-based acetabular liners for total hip joint replacement, biomaterials for the repair and regeneration of intervertebral discs, and the therapeutic role of exosomes in the field of bone repair. The advanced bone tissue engineering approaches, possible future directions for next-generation biomaterials, and therapeutic platforms for bone repair will provide new avenues to the orthopedic industries.

Each chapter includes extensive prospects about the currently available and future research options. Combining different materials and technologies, this book showcases the importance of these materials and/or composites in bone tissue engineering. The book provides an overview to researchers, professors, engineers, pharmaceutics and biotechnologist professionals, medical professionals, and anyone interested in a transdisciplinary field of study. The book will also be useful as a textbook and reference book for undergraduate, postgraduate, and doctoral program students. It is also pertinent here to express our gratitude to all our esteemed authors and contributors for their precious time and valuable efforts in contributing to this book to make it a comprehensive source of learning and creating a deep understanding of the *Emerging Materials and Technologies for Bone Repair and Regeneration.*

Ashok Kumar
Sneha Singh
Prerna Singh

I

Introduction: The Synthesis and Characterization of Biomaterials for Bone Regeneration

Introduction: The Sophists and [illegible] Rome Generation

1 Cellular and Molecular Interplay in Bone Homeostasis and Healing

Deepak Bushan Raina

1.1 BONE STRUCTURE AND THE EXTRACELLULAR MATRIX

Bone is a composite biomaterial comprising an intricately balanced organic–inorganic matrix and water that facilitates load bearing. The bone extracellular matrix (ECM) is the second-toughest structure in the human body after teeth, but what makes the bone as hard as it is and why has it been impossible to replicate such a biocomposite (at least so far) despite the advances in material fabrication technologies? The answer lies in the hierarchical structure of the bone ECM.

Approximately 60% of bone mass comprises carbonate-substituted hydroxyapatite (HA), while the rest of the ECM comprises water and organic constituents. The organic matrix comprises 90% type 1 collagen; the remaining ECM contains glycoproteins, carboxyglutamic acid (GLA) containing proteins, glycosaminoglycans (GAGs) and small amounts of growth factors and enzymes. HA provides stiffness to the bone ECM, while the collagen matrix provides elasticity. The HA crystals in bone are nanometer sized and are shaped as needles or platelets with an approximate length of 20–50 nm, width roughly 0–20 nm and a thickness of 2–4 nm. HA nucleation occurs either on top of or within the type I collagen fibers, but the process is carefully orchestrated by phosphorylated nucleation proteins including bone sialoprotein and osteopontin during the early matrix deposition (Hunter & Goldberg, 1993).

The initial amorphous calcium phosphate (CaP), which is presumed to start its journey inside mineral-producing cells (osteoblasts), is sent out in vesicles and carefully laid out on top of and within the collagen matrix (Figure 1.1). The amorphous CaP, in the presence of nucleation proteins transforms and remodels into platelet-shaped carbonated HA (Lotsari et al., 2018). Whether the platelet-like shaping of the HA crystal occurs in response to collagen fibril loading/stretching along the long axis of the fibers or whether there are other factors responsible for shaping the HA crystal remains unclear at present.

HA crystals on and within collagen type I fibrils form an intertwined collagen–HA network that Reznikov et al. (2018) quite eloquently visualized and explained in a recent study. They proposed a fractal-like structure of the bone matrix and dissected the bone structure at multiple length scales to provide a 12-level breakup of the hierarchical structure of bone. While at the very minutest level, the HA crystals were arranged as small platelets, the authors demonstrated that multiple HA crystals organize themselves into stacks, thereby acting as bridges between multiple collagen units. The stack of HA crystals combining multiple collagen helices across different length scales (from nm to cm) gave rise to a remarkable composite structure in the form of bone (Reznikov et al. 2018). It is due to this hierarchical complexity that we have not been able to replicate a biomaterial that possesses the same dynamic and adaptive mechanical properties as bone.

I have so far focused on the composition and nano-/microstructure of bone, partly to deal with the more complex structural properties of the bone early on, while I still have your attention. We can now deal with the comparatively easier part, the macrostructure of bone. Bone can be grossly

DOI: 10.1201/9781003307310-2

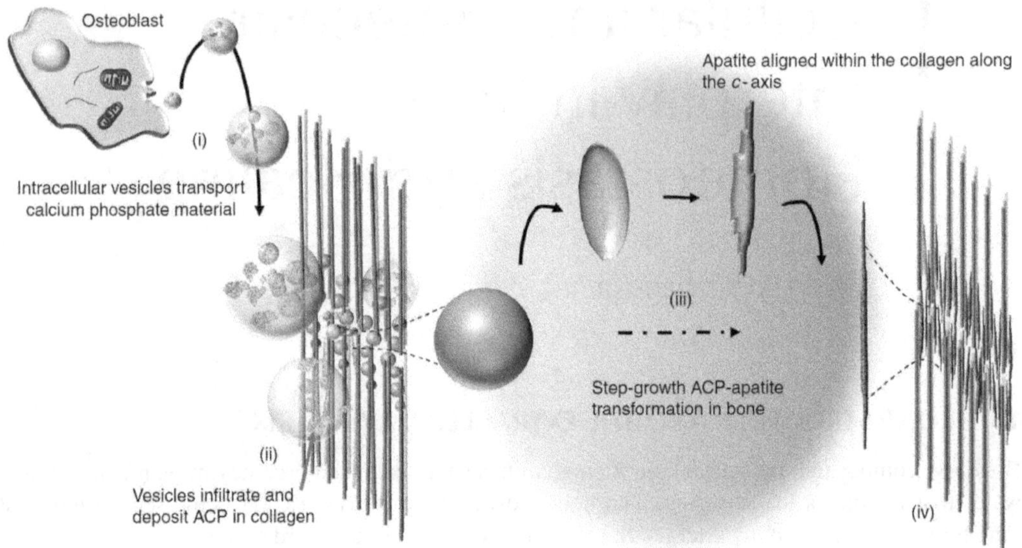

FIGURE 1.1 Proposed process of hydroxyapatite (HA) deposition and maturation by Lotsari and coworkers. Amorphous calcium phosphate (CaP) material is transported out of the osteoblasts in small vesicles, some of which penetrate the 3D fibrillar collagen network while the remaining vesicles lay the cargo on the surface of the fibril. The amorphous CaP then undergoes a step growth, transforming into crystalline HA and aligning along the c-axis of the collagen fibers, which assume a platelet-like shape. (Reproduced under the terms of CC-BY 4.0 (https://creativecommons.org/licenses/by/4.0/) International License from Lotsari, A., Rajasekharan, A. K., Halvarsson, M., & Andersson, M.: Transformation of amorphous calcium phosphate to bone-like apatite. Nat. Commun. 2018. 9. 4170. Copyright 2018 Lotsari et al., published by Springer Nature).

divided into two categories: 1) cortical and 2) cancellous or trabecular. Cortical bone is the compact/dense bone generally found away from the joints and is responsible for the toughness of the skeleton; it is organized in the form of osteons (seen as concentric mineralized rings in cross sections). In the middle of the osteons lies the Haversian canal, a narrow channel along the long axis of the bone, which is responsible for nutrient transport and mechanosensing. Cortical bone is also horizontally connected via the Volkmann's canal system. Cancellous bone, on the other hand, is found close to the joint surfaces and forms a honeycomb-like porous network of lamellae that provide the bony structure the necessary properties required for efficiently transmitting compressional forces along the longitudinal axis of the bone without fracturing. Cancellous bone is infiltrated with an intricate network of blood vessels that enables efficient nutrient and gas exchange.

1.2 BONE FROM A PHYSIOLOGICAL PERSPECTIVE

Apart from offering load bearing and mobility, bone also plays a vital role in homeostasis. But before jumping into the topic of bone-mediated homeostasis, let us take a look at the main cell types that reside within the bone ECM. It is estimated that the cortical compartment of bone remodels into a totally new unit at a rate of 3–10% every year, while the cancellous bone is replaced at a rate of 20–30%. In simpler terms, our entire skeleton is replaced by a totally new skeleton approximately every 10 years, which approximates to roughly 6–8 new skeletons during the entire lifespan.

How does the skeletal system manage to achieve this feat without taking a break? In order to replace a structure, the old structure needs to go away and a new structure needs to be laid out.

However, the challenge is to maintain an equilibrium between the demolition and construction process, and this balance is carefully orchestrated by the cells that reside in the bone matrix.

Bone comprises three main cell types, osteoclasts, osteoblasts and osteocytes (Eriksen, 2010). Osteoclasts are responsible for the break-down or resorption of bone. They are multinucleated cells that emanate from the fusion of several mononuclear hematopoietic precursors. Osteoclasts do not directly trigger bone resorption but rather are signaled by the osteocytes or the osteoblasts.

That is, osteoclastogenesis is a two-step process, wherein a stimulus from the osteocyte or the osteoblast needs to be registered before the resorption occurs. The stimulus imperative for forming and activating osteoclasts is cytokine driven and depends on two important signaling molecules; receptor activator of nuclear factor kappa B ligand (RANKL) and macrophage colony stimulating factor (M-CSF) (Anderson et al., 1997; Wong et al., 1997; Yasuda et al., 1998) (Table 1.1). Osteoclasts are thought to originate from macrophage-like cells, which possess a RANK receptor.

The binding of RANKL to the RANK receptor in the presence of M-CSF leads to osteoclastogenesis. Once an osteoclast has formed, the cell affixes itself to the bone ECM via its ruffled borders to form a tight seal with the bone surface. The osteoclasts then produce a series of proteolytic enzymes including cathepsin K and tartrate resistant acid phosphatase to digest the organic bone matrix, while the inorganic bone matrix (HA) is digested in the resulting severely acidic environment (proton pump effect) (Everts et al., 2022).

The balance between bone resorption and bone formation is sometimes affected, and a classic example is during osteoporosis, wherein the resorption process overtakes the bone formation process. The pharmacological modulation of osteoclasts and their function therefore becomes of particular importance when treating osteoporosis. There are two US FDA (Food and Drug Administration)-approved drug classes that actively target osteoclasts.

The first drug type works by actively targeting RANKL (and thereby preventing osteoclastogenesis) with an anti-RANKL antibody (commercially known as Prolia, manufactured by Amgen) (Bekker et al., 2004). By binding to the freely available RANKL, the cell surface receptor RANK on the osteoclast progenitor remains unengaged, which consequently affects the downstream signaling involved in osteoclast formation. The reduction of osteoclastogenesis has been shown to minimize bone loss associated with osteoporosis in post-menopausal women.

TABLE 1.1
Important Signaling and Growth Factors Involved in Bone Remodeling

Growth/Signaling Factor	Encoding Gene	Target Cell	Function
Receptor activator of nuclear factor kappa B ligand (RANKL)	TNFSF11	Monocyte/macrophage (Preosteoclast)	Promote osteoclast differentiation
Macrophage colony stimulating factor	CSF1	Monocyte/macrophage (preosteoclast)	Promote osteoclast differentiation
Osteoprotegrin (OPG)	TNFRSF11B	Monocyte/macrophage (preosteoclast)	Inhibit osteoclast differentiation
Bone morphogenic protein-2	BMP2	Preosteoblast/ osteoblast	Promote osteoblast differentiation
Parathyroid hormone	PTH	Osteoblast/ osteocyte	Promote both osteoblasts and osteoclasts based on RANKL/OPG ratios and sclerostin expression
Sclerostin	SOST	Osteoblast	Inhibit bone formation
Dickkopf related protein-1	DKK1	Osteoblast	Inhibit bone formation together with sclerostin

The second drug class belongs to the bisphosphonate category (Drake et al., 2008). Third-generation bisphosphonates such as zoledronic acid (ZA) do not directly affect osteoclastogenesis but instead by acting directly on mature osteoclasts. ZA preferentially binds to HA in the skeleton; when an osteoclast digests the first ZA-loaded HA crystal, ZA is released inside the cell. ZA has a strong effect on GTPases including Rho and Rab, which are responsible for the ruffled border formation in osteoclasts. Impaired ruffling prevents the osteoclasts from forming a tight seal with the underlying bone, which eventually causes osteoclast apoptosis.

Contrary to osteoclasts, osteoblasts are responsible for depositing the bone matrix (both organic and inorganic) via a tightly controlled process involving inorganic phosphate (Pi), a topic that I cover later in the chapter. They are known to possess a mesenchymal progeny, although their exact origins are not clearly understood. The role of bone morphogenic protein (BMP) signaling is of particular importance when determining the fate of mesenchymal progenitor cells that differentiate into an "osteoblastic" lineage (Rahman et al., 2015). BMP signaling has been shown to activate the downstream signaling cascade via the activation of SMADs (particularly SMAD 1, 5 and 8) and the nuclear translocation of runt-related transcription factor-2 (RUNX2), leading to an osteogenic commitment of progenitor cells. The committed progenitor cells continue to differentiate into mature osteoblasts, often seen as cuboidal cells expressing important markers including osterix, alkaline phosphatase (ALP), bone sialo protein, osteocalcin and type I collagen among others (Table 1.2).

Once fully differentiated, the osteoblasts start the mineralization process, which takes place in two phases. During the first phase, a protein-rich matrix called the osteoid is laid out in the form of lamellar structures, and the lamellae are gradually mineralized by carbonated HA when the appropriate nucleation conditions are present. Some prominent examples of drugs that modulate the osteoblast function in humans are anabolic molecules such as truncated parathyroid hormone (PTH), commercially sold as Forteo® (sold by Eli Lilly) and BMP-2 (sold as InductOS by Medtronic Inc.).

Osteocytes originate from osteoblasts that get embedded in their own ECM, generally toward the very end of their mineralization phase (Hadjidakis & Androulakis, 2006). Osteocytes are thought to be the mechano-sensors in bone, and this mechanosensing is achieved by means of an interconnected network via dendrites called canaliculi. Canaliculi respond to mechanical stimulation (excessive exercising, weight changes etc.) and inform the osteocytes to exude a biochemical response, which is capable of acting on both the osteoclasts and the osteoblasts. Osteocyte-mediated osteoclastic activation is controlled by RANKL signaling while the osteoblastic modulation is achieved via sclerostin and Dickkopf-related protein-1 (DKK-1). Osteocytes are characterized by the presence of dentin matrix protein-1 (DMP-1), fibroblast growth factor-23 and sclerostin. A schematic of the bone remodeling process is summarized in Figure 1.2.

Now that I have described the cellular composition of bone, the next step is to understand the physiological functions of bone. As stated earlier, the human skeleton undergoes constant changes,

TABLE 1.2
Some of the Important Cellular Markers Associated with Key Bone Cells

Cell	Marker(s)
Osteoclast	Cathepsin-K, tartrate-resistant acid phosphatase 5b
Osteoblast	Osterix, osteocalcin, alkaline phosphatase (ALP), RANKL, bone sialoprotein
Preosteoblast	ALP, Runt-related transcription factor-2, collagen type 1A1, connective tissue growth factor
Mesenchymal stromal cells (MSC)	STRO-1 (where STRO stands for stromal and 1 is the [1s]t isolated antibody to identify MSCs), CD-73, CD-90, CD-105
Osteocyte	DMP-1, DKK-1, fibroblast growth factor-23

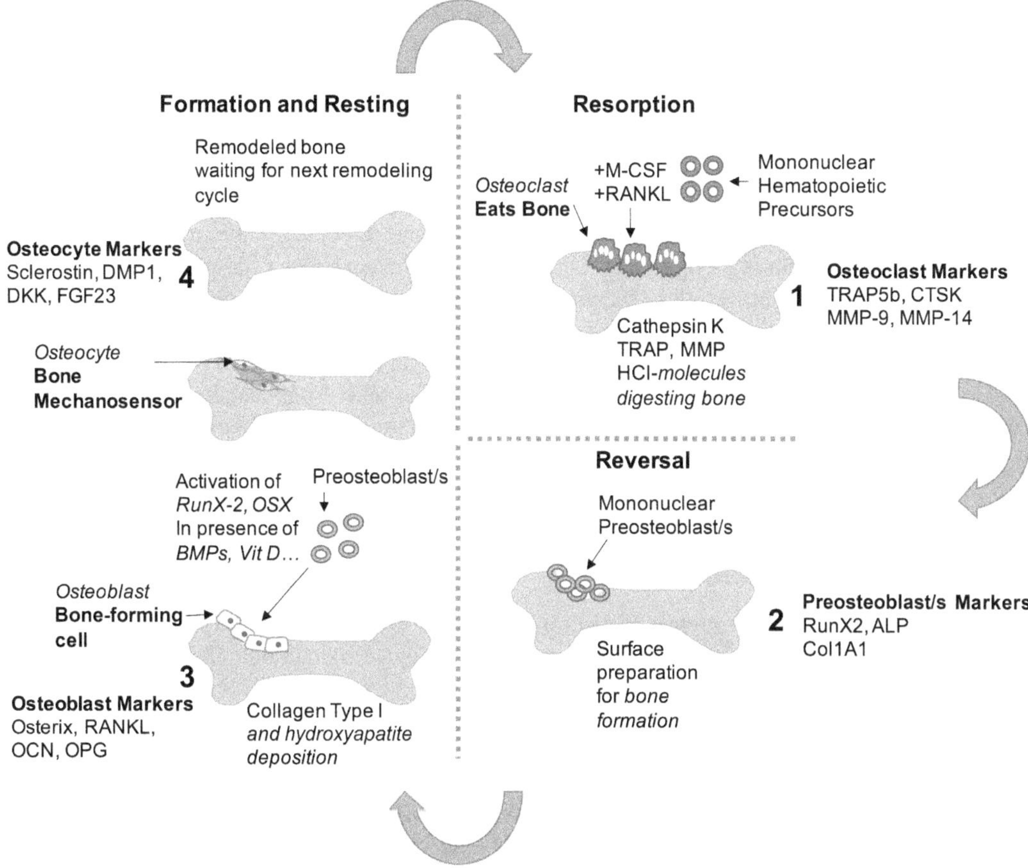

FIGURE 1.2 A simplified summary of the bone remodeling cycle. (Reproduced with permission from Raina, D.: Biomaterials as carriers for bone active molecules-An approach to create off-the-shelf bone substitutes. 2018. Doctoral Thesis, Lund University, Sweden. Copyright 2018 Deepak Bushan Raina.)

a process described as bone remodeling (Hadjidakis & Androulakis, 2006). Bone remodeling is an intricate process orchestrated by systemic and local regulators including PTH, glucocorticoids, vitamin D_3, estrogen and prostaglandin among others.

The process starts with bone resorption in response to a stimulus (e.g., an injury or mechanical stimulus) (Figure 1.2). Mononuclear cells from the blood reach the injury site and respond to RANKL/M-CSF signaling, leading to osteoclastogenesis. The osteoclasts clear the injury site of the damaged bone matrix followed by repopulation of the resorbed area by osteoblast-like cells that produce a mineralized bone matrix until the site is fully repaired.

During this process, some of the osteoblasts turn into osteocytes, and the remodeling cycle is believed to be complete, after which a resting period is initiated before remodeling at the next site begins. This remodeling process continues throughout the life of an individual, but there are instances wherein the remodeling process gets severely affected. An imbalance between the anabolic and catabolic events in the remodeling cycle leads to an altered bone turnover.

The other important role bone plays in homeostasis is regulating the Ca and PO_4 concentrations in body fluids (Al-Bari & Al Mamun, 2020; Taylor & Bushinsky, 2009). Based on the abundant HA crystals present in the bone ECM, bone is a reservoir of Ca^{2+} and PO_4- ions, which are key in carrying out important bodily functions, but where does the Ca supply come from? There are two sources: 1) dietary intake and 2) Ca released from the bone itself.

Dietary Ca is absorbed in the gastrointestinal tract and processed in both the GI system and the kidneys. The absorbed dietary Ca is then passed into the extracellular fluid, where the Ca ions are actively recruited in the skeleton. But how does the Ca then get incorporated into the bone ECM? To understand this, we need to revisit the mineralization capabilities of osteoblasts (and the effect of Ca on osteoprogenitors). It is well understood that progenitor cells such as the mesenchymal stromal cells (MSCs) from bone marrow require Ca and PO_4 ions in order to adapt an osteogenic fate.

The extracellular Ca and PO_4 ions are internalized by the osteoprogenitors differentiating into osteoblasts. The osteoblasts then process these ions to form amorphous CaP, which is transported back into the ECM in small vesicles. The amorphous CaP deposited on the collagen fibers acts as a starting material for crystalline HA, which is an integral part of the osteon. Once the HA is embedded in the osteon, no Ca or PO_4 ion release occurs until an osteoclast actively resorbs the bone matrix, leading to calcium release. This is why patients who take drugs that affect the osteoclasts (such as bisphosphonates) require dietary Ca supplements in order to avoid hypocalcemia caused by the inability of the osteoclasts to release Ca ions into the circulation.

1.3 PHYSIOLOGICAL AND PATHOLOGICAL MINERALIZATION AT THE MOLECULAR LEVEL

HA deposition is a carefully orchestrated process that mineralizes the skeleton in normal conditions and results in extraskeletal mineralization in pathological conditions, including of the soft tissues such as muscle, blood vessels and cartilage. The primary building block for crystalline HA that exists in the bone matrix arises from pyrophosphate (PP_i). PP_i performs a balancing act by 1) acting as a source of inorganic phosphate (Pi) that together with Ca^{2+} ions forms first amorphous calcium phosphate and eventually crystalline calcium phosphate and 2) simultaneously inhibiting mineralization regulated by the P_i/PP_i ratio (Figure 1.3). PP_i is a small molecule that is produced and transported outside the cell by membrane proteins encoded by the ENPP1 and ANK genes (Hessle et al., 2002; Ho et al., 2000; Okawa et al., 1998).

Mutations or knockout models of ENPP1 and ANK perturb the P_i/PP_i ratio, which affects the HA inhibition property of PP_i (due to less extracellular PP_i) and thereby leads to the ectopic ossification of blood vessels and ligaments as well as an osteoarthritis-like phenotype (mineralization of the cartilage) in mice. In order to obtain P_i from PP_i, tissue-nonspecific alkaline phosphatase (TNAP) plays a vital role. TNAP is present in various tissues, but its coexpression with collagen type I is unique to bone (Murshed et al., 2005); it is known to hydrolyze PP_i to P_i making P_i available to osteoblasts.

TNAP-mutated mice show a phenotype that resembles rickets and osteomalacia (hypophosphatasia) due to the lack of extracellular P_i (Henthorn & Whyte, 1992). EPPN1, on the other hand, is responsible for the production and transport of PP_i, and EPPN1 knockout mice show a phenotype resembling the pathological mineralization of blood vessels due to the absence of extracellular PP_i that should in normal situations block the formation of HA crystals. Hessle et al. (2002) eloquently showed that a double knockout mouse model of ENPP1 (which codes for plasma cell membrane protein 1 (PC-1) and TNAP rescues the osteomalacia phenotype of TNAP null mice and prevents ectopic ossification of blood vessels characteristic of EPPN1 knockout mice.

To further elucidate that it is indeed the dysregulation of extracellular PP_i that leads to pathologic/ectopic ossification, Murshed et al. (2005) used both ANK and EPPN1 knockout mice, which do not show pathological ossification when fed a regular diet. However, when the mice lacking extracellular PP_i were fed a diet with high phosphorus, extensive ectopic mineralization could be observed, consolidating the role of PP_i as not only the source of Pi but also as an inhibitor of mineralization. Once the P_i/PP_i ratio is balanced, P_i together with Ca ions forms amorphous HA that is transported out from the osteoblasts in matrix vesicles. The amorphous HA then undergoes a series of maturation steps before it is incorporated into the tightly knit collagen type I network.

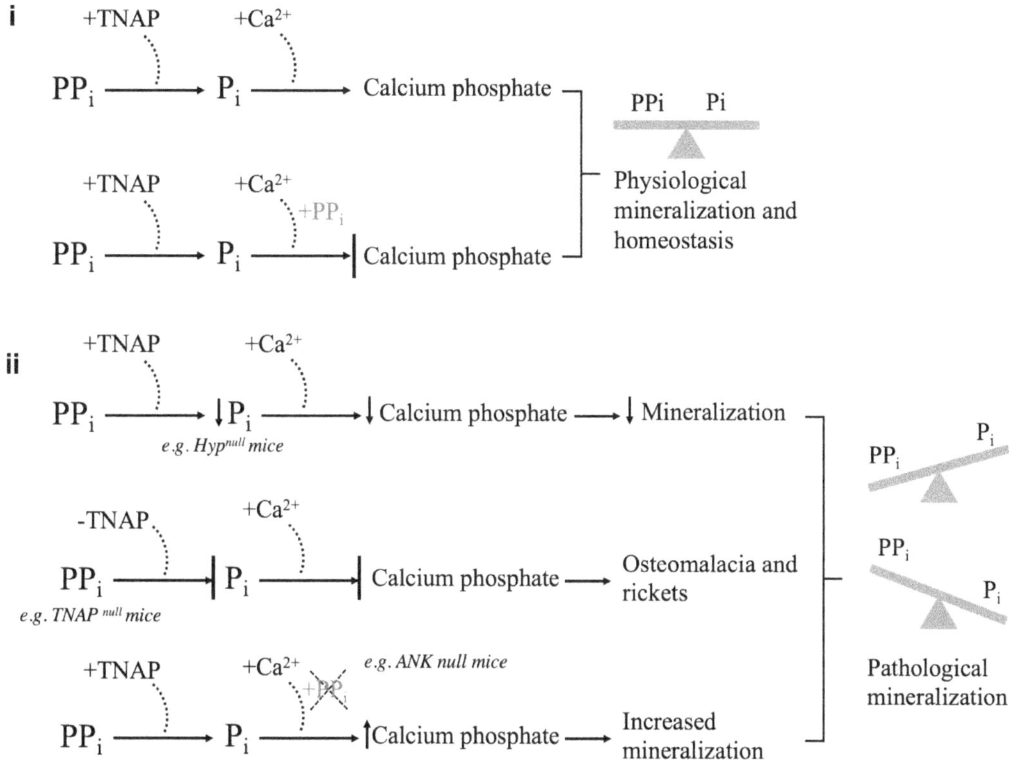

FIGURE 1.3 Mineralization in normal and pathological conditions. Notice how mineralization is a carefully orchestrated process dependent on the P_i/PP_i ratios. Imbalance in the P_i/PP_i can lead to pathological mineralization or lack of mineralization.

1.4 FRACTURE HEALING MECHANISMS AND CELLULAR INTERPLAY

Fracture healing can be considered a true regenerative process since fractures heal without forming scar tissue. There are two fundamental pathways to fracture healing; 1) direct or intramembranous ossification (IO) and 2) indirect or endochondral ossification (EO).

1.4.1 Direct Fracture Healing

Direct fracture healing occurs when the gap between the fracture ends is very small and the interfragmentary strain between the two broken bone ends is minimal. In general, fractures that are mechanically stabilized using hardware components with a fracture gap of <1 mm heal via the IO route, which is subclassified into contact or gap healing. Contact healing occurs when the distance between the fracture ends is <0.01 mm and interfragmentary strain is <2% (Shapiro, 1988).

This type of fracture healing is characterized by the formation of cutting cones characterized by the presence of osteoclasts at the tip of the cone that digest the dead bone immediately at the vicinity of the fracture line in the longitudinal direction at a speed of up to 0.1 mm/day (Marsell & Einhorn, 2011). The osteoclasts are followed by osteoblasts that subsequently lay the new mineralized bone matrix, ensuring continuity in the Haversian system in the native and new bone. As soon as a bony union is achieved, the prefracture nutrient and blood flow is restored in the bone, and the primary osteons remodel into lamellar bone over a course of several months.

Gap healing occurs when a correct anatomical reduction of the fracture ends is achieved but the gap between the fracture ends is up to 1 mm (Kaderly, 1991). Contrary to contact healing, wherein the bony union and remodeling is a one-step process, first a lamellar structure is laid out that is perpendicular (rather than parallel) to the longitudinal axis of the bone (Schenk, 1994). This structure is, however, mechanically weak and requires a second mineralization phase where the perpendicularly laid bone is resorbed and simultaneously a new longitudinally aligned bone is laid out, similar to the process in contact healing. Despite the subcategories, IO leads to the direct consolidation of the fractured bone ends without the formation of a large bony callus.

Due to the "direct" nature of healing in IO, mesenchymal progenitor cells commit to a preosteogenic and osteogenic fate rather directly and start laying out the bone matrix, hence the name direct ossification. In the context of embryogenesis and growth, only a few types of bones in the skeleton (e.g., cranium, clavicle and facial bones) undergo intramembranous ossification. It is believed that the process of IO is strongly controlled by the bone morphogenic protein (BMP) family of proteins including BMP-2, BMP-4 and BMP-7, which activate transcriptional factor CBFA1 (coding the Runx2 protein) (Hall, 1988).

This Runx2 signaling leads to a downstream cascade of events including eventually the osteogenic commitment of progenitor cells. Mice lacking the CBFA1 gene have shown to be unviable immediately after birth with a complete loss of bone involving both the IO and EO ossification sites even when cartilage development was normal (Komori et al., 1997; Otto et al., 1997). Deletion or point mutations in CBFA1 in humans has been associated with a condition called cleidocranial dysplasia, in which skull sutures are not closed, clavicles develop poorly or are absent and some misalignments of the teeth are observed (Mundlos et al., 1997).

1.4.2 Indirect Fracture Healing

The vast majority of fractures heal via indirect fracture healing or EO since obtaining complete anatomical reduction and rigidity of the fracture ends is surgically challenging and occurs only occasionally. Bone formation in EO occurs in two steps: First, a cartilaginous template is laid out in the fracture gap (some part of the gap is also directly filled with bone, but I will discuss that later). Over a course of one to two weeks), the chondrocytes in the cartilage matrix become hypertrophic and start mineralizing (Einhorn & Gerstenfeld, 2015; Marsell & Einhorn, 2011), and the processes of hypertrophy and angiogenesis in the fracture gap occur simultaneously.

In the second step, the hypertrophic cartilaginous matrix is resorbed by osteoclasts, while osteogenic progenitors populate the area with active resorption, causing a second round of mineralization by the osteoblasts forming the woven bone. In contrast, very close to the fracture ends, a different kind of a healing reaction occurs that involves lifting the periosteum and consequent direct ossification, thereby making EO a mix of both IO and EO (at least in the vast majority of the cases). This is also the reason why fracture healing is considered as a recapitulation of the embryogenic skeletal development. This IO ossification occurs until the original bone ends meet.

One might then wonder about the role of an extensive cartilaginous callus. The production of cartilage matrix is a very rapid process that occurs within the first two weeks post-fracture. It is this large oval structure that provides the required torsional stiffness and stability to the overall fracture structure. EO is an intricate balance between the EO and IO pathways wherein the EO ossification allows for rapid stabilization of the fracture and the mechanical continuity in the fracture gap (or cortical union) is achieved via the IO pathway. Once complete cortical union is achieved and the mechanosensors of the bone (i.e., osteocytes) sense that the bone is ready for complete load bearing, a remodeling process begins to resorb the fracture callus since it is not load bearing anymore. At this point, it is almost impossible to differentiate the broken bone from a healthy bone, a true regenerative hallmark of bone healing!

As Figure 1.4 shows (Pfeiffenberger et al., 2021), the healing process in EO is intricately controlled by cyto/chemokines, the immune system, and the local/systemic mesenchymal niches.

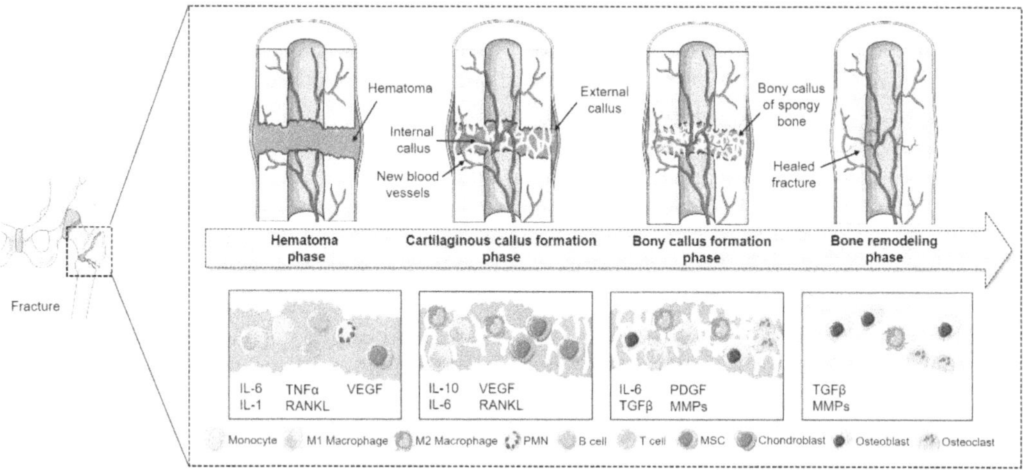

FIGURE 1.4 A schematic of EO fracture healing. (Reproduced under the terms of CC-BY 4.0 (https://creativecommons.org/licenses/by/4.0/) International License from Pfeiffenberger, M., Damerau, A., Lang, A., Buttgereit, F., Hoff, P., & Gaber, T.: Fracture Healing Research—Shift towards In Vitro Modeling? Biomedicines. 2021. 9. 748. Copyright 2021 Pfeiffenberger et al., published by MDPI).

Immediately after injury, the fracture site, which is undergoing acute inflammation, is infiltrated by a hematoma with a high pro-inflammatory drive locally at the injury site. The hematoma is a mixture of monocytes, polymorphonuclear cells, T and B cells and mesenchymal cells as well as M1 macrophages (Einhorn & Gerstenfeld, 2015).

The first step in the repair process is clearing the necrotized tissue and promoting angiogenesis in order to supply nutrients, cells and signaling molecules in the hematoma and at the fracture site. It is interesting to note that the levels of adaptive immune response are suppressed during this phase by the action of MSCs via paracrine signaling or through cell–cell communication with the T-cells, suggesting that the suppression of adaptive immunity might be a deliberate attempt to prevent the hematoma and the consequent callus from a premature attack from the immune system (Meert et al., 1998; Nauta & Fibbe, 2007). Many different cytokines are upregulated during the acute fracture healing phase, most notable of which are tumor necrosis factor (TNF)-interleukins IL-1 and IL-6, which are responsible for the homing of fracture repair cells and neo angiogenesis via IL-6 signaling, which is known to stimulate VEGF production (Glass et al., 2011; Wallace et al., 2011).

The next crucial step is to understand the source of progenitor cells in EO, and the progenitor cell origins depend on the extent of tissue trauma and which components of the bone and the surrounding tissues have been affected. This phenomenon is eloquently described by Celiné Colnot, who used transgenic mouse lines and compartmentalized tissue injury models (periosteal injury to study the contribution of the periosteum as a stem cell source and endosteal injury to study the contribution of endosteum and bone marrow as a stem cell source) to map the source of progenitor cells in bone healing (Colnot, 2009). When an injury on the periosteal side of the bone was made, lineage tracing analysis showed that the source of progenitor cells was the periosteum and that these progenitor cells undergo both chondrogenesis and osteogenesis. On the contrary, the endosteal and bone marrow progenitor cells could only differentiate into bone and not cartilage. These findings indicate that although the periosteum, endosteum and the bone marrow all contribute as the progenitor cell sources, the compartmental origin of these cells decide the final fate of these progenitor cell populations.

It is understood that the osteogenic cells undergo osteogenic differentiation and produce bone mineral. What is intriguing is what happens to the cells that adapt a chondrogenic fate and how they dedifferentiate into bone. The accepted theory was that after the vascular invasion of the cartilage template, chondrocytes undergo hypertrophy and produce a soft mineralized matrix after which all the hypertrophic chondrocytes undergo apoptosis. Osteoclasts then invade the site and clear up the soft mineralized chondrocytes for a second round of mineralization by the osteoblasts (formed by the migration of circulating progenitor cells).

This theory was recently challenged by Hu and coworkers (2017), who eloquently show that not all hypertrophic chondrocytes undergo apoptosis; rather, only some do in order to create room for more mature tissue. The remaining chondrocytes undergo dedifferentiation and regain their "stemness" by expressing key transcriptional factors including OCT4, SOX2 and NANOG (Hu et al., 2017). The dedifferentiated, original chondrocytes undergo cell division and form osteoblasts.

Although I have tried to touch upon the topic of progenitor cell source and the cell fates they adapt during the healing process, I have not yet defined the progenitor populations. What comprises a progenitor cell population is not completely clear despite all our knowledge on the origins of progenitor cells. The three classical criteria for designating a cell a MSC is their plastic adherence, expression of cluster of differentiation (CD) markers including CD105, CD73, CD90 and lack of expression of CD45, CD34, CD14, CD19 and HLA-DR, and the ability to undergo tri-lineage differentiation (Dominici et al., 2006). The definition of MSCs even after nearly 50 years of their discovery is very unclear, which arises from the heterogeneity of the cells present in the bone marrow niche and the differences in the properties of MSCs isolated from different tissues.

In order to overcome these challenges, Houlihan and coworkers described the isolation of a more potent MSC niche from the endosteal linings of long bones in mice and were characterized by the presence of SCA-1$^+$ and PDGFR-⟨$^+$ and the absence of CD45$^-$, TER-119$^-$ (SCA-1$^+$ PDGFR-⟨$^+$ CD45$^-$ TER-119- or P⟨S cells) (Houlihan et al., 2012). Although the frequency of this progenitor cell type is low (10,000 cells/mouse with a frequency of 0.05–0.08% of the total cell population), these specific MSCs have much more potent osteogenic differentiation potential than conventional MSCs. Whether a similar population of MSCs could be found on the periosteal side is unclear, but the analysis of human heterotrophic ossification samples retrieved from the muscle tissue verified the presence of a similar progenitor cell population (SCA-1$^+$ PDGFR-⟨$^+$), indicating that these cells are present beyond just the bone tissue (Wosczyna et al., 2012). Furthermore, their non-hematopoietic origins (CD31, CD45, TER-119 negativity) suggest that the cells might be present locally even inside the muscle tissue and its interstitium. More sophisticated lineage tracking studies, single-cell RNA sequencing and multimodal omics-based approaches might clarify the exact subtype of MSCs in bone healing and in different compartments of the bone in the next coming years.

1.5 NONUNIONS IN FRACTURE HEALING

A vast majority of fractures heal without forming scar tissue. Approximately 5–10% of all fractures fail to heal, but a more reasonable number applicable to the general population is close to 2% (Mills et al., 2017). Some patients and fracture types are, however, more susceptible to fracture nonunions than others; the risk of nonunion development is up to 9% (Mills et al., 2017).

The FDA defines nonunion as the combination of the failed radiographic consolidation of the fracture ends after nine months from fracture fixation and no radiographic changes in the fracture gap for three consecutive months (Wildemann et al., 2021). Fracture nonunions lead to morbidity and loss of productivity and constitute a major cost to the healthcare system. Grossly, nonunions are classified as 1) atrophic or 2) hypertrophic. Atrophic nonunions, as the name suggests, refers to the lack of biological activity at the fracture gap, and the underlying causes might or might not involve sepsis (Figure 1.5). In hypertrophic nonunions, much biological activity is observed around the fracture gap, but the fracture still fails to unite (Figure 1.5).

Gender, genetic factors, comorbidities and associated medication, infection, smoking and extent of trauma are all associated with increased risk of nonunion. Men have been shown to suffer with more frequent nonunions than females at earlier ages (<50), while the incidence is similar for men and women at later ages (>60). Smoking and associated vasoconstriction as well as the use of

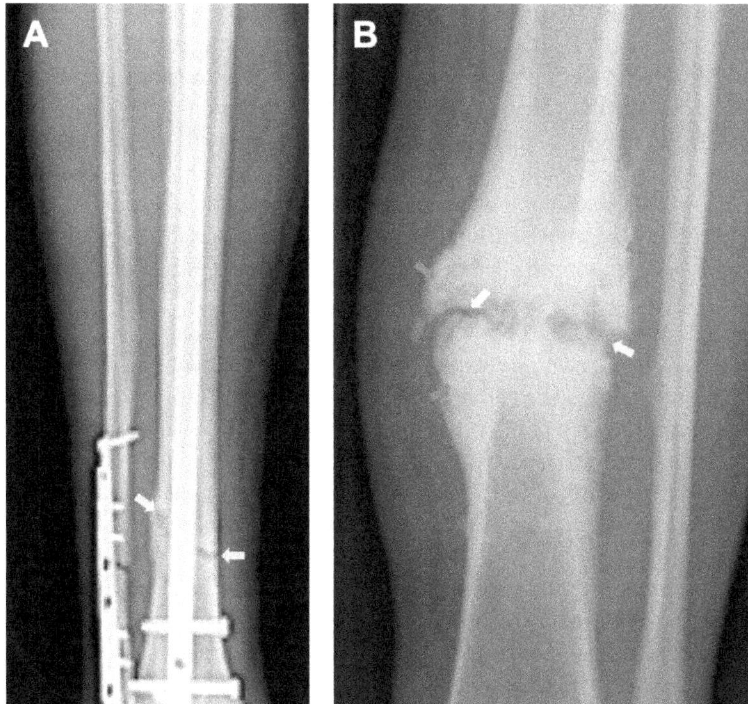

FIGURE 1.5 Clinical examples of fracture nonunions: (A) a classic example of an atrophic nonunion of the distal tibia three months postoperative; notice the lack of biological activity and fracture callus and a clear fracture line (yellow arrows), (B) a clinical case of a hypertrophic nonunion characterized by the presence of a large bony callus (red arrows) that has failed to unite due to the presence of a clear fracture gap (yellow arrows). (Reproduced under the terms of CC-BY 4.0 (https://creativecommons.org/licenses/by/4.0/) International License from Morshed, S.: Current Options for Determining Fracture Union. Advances in Medicine. 2014. 2014. Copyright 2014 S. Morshed, published by Hindawi; Reproduced under the terms of CC-BY 4.0 (https://creativecommons.org/licenses/by/4.0/) International License from Salih, S., Blakey, C., Chan, D., McGregor-Riley, J. C., Royston, S. L., Gowlett, S., Moore, D., & Dennison, M. G.: The callus fracture sign: a radiological predictor of progression to hypertrophic nonunion in diaphyseal tibial fractures. Strategies in Trauma and Limb Reconstruction. 2015. 10. 149–153. Copyright 2015 Salih et al., published by Springer Nature).

nonsteroidal anti-inflammatory medications are also known to impair fracture healing (Ding et al., 2018; Wildemann et al., 2021).

The pathogenesis of fracture nonunions is complex and multifactorial but is suggested to be linked with the basic principles of fracture healing, specifically fracture reduction and mechanical stability. Researchers have shown that cortical defects in the long bone heal if the interfragmentary movement is limited to <1 mm and the fracture gap is <3 mm (Wildemann et al., 2021), and interfragmentary movements >2 mm have been shown to impair or delay fracture healing (Claes, 2021). From a biological perspective, the inflammatory environment at the fracture site is very important, as I described earlier in this chapter. Cytokines and enzymes including TNF-(, IL-6, BMPs, IGF and MMPs are carefully orchestrated during the bridging process, and an imbalance in the spatiotemporal expression of these key regulators may influence the healing outcome. Smoking, for instance, is known to inhibit the production of TNF-(directly controlled by the nicotine in cigarette smoke and this imbalance in TNF-(production (which is known to both promote osteogenic differentiation of progenitors and assist in removing the cartilage template in endochondral ossification) early on, may explain why fractures are more challenging to treat in smokers (Gerstenfeld et al., 2003).

Another example is the local tissue levels of BMPs during fracture healing. Kloen and coworkers analyzed the expression of BMP-2, BMP-7, BMP-14 and their respective pSMADs 1/5/8 as well as the expression of BMP inhibitors chordin, gremlin and noggin in human tissues obtained from the fracture gap (Kloen et al., 2012). They concluded that the expression of BMPs in the cartilaginous component of the fracture gap was markedly reduced compared with the mineralized areas of the fracture callus, suggesting a potential role of the BMP family proteins in the process of endochondral ossification and subsequent union or nonunion. This explanation becomes particularly important in patients consuming NSAIDs since it has been shown that COX-2 inhibition reduces the BMP sensitivity of the osteoprogenitor cells and even impairs chondrocyte function (Daluiski et al., 2006; Li et al., 2014).

Another critical factor deciding the outcome of fracture treatment is vascularization. Reports have shown that nonunions tend to be hypervascularized (as seen by an increased expression of VEGF) both in experimental models and in patients indicating that rapid vascularization of the cartilage bed within the fracture gap may lead to inferior scaffolding material for new bone formation (Garcia et al., 2012; Sarahrudi et al., 2009). Wnt signaling pathway and the consequent expression of β-catenin are important regulators of MSC differentiation and bone/cartilage homeostasis. Alcohol consumption is known to affect β-catenin expression and consequently lead to impaired fracture healing (Lauing et al., 2012).

Taken together, the evidence from existing studies in the literature clearly explains the multifaceted etiology of fracture nonunion and possibly hints toward approaching and solving this problem. Since the goal of this chapter is to provide insight into the cellular and molecular interplay in bone regeneration, we now discuss various cell and molecular therapies that have been explored and applied in bone regeneration without going into the detailed topic of bone tissue engineering.

1.6 CELL-BASED THERAPIES IN FRACTURE HEALING

When fractures do not unite, or large pieces of bone are missing due to significant trauma to the bone, additional biological interventions are necessary, and a myriad of cell therapy approaches have been described to solve this problem. When it comes to cell-based technologies to improve fracture healing, MSCs have always been considered a cell population of interest. Pittenger and coworkers were the first scholars to define the antigenic signature of these cells and their ability to undergo trilineage (adipo-, chondro- and osteogenic) differentiation under controlled culture conditions (Pittenger et al., 1999).

The frequency of MSCs in bone marrow is rather low, accounting for only up to 0.001–0.01% (or about 600 cells/mL bone marrow) of the total mononuclear cells found in the bone marrow, although well-established methods exist for expanding these cell in vitro (Homma et al., 2013; Khatkar & See, 2021; Pittenger et al., 1999; Rosset et al., 2014). Herniguo and coworkers performed one of the first large studies on treating fracture nonunions with MSCs; they prepared concentrates from 300 mL bone marrow aspirates and reported a success rate of 88%, and the outcome demonstrated a positive correlation with total number of injected cells (Hernigou et al., 2005). However, the research group met with significant challenges in terms of total cell number (only about 50,000 MSCs could be isolated from 300 mL bone marrow aspirates), making the widespread use of this technique very difficult.

As a strategy to overcome inadequate cell numbers, Kitoh and coworkers prepared expanded MSC cultures in vitro for use in pediatric patients undergoing limb lengthening procedures and reported much better healing outcomes in patients who received the cell therapy than in those who did not (Kitoh et al., 2009). Others have combined MSCs with biomaterial scaffolds during either surgery or prolonged in vitro culture followed by implantation, but contributors discuss these concepts will be discussed in some of the later chapters in this book (Kim et al., 2009; Quarto et al., 2001).

Cell therapy has not only been limited to fracture nonunions but has also been tested in other bone related conditions. One of the other popular areas of use that cell therapy approach found has been the treatment of avascular necrosis (AVN) of the femoral head. Once again Hernigou and coworkers were at the forefront of treating this condition and reported that out > 500 AVN patients that were treated with standard-of-care core decompression combined with autologous MSC cell therapy, only 94 patients required a total hip replacement (Hernigou et al., 2009). These studies were soon followed by others including a randomized study by Gangji and coworkers who demonstrated that core decompression combined with MSCs was superior to core decompression alone (Gangji et al., 2004). It must however be noted that cell therapy is seen as a medicinal product and regulated by healthcare agencies across the globe, which have made the translation of the early studies into large scale randomized controlled trials cumbersome due to the risks such therapies possess to human health.

Since the first-time use of MSCs in a clinical setting in the early 2000's, several experimental approaches have also been described to overcome challenges associated with cell number, transplantation viability and potency. One of the most recent and promising attempts has been to engineer the cells to produce pro-osteogenic factors such as BMPs. This concept has been elegantly shown by Pigeot and coworkers, wherein they utilize an immortalized human MSC line overexpressing BMP-2 for in-vitro culture for a 3-week period (Pigeot et al., 2021). After the culture period of 3-weeks is complete, a cartilaginous matrix is laid out by the MSCs rich in ECM and signaling molecules. The MSCs are then devitalized by inducing death using an iCaspase based induced death system in order to ensure that the ECM product is devoid of any living cells or genetic material. Upon implantation of the devitalized ECM, the group demonstrated robust bone formation in ectopic implantation in nude mice. They even scaled up the production of this functional endochondral template in a bioreactor setup to successfully treat rat mandibular bone defects. This is just an example to show the progress cell therapy has made since the initial clinical study in the early 2000's and there is certainly more to come. However, experimental materials and cell therapies have to be translated into the clinical setting in a step-by-step manner from in-vitro studies to small and large animal proof-of-concept studies followed by feasibility studies in humans, all of which requires time and resources.

CONCLUSION

This chapter sheds light on the basics of bone biology from a cellular and molecular perspective. Bone homeostasis is an excellent example of a complex collaborative effort of several cell types, signaling molecules, growth factors, enzymes and proteins to carefully orchestrate skeletal function as well as calcium ion homeostasis. Injury to the bone tissue generally resolves without leaving a scar but 5–10% of the cases demonstrate delayed healing and this chapter provides explanations as to why such a phenomenon occurs. Finally, the potential of tissue engineering, particularly using cells as therapeutic tools to resolve the problem with bone healing using the bone tissue engineering approaches, provides a brief roadmap to future possibilities to explore in fracture healing.

LIST OF ABBREVIATIONS

ALP	Alkaline phosphatase
AVN	Avascular necrosis
BMP	Bone Morphogenic Protein
BSP	Bone sialo protein
CaP	Calcium Phosphate
CD	Cluster of differentiation
DKK-1	Dickkopf related protein-1
ECM	Extracellular matrix
EO	Endochondral ossification
GAG	Glycosaminoglycans

GLA Carboxyglutamic acid
HA Hydroxyapatite
IGF Insulin growth factor
IO Intramembranous ossification
M-CSF Macrophage colony stimulating factor
MMP Matrix metalloproteinases
MSC Mesenchymal stromal cell
OCN Osteocalcin
OPG Osteoprotegrin
PP_i Pyrophosphate
PTH Parathyroid hormone
RANK Receptor activator of nuclear factor kappa B
RANKL Receptor activator of nuclear factor kappa B ligand
RUNX-2 Runt related transcription factor-2
TNAP Tissue nonspecific alkaline phosphatase
TNF-⟨ Tumor necrosis factor
VEGF Vascular endothelial growth factor
ZA Zoledronic Acid

REFERENCES

Al-Bari, A. A., & Al Mamun, A. (2020). Current advances in regulation of bone homeostasis. *FASEB Bioadv.* 2: 668–679.

Anderson, D. M., Maraskovsky, E., Billingsley, W. L., Dougall, W. C., Tometsko, M. E., Roux, E. R., Teepe, M. C., DuBose, R. F., Cosman, D., & Galibert, L. (1997). A homologue of the TNF receptor and its ligand enhance T-cell growth and dendritic-cell function. *Nature.* 390: 175–179.

Bekker, P. J., Holloway, D. L., Rasmussen, A. S., Murphy, R., Martin, S. W., Leese, P. T., Holmes, G. B., Dunstan, C. R., & DePaoli, A. M. (2004). A single-dose placebo-controlled study of AMG 162, a fully human monoclonal antibody to RANKL, in postmenopausal women. *J. Bone Miner. Res.* 19: 1059–1066.

Claes, L. (2021). Improvement of clinical fracture healing—What can be learned from mechano-biological research? *J. Biomech.* 115: 110148.

Colnot, C. (2009). Skeletal cell fate decisions within periosteum and bone marrow during bone regeneration. *J. Bone Miner. Res.* 24: 274–282.

Daluiski, A., Ramsey, K. E., Shi, Y., Bostrom, M. P., Nestor, B. J., Martin, G., Hotchkiss, R., & Stephan, D. A. (2006). Cyclooxygenase-2 inhibitors in human skeletal fracture healing. *Orthopedics.* 29: 259–261.

Ding, Z. C., Lin, Y. K., Gan, Y. K., & Tang, T. T. (2018). Molecular pathogenesis of fracture nonunion. *J. Orthop. Translat.* 14: 45–56.

Dominici, M., Le Blanc, K., Mueller, I., Slaper-Cortenbach, I., Marini, F., Krause, D., Deans, R., Keating, A., Prockop, D., & Horwitz, E. (2006). Minimal criteria for defining multipotent mesenchymal stromal cells: The International Society for Cellular Therapy position statement. *Cytotherapy.* 8: 315–317.

Drake, M. T., Clarke, B. L., & Khosla, S. (2008). Bisphosphonates: Mechanism of action and role in clinical practice. *Mayo Clin. Proc.* 83: 1032–1045.

Einhorn, T. A., & Gerstenfeld, L. C. (2015). Fracture healing: Mechanisms and interventions. *Nat. Rev. Rheumatol.* 11: 45–54.

Eriksen, E. F. (2010). Cellular mechanisms of bone remodeling. *Rev. Endocr. Metab. Disord.* 11: 219–227.

Everts, V., Jansen, I. D. C., & de Vries, T. J. (2022). Mechanisms of bone resorption. *Bone.* 163: 116499.

Gangji, V., Hauzeur, J. P., Matos, C., De Maertelaer, V., Toungouz, M., & Lambermont, M. (2004). Treatment of osteonecrosis of the femoral head with implantation of autologous bone-marrow cells: A pilot study. *J. Bone Joint Surg. Am.* 86: 1153–1160.

Garcia, P., Pieruschka, A., Klein, M., Tami, A., Histing, T., Holstein, J. H., Scheuer, C., Pohlemann, T., & Menger, M. D. (2012). Temporal and spatial vascularization patterns of unions and nonunions: Role of vascular endothelial growth factor and bone morphogenetic proteins. *J. Bone Joint Surg. Am.* 94: 49–58.

Gerstenfeld, L. C., Cho, T. J., Kon, T., Aizawa, T., Tsay, A., Fitch, J., Barnes, G. L., Graves, D. T., & Einhorn, T. A. (2003). Impaired fracture healing in the absence of TNF-alpha signaling: The role of TNF-alpha in endochondral cartilage resorption. *J. Bone Miner. Res.* 18: 1584–1592.

Glass, G. E., Chan, J. K., Freidin, A., Feldmann, M., Horwood, N. J., & Nanchahal, J. (2011). TNF-α promotes fracture repair by augmenting the recruitment and differentiation of muscle-derived stromal cells. *Proc. Natl. Acad. Sci.* 108: 1585–1590.

Hadjidakis, D. J., & Androulakis, I. I. (2006). Bone remodeling. *Ann. N. Y. Acad. Sci.* 1092: 385–396.

Hall, B. K. (1988). The embryonic development of bone. *Am. Sci.* 76: 174–181.

Henthorn, P. S., & Whyte, M. P. (1992). Missense mutations of the tissue-nonspecific alkaline phosphatase gene in hypophosphatasia. *Clin. Chem.* 38: 2501–2505.

Hernigou, P., Poignard, A., Beaujean, F., & Rouard, H. (2005). Percutaneous autologous bone-marrow grafting for nonunions. Influence of the number and concentration of progenitor cells. *J. Bone Joint Surg. Am.* 87: 1430–1437.

Hernigou, P., Poignard, A., Zilber, S., & Rouard, H. (2009). Cell therapy of hip osteonecrosis with autologous bone marrow grafting. *Indian J. Orthop.* 43: 40–45.

Hessle, L., Johnson, K. A., Anderson, H. C., Narisawa, S., Sali, A., Goding, J. W., Terkeltaub, R., & Millan, J. L. (2002). Tissue-nonspecific alkaline phosphatase and plasma cell membrane glycoprotein-1 are central antagonistic regulators of bone mineralization. *Proc. Natl. Acad. Sci.* 99: 9445–9449.

Ho, A. M., Johnson, M. D., & Kingsley, D. M. (2000). Role of the mouse *ank* gene in control of tissue calcification and arthritis. *Science.* 289: 265–270.

Homma, Y., Zimmermann, G., & Hernigou, P. (2013). Cellular therapies for the treatment of non-union: The past, present and future. *Injury.* 44: S46–S49.

Houlihan, D. D., Mabuchi, Y., Morikawa, S., Niibe, K., Araki, D., Suzuki, S., Okano, H., & Matsuzaki, Y. (2012). Isolation of mouse mesenchymal stem cells on the basis of expression of Sca-1 and PDGFR-α. *Nat. Protoc.* 7: 2103–2111.

Hu, D. P., Ferro, F., Yang, F., Taylor, A. J., Chang, W., Miclau, T., Marcucio, R. S., & Bahney, C. S. (2017). Cartilage to bone transformation during fracture healing is coordinated by the invading vasculature and induction of the core pluripotency genes. *Development.* 144: 221–234.

Hunter, G. K., & Goldberg, H. A. (1993). Nucleation of hydroxyapatite by bone sialoprotein. *Proc. Natl. Acad. Sci.* 90: 8562–8565.

Kaderly, R. E. (1991). Primary bone healing. *Semin. Vet. Med. Surg. Small Anim.* 6: 21–25.

Khatkar, H., & See, A. (2021). Stem cell therapy in the management of fracture non-union—evaluating cellular mechanisms and clinical progress. *Cureus.* 13: e13869.

Kim, S. J., Shin, Y. W., Yang, K. H., Kim, S. B., Yoo, M. J., Han, S. K., Im, S. A., Won, Y. D., Sung, Y. B., Jeon, T. S., Chang, C. H., Jang, J. D., Lee, S. B., Kim, H. C., & Lee, S. Y. (2009). A multi-center, randomized, clinical study to compare the effect and safety of autologous cultured osteoblast (Ossron) injection to treat fractures. *BMC Musculoskelet. Disord.* 10: 20.

Kitoh, H., Kawasumi, M., Kaneko, H., & Ishiguro, N. (2009). Differential effects of culture-expanded bone marrow cells on the regeneration of bone between the femoral and the tibial lengthenings. *J. Pediatr. Orthop.* 29: 643–649.

Kloen, P., Lauzier, D., & Hamdy, R. C. (2012). Co-expression of BMPs and BMP-inhibitors in human fractures and non-unions. *Bone.* 51: 59–68.

Komori, T., Yagi, H., Nomura, S., Yamaguchi, A., Sasaki, K., Deguchi, K., Shimizu, Y., Bronson, R. T., Gao, Y. H., Inada, M., Sato, M., Okamoto, R., Kitamura, Y., Yoshiki, S., & Kishimoto, T. (1997). Targeted disruption of Cbfa1 results in a complete lack of bone formation owing to maturational arrest of osteoblasts. *Cell.* 89: 755–764.

Lauing, K. L., Roper, P. M., Nauer, R. K., & Callaci, J. J. (2012). Acute alcohol exposure impairs fracture healing and deregulates β-catenin signaling in the fracture callus. *Alcohol Clin. Exp. Res.* 36: 2095–2103.

Li, T. F., Yukata, K., Yin, G., Sheu, T., Maruyama, T., Jonason, J. H., Hsu, W., Zhang, X., Xiao, G., Konttinen, Y. T., Chen, D., & O'Keefe, R. J. (2014). BMP-2 induces ATF4 phosphorylation in chondrocytes through a COX-2/PGE2 dependent signaling pathway. *Osteoarthr. Cartil.* 22: 481–489.

Lotsari, A., Rajasekharan, A. K., Halvarsson, M., & Andersson, M. (2018). Transformation of amorphous calcium phosphate to bone-like apatite. *Nat. Commun.* 9: 4170.

Marsell, R., & Einhorn, T. A. (2011). The biology of fracture healing. *Injury.* 42: 551–555.

Meert, K. L., Ofenstein, J. P., & Sarnaik, A. P. (1998). Altered T cell cytokine production following mechanical trauma. *Ann. Clin. Lab Sci.* 28: 283–288.

Mills, L. A., Aitken, S. A., & Simpson, A. (2017). The risk of non-union per fracture: Current myths and revised figures from a population of over 4 million adults. *Acta Orthop.* 88: 434–439.

Morshed, S. (2014). Current options for determining fracture union. *Adv. Med.* 2014: 708574.

Mundlos, S., Otto, F., Mundlos, C., Mulliken, J. B., Aylsworth, A. S., Albright, S., Lindhout, D., Cole, W. G., Henn, W., Knoll, J. H., Owen, M. J., Mertelsmann, R., Zabel, B. U., & Olsen, B. R. (1997). Mutations involving the transcription factor CBFA1 cause cleidocranial dysplasia. *Cell.* 89: 773–779.

Murshed, M., Harmey, D., Millán, J. L., McKee, M. D., & Karsenty, G. (2005). Unique coexpression in osteoblasts of broadly expressed genes accounts for the spatial restriction of ECM mineralization to bone. *Genes Dev.* 19: 1093–1104.

Nauta, A. J., & Fibbe, W. E. (2007). Immunomodulatory properties of mesenchymal stromal cells. *Blood.* 110: 3499–3506.

Okawa, A., Nakamura, I., Goto, S., Moriya, H., Nakamura, Y., & Ikegawa, S. (1998). Mutation in Npps in a mouse model of ossification of the posterior longitudinal ligament of the spine. *Nat. Genet.* 19: 271–273.

Otto, F., Thornell, A. P., Crompton, T., Denzel, A., Gilmour, K. C., Rosewell, I. R., Stamp, G. W., Beddington, R. S., Mundlos, S., Olsen, B. R., Selby, P. B., & Owen, M. J. (1997). Cbfa1, a candidate gene for cleidocranial dysplasia syndrome, is essential for osteoblast differentiation and bone development. *Cell.* 89: 765–771.

Pfeiffenberger, M., Damerau, A., Lang, A., Buttgereit, F., Hoff, P., & Gaber, T. (2021). Fracture healing research—shift towards In vitro modeling? *Biomedicines.* 9: 748.

Pigeot, S., Klein, T., Gullotta, F., Dupard, S. J., Garcia, A., García-García, A., Prithiviraj, S., Lorenzo, P., Filippi, M., Jaquiery, C., Kouba, L., Asnaghi, M. A., Raina, D. B., Dasen, B., Isaksson, H., Önnerfjord, P., Tägil, M., Bondanza, A., Martin, I., & Bourgine, P. E. (2021). Manufacturing of human tissues as off-the-shelf grafts Programmed to induce regeneration. *Adv. Mater.* 33: 2103737.

Pittenger, M. F., Mackay, A. M., Beck, S. C., Jaiswal, R. K., Douglas, R., Mosca, J. D., Moorman, M. A., Simonetti, D. W., Craig, S., & Marshak, D. R. (1999). Multilineage potential of adult human mesenchymal stem cells. *Science.* 284: 143–147.

Quarto, R., Mastrogiacomo, M., Cancedda, R., Kutepov, S. M., Mukhachev, V., Lavroukov, A., Kon, E., & Marcacci, M. (2001). Repair of large bone defects with the use of autologous bone marrow stromal cells. *N. Engl. J. Med.* 344: 385–386.

Rahman, M. S., Akhtar, N., Jamil, H. M., Banik, R. S., & Asaduzzaman, S. M. (2015). TGF-β/BMP signaling and other molecular events: Regulation of osteoblastogenesis and bone formation. *Bone Res.* 3: 15005.

Raina, D. (2018). *Biomaterials as Carriers for Bone Active Molecules-An Approach to Create Off-the-Shelf Bone Substitutes.* (Doctoral Dissertation, Lund University), Lund, Sweden.

Reznikov, N., Bilton, M., Lari, L., Stevens, M. M., & Kröger, R. (2018). Fractal-like hierarchical organization of bone begins at the nanoscale. *Science.* 360: eaao2189.

Rosset, P., Deschaseaux, F., & Layrolle, P. (2014). Cell therapy for bone repair. *Orthop. Traumatol.-Sur.* 100: S107–S112.

Salih, S., Blakey, C., Chan, D., McGregor-Riley, J. C., Royston, S. L., Gowlett, S., Moore, D., & Dennison, M. G. (2015). The callus fracture sign: A radiological predictor of progression to hypertrophic non-union in diaphyseal tibial fractures. *Strategies Trauma Limb Reconstr.* 10: 149–153.

Sarahrudi, K., Thomas, A., Braunsteiner, T., Wolf, H., Vécsei, V., & Aharinejad, S. (2009). VEGF serum concentrations in patients with long bone fractures: A comparison between impaired and normal fracture healing. *J. Orthop. Res.* 27: 1293–1297.

Schenk, R. (1994). Histological and ultrastructural features of fracture healing. *Bone Form. Repair.* 117–146.

Shapiro, F. (1988). Cortical bone repair: The relationship of the lacunar-canalicular system and intercellular gap junctions to the repair process. *J. Bone Joint Surg. Am.* 70: 1067–1081.

Taylor, J. G., & Bushinsky, D. A. (2009). Calcium and phosphorus homeostasis. *Blood Purif.* 27: 387–394.

Wallace, A., Cooney, T. E., Englund, R., & Lubahn, J. D. (2011). Effects of interleukin-6 ablation on fracture healing in mice. *J. Orthop. Res.* 29: 1437–1442.

Wildemann, B., Ignatius, A., Leung, F., Taitsman, L. A., Smith, R. M., Pesántez, R., Stoddart, M. J., Richards, R. G., & Jupiter, J. B. (2021). Non-union bone fractures. *Nat. Rev. Dis. Primers.* 7: 57.

Wong, B. R., Rho, J., Arron, J., Robinson, E., Orlinick, J., Chao, M., Kalachikov, S., Cayani, E., Bartlett, F. S., 3rd, Frankel, W. N., Lee, S. Y., & Choi, Y. (1997). TRANCE is a novel ligand of the tumor necrosis factor receptor family that activates c-Jun N-terminal kinase in T cells. *J. Biol. Chem.* 272: 25190–25194.

Wosczyna, M. N., Biswas, A. A., Cogswell, C. A., & Goldhamer, D. J. (2012). Multipotent progenitors resident in the skeletal muscle interstitium exhibit robust BMP-dependent osteogenic activity and mediate heterotopic ossification. *J. Bone Miner. Res.* 27: 1004–1017.

Yasuda, H., Shima, N., Nakagawa, N., Yamaguchi, K., Kinosaki, M., Mochizuki, S., Tomoyasu, A., Yano, K., Goto, M., Murakami, A., Tsuda, E., Morinaga, T., Higashio, K., Udagawa, N., Takahashi, N., & Suda, T. (1998). Osteoclast differentiation factor is a ligand for osteoprotegerin/osteoclastogenesis-inhibitory factor and is identical to TRANCE/RANKL. *Proc. Natl. Acad. Sci.* 95: 3597–3602.

2 Choice and Selection of Biomaterials for Bone Repair

Andreas K Nüssler and Sabrina Ehnert

2.1 INTRODUCTION

In the course of everyday life, the musculoskeletal system is subjected to strong physical stresses that can lead to bone injuries and diseases. However, bone can be kept healthy, strengthened, or prevented from further deterioration by a healthy lifestyle, including continuous athletic training (Amini et al., 2012). However, large/critical defects caused by accidents, medical conditions, nonunions or other trauma, healing is impaired and therefore requires extensive clinical intervention (Hernandez et al., 2012). Interventions for serious injuries increase the economic burden on health insurance companies and society.

Bone is the second most commonly transplanted tissue after blood, with at least over two million bone transplants per year (Finkemeier, 2002); autografts are considered the state-of-the-art procedure. In this process, bone or spongiosa is harvested from the patient, the latter often from the iliac crest, and transplanted at the defect site. Although it is clinically superior, disadvantages such as donor site morbidity, long-term postoperative pain, and the need for specialized surgical procedures limit its use (Winkler et al., 2018). Therefore, in recent decades, a number of alternatives have been considered and developed to overcome the limits of autologous or cancellous bone grafting. This book chapter will summarize the alternatives and discuss their requirements and future directions.

2.2 BIOMATERIALS FOR BONE REPAIR TO REPLACE AUTOGRAFTS/ALLOGRAFTS

In the first line, bone can be repaired using autologous cells, either by augmenting the cell population at the defect site or by transplanting the autogenous grafted bone or spongiosa. For instance, in the case of a maxillofacial defect, bone repair entails enhancing local cell proliferation using a specific membrane to inhibit soft tissue infiltration, also known as guided bone regeneration (Retzepi & Donos, 2010). In this case, the cells excrete a specific matrix, resulting in the new generation of woven bone, which eventually transforms into lamellar bone. This technology is usually applicable for small defects but will most likely not be able to repair large bone defects.

Historically, three important discoveries have advanced bone research: the discovery of bone morphogenic proteins (BMPs) in 1965, the discovery of pluripotent mesenchymal stromal cells (MSCs) in 1991, and the development of bone-mimicking materials composed of calcium phosphate ceramics, collagen, and other proteins (Arvidson et al., 2011). The concept of tissue engineering using various combinations of cells and growth factors with scaffolds or other matrices has opened new avenues for the discovery of bone grafts with superior clinical outcomes (Winkler et al., 2018; Henkel et al., 2013).

2.3 BIOMATERIALS

A common way of classifying biomaterials is to distinguish between nonliving material and material that has been functionalized to achieve organic properties to better integrate into biological

 DOI: 10.1201/9781003307310-3

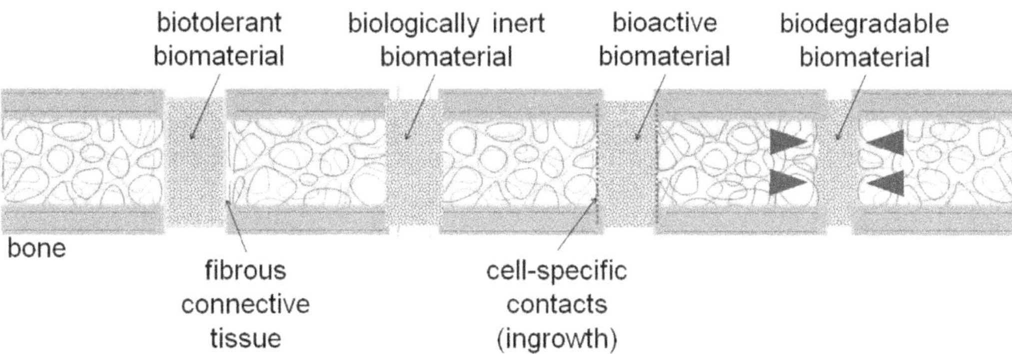

FIGURE 2.1 Schematic example for the different classes of bio- or implant materials. Depending on the characteristics of the biomaterial (dotted rectangle), there are different interactions with the bone (porous tube). Biologically inert and biotolerant biomaterials (covered with fibrous connective tissue) show no direct interaction with the bone. Bioactive biomaterials develop cell-specific contacts that can lead to degradation and replacement (biodegradable) of the biomaterials.

systems (Koons et al., 2020). Biocompatibility is critical for bone replacement materials, as they are within a living being for a long period of time. Generally, they are classified as bioactive, bioinert, or biocompatible, meaning that they do not cause unwanted side effects (Figure 2.1).

Biotolerant biomaterials may remain in the body for months to several years without decomposition, cellular alteration, or toxic effects during the period of use (in vivo). However, minor defects in tissue reaction may occur. Biotolerant materials are often encapsulated in fibrous connective tissue or demarcated from the target tissue by fibrous connective tissue so that no rejection reaction occurs. This also means that there is no direct, mechanical anchoring of the implant in the target tissue.

- Biologically inert biomaterials have no chemical or biological interaction with the surrounding tissue. In addition, the substances released from the material into the tissue/body do not exceed the specified limits at any time; this makes such materials corrosion resistant, refractory, and passivatable and gives them high thermal and mechanical stability and resistance. When implanted, often a direct, mechanical anchoring of the material in the target tissue occurs.
- Bioactive biomaterials make the tissue react to the material. This can be achieved, for example, with a coating that promotes the formation of new bone around the implant, that is, the implant has an osteoinductive or osteoanabolic effect. The material, but usually only the coating, is converted into bone material during this process. Thus, in contrast to biologically inert materials, a cohesive connection between biomaterial and tissue is formed that can only be loosened by destruction and that allows the transfer of tensile loads.
- Biodegradable materials are degraded or absorbed in the tissue. Often, these materials are also bioactive as a result.

Many materials from metals to artificial and natural polymers are used in bone tissue engineering to provide support and stiffness or to act as fillers and scaffolds to provide regenerative drug-delivery vehicles (Gautam et al., 2022). Commonly used biomaterials and their classification are shown in Figure 2.2.

Ceramics, composites, metals, plastics, or other support materials are commonly used due to their nonbioactive properties (Gautam et al., 2022). However, acrylic cements, for example, have limitations due to exothermic reactions that can lead to necrosis of the surrounding tissue at the

		biological inert	biotolerant		bioactive		biodegradable
Ceramics		aluminum oxide (Al_2O_3) zirconium oxide (ZrO_2)			bioglasses Calsil (calcium silicate / Ca_2SiO_4) Hydroxyapatite (HAP / $Ca_5(PO_4)_3$) Fluorapatite (CaF) Brushite ($CaHPO_4$) SiO_2 mesoporous materials	calcium phosphates* calcium sulfate ($CaSO_4$) Aragonite (Coral-$CaCO_3$) Magnesium (Mg)	$Ca_5(PO_4)_3$ < 10 μm
Polymers	natural	agarose alginate			gelatine chitosan	collagen hyaluronic acid	
	synthetic	PA	PMMA PE PA6 PFTE			PEAK PUR	PCL PLA PLGA
Metals		pure titanium titanium alloys (e.g. Ti-6Al-4V)	gold alloys (Co, Cr, Mo) stainless steel niobium (Nb) tantalum (Ta) zirconium (Zr)		coated metals chemically etched metallic alloys (Ti, Zr, Nb, Ta)	biodegradable metals (Ti, Co, Fe, Mg, Ta, Zn, Ni, Ir)	
Composits				Ta composites PMMA bioglass PMMA HAP	glass ceramics		

FIGURE 2.2 Commonly used biomaterials and their classification. Biomaterials can be categorized as ceramics, natural and synthetic polymers, metals, and composite materials. Within each category there are different examples for biologically inert, biotolerant, bioactive, and biodegradable biomaterials.

Notes. PMMA: polymethyl methacrylate; PE: Polyethylene; PA6: poly(hexano-6-lactam); PTFE: poly(tetra-fluor-ethylene); PEAK: poly(aryl-ether-ketone); PUR: Polyurethane; PCL: Poly-caprolactone; PLA: poly(lactic acid); PLGA: poly(lactic acid-co-glycolic acid).

graft site, accompanied by inflammatory reactions and ischemia. Metal-based bone graft substitutes are often subject to limitations such as stress reactions, increased ion secretion leading to detrimental toxicity, and their removal requires additional surgical procedures (Koons et al., 2020).

These flaws mean that for a synthetic bone graft, not only is biocompatibility required, but the biomaterial should also have mechanical strength essentially equivalent to that of bone and be osteoconductive (triggering bone formation on its surface) and osteoinductive (facilitating cell infiltration) to effectively initiate bone regeneration. Composite materials such as hydroxyapatite (HAP) and collagen type 1 are particularly relevant here (Zhou & Lee, 2011). HAP is biocompatible and osteoconductive and occurs naturally in bone, which is why it is widely used in various bone substitutes, fillers, bioactive coatings, bone composites, and drug carriers and in the fabrication of scaffolds for bone tissue engineering. In addition, calcium phosphate/sulphate cement has been widely used in the clinic because it has good bone regeneration potential. However, as it has a higher resorption rate than bone formation rate (Samavedi et al., 2013), it is today replaced with tricalcium phosphate (Yanoso-Scholl et al., 2010).

HAP, with the chemical formula $Ca_5(PO_4)_3(OH)$, is the most abundant mineral component of human bone. Approximately 50% v/v (70% w/w) of the mineralized bone matrix contains hydroxyapatite or one of its derivatives, where the OH^- ion is replaced by fluoride, chloride, or carbonate (Singh et al., 2018). Bone biomaterials containing HAP or its derivatives are often described as favoring cell attachment and proliferation and osteogenic differentiation (Jain et al., 2015; Thein-Han & Misra, 2009).

However, the way HAP is incorporated into the bone biomaterial is crucial. In its natural form, it is insoluble and can therefore be easily incorporated into bone biomaterials made from polymer cryogels, but an equal distribution of the HAP has to be guaranteed as gravitational forces may result in sedimentation and consequently gradient formation of the hydroxyapatite (Häussling et al., 2019). Furthermore, by incorporating insoluble hydroxyapatite into an aqueous polymer, direct contact of the target cells with the osteoinductive minerals is shielded. When calcium–phosphate crystallization is initiated directly after cryogels are polymerized, the mineralized crystals strengthen the stability and roughen the surface of the cryogels (Häussling et al., 2019).

Up to 95% of the bone extracellular matrix (ECM) is composed of type I, III, and IV collagen, while the remaining components consist of noncollagenous proteins such as proteoglycans (e.g., biglycan and decorin), glycoproteins (e.g., osteonectin), γ-carboxyglutamic acid-containing proteins (e.g., osteocalcin), etc. (Lin et al., 2020). The peptide chains in collagen are arranged in a triple helix structure, and these collagen fibrils interact with the nano-HAP to form an excellent composite material (Robey et al., 1993). In the same vein, Teotia et al. (2017) demonstrated that collagen and HAP combined have better regenerative bone properties than tricalcium phosphate or collagen scaffolds alone.

To facilitate the infiltration of new blood vessels and seeding of osteoprogenitor cells of a given scaffold, the optimal pore size is 100–300 μm. Conventionally, they are used in the form of foams or granules or as orthopedic defect fillers to create a scaffold structure that facilitates cellular infiltration and tissue regeneration (Koons et al., 2020). Although the structural mimicry of bone tissue is an important aspect, for tissue regeneration, the recruitment of cells to the defect site followed by their differentiation into chondrogenic and osteogenic lineages is important; otherwise their differentiation into fibroblastic lineages is favored, leading to the development of fibrous tissue (Satija et al., 2007).

2.4 BIOMECHANICAL CHARACTERISTICS OF THE BIOMATERIALS

2.4.1 Porosity and Stiffness

A vast range of synthetic ceramics and freeze-dried biomaterials exists for bone tissue engineering (Jain et al., 2015; Mayr-Wohlfart et al., 2001; Ayobian-Markazi et al., 2012; George et al., 2006). Pore size and shape, wall thickness, porosity, and stiffness are critical for the architecture of these biomaterials. The stiffness of the material can affect the differentiation of the progenitor cells in their close proximity; while materials with low stiffness are more favorable for adipogenic and chondrogenic differentiation, biomaterials with higher stiffness favor osteogenic differentiation (Zhao et al., 2014).

At the same time, bone biomaterials should retain some flexibility in order to pass on mechanical stimuli to the cells, which is required for osteogenic differentiation (Dawson & Oreffo, 2008; Chen & Jacobs, 2013). The flexibility of these materials is provided on one hand by the material itself and on the other hand by the structure of the material. Organic materials, such as collagen and gelatin provide better flexibility than inorganic materials such as bone cements, ceramics, or metals. Furthermore, porous biomaterials provide better flexibility than solid biomaterials. For example, a bone composed of only compact cortical bone would be very stiff (10–20 gPa depending on the direction of the force applied) but also brittle when external forces are applied (Zioupos & Currey, 1998; Morgan et al., 2018). The inner porous trabecular bone, in contrast, is less stiff (0.1 mPa–3 gPa depending on the direction of the force applied) but can better can better distribute or dissipate forces acting on it (Morgan et al., 2018; Oftadeh et al., 2015).

Similar to bone, porosity provides another important property for bone graft substitutes, namely reducing the weight of the material. However, the architecture of the pores is decisive for how the forces acting on the material are transmitted. Thanks to the German surgeon Julius Wolff, the best described example of force transmission in bone is the femoral head. The applied force results in areas with principal and secondary tensile stress as well as principal and secondary compressive stress in the femoral head (Boyle & Kim, 2011). This affects the structure of the trabeculae (natural pores) within the femoral head.

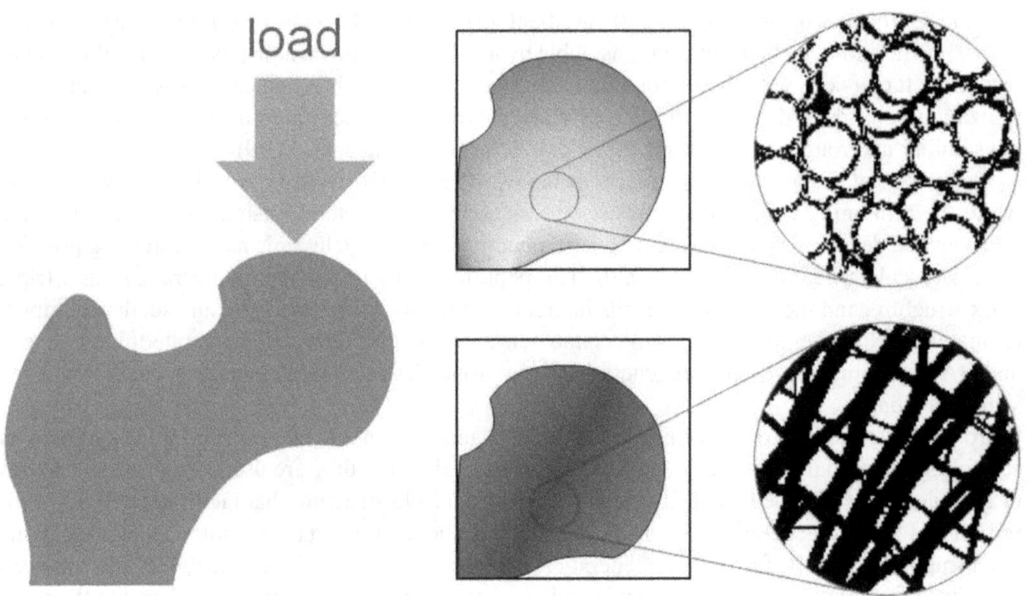

FIGURE 2.3 Relevance of the pore structure for implant stability. Simplified graphic from Jang and Kim (2008). Finite element simulation of a load applied on a femur head implant with different pore structures. The uniform circular pores result in a stress peak at the distal part of the femoral head, which makes the implant vulnerable to failure. The trabeculae-like pore structure directs the stress along the femur.

Computer-aided pixel-based finite element simulations proved that the structure or architecture of the pores is critical in pressure distribution and thus stability of the material (Jang & Kim, 2008). This is of special importance for implant development (Figure 2.3). There, pore structure and porosity also affect cell attachment to and cell infiltration into the bone biomaterial, but they also affect nutrient delivery and metabolite removal, a factor determined by the permeability of materials.

In vitro, the osteogenic differentiation of mesenchymal stem cells was improved by cultivation on three-dimensional scaffolds, which favored their cell agglomeration (Furuhata et al., 2017). This factor is also critically dependent on the scaffolds' pore size. For bone tissue engineering, a carrier pore size within the range of 20 µm to 300 µm is recommended to favor osteogenesis (Jain et al., 2015). The smaller pores, however, may hinder vascularization when transplanted in vivo (Di Luca et al., 2016). Thus, studies claim a minimum pore size of 100 µm to not only favor osteogenesis but also provide successful vascularization in vivo (Daculsi & Passuti, 1990; Murphy & O'Brien, 2010).

At present, several raw materials and production processes are under scrutiny, all providing precise advantages and disadvantages (Chocholata et al., 2019; Wubneh et al., 2018). Collagen, being the most profuse organic matrix in bone, is a popular choice as a protein carrier for bone graft substitutes. As described above, collagen in biomaterials makes the cells mostly flexible (Dawson & Oreffo, 2008), which facilitates osteogenic differentiation. However, if the scaffold is too flexible, MSCs can differentiate into adipocytes and not osteoblasts (Zhao et al., 2014).

It has been shown that carrier stiffness above 60 kPa induces the expression of osteogenic transcription factors and marker genes (Sun et al., 2018; Engler et al., 2006), and carrier stiffness below 60 kPa preserved the expression of stem cells markers, including Sox2, that can inhibit osteogenic differentiation (Ding et al., 2012; Marcellini et al., 2012; Park et al., 2012; Seo et al., 2013). Collagen or gelatin form natural hydrogels, but these hydrogels are very soft and lack a macro-porous structure. Furthermore, the noncovalent aggregations of collagen or gelatin are easily dissolved at temperatures higher than 30 to 35 °C, which destroys their physical network. Therefore, ECM proteins such as collagen or gelatin may be covalently crosslinked by glutaraldehyde. The coupling of the carboxyl and amino groups forms stable amide bonds and thus upsurges the stability and mechanical properties of the resulting gels (Ofner & Bubnis, 1996). When polymerization happens at temperatures below 0 °C, the ice crystals in the aqueous solution serve as "space holders" to form micro/macro porous gels: so-called cryogels. Apart from collagen and gelatin, a wide variety of monomers and crosslinkers exist that provide a platform for the simple and cheap production of cryogels in different shapes (see Section 2.5.1).

2.4.2 Surface Modifications

Surface roughness has been shown to have a critical influence on the osteogenic differentiation potential of osteoprogenitor cells; increasing the surface roughness of scaffolds was sufficient to trigger the spontaneous osteogenesis of cultured osteoprogenitor cells (Faia-Torres et al., 2014, 2015). It was postulated that rougher surfaces trigger that osteogenic differentiation by promoting the development of strong focal adhesions (Mathieu & Loboa, 2012). However, a rough surface is not the only property that can be achieved through surface modification. Surface modifications can provide antimicrobial effects to the bone substitute materials (Figure 2.4) (Jaggessar et al., 2017; Ivanova et al., 2012; Glinel et al., 2012).

One option is the coating of the biomaterial with anti-adhesive, super-hydrophobic, or biologically inert polymers. This more passive approach should prevent adhesion of the microbes on the surface of the bone substitute material (Glinel et al., 2012). Alternatively, the surface of the bone biomaterials can be modified to actively kill bacteria. This includes coating the material with organic substances such as antibiotics or other bactericidal and antimicrobial substances that actively kill or prevent proliferation of bacteria. Coating with bactericidal enzymes such as lysozyme (Mueller et al., 2017) or chitosan (Thein-Han & Misra, 2009; Xing et al., 2022) can also actively kill microbes that try to attach to the bone biomaterial.

Inorganic antibacterial nanomaterials can be divided into metal ions and photocatalytic oxides based on their mode of action (Han et al., 2022). Metal ions with antibacterial functions are silver (Ag^+), copper (Cu^{2+}), zinc (Zn^{2+}), nickel (Ni^{2+}), cobalt (Co^{2+}), and aluminum (Al^+). These metallic ions can be loaded on a variety of natural or synthetic substrates. When released into the peripheral tissue, they exert antibacterial and bactericidal effects. However, their release kinetics have to be tightly controlled, as for example silver ions may also interfere with the coagulation of blood (Kapadia et al., 2005; Laloy et al., 2014).

Commonly used oxide photocatalytic antimicrobial materials are, among others, titanium dioxide (TiO_2), zinc oxide (ZnO), magnesium oxide (MgO), and cadmium sulfide (CdS) (Yemmireddy & Hung, 2017; Prakash et al., 2022). These photocatalysts possess antimicrobial properties through the photocatalytic production of cytotoxic reactive oxygen species (ROS) (Liu et al., 2020). However, as the name suggests, the generation of ROS by such photocatalytic antimicrobial materials requires UV/sunlight, which makes them very useful for disinfecting surfaces, air, and water but limits their use inside the human body (Prakash et al., 2022).

These described antimicrobial strategies do not represent stand-alone techniques but can be applied in combination. For example, when lysozyme is combined with thin zwitterionic polymer films (Khlyustova et al., 2022), graphene oxide (Li et al., 2019), bioglass (Zheng et al., 2016), or chitosan-silver nanocomposites in an enzyme-responsive composite coating (Liu et al., 2018). Other examples include silver-doped or β-defensin-2-loaded mesoporous bioglass (Qian et al., 2021; Ren et al., 2021).

Nature provides another strategy to generate antibacterial properties on bone substitute materials that involves the nanostructures of the material surface. A schematic representation of the interaction of different nanostructure geometries with Gram-negative and Gram-positive bacteria is given in Figure 2.5. The leaves of lotus (*Nelumbo nucifera*) and taro (*Colocasia esculenta*) plants have characteristic microstructures that give the leaf anti-biofouling and self-cleaning properties (Jaggessar et al., 2017). The microscopic elliptical protrusions covered by nanoscale crystals result

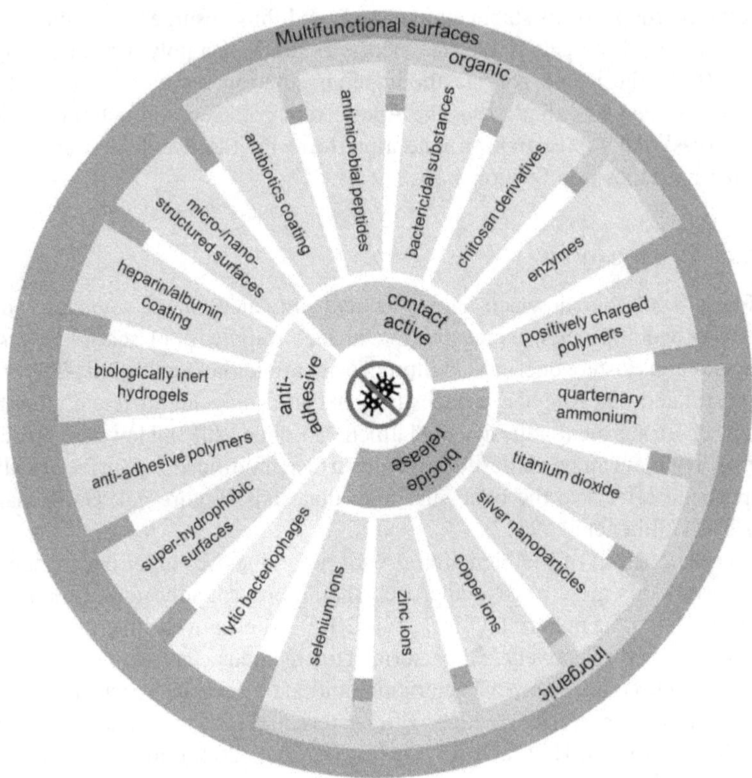

FIGURE 2.4 Overview of different surface modification strategies to gain antibacterial properties (Jaggessar et al., 2017; Ivanova et al., 2012; Glinel et al., 2012). Modifications can be roughly divided into anti-adhesive, contact active, biocide release, and other treatments, e.g., adding lytic bacteriophages.

in high contact angles, giving the surface its super-hydrophobic property (Bhushan et al., 2009). This super-hydrophobicity makes the surface anti-adhesive not only to dirt and particles but also to bacteria (Ma et al., 2011).

While lotus and taro leaves are anti-adhesive to bacteria, there exist other nanostructured surfaces in nature that actively kill bacteria, such as the skin of a gecko (*Gekkonidae*) and the wings of the cicada fly (*Cicadoidea*) and the dragonfly (*Anisoptera*). The nanostructure of the cicada wing ruptures Gram-negative bacteria, usually in the spaces between the nanopillars (Ivanova et al., 2012). Gram-positive bacteria, however, resist this effect and survive (Hasan et al., 2013).

In contrast to the relatively uniform nanostructure of the cicada wing, the nanostructure of the dragonfly wing is nanopillars with different heights, which also has a bactericidal effect against certain Gram-positive bacteria. When Gram-negative bacteria come into contact with these heterogeneous nanostructures, the larger nanopillars bend and start to secrete an extracellular polymeric substance. As a result, the bacteria strongly adhere to the nanostructures. Bacterial membranes separate when bacteria try to overcome the strong adhesion force to move away from the nanostructures (Bandara et al., 2017). The nanostructure of gecko skin consists of thin, curved (10 to 20 nm curvature) spinels from several hundred nanometers to a few micrometers in length (Watson et al., 2015). Gram-negative bacteria with a diameter greater than 500 nm are penetrated by the nanostructure of the gecko skin, while the smaller Gram-positive bacteria (<300 to 400 nm) remain undamaged on top of the nanostructure (Watson et al., 2015).

These and other natural examples have inspired the design of nanostructured antibacterial implant surfaces made of synthetic materials (Jaggessar et al., 2017; Jenkins et al., 2020) such as

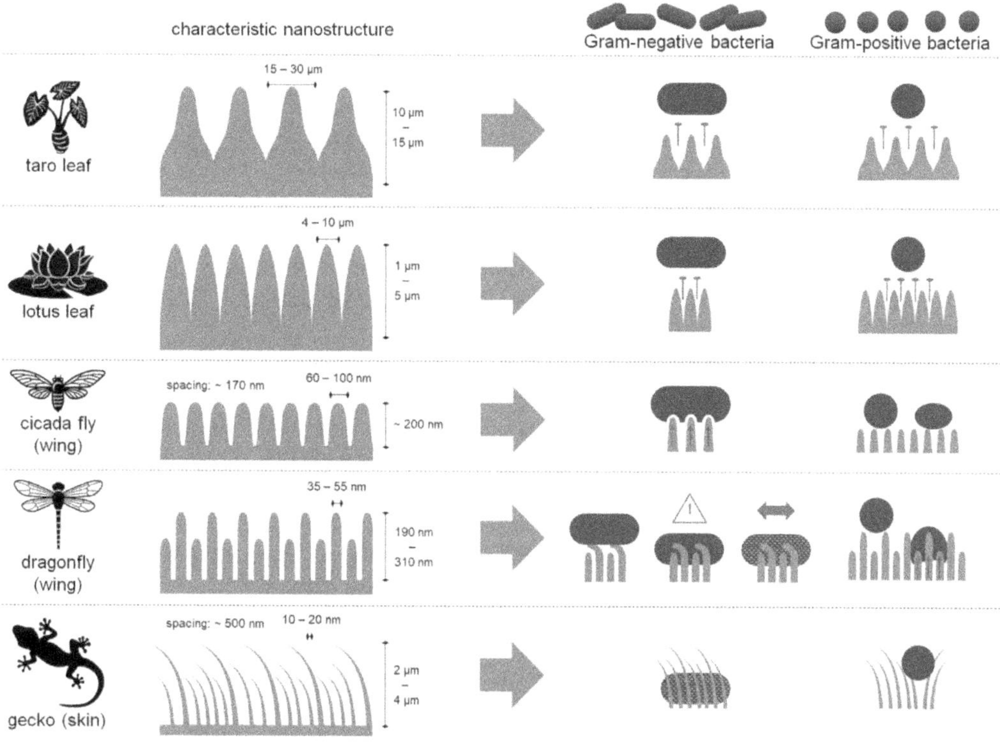

FIGURE 2.5 Schematic overview of the micro-/nanostructure of natural surfaces and their effect on Gram positive and Gram-negative bacteria. The graphical content is based on (Jaggessar et al., 2017; Ma et al., 2011; Bandara et al., 2017; Jenkins et al., 2020). The table gives an overview on the shape and size of the different surface nanostructures, as well as their interaction with gram negative and gram positive bacteria.

nanoparticles, nanowires, nanotubes, nanopillars, nanoflowers, and nanoripples (Liu et al., 2020). Ag, TiO_2, Fe_3O_4, Al_2O_3, MoO_3 and CrO nanostructures have been described for coating metal implants (Jaggessar et al., 2017). Analyzing the bactericidal effects of synthetic TiO_2 nanopillars revealed that the nanopillars do not rupture or lyse the bacteria, but by inducing deformation and penetration of the bacterial cell envelope, they can inhibit bacterial cell division and induce oxidative stress (Jenkins et al., 2020), although this effect might be dependent on the diameter and length of the nanostructures.

The clinical application of such nano- or microstructures is critically discussed. Applied in load-bearing areas, the nano- or microstructures can be destroyed by forces acting on the biomaterial, resulting in wear debris or attrition. The formed wear particles can then cause inflammatory reactions that eventually result in the loosening of the material (Hodges et al., 2021).

2.5 METHODOLOGY

The described material architecture and associated surface modification can be obtained by different methodologies. A brief overview on different production techniques is provided in this section.

2.5.1 Cryogels

In contrast to classical hydrogels, cryogels are synthesized at subzero temperatures from monomeric or polymeric precursors, of which a large variety of natural and synthetic precursors exist.

A three-dimensional network with a system of interconnected macropores, usually in the range of 1–100 μm, is formed. The advantages of the open pore structure are the efficient transport of nutrients and oxygen and the unhindered removal of metabolic end products. The choice of polymer in combination with the freezing temperature influences the pore size and stiffness of the cryogels (Hixon et al., 2017).

For example, the largest ice crystals are formed at approximately −15 °C. Further decreasing the freezing temperature reduces the size of the ice crystals that serve as space holders for the pores in the cryogel. When collagen- or gelatin-based cryogels are too flexible, other polymers might be used to increase the cryogel stiffness. These cryogels might be covalently coated with RGD peptides to improve cell attachment and support osteogenic differentiation (Bilem et al., 2016; Huettner et al., 2018; Bellis, 2011).

Cryogels are remarkable because of their porous structure, which excellently mimics the structure of cancellous bone (Hixon et al., 2017; Savina et al., 2016). Various monomers such as alginate, gelatin, collagen, fibrinogen, serum albumin, hyaluronic acid, chitosan, acrylic acid, 2-hydroxyethyl methacrylate (HEMA), ethylene glycol diglycidyl ether, 1,4-butanediol diglycidyl ether, sulfonic acid sodium salt, and 2-acrylamido-2-methylpropane acrylamide (aAm) and their derivatives can serve as building blocks for cryogels. They are interconnected with typical crosslinkers such as glutaraldehyde, N,N-methylene(bis) acrylamide (BAAm), methyl-methacrylate (MMA), poly-ethylene glycol diacrylate, and biodegradable crosslinkers (Memic et al., 2019).

HEMA polymerized with MMA or BAAm is usually the base for cryogels with tunable mechanical properties, which have already been used for tissue engineering and biomedical applications (Savina et al., 2007; Dalton et al., 2002; Ferruti et al., 2004; Štol et al., 1985; Saylan & Denizli, 2019). For example, healing of large bone defects in rabbit calvaria was improved by the application of such HEMA-based cryogels (Kim et al., 2016). However, the known toxicity of the individual building blocks (e.g., HEMA, BAAm, APS, TEMED) keeps the appropriateness of their use for bone tissue engineering in humans a subject of question, although the toxicity occurs only in the native form of the chemicals and disappears when they are crosslinked (Kumari et al., 2016; Backer et al., 2016).

2.5.2 Additive Manufacturing Techniques

Compared with classic subtractive manufacturing processes such as milling, additive manufacturing processes have several advantages. These advantages include raw material savings and the creation of more complex 3D structures. Recently, different additive manufacturing techniques have evolved (Figure 2.6) (Prakash et al., 2018; Mota et al., 2015; Charbonnier et al., 2021; Stanco et al., 2020).

- Material extrusion (ME), e.g., fused deposition modeling (FDM) or fused filament fabrication (FFF)—colloquially referred to as 3D printing—is the best known example for additive manufacturing. A filament of solid thermoplastic material is forced through a heated nozzle. As the print head moves over the surface, a thin line of the molten filament is deposited that then cools and hardens. Once the entire cross-section has been traced, the build platform lowers by one layer of thickness. Depending on the geometry of the print object, it is sometimes necessary to use additional support structures, for instance if a model has steep overhangs. For bone biomaterials, the thermoplastic material might contain ceramic or metal powders (Ortega Varela de Seijas et al., 2023; Marnot et al., 2022). The advantages of FDM or FFF are a very good surface finish and their ability to provide composite materials with different colors and materials such as polymers and even living cells (Gonzalez-Gutierrez et al., 2018).
- Material jetting (MJ) or drop-on-demand (DOD) techniques have similarities to ME. Instead of a solid thermoplastic material, a photopolymer is released from the nozzle that

hardens when exposed to UV light. Due to the liquid nature of the photopolymers, additional support structures are needed. Like ME, MJ and DOD have a very good surface finish and can generate composite materials from polymers and wax (Grottkau et al., 2020; Ng et al., 2017).

- Binder jetting (BJ) releases a binder from the nozzle that binds or fixes the powdered metal of ceramic raw material within the powder bed. Like ME and MJ, this allows the production of complex geometries, although the manufactured structures have poor mechanical properties. Furthermore, metal structures require secondary processes such as infiltration or sintering. During secondary infiltration, the formed structures are sintered in a furnace after curing and cleaning, which burns out the binder. The resulting voids (densityapabilx. 60%) will be infiltrated with bronze via capillary forces. During secondary sintering, the parts are cured in the furnace and sintered directly afterward. This way, a high density apabilx. 97%) can be achieved, although uneven shrinkage of the material can occur (Marnot et al., 2022; Meenashisundaram et al., 2020; Gokuldoss et al., 2017).
- Direct energy deposition (DED) is a rapid method that is also suitable for generating metal and ceramic materials. In contrast to BJ, the metal or ceramic powder and a photopolymer are forced through nozzles. Upon release they are melted by a focused heat source (most commonly laser) and successively added to the build platform. The process takes place in a hermetically sealed chamber filled with inert gas to control the material properties and protect the material from oxidation. Due to the lack of the powder reservoir, additional support structures are required, which limits the resolution and surface finish of the generated materials. Similar to BJ, metal structures by DED require secondary processes that can cause shrinkage of the material (Avila et al., 2021).
- Powder bed fusion techniques, which include selective laser sintering (SLS), selective laser melting (SLM), and electron beam melting (EBM), can be used to generate polymer and metal materials with excellent mechanical properties and complex geometries. During SLS, the polymer powder is heated to just below the melting point, which results in metal alloys (Kamboj et al., 2020, 2021; Shi et al., 2020). In contrast, during SLM, the polymer powder is heated to the melting point, which results in more homogeneous materials. EBM uses a targeted high-energy or electron beam to melt the metal powder locally, which requires a vacuum and can only be used for melting conductive materials. The higher energy density allows a higher pressure speed than SLS or SLM but at the expense of the layer thickness and surface finish (Gokuldoss et al., 2017).
- VAT polymerization processes, namely stereolithography (SLA), masked SLA (MSLA), and digital light processing (DLP), use a reservoir (vat) of liquid photopolymer resin or powdered metal out of which the model is constructed layer by layer; UV light is used to cure or harden the material where required. In SLA, the light source is a laser from the top; in MSLA, the light sources are LEDs behind an LCD screen ("mask") from above, which is faster than SLA. In both SLA and MSLA, the formed material is immersed in the vat. In DLP, a digital light projector projects voxels (square pixels) from below, which makes the formed product emerge from the vat (Piedra-Cascón et al., 2021; Marsico et al., 2022).
- Sheet lamination (SL) comprises processes such as layer-laminated manufacturing (LLM) and laminated object manufacturing (LOM) in which the material is applied in layers as film. In case of paper or polymers, the thin film layers are then bonded or polymerized. In case of metals, the thin film layers are then welded by laser, diffusion, or ultrasound. Although LLM and LOM can rapidly generate products with little stress or distortion that require no post-hardening processes, the generated materials requires postprocessing and are limited in complexity. The major disadvantage of SL is the accumulating rest material.

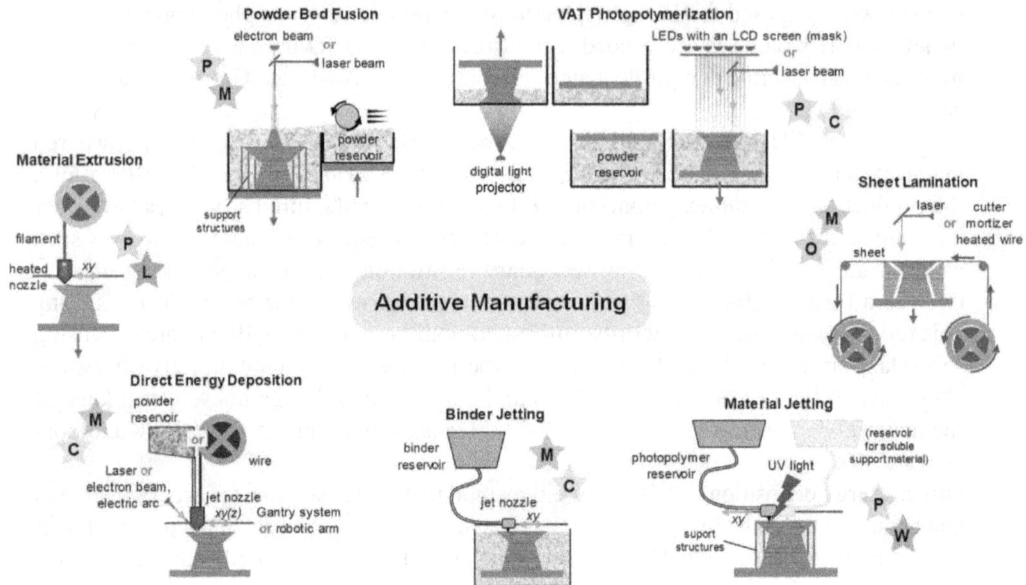

FIGURE 2.6 Overview and simplified graphics of the production process for each of the seven additive manufacturing techniques. The colored stars indicate the materials the method is suited for. P = polymers, M = metal, C = ceramics, W = wax, O = organic materials, L = living cells.

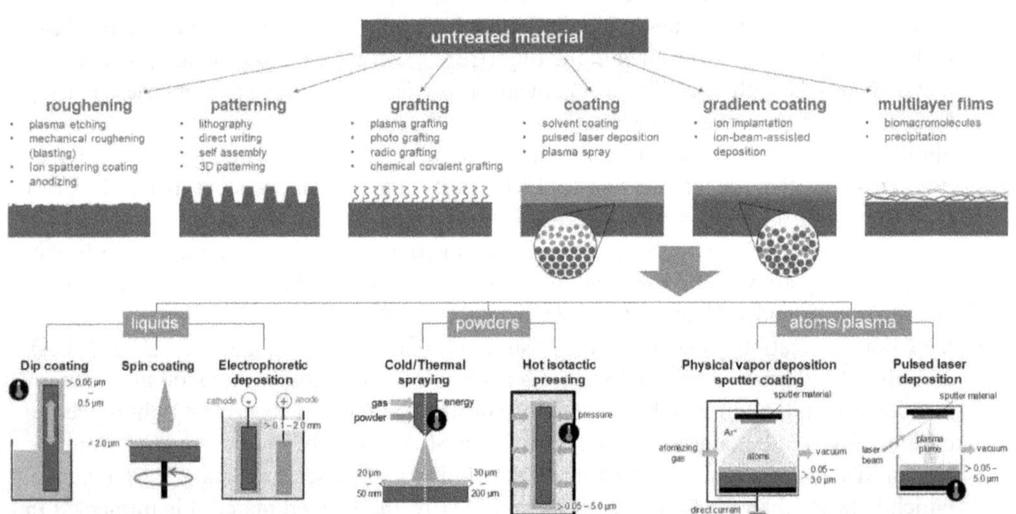

FIGURE 2.7 Overview of different surface modification techniques. With gradient coating the material and coating mix, while in classical coating the material remains unaltered. In the lower panel simplified graphics of different coating techniques (including coating thickness) for liquids, powders, and atoms/plasma are provided.

2.5.3 Surface Modification and Coating Techniques

To achieve biological activity of biomaterials, their surface is often processed or coated. Depending on the source material and the targeted surface modification, there are different techniques available (Figure 2.7).

- A rough surface improves the osseointegration of the biomaterial and the bond strength between the tissue and the material. The biomaterial surface can be roughened mechanically by blasting, chemically by etching or anodizing, or by ion sputtering coating. For blasting techniques such as sandblasting, 3D-printer construction kits exist for custom-made, automated sandblasting machines (e.g., Reptile, Locxess, Germany). The obtained results (micro to macro-scale roughness) depend on the blasting material, the blasting angle, the blasting pressure, and the working distance between blasting jet and material (Finger et al., 2020).
- With etching or anodizing, nano-scale to pico-scale roughness is obtained. Etching is the process of removing one material from the surface of another (Bright et al., 2022; Shapira & Halabi, 2009). There are two main types of etching: wet and dry, also known as plasma etching. Plasma etching involves the physical removal of the surface due to ion bombardment. In wet etching, the solid material is converted into liquid compounds using a chemical solution. Anodizing is an electrochemical process for metallic materials. With anodizing, the surface is converted into a corrosion-resistant, anodic oxide (Merlo et al., 2021; Ross & Webster, 2013). The selectivity of wet etching and anodizing is very high, as the chemicals used can be precisely matched to material. In ion sputter deposition, a thin film (magnesium or calcium-phosphate) is deposited or sputtered onto the target material using an ion source to create a dielectric layer (Balasubramanian, 2021; Qadir et al., 2019; Berube et al., 2005).
- Patterning provides the biomaterial with a structured surface geometry that can be obtained by processes like lithography, direct-writing, self-assembly, or 3D patterning (Kiyama et al., 2018). Lithography is the transfer of a pattern onto a light-sensitive material by selective exposure to a radiation source. Direct writing (also known as mask-less lithography) can be compared with additive manufacturing techniques with regard to the computer-controlled patterning source. Self-assembly and 3D patterning are frequently used to generate nano- or micro-patterned surfaces, with the difference being that during self-assembly, the pattern formation occurs autonomously (Murphy et al., 2021; Song et al., 2018; Ivanova et al., 2017).
- Grafting techniques to obtain structure surfaces include plasma-, photo-, radio-, and chemical covalent grafting, named after the underlying reaction mechanism. Grafting summarizes polymerization reactions induced by plasma, UV-light, radiofrequency, or some chemical (Minko, 2008).
- In classical coating procedures, the coating material is added on top of the biomaterial. The large variety of coating techniques include solvent or sol coatings and plasma spraying; they are chosen depending on the material to be coated and the desired coating thickness. Soluble coating substrates are frequently applied by solvent or sol (e.g., dip coating, spin coating, or electrophoretic deposition). Powders are applied by cold or thermal spray or hot isotactic pressing. Solid materials may be ionized or atomized for coating with plasma spray techniques such as physical vapor deposition, sputter coating, and pulsed laser deposition (Hildebrand et al., 2006; Erkoc & Ulucan-Karnak, 2021).
- While in classical coating procedures, the coated biomaterial is not altered, gradient coatings gradually permeate the surface of the biomaterial, resulting in a gradient of biomaterial and coating material. Typical methods for gradient coating are ion implantation and ion-beam-assisted deposition. As implied by the name, these methods accelerate ions of one element into the target material, thereby changing the physical, chemical, or electrical properties of the target (Tseng, 2005).
- Organic bioactive substances to kill bacteria, such as antibiotics or antimicrobial peptides; to induce osteogenesis, such as BMPs, vascular endothelial growth factor, parathyroid hormone, or hypoxia-inducible factor 1-alpha (Majidinia et al., 2018); or to inhibit osteoclastogenesis, such as statins (Bjelic & Finsgar, 2022), require special conditions for the

coatings not to lose their functionality. For example, the temperature must not exceed 40 °C to avoid denaturing the peptides and organic macromolecules. In addition, physiological pH and osmolarity must be provided. Therefore, such substances are usually applied as multilayered films or precipitates.

CONCLUSION

Given that materials for bone repair have to be biocompatible, the presented chapter clearly shows that not only the material composition is critical when designing such biomaterials but also the materials' stiffness and their micro and macro-architectures. The choice of material will affect the physical properties of the biomaterial such as its stiffness and porosity, which in turn will affect the cells' behavior on the material. A crucial point is the functionalization of the biomaterials, which can provide advantages for the bone cells (being osteoinductive or osteoanabolic) and can repel or kill bacteria to prevent infections.

Overall, the choice of techniques to generate a bone biomaterial and, if required, its functionalization strongly depends on the bones targeted for replacement. Weight bearing, stability, and bacterial load play a crucial role. The presented techniques here allow for developing individual strategies to generate porous bone biomaterials by cryogels or more planned by additive manufacturing. The different surface modifications techniques described further allow functionalization of the generated bone biomaterials.

LIST OF ABBREVIATIONS

aAm	2-Acrylamido-2-Methylpropane Acrylamide
BAAm	N,N-Methylene(Bis) Acrylamide
BMPs	Bone Morphogenic Proteins
DLP	Digital Light Processing
DOD	Drop-On-Demand
HAP	Hydroxyapatite
HEMA	2-Hydroxyethyl Methacrylate
ME	Material Extrusion
MJ	Material Jetting
MSCs	Mesenchymal Stromal Cells
MSLA	Masked Stereolithography
SL	Sheet Lamination
SLA	Stereolithography
SLM	Selective Laser Melting
SLS	Selective Laser Sintering

REFERENCES

Amini, A. R., Laurencin, C. T., & Nukavarapu, S. P. (2012). Bone tissue engineering: Recent advances and challenges. *Crit. Rev. Biomed. Eng*. 40: 363–408.

Arvidson, K., Abdallah, B. M., Applegate, L. A., Baldini, N., Cenni, E., Gomez-Barrena, E., Granchi, D., Kassem, M., Konttinen, Y. T., Mustafa, K., & Pioletti, D. P. (2011). Bone regeneration and stem cells. *J. Cell. Mol. Med*. 15: 718–746.

Avila, J. D., Stenberg, K., Bose, S., & Bandyopadhyay, A. (2021). Hydroxyapatite reinforced ti6al4v composites for load-bearing implants. *Acta Biomater*. 123: 379–392.

Ayobian-Markazi, N., Fourootan, T., & Kharazifar, M. J. (2012). Comparison of cell viability and morphology of a human osteoblast-like cell line (saos-2) seeded on various bone substitute materials: An in vitro study. *Dent. Res. J*. 9: 86–92.

Backer, A., Goppert, B., Sturm, S., Abaffy, P., Sollich, T., & Gruhl, F. J. (2016). Impact of adjustable cryogel properties on the performance of prostate cancer cells in 3d. *Springerplus*. 5: 902.

Balasubramanian, S. (2021). Magnetron sputtered magnesium-based thin film metallic glasses for bioimplants. *Biointerphases*. 16: 011005.

Bandara, C. D., Singh, S., Afara, I. O., Wolff, A., Tesfamichael, T., Ostrikov, K., & Oloyede, A. (2017). Bactericidal effects of natural nanotopography of dragonfly wing on Escherichia coli. *ACS Appl. Mater. Interfaces*. 9: 6746–6760.

Bellis, S. L. (2011). Advantages of rgd peptides for directing cell association with biomaterials. *Biomaterials*. 32: 4205–4210.

Berube, P., Yang, Y., Carnes, D. L., Stover, R. E., Boland, E. J., & Ong, J. L. (2005). The effect of sputtered calcium phosphate coatings of different crystallinity on osteoblast differentiation. *J. Periodontol*. 76: 1697–1709.

Bhushan, B., Jung, Y. C., & Koch, K. (2009). Micro-, nano- and hierarchical structures for superhydrophobicity, self-cleaning and low adhesion. *Philos. Trans. A: Math. Phys. Eng. Sci*. 367: 1631–1672.

Bilem, I., Chevallier, P., Plawinski, L., Sone, E. D., Durrieu, M. C., & Laroche, G. (2016). Rgd and bmp-2 mimetic peptide crosstalk enhances osteogenic commitment of human bone marrow stem cells. *Acta Biomater*. 36: 132–142.

Bjelic, D., & Finsgar, M. (2022). Bioactive coatings with anti-osteoclast therapeutic agents for bone implants: Enhanced compliance and prolonged implant life. *Pharmacol. Res*. 176: 106060.

Boyle, C., & Kim, I. Y. (2011). Three-dimensional micro-level computational study of wolff's law via trabecular bone remodeling in the human proximal femur using design space topology optimization. *J. Biomech*. 44: 935–942.

Bright, R., Fernandes, D., Wood, J., Palms, D., Burzava, A., Ninan, N., Brown, T., Barker, D., & Vasilev, K. (2022). Long-term antibacterial properties of a nanostructured titanium alloy surface: An in vitro study. *Mater. Today Bio*. 13: 100176.

Charbonnier, B., Hadida, M., & Marchat, D. (2021). Additive manufacturing pertaining to bone: Hopes, reality and future challenges for clinical applications. *Acta Biomater*. 121: 1–28.

Chen, J. C., & Jacobs, C. R. (2013). Mechanically induced osteogenic lineage commitment of stem cells. *Stem Cell Res. Ther*. 4: 107.

Chocholata, P., Kulda, V., & Babuska, V. (2019). Fabrication of scaffolds for bone-tissue regeneration. *Materials*. 12: 568.

Daculsi, G., & Passuti, N. (1990). Effect of the macroporosity for osseous substitution of calcium phosphate ceramics. *Biomaterials*. 11: 86–87.

Dalton, P. D., Flynn, L., & Shoichet, M. S. (2002). Manufacture of poly(2-hydroxyethyl methacrylate-co-methyl methacrylate) hydrogel tubes for use as nerve guidance channels. *Biomaterials*. 23: 3843–3851.

Dawson, J. I., & Oreffo, R. O. (2008). Bridging the regeneration gap: Stem cells, biomaterials and clinical translation in bone tissue engineering. *Arch. Biochem. Biophys*. 473: 124–131.

Di Luca, A., Ostrowska, B., Lorenzo-Moldero, I., Lepedda, A., Swieszkowski, W., Van Blitterswijk, C., & Moroni, L. (2016). Gradients in pore size enhance the osteogenic differentiation of human mesenchymal stromal cells in three-dimensional scaffolds. *Sci. Rep*. 6: 1–13.

Ding, D., Xu, H., Liang, Q., Xu, L., Zhao, Y., & Wang, Y. (2012). Over-expression of sox2 in c3h10t1/2 cells inhibits osteoblast differentiation through wnt and mapk signalling pathways. *Int. Orthop*. 36: 1087–1094.

Engler, A. J., Sen, S., Sweeney, H. L., & Discher, D. E. (2006). Matrix elasticity directs stem cell lineage specification. *Cell*. 126: 677–689.

Erkoc, P., & Ulucan-Karnak, F. (2021). Nanotechnology-based antimicrobial and antiviral surface coating strategies. *Prosthesis*. 3: 25–52.

Faia-Torres, A. B., Charnley, M., Goren, T., Guimond-Lischer, S., Rottmar, M., Maniura-Weber, K., Spencer, N. D., Reis, R. L., Textor, M., & Neves, N. M. (2015). Osteogenic differentiation of human mesenchymal stem cells in the absence of osteogenic supplements: A surface-roughness gradient study. *Acta Biomater*. 28: 64–75.

Faia-Torres, A. B., Guimond-Lischer, S., Rottmar, M., Charnley, M., Goren, T., Maniura-Weber, K., Spencer, N. D., Reis, R. L., Textor, M., & Neves, N. M. (2014). Differential regulation of osteogenic differentiation of stem cells on surface roughness gradients. *Biomaterials*. 35: 9023–9032.

Ferruti, P., Grigolini, M., & Ranucci, E. (2004). Phema hydrogels obtained by a novel low-heat curing procedure with a potential for in situ preparation. *Macromol. Biosci*. 4: 591–600.

Finger, C., Stiesch, M., Eisenburger, M., Breidenstein, B., Busemann, S., & Greuling, A. (2020). Effect of sandblasting on the surface roughness and residual stress of 3y-tzp (zirconia). *SN App. Sci.* 2: 1700.

Finkemeier, C. G. (2002). Bone-grafting and bone-graft substitutes. *J. Bone Joint Surg. Am.* 84: 454–464.

Furuhata, Y., Yoshitomi, T., Kikuchi, Y., Sakao, M., & Yoshimoto, K. (2017). Osteogenic lineage commitment of adipose-derived stem cells is predetermined by three-dimensional cell accumulation on micropatterned surface. *ACS Appl. Mater. Interfaces.* 9: 9339–9347.

Gautam, G., Kumar, S., & Kumar, K. (2022). Processing of biomaterials for bone tissue engineering: State of the art. *Mater. Today: Proc.* 50: 2206–2217.

George, J., Kuboki, Y., & Miyata, T. (2006). Differentiation of mesenchymal stem cells into osteoblasts on honeycomb collagen scaffolds. *Biotechnol. Bioeng.* 95: 404–411.

Glinel, K., Thebault, P., Humblot, V., Pradier, C. M., & Jouenne, T. (2012). Antibacterial surfaces developed from bio-inspired approaches. *Acta Biomater.* 8: 1670–1684.

Gokuldoss, K. P., Kolla, S., & Eckert, J. (2017). Additive manufacturing processes: Selective laser melting, electron beam melting and binder jetting-selection guidelines. *Materials.* 10: 672.

Gonzalez-Gutierrez, J., Cano, S., Schuschnigg, S., Kukla, C., Sapkota, J., & Holzer, C. (2018). Additive manufacturing of metallic and ceramic components by the material extrusion of highly-filled polymers: A review and future perspectives. *Materials.* 11: 840.

Grottkau, B. E., Hui, Z., & Pang, Y. (2020). A novel 3d bioprinter using direct-volumetric drop-on-demand technology for fabricating micro-tissues and drug-delivery. *Int. J. Mol. Sci.* 21: 3482.

Han, D., Liu, X., & Wu, S. (2022). Metal organic framework-based antibacterial agents and their underlying mechanisms. *Chem. Soc. Rev.* 51: 7138–7169.

Hasan, J., Webb, H. K., Truong, V. K., Pogodin, S., Baulin, V. A., Watson, G. S., Watson, J. A., Crawford, R. J., & Ivanova, E. P. (2013). Selective bactericidal activity of nanopatterned superhydrophobic cicada psaltoda claripennis wing surfaces. *Appl. Microbiol. Biotechnol.* 97: 9257–9262.

Häussling, V., Deninger, S., Vidoni, L., Rinderknecht, H., Ruoß, M., Arnscheidt, C., Athanasopulu, K., Kemkemer, R., Nussler, A. K., & Ehnert, S. (2019). Impact of four protein additives in cryogels on osteogenic differentiation of adipose-derived mesenchymal stem cells. *Bioengineering.* 6: 67.

Henkel, J., Woodruff, M. A., Epari, D. R., Steck, R., Glatt, V., Dickinson, I. C., Choong, P. F., Schuetz, M. A., & Hutmacher, D. W. (2013). Bone regeneration based on tissue engineering conceptions—A 2[1s]t century perspective. *Bone Res.* 1: 216–248.

Hernandez, R. K., Do, T. P., Critchlow, C. W., Dent, R. E., & Jick, S. S. (2012). Patient-related risk factors for fracture-healing complications in the United Kingdom general practice research database. *Acta Orthop.* 83: 653–660.

Hildebrand, H. F., Blanchemain, N., Mayer, G., Chai, F., Lefebvre, M., & Boschin, F. (2006). Surface coatings for biological activation and functionalization of medical devices. *Surf. Coat. Technol.* 200: 6318–6324.

Hixon, K. R., Lu, T., & Sell, S. A. (2017). A comprehensive review of cryogels and their roles in tissue engineering applications. *Acta Biomater.* 62: 29–41.

Hodges, N. A., Sussman, E. M., & Stegemann, J. P. (2021). Aseptic and septic prosthetic joint loosening: Impact of biomaterial wear on immune cell function, inflammation, and infection. *Biomaterials.* 278: 121127.

Huettner, N., Dargaville, T. R., & Forget, A. (2018). Discovering cell-adhesion peptides in tissue engineering: Beyond RGD. *Trends Biotechnol.* 36: 372–383.

Ivanova, E. P., Hasan, J., Webb, H. K., Truong, V. K., Watson, G. S., & Watson, J. A. (2012). Natural bactericidal surfaces: Mechanical rupture of pseudomonas aeruginosa cells by cicada wings. *Small.* 8: 2489–2494.

Ivanova, E. P., Nguyen, S. H., Guo, Y., Baulin, V. A., Webb, H. K., Truong, V. K., Wandiyanto, J. V., Garvey, C. J., Mahon, P. J., Mainwaring, D. E., & Crawford, R. J. (2017). Bactericidal activity of self-assembled palmitic and stearic fatty acid crystals on highly ordered pyrolytic graphite. *Acta Biomater.* 59: 148–157.

Jaggessar, A., Shahali, H., Mathew, A., & Yarlagadda, P. K. (2017). Bio-mimicking nano and micro-structured surface fabrication for antibacterial properties in medical implants. *J. Nanobiotechnol.* 15: 1–20.

Jain, K. G., Mohanty, S., Ray, A. R., Malhotra, R., & Airan, B. (2015). Culture & differentiation of mesenchymal stem cell into osteoblast on degradable biomedical composite scaffold: In vitro study. *Indian J. Med. Res.* 142: 747–758.

Jang, I. G., & Kim, I. Y. (2008). Computational study of wolff's law with trabecular architecture in the human proximal femur using topology optimization. *J. Biomech.* 41: 2353–2361.

Jenkins, J., Mantell, J., Neal, C., Gholinia, A., Verkade, P., Nobbs, A. H., & Su, B. (2020). Antibacterial effects of nanopillar surfaces are mediated by cell impedance, penetration and induction of oxidative stress. *Nat. Commun.* 11: 1626.

Kamboj, N., Kazantseva, J., Rahmani, R., Rodríguez, M. A., & Hussainova, I. (2020). Selective laser sintered bio-inspired silicon-wollastonite scaffolds for bone tissue engineering. *Mater. Sci. Eng.: C.* 116: 111223.

Kamboj, N., Ressler, A., & Hussainova, I. (2021). Bioactive ceramic scaffolds for bone tissue engineering by powder bed selective laser processing: A review. *Materials.* 14: 5338.

Kapadia, N. P., Kristol, D., & Spillert, C. R. (2005). Effect of endotoxin and silver ion on the clotting time of blood. *Proceedings of the IEEE 3[1s]t Annual Northeast Bioengineering Conference*, IEEE, Hoboken, NJ, pp. 161–162.

Khlyustova, A., Kirsch, M., Ma, X., Cheng, Y., & Yang, R. (2022). Surfaces with antifouling-antimicrobial dual function via immobilization of lysozyme on zwitterionic polymer thin films. *J. Mater. Chem. B.* 10: 2728–2739.

Kim, S., Hwang, Y., Kashif, M., Jeong, D., & Kim, G. (2016). Evaluation of bone regeneration on polyhydroxyethyl-polymethyl methacrylate membrane in a rabbit calvarial defect model. *In Vivo.* 30: 587–591.

Kiyama, R., Nonoyama, T., Wada, S., Semba, S., Kitamura, N., Nakajima, T., Kurokawa, T., Yasuda, K., Tanaka, S., & Gong, J. P. (2018). Micro patterning of hydroxyapatite by soft lithography on hydrogels for selective osteoconduction. *Acta Biomater.* 81: 60–69.

Koons, G. L., Diba, M., & Mikos, A. G. (2020). Materials design for bone-tissue engineering. *Nat. Rev. Mater.* 5: 584–603.

Kumari, J., Karande, A. A., & Kumar, A. (2016). Combined effect of cryogel matrix and temperature-reversible soluble—Insoluble polymer for the development of in vitro human liver tissue. *ACS Appl. Mater. Interfaces.* 8: 264–277.

Laloy, J., Minet, V., Alpan, L., Mullier, F., Beken, S., Toussaint, O., Lucas, S., & Dogné, J. M. (2014). Impact of silver nanoparticles on haemolysis, platelet function and coagulation. *Nanobiomedicine.* 1: 1–4.

Li, M., Li, H., Pan, Q., Gao, C., Wang, Y., Yang, S., Zan, X., & Guan, Y. (2019). Graphene oxide and lysozyme ultrathin films with strong antibacterial and enhanced osteogenesis. *Langmuir.* 35: 6752–6761.

Lin, X., Patil, S., Gao, Y. G., & Qian, A. (2020). The bone extracellular matrix in bone formation and regeneration. *Front. Pharmacol.* 11: 757.

Liu, J., Liu, J., Attarilar, S., Wang, C., Tamaddon, M., Yang, C., Xie, K., Yao, J., Wang, L., Liu, C., & Tang, Y. (2020). Nano-modified titanium implant materials: A way toward improved antibacterial properties. *Front. Bioeng. Biotech.* 8: 576969.

Liu, P., Hao, Y., Ding, Y., Yuan, Z., Liu, Y., & Cai, K. (2018). Fabrication of enzyme-responsive composite coating for the design of antibacterial surface. *J. Mater. Sci. Mater. Med.* 29: 160.

Ma, J., Sun, Y., Gleichauf, K., Lou, J., & Li, Q. (2011). Nanostructure on taro leaves resists fouling by colloids and bacteria under submerged conditions. *Langmuir.* 27: 10035–10040.

Majidinia, M., Sadeghpour, A., & Yousefi, B. (2018). The roles of signaling pathways in bone repair and regeneration. *J. Cell. Physiol.* 233: 2937–2948.

Marcellini, S., Henriquez, J. P., & Bertin, A. (2012). Control of osteogenesis by the canonical wnt and bmp pathways in vivo: Cooperation and antagonism between the canonical wnt and bmp pathways as cells differentiate from osteochondroprogenitors to osteoblasts and osteocytes. *Bioessays.* 34: 953–962.

Marnot, A., Dobbs, A., & Brettmann, B. (2022). Material extrusion additive manufacturing of dense pastes consisting of macroscopic particles. *MRS Commun.* 12: 483–494.

Marsico, C., Carpenter, I., Kutsch, J., Fehrenbacher, L., & Arola, D. (2022). Additive manufacturing of lithium disilicate glass-ceramic by vat polymerization for dental appliances. *Dent. Mater.* 38: 2030–2040.

Mathieu, P. S., & Loboa, E. G. (2012). Cytoskeletal and focal adhesion influences on mesenchymal stem cell shape, mechanical properties, and differentiation down osteogenic, adipogenic, and chondrogenic pathways. *Tissue Eng. Part B Rev.* 18: 436–444.

Mayr-Wohlfart, U., Fiedler, J., Günther, K. P., Puhl, W., & Kessler, S. (2001). Proliferation and differentiation rates of a human osteoblast-like cell line (saos-2) in contact with different bone substitute materials. *J. Biomed. Mater. Res.* 57: 132–139.

Meenashisundaram, G. K., Xu, Z., Nai, M. L. S., Lu, S., Ten, J. S., & Wei, J. (2020). Binder jetting additive manufacturing of high porosity 316l stainless steel metal foams. *Materials.* 13: 3744.

Memic, A., Colombani, T., Eggermont, L. J., Rezaeeyazdi, M., Steingold, J., Rogers, Z. J., Navare, K. J., Mohammed, H. S., & Bencherif, S. A. (2019). Latest advances in cryogel technology for biomedical applications. *Adv. Ther.* 2: 1800114.

Merlo, J. L., Katunar, M. R., Tano de la Hoz, M. F., Carrizo, S., Salemme Alonso, L., Otaz, M. A., Ballarre, J., & Ceré, S. (2021). Short-term in vivo response to anodized magnesium alloy as a biodegradable material for bone fracture fixation devices. *ACS Appl. Bio. Mater.* 4: 7123–7133.

Minko, S. (2008). Grafting on solid surfaces: "Grafting to" and "grafting from" methods. In *Polymer Surfaces and Interfaces: Characterization, Modification and Applications*. M. Stamm, Ed. Berlin Heidelberg: Springer, pp. 215–234.

Morgan, E. F., Unnikrisnan, G. U., & Hussein, A. I. (2018). Bone mechanical properties in healthy and diseased states. *Annu. Rev. Biomed. Eng.* 20: 119–143.

Mota, C., Puppi, D., Chiellini, F., & Chiellini, E. (2015). Additive manufacturing techniques for the production of tissue engineering constructs. *J. Tissue Eng. Regen. Med.* 9: 174–190.

Mueller, B., Treccani, L., & Rezwan, K. (2017). Antibacterial active open-porous hydroxyapatite/lysozyme scaffolds suitable as bone graft and depot for localized drug delivery. *J. Biomater. Appl.* 31: 1123–1134.

Murphy, C. M., Cao, Y., Sepúlveda, N., & Li, W. (2021). Quick self-assembly of bio-inspired multi-dimensional well-ordered structures induced by ultrasonic wave energy. *pLoS One*. 16: e0246453.

Murphy, C. M., & O'Brien, F. J. (2010). Understanding the effect of mean pore size on cell activity in collagen-glycosaminoglycan scaffolds. *Cell Adh. Migr.* 4: 377–381.

Ng, W. L., Yeong, W. Y., & Naing, M. W. (2017). Polyvinylpyrrolidone-based bio-ink improves cell viability and homogeneity during drop-on-demand printing. *Materials*. 10: 190.

Ofner, III, C. M., & Bubnis, W. A. (1996). Chemical and swelling evaluations of amino group crosslinking in gelatin and modified gelatin matrices. *Pharm. Res.* 13: 1821–1827.

Oftadeh, R., Perez-Viloria, M., Villa-Camacho, J. C., Vaziri, A., & Nazarian, A. (2015). Biomechanics and mechanobiology of trabecular bone: A review. *J. Biomech. Eng.* 137.

Ortega Varela de Seijas, M., Bardenhagen, A., Rohr, T., & Stoll, E. (2023). Indirect induction sintering of metal parts produced through material extrusion additive manufacturing. *Materials*. 16: 885.

Park, S. B., Seo, K. W., So, A. Y., Seo, M. S., Yu, K. R., Kang, S. K., & Kang, K. S. (2012). Sox2 has a crucial role in the lineage determination and proliferation of mesenchymal stem cells through dickkopf-1 and c-myc. *Cell Death Differ.* 19: 534–545.

Piedra-Cascón, W., Krishnamurthy, V. R., Att, W., & Revilla-León, M. (2021). 3d printing parameters, supporting structures, slicing, and post-processing procedures of vat-polymerization additive manufacturing technologies: A narrative review. *J. Dent.* 109: 103630.

Prakash, J., Krishna, S. B. N., Kumar, P., Kumar, V., Ghosh, K. S., Swart, H. C., Bellucci, S., & Cho, J. (2022). Recent advances on metal oxide based nano-photocatalysts as potential antibacterial and antiviral agents. *Catalysts*. 12: 1047.

Prakash, K. S., Nancharaih, T., & Rao, V. S. (2018). Additive manufacturing techniques in manufacturing -an overview. *Mater. Today: Proc.* 5: 3873–3882.

Qadir, M., Li, Y., & Wen, C. (2019). Ion-substituted calcium phosphate coatings by physical vapor deposition magnetron sputtering for biomedical applications: A review. *Acta Biomater.* 89: 14–32.

Qian, G., Zhang, L., Liu, X., Wu, S., Peng, S., & Shuai, C. (2021). Silver-doped bioglass modified scaffolds: A sustained antibacterial efficacy. *Mater. Sci. Eng.: C*. 129: 112425.

Ren, L., Zhang, Z., Deng, C., Zhang, N., & Li, D. (2021). Antibacterial and pro-osteogenic effects of beta-defensin-2-loaded mesoporous bioglass. *Dent. Mater. J.* 40: 464–471.

Retzepi, M., & Donos, N. (2010). Guided bone regeneration: Biological principle and therapeutic applications. *Clin. Oral Implants Res.* 21: 567–576.

Robey, P. G., Fedarko, N. S., Hefferan, T. E., Bianco, P., Vetter, U. K., Grzesik, W., Friedenstein, A., van der Pluijm, G., Mintz, K. P., Young, M. F., & Kerr, J. M. (1993). Structure and molecular regulation of bone matrix proteins. *J. Bone Miner. Res.* 8: S483–S487.

Ross, A. P., & Webster, T. J. (2013). Anodizing color coded anodized ti6al4v medical devices for increasing bone cell functions. *Int. J. Nanomed.* 8: 109–117.

Samavedi, S., Whittington, A. R., & Goldstein, A. S. (2013). Calcium phosphate ceramics in bone tissue engineering: A review of properties and their influence on cell behavior. *Acta Biomater.* 9: 8037–8045.

Satija, N. K., Gurudutta, G. U., Sharma, S., Afrin, F., Gupta, P., Verma, Y. K., Singh, V. K., & Tripathi, R. P. (2007). Mesenchymal stem cells: Molecular targets for tissue engineering. *Stem Cells Dev*. 16: 7–23.
Savina, I. N., Cnudde, V., D'hollander, S., Van Hoorebeke, L., Mattiasson, B., Galaev, I. Y., & Du Prez, F. (2007). Cryogels from poly(2-hydroxyethyl methacrylate): Macroporous, interconnected materials with potential as cell scaffolds. *Soft Matter*. 3: 1176–1184.
Savina, I. N., Ingavle, G. C., Cundy, A. B., & Mikhalovsky, S. V. (2016). A simple method for the production of large volume 3D macroporous hydrogels for advanced biotechnological, medical and environmental applications. *Sci. Rep*. 6: 1–9.
Saylan, Y., & Denizli, A. (2019). Supermacroporous composite cryogels in biomedical applications. *Gels*. 5: 20.
Seo, E., Basu-Roy, U., Gunaratne, P. H., Coarfa, C., Lim, D. S., Basilico, C., & Mansukhani, A. (2013). Sox2 regulates yap1 to maintain stemness and determine cell fate in the osteo-adipo lineage. *Cell Rep*. 3: 2075–2087.
Shapira, L., & Halabi, A. (2009). Behavior of two osteoblast-like cell lines cultured on machined or rough titanium surfaces. *Clin. Oral Implants Res*. 20: 50–55.
Shi, Y., Pan, T., Zhu, W., Yan, C., & Xia, Z. (2020). Artificial bone scaffolds of coral imitation prepared by selective laser sintering. *J. Mech. Behav. Biomed. Mater*. 104: 103664.
Singh, A., Tiwari, A., Bajpai, J., & Bajpai, A. (2018). Polymer-based antimicrobial coatings as potential biomaterials: From action to application. In *Handbook of Antimicrobial Coatings*. A. Tiwari, Ed. Amsterdam: Elsevier, pp. 27–61.
Song, Y., Ma, A., Ning, J., Zhong, X., Zhang, Q., Zhang, X., Hong, G., Li, Y., Sasaki, K., & Li, C. (2018). Loading icariin on titanium surfaces by phase-transited lysozyme priming and layer-by-layer self-assembly of hyaluronic acid/chitosan to improve surface osteogenesis ability. *Int. J. Nanomed*. 13: 6751–6767.
Stanco, D., Urbán, P., Tirendi, S., Ciardelli, G., & Barrero, J. (2020). 3d bioprinting for orthopaedic applications: Current advances, challenges and regulatory considerations. *Bioprinting*. 20: e00103.
Štol, M., Tolar, M., & Adam, M. (1985). Poly(2-hydroxyethyl methacrylate)—Collagen composites which promote muscle cell differentiation in vitro. *Biomaterials*. 6: 193–197.
Sun, M., Chi, G., Xu, J., Tan, Y., Xu, J., Lv, S., Xu, Z., Xia, Y., Li, L., & Li, Y. (2018). Extracellular matrix stiffness controls osteogenic differentiation of mesenchymal stem cells mediated by integrin alpha5. *Stem Cell Res. Ther*. 9: 1–13.
Teotia, A. K., Raina, D. B., Singh, C., Sinha, N., Isaksson, H., Tagil, M., Lidgren, L., & Kumar, A. (2017). Nano-hydroxyapatite bone substitute functionalized with bone active molecules for enhanced cranial bone regeneration. *ACS Appl. Mater. Interfaces*. 9: 6816–6828.
Thein-Han, W. W., & Misra, R. D. K. (2009). Biomimetic chitosan-nanohydroxyapatite composite scaffolds for bone tissue engineering. *Acta Biomater*. 5: 1182–1197.
Tseng, A. A. (2005). Recent developments in nanofabrication using focused ion beams. *Small*. 1: 924–939.
Watson, G. S., Green, D. W., Schwarzkopf, L., Li, X., Cribb, B. W., Myhra, S., & Watson, J. A. (2015). A gecko skin micro/nano structure—A low adhesion, superhydrophobic, anti-wetting, self-cleaning, biocompatible, antibacterial surface. *Acta Biomater*. 21: 109–122.
Winkler, T., Sass, F. A., Duda, G. N., & Schmidt-Bleek, K. (2018). A review of biomaterials in bone defect healing, remaining shortcomings and future opportunities for bone tissue engineering: The unsolved challenge. *Bone Joint Res*. 7: 232–243.
Wubneh, A., Tsekoura, E. K., Ayranci, C., & Uludağ, H. (2018). Current state of fabrication technologies and materials for bone tissue engineering. *Acta Biomater*. 80: 1–30.
Xing, X., Su, J., Liu, Y., Lin, H., Wang, Y., & Cheng, H. (2022). A novel visible light-curing chitosan-based hydrogel membrane for guided tissue regeneration. *Colloids Surf. B: Biointerfaces*. 218: 112760.
Yanoso-Scholl, L., Jacobson, J. A., Bradica, G., Lerner, A. L., O'Keefe, R. J., Schwarz, E. M., Zuscik, M. J., & Awad, H. A. (2010). Evaluation of dense polylactic acid/beta-tricalcium phosphate scaffolds for bone tissue engineering. *J. Biomed. Mater. Res. A*. 95: 717–726.
Yemmireddy, V. K., & Hung, Y. C. (2017). Using photocatalyst metal oxides as antimicrobial surface coatings to ensure food safety-opportunities and challenges. *Compr. Rev. Food Sci. Food Saf*. 16: 617–631.
Zhao, W., Li, X., Liu, X., Zhang, N., & Wen, X. (2014). Effects of substrate stiffness on adipogenic and osteogenic differentiation of human mesenchymal stem cells. *Mater. Sci. Eng.: C*. 40: 316–323.

Zheng, K., Lu, M., Liu, Y., Chen, Q., Taccardi, N., Hüser, N., & Boccaccini, A. R. (2016). Monodispersed lysozyme-functionalized bioactive glass nanoparticles with antibacterial and anticancer activities. *Biomed. Mater.* 11: 035012.

Zhou, H., & Lee, J. (2011). Nanoscale hydroxyapatite particles for bone tissue engineering. *Acta Biomater.* 7: 2769–2781.

Ziuopos, P., & Currey, J. D. (1998). Changes in the stiffness, strength, and toughness of human cortical bone with age. *Bone*. 22: 57–66.

3 Synthetic Bone Analogue Materials and Design for Skeletal Tissue Healing

Samir Das, Mitali Mishra, Kanta Chakraborty, Sayan Das, Baisakhee Saha, and Santanu Dhara

3.1 INTRODUCTION

Trauma and disease cause tissue loss and damage; in severe injuries, body movement is hampered due to discontinuity in vital long bone tissue. Fabricating bone analogues and harvesting them at the damage site is the last resort for skeletal tissue regeneration, especially for load-bearing tissue damage with critical-size defects. Orthopaedic implant is the most common transplantation technique after blood transfusion (Campana et al., 2014).

Transplantation of xenogeneic or allogenic bone substitutes is an early option to address the shortage of organs and avoid donor site comorbidity. Different inorganic and organic synthetic, semisynthetic or combined hybrid graft substitutes can be used to treat skeletal tissue defects while avoiding autologous or allogeneic bone (Burwell, 1994; Donati et al., 2007). Autologous bone is considered the benchmark among bone grafts since all significant features required in bone regeneration are present and meet the biological and mechanical requisites for a filling material (Saikia et al., 2008); however, in addition to cost, donor site comorbidity and shortage of donor tissues limit its applications.

Allogeneic bone is one of the alternatives of autologous bone, but there is always a risk of disease transmission in addition to rejected immune response related to foreign body reaction (Gunzburg et al., 2002). Another alternative to autograft is xenogeneic bone grafting; however, the same limitations persist, with higher chances of immunogenicity problems and disease transmission (Busch et al., 2021). The ideal material for bone implants should have biocompatibility and bioresorbability with osteoconductive, osteoinductive and biomimicking skeletal tissue. In addition to microporosity, mechanical integrity and cost effectiveness are the prerequisites for the success of bone implants (Faour et al., 2011).

To avoid these existing limitations in providing structural and functional support to damaged bone, there is an imperative need for synthetic bone analogues (Evaniew et al., 2013). Customized implants that are close in size and shape to the defect size are important for the success of bone regeneration via tissue engineering utilizing hybrid materials. Several parameters must be considered to construct an ideal bone graft substitute that mimics the microstructure of bone hierarchical architecture, complexity, and functionality. Architecture-based parameters such as pore size, pore distribution, and surface characteristics influence cellular response, cell seeding potential, angiogenesis, and ultimately osteogenesis are important as well (Bobbert et al., 2017).

Being an anisotropic material, bone exhibits differences in mechanical properties based on anatomical location and loading direction (Rho et al., 1998). Therefore, different mathematical bone modelling is needed based on geometrical irregularity and mechanical properties between cancellous bone and cortical bone (Ait Oumghar et al., 2020). Along with the chronological development of biomaterials, the concept of synthetic bone tissue substitute has changed from bioinert to bioresorbable materials (Sheikh et al., 2015). Here, we draft the recent practices for developing skeletal

DOI: 10.1201/9781003307310-4

tissue in terms of the most-used clinically available bone substitutes that can match natural bone tissues, according to the literature. Along with giving a brief description of the design morphology, we highlight different techniques used in developing synthetic bone analogues.

3.2 STRUCTURAL AND FUNCTIONAL PROPERTIES OF SKELETAL TISSUES

3.2.1 Hard Skeletal Tissues

Hard skeletal tissue consists of the bone tissues that provide support, protection, and structural integrity to the human body. It exhibits different mechanical properties based on anatomical location and loading direction. Bone tissue is broadly classified as compact or spongy. Some of is physicochemical properties are listed in Table 3.1.

Calcium phosphate apatite is the major component of hard tissues; in addition to pH buffering, its functions include structural protection, mastication, and motion. Their construction and adaptations are induced by complicated physiochemical and cellular activity. Having a closed hexagonal crystal structure, hydroxyapatite (HAP) induces mechanotransduction to skeletal tissue cells by generating piezoelectricity.

3.2.1.1 Physicochemical Element

Human long bone is basically a functionally graded anisotropic structure (Figure 3.1) in which the dense outer layer (cortex) is a nanohybrid of collagen and apatite mineral and the innermost layer is porous or cancellous and the density varies according to age and site. Both the materials are piezoelectric in nature, thereby causing mechanotransduction to the tissue under movement. The chemical assembly of calcium phosphate apatite present in biominerals can be expressed as (Barrère et al., 2008):

$$Ca_{10-(x-u)}(PO_4)_{6-x}(HPO_4 \text{ or } CO_3)_x(OH, F\ldots)_{2-(x-2u)}$$

where $0 <= x <= 2$ and $0 <= 2u <= x$ and u can be neglected. The inorganic natural component and the calcification mechanism of skeletal tissue is described in various studies in the literature (Rhee et al., 2000), and the entire collagen network of bone is described as a thin plate with irregular shape (20 Å to 1100 Å) (Kim et al., 1995) and crystallinity (Lambert et al., 2013).

3.2.1.2 Biological Properties of Hard Skeletal Tissue

Generally, modelling denotes modification of shape; in contrast, bone remodelling signifies maintenance of structural integrity and calcium phosphate balance; these two procedures take place simultaneously, and differences among them are fairly clear. Throughout the growth, subtraction, and replacement of skeletal bone, different types of skeletal tissues and related markers play a vital role in facilitating osteogenesis and osseointegration as in Table 3.2.

TABLE 3.1
Mechanical Characteristics of Compact and Spongy Bone Tissue

Bone Type and Loading	Bone Density (g/cm³)	Elastic Modulus (gPa)	Compressive Strength (mPa)	Reference
Compact bone, Longitudinal	1.99	17–20	131–224	Roach et al. (2007)
Compact bone, Transverse	1.99	6–13	106–133	Roach et al. (2007)
Spongy bone, Longitudinal	0.05–1.0	20	2–5	Wang et al. (2007)
Spongy bone, Transverse	0.05–1.0	14.7	0.8	Wang et al. (2007)

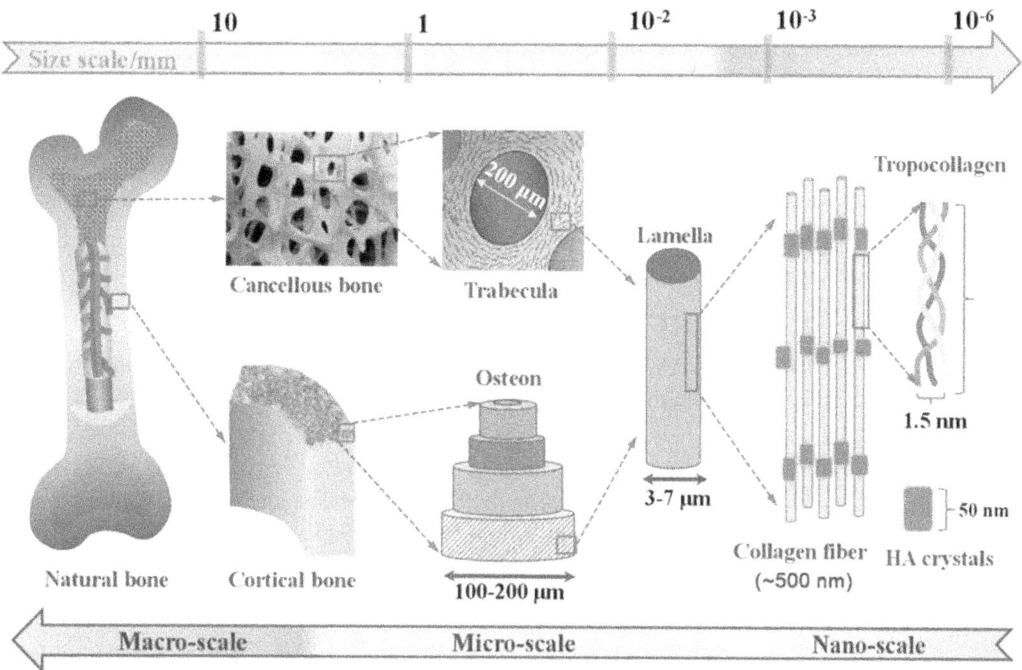

FIGURE 3.1 Schematic of skeletal tissue architecture. (Reproduced under the terms of CC-BY 4.0 (https://creativecommons.org/licenses/by/4.0/) International License from Gao, C., Peng, S., Feng, P., & Shuai, C.: Bone biomaterials and interactions with stem cells. Bone Res. 2017. 5. 1–33. Copyright 2017 Gao et al., published by Springer Nature).

TABLE 3.2
Different Types of Bone Cells, Their Functions, and Their Associated Markers

Bone cell	Function	Marker
Osteoprogenitor	• High growth and differentiation potential	• Alkaline phosphatase activity • Collagen type 1 • Sialoprotein • Osteocalcin
Osteoblast	• Nonproliferative cells • Highly differentiated • Bone mineralization	• Alkaline phosphatase activity • Calcium phosphate • Osteocalcin • Osteopontin • Bone sialoprotein
Osteoclast	• Bone resorption encourages osteoblast cells to form new bone	• Tartrate-resistant acid phosphatase

3.2.2 Soft Skeletal Tissues

One of the most crucial soft skeletal tissues is the normal articular cartilage that is a part of hyaline cartilage (Fawcett & Bloom, 1986). The extracellular matrix (ECM) of cartilage involves proteoglycan molecules with sulphated glycosaminoglycan, along with collagen type II fibrils, collagen types IX and X, fibronectin, and tenascin-C (Hunziker, 2002; Reinholz et al., 2004; Ghert et al., 2002).

As the bone and cartilage are linked with each other at the developmental stage, cartilage mediates osteogenesis in a process called endochondral ossification (Mackie et al., 2008).

The collagenous system with water-bound glycosaminoglycans, facilitates articular cartilage for bearing mechanical tension as well as providing specific tissue function (Armstrong et al., 1984). Collagen with glycosaminoglycans showed limited self-healing potential with chondral lesions (Campbell, 1969). These bone tissues do not possess inflammatory responses or form blood vessels, and the migration of bone marrow cells through drilling is used to treat chondral defects (Chen et al., 1999; Mankin & Buckwalter, 1996).

3.2.3 Skeletal Tissue Regeneration

Due to the intrinsic tissue regenerative capacity of bone, minor cracks, fractures, and injuries heal themselves. Natural bone remodelling follows the process shown Figure 3.2.

3.2.3.1 Hematoma Formation

When a bone fractures, blood vessels connecting the bone and periosteum rupture, forming hematomas and thereby causing hypoxic condition. Initially, hematoma is in a liquid state and diffuses within the surrounding tissues, but it eventually solidifies before being resorbed. This process forms the temporary frame for subsequent healing.

3.2.3.2 Soft and Hard Callus Formation

Soft calluses form within two to six weeks after bone fractures; soft bone substitutes the blood clot that formed during the inflammatory stage of bone healing. Soft calluses are not mechanically strong enough to hold bones together and eventually transform into hard calluses. Callus formation heals fractures via endochondral or intramembranous ossification, a bone remodelling process to form new bone material mediated by osteoblasts. Flat bones such as the bone of skulls and mandibles are developed by intramembranous ossification, where mesenchymal stem cells (MSCs) directly differentiate and proliferate into osteoblasts that mediate the formation of collagen fibrils and the mineralization process. The various stages of intramembranous ossification are described in Figure 3.3.

Long bones such as the femur, humerus, and ulna develop by endochondral ossification, in which MSCs differentiate into chondroblasts that further form the membrane called the perichondrium that covers cartilaginous template. Eventually, these chondroblasts differentiate to form chondrocytes. These cells mediate the process of mineralization on the cartilaginous template as well as vascularization (Sheehy et al., 2019). The process of endochondral ossification is described in Figure 3.4.

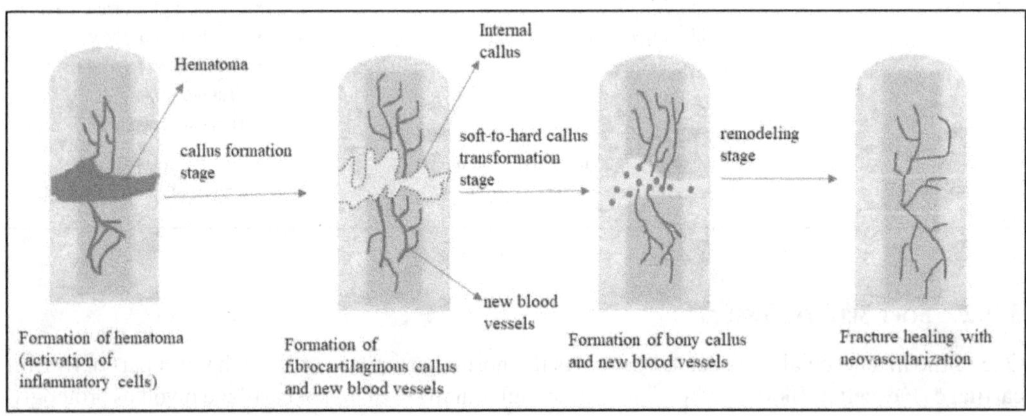

FIGURE 3.2 Phases of skeletal tissue regeneration.

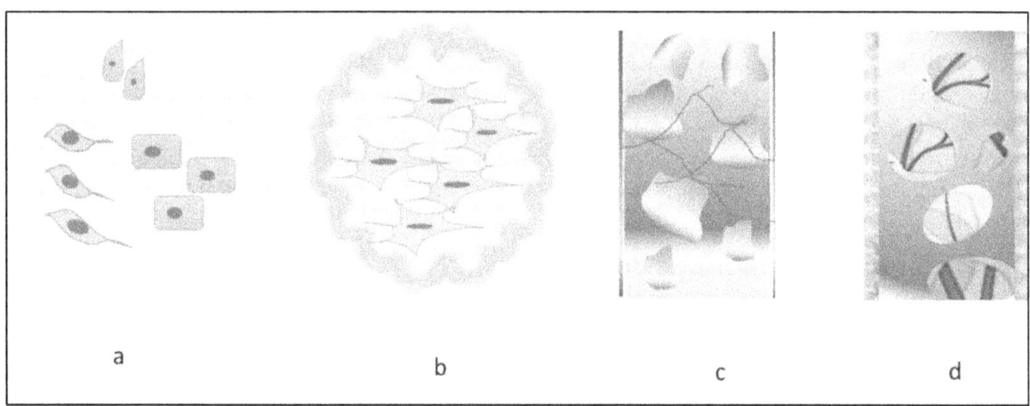

FIGURE 3.3 Phases of intramembranous ossification: (a) mesenchymal cells clustering to form ossification centres; (b) calcification; (c) trabecular matrix; and (d) periosteum formation regeneration.

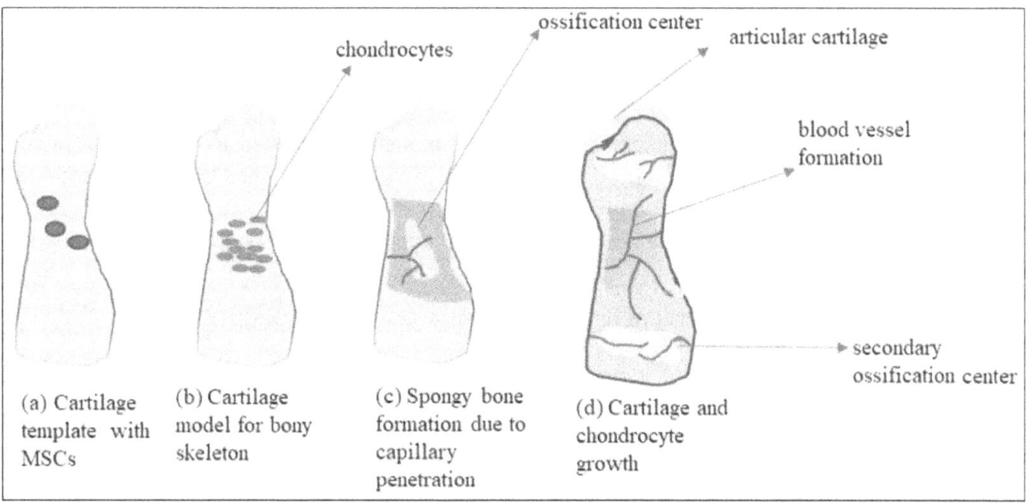

FIGURE 3.4 Different phases of endochondral ossification: (a) differentiation of MSCs into chondrocytes; (b) intermediate cartilage formation; (c) penetration of capillaries in cartilage and periosteum formation; (d) cartilage and chondrocyte growth phase.

Bone fractures will not heal on their own if the defect size exceeds the critical limit (generally >2 cm, based on the fracture site) (Schemitsch, 2017; Annamalai et al., 2019); clinical intervention is a promising way to exogenously regenerate large-scale bone defects. Scaffolds with cells, materials, and growth factors are the key elemental requirements for making bone constructs (Amini et al., 2012). However, the in vitro osteogenic priming of an engineered tissue can prevent the vascularization of the bone analogue by closing up the pores present in the scaffold with a calcified matrix, resulting in bone analogue degradation (Freeman et al., 2020).

Recent advancements in bone tissue engineering generally employ the potential of chondrogenically differentiated cells that can mediate endochondral ossification on grafted implants. A significant advantage of this pathway is that the grafted implant comprises cartilage, a tissue that needs very little oxygen tension in given physiological conditions. As a result, the cellular portion of the implanted construct can live in hypoxic conditions for extended periods of time before angiogenic processes from the surrounding tissues can induce vascularization at the implantation site (Filippi et al., 2023; Farrell et al., 2009) to mimic the native tissue microenvironment.

3.2.3.3 Three-Dimensional Structure Reconstruction during Bone Remodelling

Remodelling is the final phase of fracture healing, and it continues for more than a few months. In regeneration, bone regenerates and eventually condenses towards its original form through maintaining balance between activity of osteoclast and osteoblast. Biological cues such as vascular endothelial growth factor and bone morphogenetic proteins (BMPs) are the key players in promoting the differentiation and metabolism of preosteoblasts toward three-dimensional (3D) bone formation.

3.2.4 Ectopic vs. Orthotropic Bone Formation

One of the tissue regeneration approaches is ectopic bone formation, which is most often experimentally induced outside their typical origins but does also have clinical relevance. One of the disease entities in which ectopic bone formation can be found is fibrodysplasia ossificans progressive. Different ectopic locations are used for tissue engineering purposes including subcutaneous, intramuscular, and kidney capsule implantation. These ectopic models are significant in the evaluation of novel osteoinductive materials, osteogenic stem cells, growth factors, and relevant pathways for signalling molecules (Scott et al., 2012).

In contrast, orthotropic bone formation refers to developing bone tissues at their correct anatomical origin. In bone tissue engineering, different orthotropic-based models are created and utilized for evaluating bone structure as well as mechanical properties. These models generally utilize different types of simulation methods to understand the mechanical behaviour of bone or bone grafts under loading conditions. The studies based on these models contributed to improving fracture prediction, orthopaedic implant design, fracture fixation device performance, and device activities under dynamic mechanical stimulation (Geraldes & Phillips, 2014; Mathai et al., 2021). Therefore, evaluating ectopic bone formation is favourable for developing improved skeletal tissue analogues.

3.2.5 Tissue Engineering Approaches to Bone Analogue Development

In the last few decades, there has been a growing need for orthopaedic hip, knee, shoulder, phalanx, and other implants. Bone analogues with ordered structures and significant functionality could be engineered by amalgamating biomaterials with suitable pore size, porosity, and mechanical strength with cells and bioactive agents. The optimal pore dimensions are important for enhanced osteogenic differentiation as well as cellular activities.

For instance, Hulbert et al. (1970) proposed that at least 100 μm pore size is necessary for tissue mineralization as porosity of 75 to 100 μm promoted unmineralized ingrowth of osteoid tissue; however, there was an absence of nonadherent fibrous capsules formed on the surface of the osteoid tissue, indicating a lack of new tissue growth. Hench and colleagues developed bioactive silicate glass in 1971 that enabled tissue on-growth after implantation. The microporous bioactive materials with pores offered a template for both fibrous and vascular tissue in growth, which facilitates osteoblast differentiation toward new lamellar bone deposition. Bone analogues with pores of at least 100 μm and interconnectivity offer large surface area and a framework for tissue growth with proper vascularization toward improving tissue-integration properties (Hench et al., 1971). However, the insufficient mechanical strength of porous templates limits their applications in fabricating implants for load-bearing applications. To develop successful bone analogues, efforts have been made to employ interdisciplinary approaches that could relate engineering and biological principles to restore functional bones.

3.2.6 Materials for Skeletal Bone Tissue Engineering

Biomaterials with unique properties have crucial aspects for consideration during designing and fabricating bone analogues. Various biomaterials have been used for dental fillings and intraocular lens replacement. The developments in the fields of cell and molecular biology, materials science, chemistry, and engineering have provided extensive opportunities to explore different biomaterials for medical use. Considering the trends, challenges, and demands related to biomaterials, we provide in this section insights into biomaterials used for skeletal tissue regeneration.

3.2.7 The Chronobiological Development of Biomaterials

Nonbiological materials have been successfully applied in the human body toward osseointegration since ancient times (Ratner & Zhang, 2020). However, there have been very few scientific explanations of the biological and medicinal science behind these successes (and longevity). Notably and impressively, however, research established that the human body can adapt certain implants and that it is possible to meet the demand to reestablish the missing functions of physiologic and anatomic body parts with a graft. There are five different generations of materials, clearly marked in Table 3.3, based on developmental time, application, and advancement to improve tissue ingrowth and growth properties.

3.2.8 Commercially Available Products for Skeletal Tissue Regeneration

Biomaterials for generating successful synthetic bone analogues should have certain properties like biocompatibility following International Organization for Standardization 10993 test protocols,

TABLE 3.3
Generations of Biomaterials and Their Mechanisms

Generation	Motivation	Properties	Example	References
First	• Perfect physical properties for matching the replaced tissue • Minimize toxicity and interaction with the surrounding tissue	Inert materials provoke a rubbery foreign capsule around the implant	Metals: cobalt and chrome-based alloys, stainless steels Ceramics: alumina, zirconia Polymers: silicon rubbers, ultra-high-molecular weight polyethylene	Ratner & Zhang (2020)
Second	• Ability to interact with the biological system • Enhanced tissue-to-surface bonding	Bioresorbable	Polymers: polyglycolide, polylactic acid Ceramics: bioglass calcium phosphates	Lee et al. (2010); Hench & Thompson (2010)
Third	• Stimulation of particular cellular response at the molecular level	Resorption and bioactivity Osteoconduction	Titanium and titanium alloys (these can encourage embryonic stem cells to create bone nodules)	Hench & Thompson (2010)
Fourth	• Highly biocompatible • Accelerate transportation of nutrients within the tissue • No inflammatory response • Prolonged plasma stability and prevent outward migration of reactive species	Biomolecules act synergically with cells The structure–function association of tissue analogue with the living systems	Proteins: silk, gelatine, keratin, collagen Peptides: amphiphiles, amino acids Carbohydrates: glycodendrimer, cyclodextrin Nucleic acids: DNA, RNA, PNA Lipids: fatty acid, cholesterol	Hench & Thompson, 2010)
Fifth	• Porous 3D templates of various biomaterials for proliferation, attachment, and ECM formation and differentiation of cells	Replicate micro-environmental structures that activate the regeneration of new tissues	Porous gelatine, HAP, titanium-based alloys	Hench & Thompson (2010)

TABLE 3.4
Commercially Available Products for Developing Synthetic Skeletal Tissue Analogue

Product	Description/Constituents	References
Osbone	Pure synthetic HAP	Guarino et al. (2015)
Bonesave	HA/ß-TCP (60/40)	Carrel et al. (2014)
NovaBone dental putty	70% calcium phospho-silicate, with added polyethylene glycol, embedded in glycerine	Kapur et al. (2010)
Ostim paste	35% nanohydroxyapatite in water	Huwais & Meyer (2017)
NanoBone	Nanohydroxyapatite (as particulate or as paste with silica gel)	Hinze et al. (2010)
Biobon	Low crystalline apatite	Konermann et al. (2014)
ActiFuse/Pore-Si	Si-HA	Linhart et al. (2003)
OsSatura BCP	HA/ß-TCP (80/20)	Hing (2005)

β-TCP: β-tricalcium phosphate

satisfactory mechanical compatibility, and high corrosion and wear resistance to mimic the native skeletal tissue after implantation. Some of the biomaterial-based commercially available products for developing synthetic skeletal tissue analogue are described in Table 3.4.

3.2.9 Tissue Engineering Strategies: Design and Fabrication

Designing and fabrication using different materials are also crucial for developing successful synthetic bone analogues through tissue engineering. In designing a scaffold construct, the topographical aspect also needs to be considered. It has been evidenced that macro-topography can promote and modulate cell attachment, migration, proliferation, ECM deposition, and protein abundance by physical confinement (Xie et al., 2023). Macroporous bioactive scaffold is important for achieving osteoinduction and osteoconduction after implantation.

During bone healing, osteoinduction plays an important role by promoting osteogenesis. Osseointegration can be achieved by direct bone-to-implant contact. Due to stress shielding and interfacial failure, osseointegration is difficult to incorporate at the defect site after implantation. In this view, Hulbert et al. (1970) developed an interconnected bioinert porous architecture that influences cell adhesion and tissue ingrowth. On the other hand, Hench's concept emphasized bioactive implants with direct bone bonding, as described in Figure 3.5.

Addressing the complex loading issue, macroporous and bioactive interfacial architecture improves interfacial bone bonding via tissue on-growth and ingrowth. A higher volume of materials interacts with a higher volume of bone; minimizes stress shielding; and facilitates cell expansion, vascularization, and nutrient transport. Advanced fabrication modalities such as rapid prototyping via 3D printing provide controlled porosity with customized designs and tailorable properties. However, uniformly porous, 3D-printed scaffolds made up of a single material display modulus mismatch (metal) or mechanically brittle or weak (ceramic or polymer) interfaces. Therefore, combinations of different transient and permanent materials need to be explored for generating successful synthetic tissue analogues. In this context, ceramic–polymer combinations are well explored, but the degradation kinetics of both the materials need to be complementary to achieve a balance between physical support, bioactivity, and mechanical properties that make them amenable for better cell anchorage and differentiation (Trappmann et al., 2012). Being an anisotropic material, bone exhibits different mechanical properties that can be taken care of by proper design optimization, as shown in Figure 3.6.

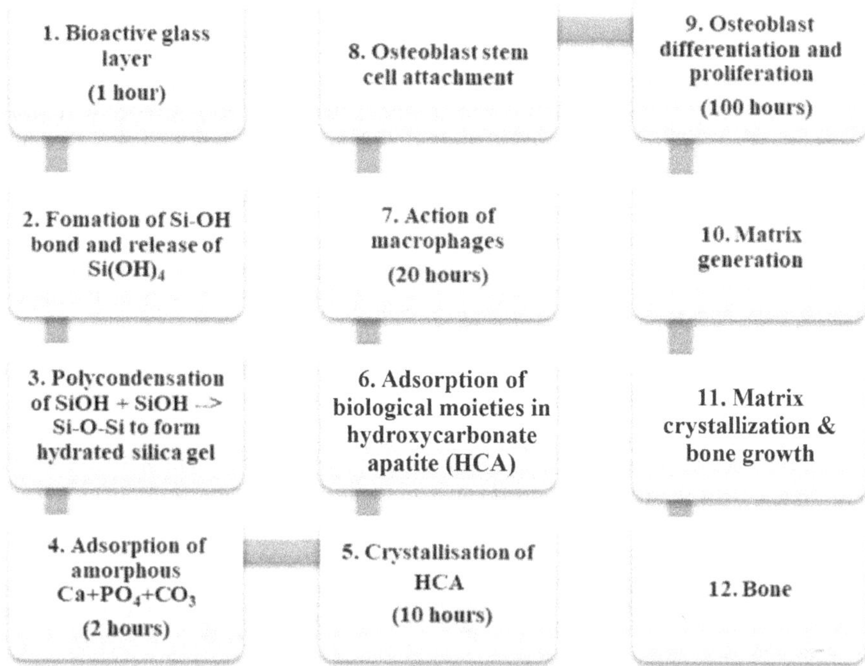

FIGURE 3.5 Sequence and rates of surface reaction stages to grow new bone at the interface with 45S5 bioglass.

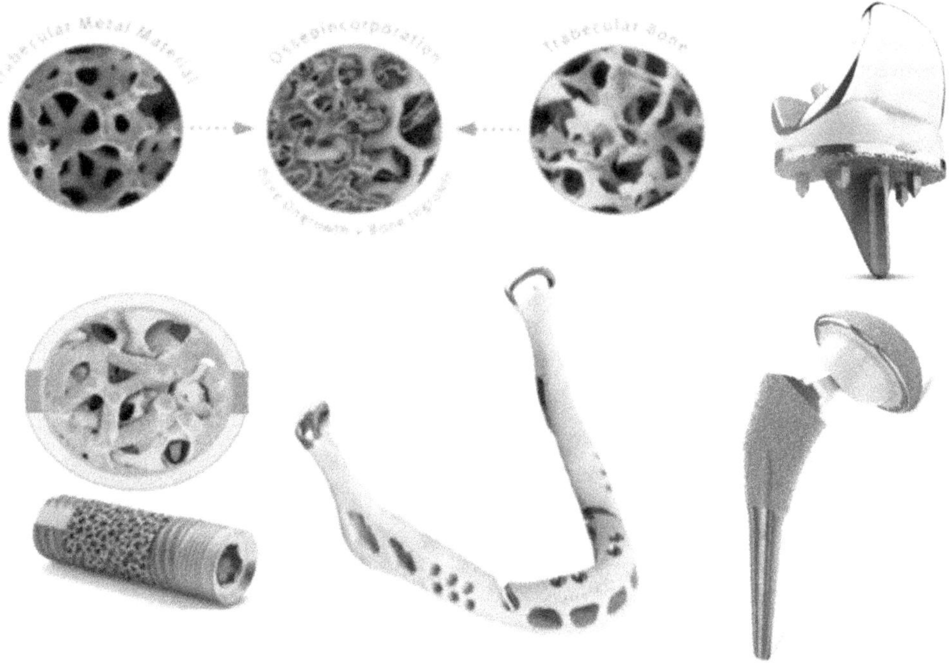

FIGURE 3.6 Example of hybrid design template based on Hulbert and Hench for better tissue ingrowth and on-growth after implantation causing interfacial bonding with minimal stress shielding. (Courtesy of ®Zimmer Biomet, Warsaw, Indiana, United States).

3.3 DEVELOPING SYNTHETIC BONE TISSUE ANALOGUES

Today, researchers have adopted hybrid design modification techniques that combine porous and dense structural morphology, as shown in Figure 3.7, so that the bone ingrowth and on-growth can be seen simultaneously through osteoincorporation in a shorter period of time. A suitable design strategy is crucial for orchestrating crosstalk among cells, growth factors, and materials for making synthetic bone constructs (Bose et al., 2012). However, designing is not an easy task given the huge number of variables that need to be considered (Figure 3.7).

Tan and van Arkel (2021) developed a topology optimization technique that involved using a porous and selectively hollow femoral hip stem with increased compliance to reduce the stress-shielding effect. Another group of researchers used a lattice-based porous trabecular stem design to optimize the fatigue life of the implant by enabling natural bone anisotropy (Hossain et al., 2021). De Martino et al. (2016) studied a total knee arthroplasty using cementless porous tantalum monoblocks to minimize aseptic loosening during postimplantation and Zhang et al. (2021) proposed a novel design methodology by merging the diamond-shaped porous structure with traditional tapped dental thread to reduce stiffness, in contrast with solid implant, for better biomechanical behaviour. Along with topological modification, different numerical optimization techniques like finite element analysis and sequential quadratic programming have been developed by different research groups to minimize the stress-shielding effect under dynamic loading conditions. So apart from material selection, the successful fabrication of synthetic tissue analogues largely depends on design optimization to mimic the exact structural hierarchy of the defect model (Karakurt & Lin, 2020).

3.3.1 Factors Involved in Designing Scaffolds for Skeletal Tissue Regeneration

3.3.1.1 Mechanical Property of Scaffolding Material

The mechanical properties of biomaterials are a crucial aspect to consider when choosing them for scaffold fabrication (Shoichet, 2010). Certain factors such as the elastic modulus, flexural modulus, tensile strength, and compressive strength of scaffold constructs need to be quantified before selecting them for tissue fabrication (Dhandayuthapani et al., 2011; Niu et al., 2012).

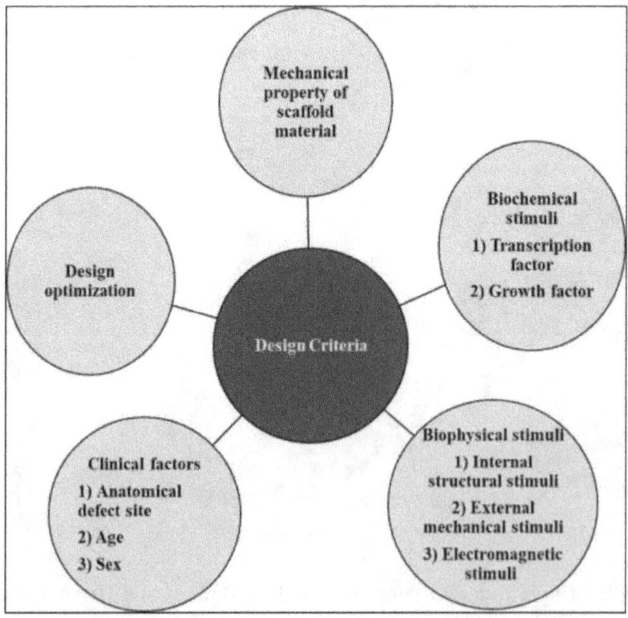

FIGURE 3.7 Essential factors for designing bone scaffolds.

3.3.1.2 Biochemical Stimulation

The integrated expression of diverse biomolecules including transcription factors and growth factors is essential for facilitating cellular commitment and differentiation. Thus, amalgamating these key factors into tissue engineering is a promising approach to enhancing osteogenic cell function during the healing process. Transforming growth factor beta, BMPs, fibroblast growth factors, insulin-like growth factors, platelet-derived growth factor, and Sonic hedgehog are prominent among growth factors. Different transcription factors such as transcriptional coactivator with a PDZ-binding domain, Runt-related transcription factor 2, and osterix are key players in osteogenesis and during bone repair and regeneration (Polo-Corrales et al., 2014).

3.3.1.3 Biophysical Stimulation

Inherent structural stimuli, exogenous mechanical stimuli, and electromagnetic stimuli are important biophysical cues based on the physical properties of the scaffolds (Hao et al., 2021). Structural stimulation is generated by matrix stiffness and topography, which govern the fate of MSCs toward either neurogenic, myogenic, or osteogenic cell lineage (Engler et al., 2006). However, the stimulus from surface topography of material influences cellular behaviour and cell adhesion property (Park & Im, 2015; Dobbenga et al., 2016; Dalby et al., 2014).

Mechanical stimulus generated from compressive or tensile loading can trigger 3D scaffolds seeded with osteoprogenitor cells. In tissue engineering, bioreactors are the preferred choice to mimic the in vivo mechanical stimuli outside the body environment before the actual implantation (Yeatts et al., 2013). Electrical stimuli like direct current and inductive and capacitive coupling also influence osteogenic fate (Bassett et al., 1974; Evans et al., 2001). Therefore, combining different biochemical and biophysical cues facilitates osteogenic induction of MSCs toward bone healing.

3.3.2 Topological and Numerical Design Optimization toward Skeletal Tissue Development

Scaffolding is an essential step in bone tissue remodelling and development that is aided by additive manufacturing techniques. Methods involved in design optimization for developing synthetic bone analogue include computer-aided design (CAD), topology optimization, reverse modelling, and mathematical modelling. Porosity and pore interconnectivity of the scaffold constructs dictate geometrical morphology, mechanical features as well as biological performance (Song et al., 2017; Hollister et al., 2016; Shuai et al., 2018).

Though increasing scaffold porosity can stimulate more bone ingrowth in a shorter time period, it can compromise mechanical strength; therefore, it is necessary to maintain the optimum porosity, which can be achieved through different design optimization techniques. Not only the scaffold design but also the dynamic changes in the mechanical functions after implantation should be considered. Moreover, the outer morphology of the scaffolds should mimic the defect site hierarchy in accordance with the patient-specific tissue model.

3.3.2.1 CAD

CAD is the most common approach for customized patient-specific skeletal tissue design. UG, CATIA, and Pro/E are different CAD tools that construct models based on two basic principles (Landers & Mülhaupt, 2000; Ovsianikov et al., 2011).

A. Constructive solid geometry

In this method, particular model construction is based on various Boolean operations. Constructive solid geometry (CSG) modellers are used to fabricate complex objects or surfaces by combining simple objects such as cubes, spheres, and cylinders. The user may alter their convoluted geometry when CSG is procedural or parametric by modifying the items' positions or the Boolean algorithm which was employed to combine primitive components.

B. Boundary representation

This method represents different model constructs based on their boundary conditions (Naing et al., 2005; Chiu et al., 2006). The models obtained by this method have much higher storage requirements than the CSG method. The file contains the blueprint of the derived construct, and its size increases dramatically as model size or internal complexity increase. According to the aforementioned principles, CAD tools can be used to create different unit cells followed by their assembly to obtain the whole construct. Some software has successfully evolved to simplify the CAD. For example, MATERIALISE can build scaffolds quickly using various elements like cross 1, G6, G7, and dode thin. Preferred synthetic tissue analogues with appropriate porosity can be obtained by incorporating different parameters in a computer-aided system for tissue scaffolds (Naing et al., 2005; Cheah et al., 2004). CAD-based methods for designing bone constructs have many benefits, but they also have certain drawbacks and limitations:

- The method is only able to design scaffold templates with periodic and regular structure.
- The method has less control over mechanical properties and the structural integrity of designed scaffolds.
- Mechanical instability inevitably arises due to external model contour (Lu et al., 2013).

3.3.2.2 Topology Optimization

Although scaffold porosity facilitates nutrient and metabolite transport, it unavoidably impairs the porosity (Yu et al., 2017; Kerativitayanan et al., 2017). Thus, in design, these two conflicting parameters should be considered to achieve optimal performance. Topology optimization helps to achieve optimum material distribution in a defined area on the basis of specific load and constraint conditions (Al-Tamimi et al., 2017). Thus, the designed scaffold is expected to show optimum mechanical properties as well as comprehensive nutrient, metabolite, and growth factor transport. In scaffold designing, first, a topological algorithm is used for unit cell design followed by a periodic repetition of the same process to get the whole scaffold. The optimization algorithms are as follows:

- Solid isotropic material with penalization is used in the initial phase of the design to predict the optimal material distribution within a given designed space of a construct.
- Evolutionary structural optimization is a design method in which inefficient materials are removed from a structure that has to be constructed.
- Level-set algorithm: This algorithm focuses on locating the phase boundaries to efficiently control the topology changes in the designed construct (Osher & Fedkiw, 2001).

However, topology optimization can only achieve regular porous architecture; it is unable to mimic the actual asymmetrical structure of native bone (Yang et al., 2019).

3.3.2.3 Reverse Modelling

Reverse engineering, or back engineering, involves determining how a part was designed so it can be re-created without knowing its exact design specifications. Using different porous structure-based scaffolds with specific design criteria, reverse modelling can help to achieve a scaffold construct that matches the native bone, although the model accuracy generally depends on the image resolution device. The process (see the schematic representation in Figure 3.8) also involves a highly involved computational setup and high storage space (Hollister et al., 2000).

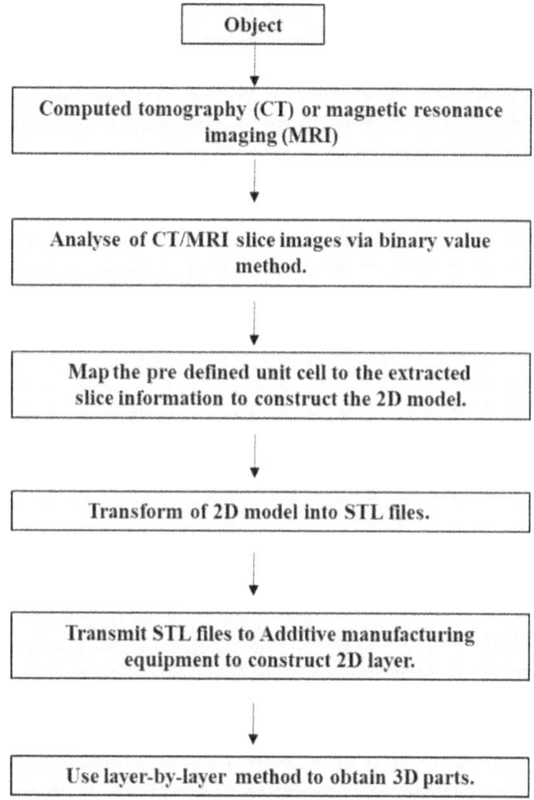

FIGURE 3.8 Schematic representation of using reverse modelling for design optimization.

Capturing and converting physical data into electronic data for reverse modelling primarily involves a 3D scanner and a coordinate measuring machine (CMM). The CMM consists of an automatic three-axis motor detection system with a sensor probe that receives the externally generated data and helps to quantify an element with accuracy. The machine also holds a shape pattern as a reference so it can be drawn in 3D software (Manzoor Hussain et al., 2008). The 3D scanner captures shapes and ensures that the proposed drawing exactly matches the product to be re-created.

3.3.2.4 Mathematical Modelling

To overcome the geometrical limitations of the traditional porous elements, mathematical modelling is used for shape-related functions to fabricate porous constructs with inherent functional surfaces or asymmetrical polygonal models. The most common methods are as follows.

A. Triply periodic minimal surface (TPMS)

TPMS mainly utilizes trigonometric functions to obtain a composite porous structure with minimal surface having zero curvature at any point. Scaffolds with minimal surfaces are more prone to higher permeability and wettability with deeper cells in growth (Melchels et al., 2010a). Different TPMS models can be characterized with implicit functions as follows (Strano et al., 2013):

Schwartz surface: $$cos\left(\frac{2\pi}{l}x\right)+coscos\left(\frac{2\pi}{l}y\right)+coscos\left(\frac{2\pi}{l}z\right)=K,$$

Gyroid surface:

$$cos\left(\frac{2\pi}{l}x\right)sin\left(\frac{2\pi}{l}y\right)+coscos\left(\frac{2\pi}{l}y\right)sin\left(\frac{2\pi}{l}z\right)+ coscos\left(\frac{2\pi}{l}z\right)sin\left(\frac{2\pi}{l}x\right)=K,$$

Diamond su-rface:

$$sin\left(\frac{2\pi}{l}x\right)sin\left(\frac{2\pi}{l}y\right)sin\left(\frac{2\pi}{l}z\right)+sin\left(\frac{2\pi}{l}x\right)cos\left(\frac{2\pi}{l}y\right)cos\left(\frac{2\pi}{l}z\right)+ cos\left(\frac{2\pi}{l}x\right)sin\left(\frac{2\pi}{l}y\right)cos\left(\frac{2\pi}{l}z\right)+cos\left(\frac{2\pi}{l}x\right)cos\left(\frac{2\pi}{l}y\right)sin\left(\frac{2\pi}{l}z\right)=K,$$

Here, l is the periodic length and K is the offset parameter. In addition to the regular structures, heterogeneous, gradient, hybrid, and irregular porous structures can also be obtained via TPMS. Melchels et al. (2010b) also reported on using TPMS to design a gradation in porosity.

B. Voronoi Tessellation

In this method, the design volume is randomly filled with a set of points (or seeds) to segregate different areas, followed by specifying a thickness to the edges of those areas to attain a porous scaffold. A bone-like trabecular structure was designed using micro-CT-guided images of the trabecular bone, and the final features of the construct could be customized by changing the trabecular thickness and separation during the design stage (Gómez et al., 2016). For the successful balance between irregularity and controllability, Wang et al. (2018) introduced a scale coefficient with controlled porosity and strut thickness. Thus, by combining beneficial aspects of topology optimization and reverse modelling, Voronoi tessellation can achieve sufficient porosity, permeability, and mechanical strength for synthetic bone analogues with varying load-bearing capacity.

In short, biomimetic synthetic tissue analogues can be developed by merging suitable materials with bioactive cues through optimized design strategy. The improved bioactivity leads to enhanced osteoconduction, osseointegration, and osteoinduction with increased angiogenesis (Turnbull et al., 2018). The most promising strategy could be integrating the bioactive materials with suitable fabrication techniques for providing mechanical and structural properties to synthetic tissue analogues that are comparable with those of native bone (Castilho et al., 2020; Peppas & Langer, 1994).

3.4 FABRICATING BONE ANALOGUES

Bone tissue engineering has delivered many alternatives for repairing and remodelling critically injured bones. In developing ideal biomimetic bone grafts, fabrication methods must incorporate all the parameters we have discussed (porosity, load-bearing capacity, etc.). Many technologies for bone analogue fabrications have been developed so far. The selection of fabrication method is dependent on the prerequisite form and architecture of the biomaterial and important factors (solubility and melting temperature) that affect material processing.

There are several conventional approaches like solvent casting, sol-gel process, microsphere sintering, and thermal-induced phase separation. Some of their key features, advantages, and limitations are described in Table 3.5. Electrospinning is a recently developed yet simple and cost-effective technique for nanomaterial fabrication. CAD and computer-aided manufacturing are making possible customized implants and devices for healthcare industries developed based on top-down reverse engineering and bottom-up 3D printing. The schematics of top-down and bottom-up approaches are presented in Figure 3.9. In this section, we will provide insight into conventional as well as advanced techniques and a comparative overview of benefits and limitations of each fabrication technique (Ghelich et al., 2022).

TABLE 3.5
Conventional Bottom-Up Approaches to Skeletal Tissue Fabrication

Techniques	Key Features	Advantages	Limitations	References
Solvent casting	Porosity: 20–30%, Pore size: 30–300 μm Pore interconnectivity: high	Simple process Suitable for strong bone analogue fabrication	Less control over pore size Low reproducibility	Rhim et al. (2006)
Sol-gel process	Porosity: 85–95 % Pore size: 200–1000 μm Pore interconnectivity: medium	Low cost Suitable for wide range of materials	Shape of structure is limited to mould shape	Hench (1990)
Microsphere sintering	Porosity: 40% Pore size: 90 μm Pore interconnectivity: medium	Scaffold with good mechanical property Pore connectivity is high by CO_2-mediated sintering	High-temperature process Limited to mould shape	Gupta et al. (2017)
Thermal-induced phase separation	Porosity: 73.5–97.5% Pore size: 0.03–420μm Pore interconnectivity: medium	Uniform porosity, Defect free, Anisotropy	Not suitable for osteoblast seeding	Lee et al. (2004)
Electrospinning	Porosity: 40% Pore size: 90μm Pore interconnectivity: medium	Porosity is high, Facilitates cell attachment	High voltage causes cell damage Difficult to control fibre morphology and orientation	Teo & Ramakrishna (2006)

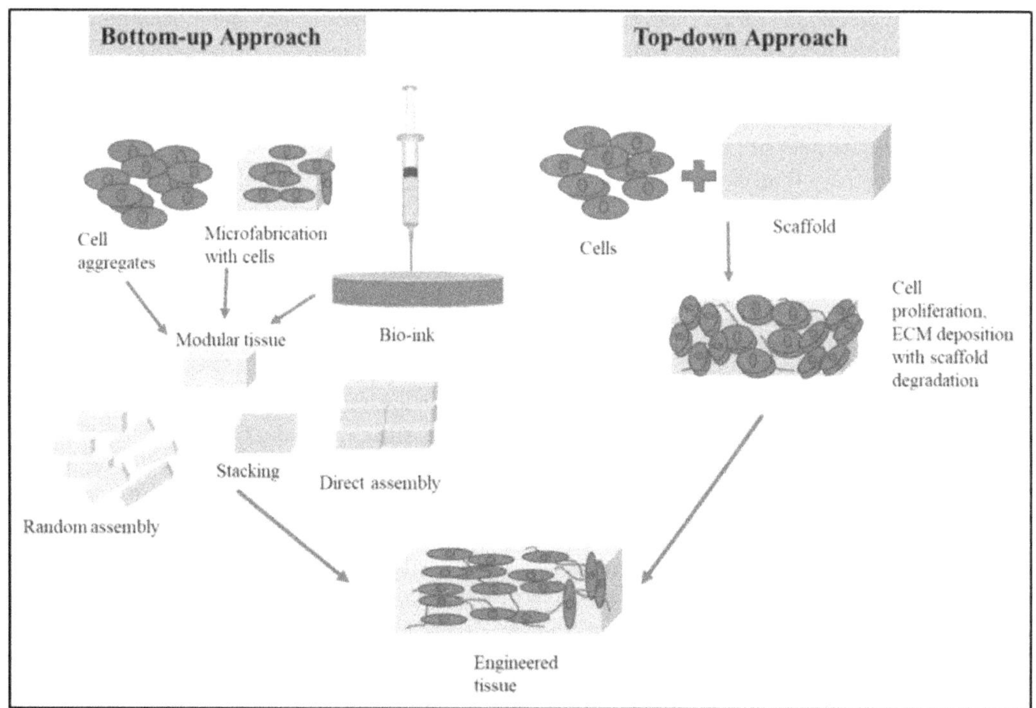

FIGURE 3.9 Schematic comparison between bottom-up and top-down approaches.

3.4.1 Top-Down Approaches

This type of tissue engineering approach includes the fabrication of templates or synthetic bone constructs of the required architecture on which cells are seeded. These cells are anticipated to get attached and proliferate to populate scaffolds as well as form an extracellular matrix (ECM) simultaneously. Different signals like growth factors, and mechanical/electrical stimuli are delivered to regulate cell activity and mimic *in vivo* tissue microenvironments, biomolecule-based signalling and mechanobiology (Li et al., 2017). Top-down methods include computer numerical control machines that have been used to custom design dental crowns, mandibles, cranial plates, tibia trays, and femoral knee implants.

3.4.2 Bottom-Up Approaches

The fabrication methods we have been briefly described so far usually offer only limited control over porosity, architecture, and interconnectivity. Cell immobilization on ECM-supporting scaffolds is quite challenging, leading to less cell seeding and uneven distribution on the scaffold. To overcome the limitations of previously discussed methods, several advanced and emerging bottom-up approaches are employed to mimic in vivo bone tissue architecture, microenvironment, and function (Santoliquido et al., 2019).

In bottom-up techniques, micro-level tissue building blocks (cell-seeded modules) are arranged into 3D structures to replicate the natural intricacies of native bone (Shirinzadeh et al., 2004). Fibre fabrication is one of the key bottom-up fabrication techniques, which include technologies such as wet spinning, microfluidic spinning, interfacial polyelectrolyte complexation, and melt spinning.

3.5 RECENT ADVANCEMENTS IN FABRICATION TECHNIQUES

3.5.1 Additive Manufacturing: 3D Printing

The standard techniques for fabricating scaffolds, which have been briefly mentioned so far, typically provide little regulation over void/pore size, shape, and connectivity between pores. With the development of 3D printing, it has been easier to spatially regulate scaffold microarchitecture and spatial features (Zhang et al., 2023). The advancement of 3D printing has made it possible to create complex structures with greater regulation over geometrical parameters, void/pore size, morphology, and connectivity than conventional top-down methods (Gross et al., 2014).

In 3D printing, a bone defect or fracture site is scanned or imaged using computer tomography or magnetic resonance imaging, a model of the bone construct is created using CAD, and the desired construct is typically printed layer-wise using ink. The cross-sections of the various complex structures are accessible using CAD models. As a result, it is possible to build gradually porous, hierarchical 3D structures with high regulation over the size of pores and interconnectivity on every cross-section (Zhang et al., 2015).

Large segmental bone lesions can be repaired with additive manufacturing (AM)/3D printing, which can create scaffolds with both a porous interior structure and a tailored external shape. Benefits of 3D printing include strong control over structure and porosity; reproducibility; a large variety of printable materials including natural and synthetic polymers (Sears et al., 2017), ceramics (Becker et al., 2012), metals (Pei et al., 2017), and composites (Corcione et al., 2017); and a simple process. Another term for 3D printing is rapid prototyping due to the processing time's short duration. Costly equipment and printable object dimensions are constraints on 3D printing in bone tissue fabrication.

The different AM techniques used in bone tissue engineering can be divided into three major groups: i) extrusion based, ii) powder based, and iii) vat photo polymerization. A critical overview of different additive manufacturing processes; their key features, advantages, and limitations; and their potential applications (Garot et al., 2021) is provided in Table 3.6.

TABLE 3.6
Additive Fabrication Techniques in Bone Tissue Engineering

Process		Brief Description	Materials Used	Pros	Cons	Application	References
Extrusion based	Fused deposition modelling	Theapabilr releases material followed by heating and further deposition of ink in a layered fashion.	Polymers (ABS, PC, PLA, etc.) Metals/ceramics with binders	Cost-effective, Patient specific Generates suitable voids in scaffold for bone tissue ingrowth	Anisotropy, Poor surface morphology Only suitable for some thermoplastic polymers Medium resolution Difficult to fabricate small-diameter structures	PCL/hydroxyapatite (HA)-based analogues of goat femur with good biocompatibility and osteogenic potential	Garot et al. (2021)
	Robocasting	Polymericapabils released through micro-nozzles are deposited on a substrate in a layered fashion per the CAD model.	Metal-based slurry and ceramics Polymers including fibrin, chitosan, hyaluronic acid, GelMA, etc.	Supports processing at a range of temperatures Suitable for live cell printing	Limited resolution and printing accuracy Inferior built speed compared with SLA and other fabrication methods	Beta TCP-based mandibles Skull implant in rabbit	Kim et al. (2016)
Powder based	Selective laser machining(SLM)	Using a high-energy laser, selective fusion deposits a thin metallic biomaterial powder in a layered manner under a high vacuum.	Metal-based biomaterials	Post-processing is not required Feasible at the industrial level Less porosity in printed material	Nonuniform microstructure Rough topology Costly Bulky machines take up space	Titanium and Ti6Al4V-based maxillofacial alveolar orbital wall implanted in a human	Tovar et al. (2018)
	Electron beam melting	Similar to SLM except it provided an energy source as a collimated electron	Metallic biomaterials	High mechanical strength	Average ductility Expensive Bulky machines	Ti and Ti6Al4V-based skull and chest implanted in a human	Ma et al. (2017)
	Inkjet printing	Head releases droplets of biomaterials on the substrate per CAD model followed by liquid-to-solid transient phase conversion until the whole structure is built.	Polymer Ceramics	Remarkable cell adhesion and proliferation as well as osteogenic potential	Cannot print metals Generates brittle structures Inappropriate for load-bearing applications	α-TCP-based construct for craniofacial bone defects, bone bridging, PEEK-based scapula in a human	Aragón & Méndez (2016)

(Continued)

TABLE 3.6 (*Continued*)
Additive Fabrication Techniques in Bone Tissue Engineering

Process		Brief Description	Materials Used	Pros	Cons	Application	References
Vat polymerization	Stereolithography (SLA)	A collector is loaded with a resin-based UV-cured material with a movable building plate. Post-processing step is required for removal of resin and curing of material.	Photosensitive polymers and ceramics	Remarkable resolution at ~25 µm with accuracy Suitable for printing small or medium-sized single parts with biological cues and live cells	Unreacted monomer Resin causes photoinitiator-related contamination Limited availability of photo resins	HA-based skull implants in a human	Dong et al. (2018)
	Digital light processing (DLP)	DLP differs from SLA in terms of the curing method. For reflecting laser, a digital light projector is used in place of a mirror.	Photosensitive polymers and ceramics	Vulnerability of live cells is maintained High Resolution and precision	Time-consuming post-processing Comparatively slower than SLA Availability of photo initiators is significantly limited	Bioglass-based mandibles in rabbit	Brie et al. (2013)

3.5.2 3D Bioprinting

In the process of 3D bioprinting, bioinks with cells, bioactive agents, and growth factors are printed to form a 3D hierarchical construct (Samandari et al., 2021). The schematics of the 3D printer and 3D bioprinter are presented in Figure 3.10. The initial steps in 3D bioprinting are the same as 3D printing except for the last step, in which cell proliferation and development take place in bioreactors (Yin et al., 2019). The process is an emerging tissue engineering fabrication method in critical bone defect repair and replacement (Zhang et al., 2023). It provides unique design flexibility in fabricating hierarchical bone constructs which support cell differentiation and growth and have control over the distribution of cells and fine resolution. Moreover, its ease of scale-up and cost-effectiveness are some of the attractive features that make this method feasible for bone graft manufacturing. The major limitation of bioprinting techniques is the low mechanical integrity of the 3D-printed structure (Cheng et al., 2021).

3.5.3 Next-Generation 3D Bioprinting

Bioprinting in 3D is one of the most sophisticated techniques for bone tissue fabrication with cells, biomaterials, and bioactive cues to promote osteogenesis and replicate natural intricacies. The whole process is highly regulated and remains active throughout the lifetime of the part in response to biological and environmental cues as well as tissue damage (Bonnans et al., 2014). Designing grafts for mimicking complete 3D architecture is necessary. Scaffolds printed in 3D are nonresponsive to dynamic changes that happen naturally in the body micro-environment. With the advent of shape memory biomaterials, 4D bioprinting aims to develop tissue constructs that can change their morphology and mechanical characteristics in response to dynamic signals (temperature, chemical, light, ultrasound, electrical, and biological signals).

Tissue-specific 3D designs along with 4D bioprinting will advance more robust and biologically active humanized tissues for healing and disease models, as well as tools for fundamental biological studies (Gaspar et al., 2020). For instance, Sawkins et al. (2015) fabricated a mechanically strong analogue for cancellous bone from aapabilo-responsive material polylactic-co-glycolic acid that

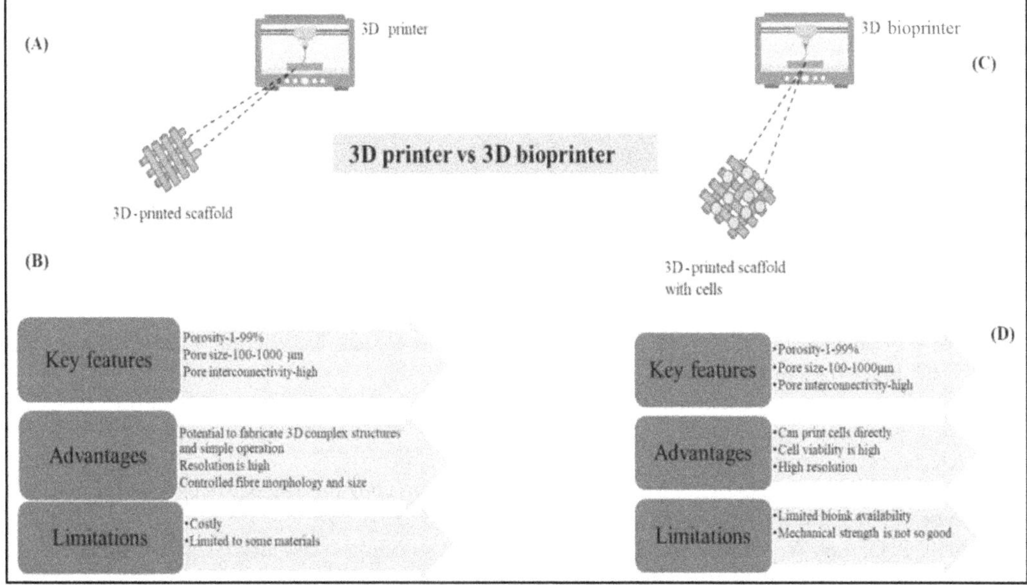

FIGURE 3.10 Comparison between (A)(B) 3D printer and (C)(D)3D bioprinter.

facilited the integration of thermal sensitive cells, growth factors, and proteins. This method has opened vistas for fabricating patient-specific customized organs and tissues. From a tissue engineering perspective, constructing specific biologically active cell-rich modules is more advantageous and effective than designing the whole complex structures of native tissues. Hence, hybrid technologies are increasingly being used; in the near future, their products will be a boon in the healthcare sector for novel innovative materials for treating bone defects. However, there is an imperative need to fill gaps between research results and translational biomedical applications (Sawkins et al., 2015).

CONCLUSION

Current approaches for repairing and remodelling defective bone tissues have intrinsic limitations. With demand, there is an urge for innovative treatment modalities. Advanced design using macroporous bioactive materials and combinations of various fabrication techniques are necessary for the successful development of skeletal tissue analogues. Implementing these novel techniques gives us an opportunity to aid the development of tissue-engineering approaches in clinical practice; however, today's treatment approaches are inadequate.

In the near future, it will be necessary to analyse and validate the development of bone and its surrounding tissues to understand the interaction between cells with their local microenvironment and growth factors. The development of patient-specific tissue constructs is the prime concern in tissue engineering. Such analogues clearly need a multidisciplinary approach, including efforts from cell scientists, biomedical engineers, clinicians, and patients. Ultimately, clinical success will rely on combining the factors we have discussed here and their proper implementation in the development of artificial bone tissue analogues.

LIST OF ABBREVIATIONS

3D	Three-dimensional
AM	Additive manufacturing
BMPs	Bone morphogenetic proteins
CAD	Computer aided design
CSG	Constructive solid geometry
ECM	Extracellular matrix
MSCs	Mesenchymal stem cells
TPMS	Triply periodic minimal surface

REFERENCES

Ait Oumghar, I., Barkaoui, A., & Chabrand, P. (2020). Toward a mathematical modeling of diseases' impact on bone remodeling: Technical review. *Front. Bioeng. Biotech.* 8: 584198.

Al-Tamimi, A. A., Fernandes, P. R. A., Peach, C., Cooper, G., Diver, C., & Bartolo, P. J. (2017). Metallic bone fixation implants: A novel design approach for reducing the stress shielding phenomenon. *Virtual Phys. Prototyp.* 12: 141–151.

Amini, A. R., Laurencin, C. T., & Nukavarapu, S. P. (2012). Bone tissue engineering: Recent advances and challenges. *Crit. Rev. Biomed. Eng.* 40: 363–408.

Annamalai, R. T., Hong, X., Schott, N. G., Tiruchinapally, G., Levi, B., & Stegemann, J. P. (2019). Injectable osteogenic microtissues containing mesenchymal stromal cells conformally fill and repair critical-size defects. *Biomaterials.* 208: 32–44.

Aragón, J., & Méndez, I. P. (2016). Dynamic 3D printed titanium copy prosthesis: A novel design for large chest wall resection and reconstruction. *J. Thorac. Dis.* 8: E385–E389.

Armstrong, C. G., Lai, W. M., & Mow, V. C. (1984). An analysis of the unconfined compression of articular cartilage. *J. Biomech. Eng.* 106: 165–173.

Barrère, F., Mahmood, T. A., de Groot, K., & van Blitterswijk, C. A. (2008). Advanced biomaterials for skeletal tissue regeneration: Instructive and smart functions. *Mater. Sci. Eng. R Rep.* 59: 38–71.

Bassett, C. A. L., Pawluk, R. J., & Pilla, A. A. (1974). Acceleration of fracture repair by electromagnetic fields: A surgically noninvasive method. *Ann. N. Y. Acad. Sci.* 238: 242–262.

Becker, S. T., Bolte, H., Schünemann, K., Seitz, H., Bara, J. J., Beck-Broichsitter, B. E., Russo, P. A. J., Wiltfang, J., & Warnke, P. H. (2012). Endocultivation: The influence of delayed vs. simultaneous application of BMP-2 onto individually formed hydroxyapatite matrices for heterotopic bone induction. *Int. J. Oral Maxillofac. Surg.* 41: 1153–1160.

Bobbert, F. S. L., Lietaert, K., Eftekhari, A. A., Pouran, B., Ahmadi, S. M., Weinans, H., & Zadpoor, A. A. (2017). Additively manufactured metallic porous biomaterials based on minimal surfaces: A unique combination of topological, mechanical, and mass transport properties. *Acta Biomater.* 53: 572–584.

Bonnans, C., Chou, J., & Werb, Z. (2014). Remodelling the extracellular matrix in development and disease. *Nat. Rev. Mol. Cell Biol.* 15: 786–801.

Bose, S., Roy, M., & Bandyopadhyay, A. (2012). Recent advances in bone tissue engineering scaffolds. *Trends Biotechnol.* 30: 546–554.

Brie, J., Chartier, T., Chaput, C., Delage, C., Pradeau, B., Caire, F., Boncoeur, M. P., & Moreau, J. J. (2013). A new custom made bioceramic implant for the repair of large and complex craniofacial bone defects. *J. Cranio-Maxillofac. Surg.* 41: 403–407.

Burwell, R. (1994). History of bone grafting and bone substitutes with special reference to osteogenic induction. In *Bone Grafts, Derivatives and Substitutes*. M. R. Urist, and R. G. Burwell, Eds. Oxford: Butterworth-Heinemann, pp. 3–102.

Busch, A., Wegner, A., Haversath, M., & Jäger, M. (2021). Bone substitutes in orthopaedic surgery: Current status and future perspectives. *Z. Orthop. Unfall.* 159: 304–313.

Campana, V., Milano, G., Pagano, E., Barba, M., Cicione, C., Salonna, G., Lattanzi, W., & Logroscino, G. (2014). Bone substitutes in orthopaedic surgery: From basic science to clinical practice. *J. Mater. Sci. Mater. Med.* 25: 2445–2461.

Campbell, C. J. (1969). The healing of cartilage defects. *Clin. Orthop. Relat. Res.* 64: 45–63.

Carrel, J. P., Dent, M., Buser, D., Dent, M., Bernard, J. P., & Dent, M. (2014). Maxillary sinus grafting with a synthetic, nanocrystalline hydroxyapatite-silica gel in humans: Histologic and histomorphometric results. *Periodontics.* 34: 259–267.

Castilho, M., de Ruijter, M., Beirne, S., Villette, C. C., Ito, K., Wallace, G. G., & Malda, J. (2020). Multitechnology biofabrication: A new approach for the manufacturing of functional tissue structures? *Trends Biotechnol.* 38: 1316–1328.

Cheah, C. M., Chua, C. K., Leong, K. F., Cheong, C. H., & Naing, M. W. (2004). Automatic algorithm for generating complex polyhedral scaffold structures for tissue engineering. *Tissue Eng.* 10: 595–610.

Chen, F. S., Frenkel, S. R., & Di Cesare, P. E. (1999). Repair of articular cartilage defects: Part I: Basic science of cartilage healing. *Am. J. Orthop.* 28: 31–33.

Cheng, L., He, H., Rajput, R. S., Feng, Q., Ramesh, S., Wang, Y., Krishnan, S., Ostrovidov, S., Camci-Unal, G., & Ramalingam, M. (2021). 3D printing of micro-and nanoscale bone substitutes: A review on technical and translational perspectives. *Int. J. Nanomed.* 16: 4289.

Chiu, W. K., Yeung, Y. C., & Yu, K. M. (2006). Toolpath generation for layer manufacturing of fractal objects. *Rapid Prototyp. J.* 12: 214–221.

Corcione, C. E., Gervaso, F., Scalera, F., Montagna, F., Maiullaro, T., Sannino, A., & Maffezzoli, A. (2017). 3D printing of hydroxyapatite polymer-based composites for bone tissue engineering. *J. Polym. Eng.* 37: 741–746.

Dalby, M. J., Gadegaard, N., & Oreffo, R. O. C. (2014). Harnessing nanotopography and integrin—Matrix interactions to influence stem cell fate. *Nat. Mater.* 13: 558–569.

De Martino, I., D'Apolito, R., Sculco, P. K., Poultsides, L. A., & Gasparini, G. (2016). Total knee arthroplasty using cementless porous tantalum monoblock tibial component: A minimum 10-year follow-up. *J. Arthroplasty.* 31: 2193–2198.

Dhandayuthapani, B., Yoshida, Y., Maekawa, T., & Kumar, D. S. (2011). Polymeric scaffolds in tissue engineering application: A review. *Int. J. Polym. Sci.* 2011: 290602.

Dobbenga, S., Fratila-Apachitei, L. E., & Zadpoor, A. A. (2016). Nanopattern-induced osteogenic differentiation of stem cells—A systematic review. *Acta Biomater.* 46: 3–14.

Donati, D., Zolezzi, C., Tomba, P., & Viganò, A. (2007). Bone grafting: Historical and conceptual review, starting with an old manuscript by Vittorio Putti. *Acta Orthop*. 78: 19–25.

Dong, L., Jun, F., Hongbin, F., Dichen, L., Enchun, D., Xin, X., Ling, W., & Zheng, G. (2018). Application of 3D-printed PEEK scapula prosthesis in the treatment of scapular benign fibrous histiocytoma: A case report. *J. Bone Oncol*. 12: 78–82.

Engler, A. J., Sen, S., Sweeney, H. L., & Discher, D. E. (2006). Matrix elasticity directs stem cell lineage specification. *Cell*. 126: 677–689.

Evaniew, N., Tan, V., Parasu, N., Jurriaans, E., Finlay, K., Deheshi, B., & Ghert, M. (2013). Use of a calcium sulfate—Calcium phosphate synthetic bone graft composite in the surgical management of primary bone tumors. *Orthopedics*. 36: e216–e222.

Evans, R. D., Foltz, D., & Foltz, K. (2001). Electrical stimulation with bone and wound healing. *Clin. Podiatr. Med. Surg*. 18: 79–95.

Faour, O., Dimitriou, R., Cousins, C. A., & Giannoudis, P. V. (2011). The use of bone graft substitutes in large cancellous voids: Any specific needs? *Injury*. 42: S87–S90.

Farrell, E., van der Jagt, O. P., Koevoet, W., Kops, N., Van Manen, C. J., Hellingman, C. A., Jahr, H., O'Brien, F. J., Verhaar, J. A. N., & Weinans, H. (2009). Chondrogenic priming of human bone marrow stromal cells: A better route to bone repair? *Tissue Eng. Part C*. 15: 285–295.

Fawcett, D. W., & Bloom, W. (1986). *A Textbook of Histology*. New York: Chapman & Hall.

Filippi, M. E., Barcena, A., Trogrlić, R. Š., Cremen, G., Menteşe, E. Y., Gentile, R., Creed, M. J., Jenkins, L. T., Kalaycioglu, M., & Poudel, D. P. (2023). Interdisciplinarity in practice: Reflections from early-career researchers developing a risk-informed decision support environment for tomorrow's cities. *Int. J. Disaster Risk Reduct*. 85: 103481.

Freeman, F. E., Pitacco, P., van Dommelen, L. H. A., Nulty, J., Browe, D. C., Shin, J. Y., Alsberg, E., & Kelly, D. J. (2020). 3D bioprinting spatiotemporally defined patterns of growth factors to tightly control tissue regeneration. *Sci. Adv*. 6: eabb5093.

Garot, C., Bettega, G., & Picart, C. (2021). Additive manufacturing of material scaffolds for bone regeneration: Toward application in the clinics. *Adv. Funct. Mater*. 31: 2006967.

Gaspar, V. M., Lavrador, P., Borges, J., Oliveira, M. B., & Mano, J. F. (2020). Advanced bottom-up engineering of living architectures. *Adv. Mater*. 32: 1903975.

Geraldes, D. M., & Phillips, A. T. M. (2014). A comparative study of orthotropic and isotropic bone adaptation in the femur. *Int. J. Num. Meth. Biomed. Eng*. 30: 873–889.

Ghelich, P., Kazemzadeh-Narbat, M., Hassani Najafabadi, A., Samandari, M., Memić, A., & Tamayol, A. (2022). (Bio) manufactured solutions for treatment of bone defects with an emphasis on US-FDA regulatory science perspective. *Adv. NanoBiomed. Res*. 2: 2100073.

Ghert, M. A., Qi, W., Erickson, H. P., Block, J. A., & Scully, S. P. (2002). Tenascin-C expression and distribution in cultured human chondrocytes and chondrosarcoma cells. *J. Orthop. Res*. 20: 834–841.

Gómez, S., Vlad, M. D., López, J., & Fernández, E. (2016). Design and properties of 3D scaffolds for bone tissue engineering. *Acta Biomater*. 42: 341–350.

Gross, B. C., Erkal, J. L., Lockwood, S. Y., Chen, C., & Spence, D. M. (2014). Evaluation of 3D printing and its potential impact on biotechnology and the chemical sciences. *Anal. Chem*. 86: 3240–3253.

Guarino, V., Galizia, M., Alvarez-Perez, M., Mensitieri, G., & Ambrosio, L. (2015). Improving surface and transport properties of macroporous hydrogels for bone regeneration. *J. Biomed. Mater. Res. A*. 103: 1095–1105.

Gunzburg, R., Szpalski, M., Passuti, N., & Aebi, M. (2002). *The Use of Bone Substitutes in Spine Surgery: A State of the Art Review*. Berlin, Heidelberg: Springer.

Gupta, V., Khan, Y., Berkland, C. J., Laurencin, C. T., & Detamore, M. S. (2017). Microsphere-based scaffolds in regenerative engineering. *Annu. Rev. Biomed. Eng*. 19: 135–161.

Hao, Z., Xu, Z., Wang, X., Wang, Y., Li, H., Chen, T., Hu, Y., Chen, R., Huang, K., & Chen, C. (2021). Biophysical stimuli as the fourth pillar of bone tissue engineering. *Front. Cell Dev. Biol*. 9: 3229.

Hench, L. L. (1990). JK West the sol-gel process. *Chem. Rev*. 90: 33–72.

Hench, L. L., Splinter, R. J., Allen, W. C., & Greenlee, T. K. (1971). Bonding mechanisms at the interface of ceramic prosthetic materials. *J. Biomed. Mater. Res*. 5: 117–141.

Hench, L. L., & Thompson, I. (2010). Twenty-first century challenges for biomaterials. *J. R. Soc. Interface*. 7: S379–S391.

Hing, K. A. (2005). Bioceramic bone graft substitutes: Influence of porosity and chemistry. *Int. J. Appl. Ceram. Technol*. 2: 184–199.

Hinze, M. C., Wiedmann-Al-Ahmad, M., Glaum, R., Gutwald, R., Schmelzeisen, R., & Sauerbier, S. (2010). Bone engineering-vitalisation of alloplastic and allogenic bone grafts by human osteoblast-like cells. *British J. Oral Maxillofac. Surg*. 48: 369–373.

Hollister, S. J., Flanagan, C. L., Morrison, R. J., Patel, J. J., Wheeler, M. B., Edwards, S. P., & Green, G. E. (2016). Integrating image-based design and 3D biomaterial printing to create patient specific devices within a design control framework for clinical translation. *ACS Biomater. Sci. Eng*. 2: 1827–1836.

Hollister, S. J., Levy, R. A., Chu, T., Halloran, J. W., & Feinberg, S. E. (2000). An image-based approach for designing and manufacturing craniofacial scaffolds. *Int. J. Oral Maxillofac. Surg*. 29: 67–71.

Hossain, U., Ghouse, S., Nai, K., & Jeffers, J. R. T. (2021). Controlling and testing anisotropy in additively manufactured stochastic structures. *Addit. Manuf*. 39: 101849.

Hulbert, S. F., Young, F. A., Mathews, R. S., Klawitter, J. J., Talbert, C. D., & Stelling, F. H. (1970). Potential of ceramic materials as permanently implantable skeletal prostheses. *J. Biomed. Mater. Res*. 4: 433–456.

Hunziker, E. B. (2002). Articular cartilage repair: Basic science and clinical progress: A review of the current status and prospects. *Osteoarthr. Cartil*. 10: 432–463.

Huwais, S., & Meyer, E. G. (2017). A novel osseous densification approach in implant osteotomy preparation to increase biomechanical primary stability, bone mineral density, and bone-to-implant contact. *Int. J. Oral Maxillofac. Impl*. 32: 27–36.

Kapur, R. A., Amirfeyz, R., Wylde, V., Blom, A. W., Nelson, I. W., & Hutchinson, J. (2010). Clinical outcomes and fusion success associated with the use of BoneSave in spinal surgery. *Arch. Orthop. Trauma Surg*. 130: 641–647.

Karakurt, I., & Lin, L. (2020). 3D printing technologies: Techniques, materials, and post-processing. *Curr. Opin. Chem. Eng*. 28: 134–143.

Kerativitayanan, P., Tatullo, M., Khariton, M., Joshi, P., Perniconi, B., & Gaharwar, A. K. (2017). Nanoengineered osteoinductive and elastomeric scaffolds for bone tissue engineering. *ACS Biomater. Sci. Eng*. 3: 590–600.

Kim, H. M., Rey, C., & Glimcher, M. J. (1995). Isolation of calcium-phosphate crystals of bone by non-aqueous methods at low temperature. *J. Bone Miner. Res*. 10: 1589–1601.

Kim, J. A., Lim, J., Naren, R., Yun, H., & Park, E. K. (2016). Effect of the biodegradation rate controlled by pore structures in magnesium phosphate ceramic scaffolds on bone tissue regeneration in vivo. *Acta Biomater*. 44: 155–167.

Konermann, A., Staubwasser, M., Dirk, C., Keilig, L., Bourauel, C., Götz, W., Jäger, A., & Reichert, C. (2014). Bone substitute material composition and morphology differentially modulate calcium and phosphate release through osteoclast-like cells. *Int. J. Oral Maxillofac. Surg*. 43: 514–521.

Lambert, F., Léonard, A., Lecloux, G., Sourice, S., Pilet, P., & Rompen, E. (2013). A comparison of three calcium phosphate-based space fillers in sinus elevation: A study in rabbits. *Int. J. Oral Maxillofac. Impl*. 28: 393–402.

Landers, R., & Mülhaupt, R. (2000). Desktop manufacturing of complex objects, prototypes and biomedical scaffolds by means of computer-assisted design combined with computer-guided 3D plotting of polymers and reactive oligomers. *Macromol. Mater. Eng*. 282: 17–21.

Lee, J., Guarino, V., Gloria, A., Ambrosio, L., Tae, G., Kim, Y. H., Jung, Y., Kim, S. H., & Kim, S. H. (2010). Regeneration of Achilles' tendon: The role of dynamic stimulation for enhanced cell proliferation and mechanical properties. *J. Biomater. Sci. Polym. Ed*. 21: 1173–1190.

Lee, K. W. D., Chan, P. K., & Feng, X. (2004). Morphology development and characterization of the phase-separated structure resulting from the thermal-induced phase separation phenomenon in polymer solutions under a temperature gradient. *Chem. Eng. Sci*. 59: 1491–1504.

Li, L., Eyckmans, J., & Chen, C. S. (2017). Designer biomaterials for mechanobiology. *Nat. Mater*. 16: 1164–1168.

Linhart, W., Briem, D., Schmitz, N. D., Priemel, M., Lehmann, W., & Rueger, J. M. (2003). Treatment of metaphyseal bone defects after fractures of the distal radius: Medium-term results using a calcium-phosphate cement (BIOBON®) Mittelfristige Ergebnisse mit einem Kalziumphosphatzement (BIOBON®). *Unfallchirurg*. 106: 618–624.

Lu, G., Xu, S., Yan, Q. S., Xiong, X., & Yu, H. (2013). Study on dimension change law from CAD model to prototype of rapid investment casting based on selective laser sintering. *Adv. Mat. Res*. 774: 1046–1050.

Ma, J., Ma, L., Wang, Z., Zhu, X., & Wang, W. (2017). The use of 3D-printed titanium mesh tray in treating complex comminuted mandibular fractures: A case report. *Medicine*. 96: e7250.

Mackie, E., Ahmed, Y. A., Tatarczuch, L., Chen, K. S., & Mirams, M. (2008). Endochondral ossification: How cartilage is converted into bone in the developing skeleton. *Int. J. Biochem. Cell Biol.* 40: 46–62.

Mankin, H. J., & Buckwalter, J. A. (1996). Restoration of the osteoarthrotic joint. *J. Bone Joint Surg*. 78: 1–2.

Manzoor Hussain, M., Sambasiva Rao, C. H., & Prasad, K. E. (2008). Reverse engineering: Point cloud generation with CMM for part modeling and error analysis. *ARPN J. Eng. Appl. Sci.* 3: 37–40.

Mathai, B., Dhara, S., & Gupta, S. (2021). Orthotropic bone remodelling around uncemented femoral implant: A comparison with isotropic formulation. *Biomech. Model. Mechanobiol.* 20: 1115–1134.

Melchels, F. P. W., Barradas, A. M. C., Van Blitterswijk, C. A., De Boer, J., Feijen, J., & Grijpma, D. W. (2010a). Effects of the architecture of tissue engineering scaffolds on cell seeding and culturing. *Acta Biomater.* 6: 4208–4217.

Melchels, F. P. W., Bertoldi, K., Gabbrielli, R., Velders, A. H., Feijen, J., & Grijpma, D. W. (2010b). Mathematically defined tissue engineering scaffold architectures prepared by stereolithography. *Biomaterials*. 31: 6909–6916.

Naing, M. W., Chua, C. K., Leong, K. F., & Wang, Y. (2005). Fabrication of customised scaffolds using computer-aided design and rapid prototyping techniques. *Rapid Prototyp. J.* 11: 249–259.

Niu, L. N., Jiao, K., Qi, Y. P., Nikonov, S., Yiu, C. K. Y., Arola, D. D., Gong, S. Q., El-Marakby, A., Carrilho, M. R. O., & Hamrick, M. W. (2012). Intrafibrillar silicification of collagen scaffolds for sustained release of stem cell homing chemokine in hard tissue regeneration. *FASEB J.* 26: 4517.

Osher, S., & Fedkiw, R. P. (2001). Level set methods: An overview and some recent results. *J. Comput. Phys.* 169: 463–502.

Ovsianikov, A., Deiwick, A., Van Vlierberghe, S., Dubruel, P., Möller, L., Dräger, G., & Chichkov, B. (2011). Laser fabrication of three-dimensional CAD scaffolds from photosensitive gelatin for applications in tissue engineering. *Biomacromolecules*. 12: 851–858.

Park, S., & Im, G. (2015). Stem cell responses to nanotopography. *J. Biomed. Mater. Res. A*. 103: 1238–1245.

Pei, X., Zhang, B., Fan, Y., Zhu, X., Sun, Y., Wang, Q., Zhang, X., & Zhou, C. (2017). Bionic mechanical design of titanium bone tissue implants and 3D printing manufacture. *Mater. Lett.* 208: 133–137.

Peppas, N. A., & Langer, R. (1994). New challenges in biomaterials. *Science*. 263: 1715–1720.

Polo-Corrales, L., Latorre-Esteves, M., & Ramirez-Vick, J. E. (2014). Scaffold design for bone regeneration. *J. Nanosci. Nanotechnol.* 14: 15–56.

Ratner, B. D., & Zhang, G. (2020). A history of biomaterials. In *Biomaterials Science*. W. R. Wagner, G. Zhang, S. E. S-Elbert, and M. J. Yaszemski, Eds. San Diego, CA: Elsevier, pp. 21–34.

Reinholz, G. G., Lu, L., Saris, D. B. F., Yaszemski, M. J., & O'driscoll, S. W. (2004). Animal models for cartilage reconstruction. *Biomaterials*. 25: 1511–1521.

Rhee, S. H., Lee, J. D., & Tanaka, J. (2000). Nucleation of hydroxyapatite crystal through chemical interaction with collagen. *J. Am. Ceram. Soc.* 83: 2890–2892.

Rhim, J., Mohanty, A. K., Singh, S. P., & Ng, P. K. W. (2006). Effect of the processing methods on the performance of polylactide films: Thermocompression versus solvent casting. *J. Appl. Pol. Sci.* 101: 3736–3742.

Rho, J. Y., Kuhn-Spearing, L., & Zioupos, P. (1998). Mechanical properties and the hierarchical structure of bone. *Med. Eng. Phys.* 20: 92–102.

Roach, P., Eglin, D., Rohde, K., & Perry, C. C. (2007). Modern biomaterials: A review—Bulk properties and implications of surface modifications. *J. Mater. Sci. Mater. Med.* 18: 1263–1277.

Saikia, K. C., Bhattacharya, T. D., Bhuyan, S. K., Talukdar, D. J., Saikia, S. P., & Jitesh, P. (2008). Calcium phosphate ceramics as bone graft substitutes in filling bone tumor defects. *Indian J. Orthop.* 42: 169–172.

Samandari, M., Alipanah, F., Majidzadeh-A, K., Alvarez, M. M., Trujillo-de Santiago, G., & Tamayol, A. (2021). Controlling cellular organization in bioprinting through designed 3D microcompartmentalization. *Appl. Phy. Rev.* 8: 21404.

Santoliquido, O., Colombo, P., & Ortona, A. (2019). Additive manufacturing of ceramic components by digital light processing: A comparison between the "bottom-up" and the "top-down" approaches. *J. Eur. Ceram. Soc.* 39: 2140–2148.

Sawkins, M. J., Mistry, P., Brown, B. N., Shakesheff, K. M., Bonassar, L. J., & Yang, J. (2015). Cell and protein compatible 3D bioprinting of mechanically strong constructs for bone repair. *Biofabrication*. 7: 35004.

Schemitsch, E. H. (2017). Size matters: Defining critical in bone defect size! *J. Orthop. Trauma*. 31: S20–S22.

Scott, M. A., Levi, B., Askarinam, A., Nguyen, A., Rackohn, T., Ting, K., Soo, C., & James, A. W. (2012). Brief review of models of ectopic bone formation. *Stem Cells Dev.* 21: 655–667.

Sears, N., Dhavalikar, P., Whitely, M., & Cosgriff-Hernandez, E. (2017). Fabrication of biomimetic bone grafts with multi-material 3D printing. *Biofabrication*. 9: 25020.

Sheehy, E. J., Kelly, D. J., & O'Brien, F. J. (2019). Biomaterial-based endochondral bone regeneration: A shift from traditional tissue engineering paradigms to developmentally inspired strategies. *Mater. Today Bio*. 3: 100009.

Sheikh, Z., Najeeb, S., Khurshid, Z., Verma, V., Rashid, H., & Glogauer, M. (2015). Biodegradable materials for bone repair and tissue engineering applications. *Materials*. 8: 5744–5794.

Shirinzadeh, B., Alici, G., Foong, C. W., & Cassidy, G. (2004). Fabrication process of open surfaces by robotic fibre placement. *Robot Comput. Integr. Manuf.* 20: 17–28.

Shoichet, M. S. (2010). Polymer scaffolds for biomaterials applications. *Macromolecules*. 43: 581–591.

Shuai, C., Guo, W., Gao, C., Yang, Y., Wu, P., & Feng, P. (2018). An nMgO containing scaffold: Antibacterial activity, degradation properties and cell responses. *Int. J. Bioprint*. 4: 120.

Song, W., Chen, L., Seta, J., Markel, D. C., Yu, X., & Ren, W. (2017). Corona discharge: A novel approach to fabricate three-dimensional electrospun nanofibers for bone tissue engineering. *ACS Biomater. Sci. Eng*. 3: 1146–1153.

Strano, G., Hao, L., Everson, R. M., & Evans, K. E. (2013). A new approach to the design and optimisation of support structures in additive manufacturing. *Int. J. Adv. Manuf. Technol*. 66: 1247–1254.

Tan, N., & van Arkel, R. J. (2021). Topology optimisation for compliant hip implant design and reduced strain shielding. *Materials*. 14: 7184.

Teo, W. E., & Ramakrishna, S. (2006). A review on electrospinning design and nanofibre assemblies. *Nanotechnology*. 17: R89–R106.

Tovar, N., Witek, L., Atria, P., Sobieraj, M., Bowers, M., Lopez, C. D., Cronstein, B. N., & Coelho, P. G. (2018). Form and functional repair of long bone using 3D-printed bioactive scaffolds. *J. Tissue Eng. Regener. Med*. 12: 1986–1999.

Trappmann, B., Gautrot, J. E., Connelly, J. T., Strange, D. G. T., Li, Y., Oyen, M. L., Cohen Stuart, M. A., Boehm, H., Li, B., & Vogel, V. (2012). Extracellular-matrix tethering regulates stem-cell fate. *Nat. Mater*. 11: 642–649.

Turnbull, G., Clarke, J., Picard, F., Riches, P., Jia, L., Han, F., Li, B., & Shu, W. (2018). 3D bioactive composite scaffolds for bone tissue engineering. *Bioact. Mater*. 3: 278–314.

Wang, G., Shen, L., Zhao, J., Liang, H., Xie, D., Tian, Z., & Wang, C. (2018). Design and compressive behavior of controllable irregular porous scaffolds: Based on voronoi-tessellation and for additive manufacturing. *ACS Biomater. Sci. Eng*. 4: 719–727.

Wang, X. J., Li, Y. C., Hodgson, P. D., & Wen, C. E. (2007). Nano-and macro-scale characterisation of the mechanical properties of bovine bone. *Mater. Forum*. 31: 156–159.

Xie, W., Wei, X., Kang, H., Jiang, H., Chu, Z., Lin, Y., Hou, Y., & Wei, Q. (2023). Static and dynamic: Evolving biomaterial mechanical properties to control cellular mechanotransduction. *Adv. Sci*. 10: 2204594.

Yang, Y., Wang, G., Liang, H., Gao, C., Peng, S., Shen, L., & Shuai, C. (2019). Additive manufacturing of bone scaffolds. *Int. J. Bioprint*. 5: 148.

Yeatts, A. B., Choquette, D. T., & Fisher, J. P. (2013). Bioreactors to influence stem cell fate: Augmentation of mesenchymal stem cell signaling pathways via dynamic culture systems. *Biochim. Biophys. Acta—Gen. Subj*. 1830: 2470–2480.

Yin, S., Zhang, W., Zhang, Z., & Jiang, X. (2019). Recent advances in scaffold design and material for vascularized tissue-engineered bone regeneration. *Adv. Healthc. Mater*. 8: 1801433.

Yu, G. Z., Chou, D. T., Hong, D., Roy, A., & Kumta, P. N. (2017). Biomimetic rotated lamellar plywood motifs by additive manufacturing of metal alloy scaffolds for bone tissue engineering. *ACS Biomater. Sci. Eng*. 3: 648–657.

Zhang, J., Zhang, X., Chen, Y., Feng, W., & Chen, X. (2021). Novel design and finite element analysis of diamond-like porous implants with low stiffness. *Materials*. 14: 6918.

Zhang, Q., Zhou, J., Zhi, P., Liu, L., Liu, C., Fang, A., & Zhang, Q. (2023). 3D printing method for bone tissue engineering scaffold. *Med. Nov. Technol. Devices*. 17: 100205.

Zhang, Y., Xia, L., Zhai, D., Shi, M., Luo, Y., Feng, C., Fang, B., Yin, J., Chang, J., & Wu, C. (2015). Mesoporous bioactive glass nanolayer-functionalized 3D-printed scaffolds for accelerating osteogenesis and angiogenesis. *Nanoscale*. 7: 19207–19221.

4 Integrating 3D Printing and Electrospinning to Fabricate Scaffolds for Bone Regeneration

Didem Demir, Ashok Vaseashta, and Nimet Bölgen

4.1 INTRODUCTION

One of the most important challenges of modern medicine is tissue/organ failure or loss. In clinical practice, the gold standard for regeneration is still organ/tissue transplantation, and issues such as shortage of donors, donor-site morbidity, ethical issues in organ and tissue transplantation, the risk of infections, disease transmission, and transplant rejections have inspired the launch of a new interdisciplinary field called tissue engineering—a combination of engineering science, medicine, and biology. In this approach, medical doctors and scientists work together to repair or replace damaged or unhealthy tissue and improve the growth and function of new healthy tissue.

Bone, unlike most other tissues, has the ability to heal itself. As a living tissue that is constantly renewing itself, it can remodel. However, in cases where the tissue's self-renewal capacity is not sufficient, in the absence of common joints or in the presence of defects of critical dimensions, various tissue engineering approaches can increase and support bone healing and bone formation. Today, bone tissue engineering is the most commonly used approach. By using certain biomaterials in combination with bioactive molecules, it is possible to stimulate and improve the body's regenerative pathways, similar to natural bone formation and remodeling. In this approach, new tissue formation can be accomplished by expanding the cells collected from patients themselves in a bioreactor in vitro and seeding them in three-dimensional (3D) cell carriers, so-called scaffolds.

Alternatively, the body can be used as a bioreactor when the scaffold is implanted at the defect site and after a certain period of time surrounding cells infiltrate the scaffold. The three essential factors for successful bone regeneration are cells (osteogenic), a scaffold (osteoconductive), and growth factors (osteoinductive). Cells produce new tissue on a scaffold that provides the necessary framework, while growth factors enhance tissue regeneration and provide appropriate guidance to the desired differentiation. The cell and growth factors required for bone regeneration are the most important factor in developing new materials and production methods and scaffold manufacturing processes.

It is very important to choose a suitable material for producing bone scaffolds that provide the appropriate environment for cell growth and bone regeneration. Scaffolds made from polymer-based materials can be fabricated using traditional methods such as electrospinning, freeze drying, 3D printing or additive manufacturing, phase separation, gas foaming, and particulate leaching. Scaffolds can be designed into a wide range of structures with acceptable mechanical stability, topography, geometry, and architecture required for different applications in the field of bone tissue engineering (Figure 4.1). New technologies are presenting new pathways for producing new kinds of scaffolds that are very similar to natural bone structures. For this reason, it is very important to know the existing production methods and to combine them with new technologies to obtain biomimetic scaffolds that better simulate the native tissue structure.

DOI: 10.1201/9781003307310-5

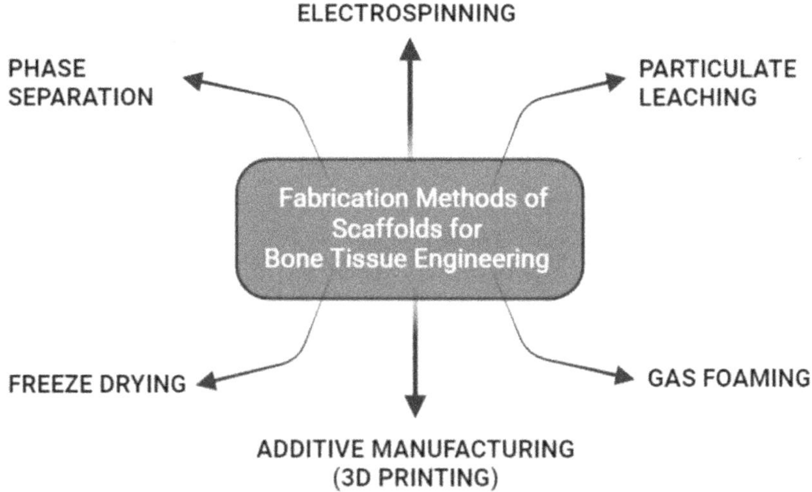

FIGURE 4.1 Conventional methods for producing bone tissue scaffolds.

One possible combination is integrating electrospinning and additive manufacturing, which allows for mimicking the complex and gradual structure of bone by designing and fabricating scaffolds with multilayer structures. Additive manufacturing and nanotechnology are two advancing frontiers of science and technology that have recently been moving toward integration to leverage their individual advantages and achieve new favorable material characteristics and applications that will help us create highly functional materials and devices.

Furthermore, additive manufacturing allows for producing scaffolds with precisely defined engineered designs that can combine multiple material structures. In addition, conventional manufacturing methods pose difficulties, especially in the manufacture of materials with heterogeneous structures, where the entire structure must be separated into its components and processed individually. Many of the limitations of additive processing are in determining how best to position the print to be designed to reduce support dependency and the possibility of misprints. This allows for design freedom on a large scale and the designing of multiple geometries with relative ease. Electrospinning is a reproducible processing technique with a simple installation that can produce fibers in one-dimensional structures in a wide range of diameters between mm and nm. While 3D printing allows the general structure of the bone extracellular matrix (ECM) to be formed at the micro scale, combining it with electrospinning imitates the nanoscale fibers of the bone matrix (Vaseashta et al., 2022).

To understand the necessity of the combination approach here, it is first essential to understand the composition of the bone. Therefore, in the first section, we give information about the general definition of bone including its chemical, morphological, and cellular compositions, followed by bone tissue engineering and its expectations, current methods and any revision to already developed methods. We specify the materials and design of architecture for bone regeneration.

We also discuss the basic working principles of both methods, which are the main subject of the chapter, and examine new scaffolds produced by combining these two methods or materials that were separately manufactured with these methods. Finally, we compile and summarize studies about using both technologies to produce hybrid scaffolds for different bone defects.

4.2 BONE

Bone is a vital, dynamic, and complex organ that continues to regenerate throughout life with a self-growing, transforming, and repairing structure. As the basic unit of the skeletal system, it is a richly vascularized connective tissue and nerve-equipped organ that comprises bone tissue, bone marrow, and periosteum (Filipowska et al., 2017). Moreover, it also has an important place in the control of the body's ion balance. To keep the concentrations of calcium, phosphate, and other ions in body fluids at a constant level, bone also provides controlled release or storage of these important ions (Florencio-Silva et al., 2015).

4.2.1 Chemical Composition

Knowing the structure of bone is very important for understanding the diseases and treatments related to it. Like other connective tissues, bone tissue contains an abundant ECM. Table 4.1 lists the chemical composition of the bone matrix. As shown, the ECM comprises organic and inorganic matter consisting of an average of 20–40% organic phase and 60–70% inorganic phase.

The organic component of bone contains more than 30 proteins, with the highest amount of type I collagen (>90% of the organic matrix) (Feng, 2009). The collagen forms triple helices of polypeptides that make up collagen fibrils, which deal with collagenous and noncollagenous proteins to form higher-order fibril bundles and fibers. Its main function is to provide mechanical support by providing flexibility and resistance and to behave like a scaffold for bone cells (Lin et al., 2020).

In contrast, the noncollagenous proteins (10% of the organic matrix) in bone consist of four main types: glycoproteins (alkaline phosphatase, ALP; osteonectin, ON; arginine–glycine–aspartic acid, RGD; etc.), proteoglycans (biglycan, decorin, keratocan, and asporin), proteins containing gamma-carboxyglutamic acid (osteocalcin-OC, periostin), and small integrin-binding ligands N-linked glycoproteins-SIBLINs (BSP, OPN) (Carvalho et al., 2021; Lin et al., 2020; Paiva & Granjeiro, 2017). The inorganic components of bone mainly comprise calcium (Ca) and phosphorus (P) in the form of spherical hydroxyapatite crystals (hAp, $Ca_{10}(PO_4)_6(OH)_2$) and create the major characteristic function by giving the matrix compression strength and bone regeneration (Jeong et al., 2019).

4.2.2 Cellular Composition

Bone consists of four basic cells that constantly interact with the matrix (Figure 4.1). The first of these are osteoprogenitor cells (mesenchymal stem cells, MSCs), which can be divided and differentiated into osteoblasts, cells that synthesize and secrete collagen under osteogenic conditions for bone formation. Moreover, they carry out the mineralization of the bone matrix; when the matrix surrounding osteoblasts calcifies, these cells become trapped within it, their morphology changes, and they become osteocytes, the primary cell of mature bone that protects bone tissue. The fourth

TABLE 4.1
The Chemical Composition of Bone Matrix and Constituents' Roles in Bone Formation

Inorganic	wt%	Function	Organic	wt%	Function
hAp	≈ 60	structural strength and bone regeneration	Collagenous protein *Type I, type III, and type V collagen*	≈ 90	mechanical support and scaffold for bone cells
Water	≈ 9	integration between hydroxyapatite and collagen			
Carbonate	≈ 4	contributes to the strength and flexibility of the skeleton	Noncollagenous protein Glycoproteins *Proteoglycans* *γ-carboxyglutamic acid containing proteins* *small integrin-binding ligands N-linked glycoproteins*	≈ 10	regulating bone matrix and mineralization osteoblast/ osteoclast activities
Sodium	≈ 0.7				
Magnesium	≈ 0.5				
Chloride	≈ 0.13				
Others *K^+, F^-, Zn^{2+}, Fe^{2+}, Cu^{2+}, Sr^{2+}, Pb^{2+}*					

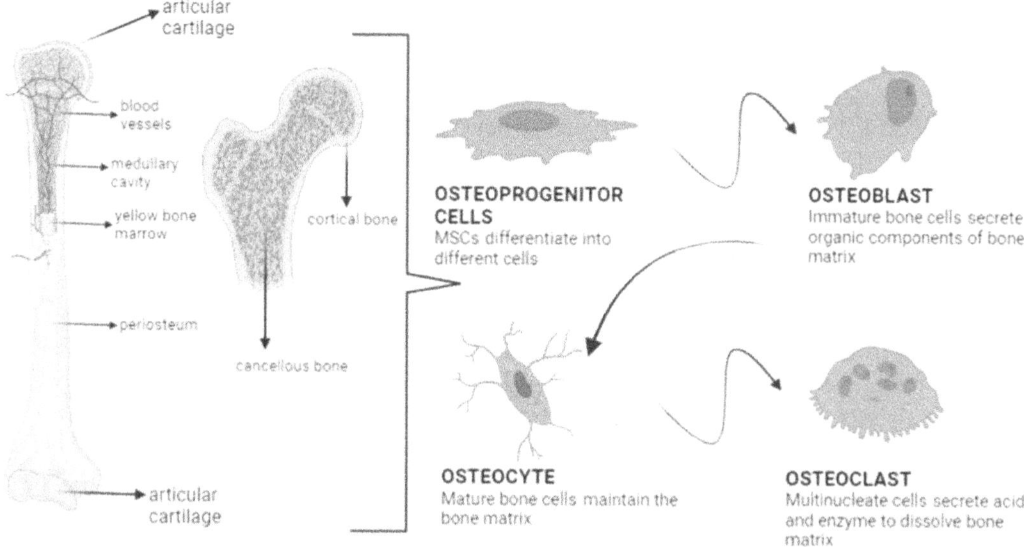

FIGURE 4.2 Anatomical division of bone including the four different cell types that interact with the bone matrix.

cell type is osteoclasts, which are responsible for tissue deterioration. Bone remodeling is tightly managed by both osteoblasts and osteoclasts: Osteoblasts are involved in the formation of new bone, while osteoclasts, as large and multinucleated cells, are responsible for the dissolution and resorption of bone (Alcorta-Sevillano et al., 2020; Florencio-Silva et al., 2015).

4.2.3 Bone Architecture

An adult human body contains a total of 213 bones divided into two different architectural types, cortical and cancellous, as well as four groups: short, long, irregular, and flat. Figure 4.2 displays the two types of bone as layers and shows their cellular makeup. The external layer consists of cortical bone, which corresponds to 80% of the total adult bone mass, while the inner layer consists of cancellous bone, which corresponds to 20% of the skeletal mass. There are also the Haversian canals along the cortical bone that are rich in blood vessels and nerves and the Volkmann tube, in which the vessels in the canals are transversely interconnected (Ng et al., 2017).

The cortical bone, also called compact bone, is a relatively dense tissue that has a porosity of 3–5% and supports most of the mechanical function. It is found predominantly in the appendicular skeleton, particularly in the diaphysis of long bones, and it is essential for physical support, structural integrity, and weight bearing. The cancellous (trabecular/spongy) bone has a light and highly porous structure with a porosity of about 80–90% surrounding numerous large cavities, giving it a honeycomb-like appearance (Xue et al., 2022). It is a reticular structure consisting of a plate or rod structure about 200 microns thick, located mainly in the axial skeleton, between the cortices of smaller flat and short bones such as the scapula, vertebrae, and pelvis (Monier-Faugere et al., 1998). Metabolic activity such as bone cell production and mineral exchange is higher in trabecular bone than in cortical bone (Bilgiç et al., 2020).

4.3 BONE TISSUE ENGINEERING

To design functional and effective techniques for bone regeneration, we need to learn more about the existing bone defects, the regeneration process, and the bone tissue engineering approach—that is, the treatment method—after acquiring basic information about the general structure of the bone. Therefore, in this section, these topics will be discussed in sequence.

4.3.1 Bone Defects

A bone defect can be defined as a lack of bone tissue where it should normally be. These defects caused by diseases, old age, infections, accidents, trauma, musculoskeletal tumor, functional atrophy, or congenital causes are one of the main problems of today's medical world. Moreover, the repair of bone defects is one of the most widely applied regenerative procedures, with more than two million bone grafts performed every year worldwide (Kiernan et al., 2018; Zhao et al., 2021b).

Although bone is a living organ with self-renewal capacity, nonunion results in poor union or pathological fracture when the bone defect exceeds the critical size threshold or when there is more than 50% loss of bone circumference (Xue et al., 2022). This size is generally expressed as 2 cm or above, and bone defects greater than this size cannot heal spontaneously, necessitating reconstruction surgery (Annamalai et al., 2019; Lu et al., 2021). Treatment modalities include allograft or autograft bones used to replace the defect and restore its function; the Masquelet technique, which uses the body's foreign body response to create a membrane of fibrous tissue around the defect site; and distraction osteogenesis, which uses the natural healing properties of bone to fill the defect (Alonzo et al., 2021; Smrke et al., 2013). With the recent advances in materials science and technologies, bone tissue engineering, which provides bone repair or new bone formation, is a significant improvement over the existing options. In recent years, cell and gene-activating materials, also known as scaffolds, have been developed as third-generation bone repair materials.

4.3.2 Scaffolds to Repair Bone Defects

The living body exhibits a 3D structure with all its tissues and organs. To repair/regenerate the lost/damaged tissues or organs, 3D scaffolds are designed and fabricated to regenerate tissues that are both anatomically and functionally similar to the native tissue or organ to be replaced/repaired. The basic approach applied here is tissue engineering, which aims to assemble functional structures that maintain, restore, and regenerate damaged tissues or organs.

Bone tissue engineering aims to regenerate new functional bone through the synergistic combination of scaffolds, cells, and growth factors/drugs/bioactive agents (Alonzo et al., 2021). Scaffolds are a critical substrate that can mimic the native bone ECM. The properties of scaffolds have been shown to affect cell behavior such as cell attachment, proliferation, and differentiation. For this reason, the design, fabrication, and characterization of scaffolds for bone regeneration is considered to be one of the fundamental steps.

As all other biomaterials will be in contact with the living body, scaffolds must first be prepared from biocompatible materials (O'Brien, 2011). To achieve this, natural (chitin, chitosan, gelatin, collagen, starch, silk, cellulose, pectin, gums, etc.) and synthetic polyethylene glycol (PEG), polyvinyl alcohol, polyglycolic acid, poly(lactic-co-glycolic) acid (PLGA), and poly[2-(dimethylamino) ethyl methacrylate] polymers considered safe by the US Food and Drug Administration can be used easily. In addition to biocompatibility, biodegradability is the second desired feature. The scaffolds must be biodegradable in parallel with the cells producing their extracellular matrices. Degradation products should be able to be removed by metabolic pathways without the need for a second surgical operation. At the same time, the by-products of this degradation should not be toxic (Bitar & Zakhem, 2014; O'Brien, 2011). Mechanical stability, easy processability, low cost, and functionality are the other features that a scaffold must have (Suamte et al., 2023; Thavornyutikarn et al., 2014).

Bone tissue engineering requires some additional properties from scaffolds to enhance the osteoconductivity, osteoinductivity, and osseointegration for bone regeneration (He et al., 2013; Qu et al., 2019). Figure 4.3 provides an overview of the other specific properties that an ideal scaffold for bone tissue engineering should have. These properties include stiffness within the scope of mechanical properties, porosity, pore size, surface topography within the scope of morphological properties, and load-bearing capacity (Lee et al., 2022). It should be noted that the natural bone has a complex hierarchical structure based on the length and width, and scaffolds should imitate that native structure.

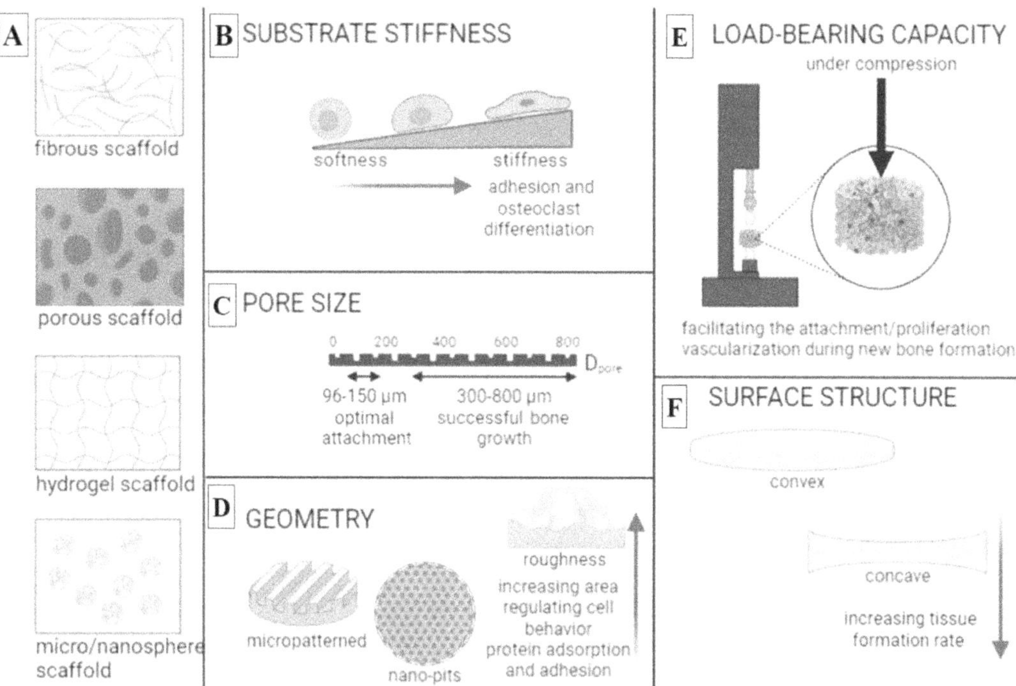

FIGURE 4.3 An overview of the mechanical and structural properties that an ideal scaffold for bone tissue engineering must possess for accelerated bone regeneration, showing the scaffolds fabricated in different structures and some of the requirements.

Studies to date have shown that the geometry and topography of the scaffolds have a profound effect on the cellular response and the rate of bone tissue regeneration. Zhao et al. (2015) investigated osteogenic differentiation on scaffolds with a micropattern structure produced using PLGA and integrating hAp ceramics. The authors observed that the micropatterning possessed better wettability and higher surface energy, which significantly enhanced the adhesion, proliferation, and osteogenic differentiation of rat bone marrow stromal cells (Zhao et al., 2015).

In another study, the influence of different-patterned piezoelectric poly(vinylidene fluoride-co-trifluoroethylene) scaffolds in the proliferation and differentiation of the preosteoblasts were investigated. It was reported that isotropic hexagonal surface topography induced the MC3T3-E1 cell differentiation and bone cell differentiation positively affected by this kind of geometry-oriented secretion of the ECM without the need of using a chemical inducer (Marques-Almeida et al., 2020). Based on the surface properties, the tissue formation rate increases with curvature and is much higher on concave surfaces than on convex and planar surfaces (Zadpoor, 2015).

In terms of mechanical properties, the scaffold stiffness plays a significant regulatory role in stem cell differentiation and cell migration, which is important for the infiltration of host tissue cells. Studies have shown that appropriate matrix stiffness can effectively induce osteogenic differentiation of MSCs and promote bone regeneration (Li et al., 2022). Furthermore, scaffolds are designed to match the mechanical properties of cancellous bone, which has a compressive strength between 2 and 12 mPa and an elastic modulus between 0.1 and 5 gPa (Wu et al., 2014).

The maintenance of cellular activity and transformation of cartilage and bone cells is highly dependent on the internal morphology and surface properties of scaffolds, including pore shape, pore size, and porosity (Zhao et al., 2021a). Adequate porosity, appropriate pore size, and interconnection of pores provide a suitable environment to support cell infiltration, nutrient and oxygen flow, waste material removal, migration, and vascularization (Abbasi et al., 2020). Osteoblasts range in size from

10 to 50 μm, but they require larger pores to regenerate mineralized bone after implantation (Abbasi et al., 2020). The maximum pore size for cell attachment is 300 μm (the optimum range is around 96–150 μm) (Murphy & O'Brien, 2010); pores larger than ~300 μm are necessary for vascularization and bone growth, thereby improving bone regeneration, and pores smaller than ~300 μm promote osteochondral ossification (Mantila Roosa et al., 2010). It has also been noted that smaller pores are suitable for controlling cell aggregation/proliferation (Chen et al., 2018) and are associated with the formation of nonmineralized osteoid or fibrous tissue (Mantila Roosa et al., 2010).

4.3.3 Scaffold Fabrication Methods for Bone Tissue Engineering

Scaffolds for bone tissue engineering can be categorized into fibrous, porous, hydrogel, or micro/nanosphere. Several processing techniques allow for fabricating scaffolds in these morphologies for bone regeneration, among which commonly used methods are solvent casting and salt particulate leaching (Thadavirul et al., 2014), gas foaming (Kim et al., 2012), emulsification (Paljevac et al., 2018), freeze-drying (Kumar et al., 2020), cryotropic gelation (Kemençe & Bölgen, 2017), electrospinning (Miszuk et al., 2021), and 3D printing (Iglesias-Mejuto & García-González, 2021). However, due to the complex and hierarchical architecture of bone consisting of spongy (cancellous bone) and hard (compact bone) tissues, it is known that a scaffold architecture to be produced in a single morphology using only one method does not provide successful bone regeneration. Therefore, the design of multiphase biomaterial structures capable of mimicking tissues in such complex construction is required. A scaffold architecture consisting of a dense layer to mimic the compact structure of bone and a porous structure to mimic its spongy part can be promising for bone regeneration.

In this context, an important scaffold design technique is manipulating micro/nanopatterning to provide contact guidance. Among the many approaches to trigger contact guidance, electrospinning shows promising potential for aligning micro/nanofibers due to its simple and versatile fabrication structure. In the electrospinning process, nanofibers are formed by forming and elongating a polymer jet under a high electrical field (Reneker & Yarin, 2008; Bölgen et al., 2022; Vaseashta, 2007).

The setup generally consists of a nozzle the polymer solution emerges from, a high-voltage power source that generates an electric field, and a collector plate that collects the fibers formed (Figure 4.4). Electrospun fibers have gained considerable attention as scaffolds for bone tissue engineering applications since these materials exhibit advantageous features including mechanical flexibility, high surface area relative to total volume ratio, and the ability to architecturally mimic the native ECM (Chen et al., 2020).

In addition, electrospinning scaffolds with different morphologies can be successfully prepared as controlled drug delivery systems by controlling the material composition by manipulating the electrospinning set-up and changing the operating parameters. Such combinations are very useful in applying bioactive molecules directly to the bone defect area, which aims to stimulate tissue regeneration while preventing infections. As an example, Zhang et al. (2022) developed nanofiber membranes in a core-sheath structure loading with nanoparticles and bioactive agents for bone tissue repair. Rezk et al. (2018) fabricated a trilayered fibrous scaffold with layers to provide mechanical stability, osteogenic drug delivery for osteoblast adhesion and proliferation, and stimulating the biomineralization process. In a separate study, Xie et al. (2021) fabricated aligned and random poly (L-lactic acid) electrospun fiber membranes in nano- and micro-scale sizes to determine the cellular responses of bone marrow MSCs. More studies are summarized in Table 4.2.

Despite the advantages we have discussed, there are difficulties in using scaffolds produced by electrospinning for regenerative medicine. Conventional two-dimensional electrospun membranes composed of densely packed fibers inhibit both cell infiltration and growth along the scaffolds. Specifically for bone tissue engineering, the small pore size of electrospun structures can restrict bone cell infiltration, limit tissue ingrowth, and partially mimic the ECM on a planar rather than 3D structure. (Belgheisi et al., 2022). Especially for load-bearing applications, the electrospun structures possess insufficient mechanical strength (Khorshidi et al., 2016). In addition, this homogeneous structure, which consists of fibers stacked on top of each other and exhibits a single morphology, is not suitable on its own to mimic the heterogeneous structure of bone. For these reasons,

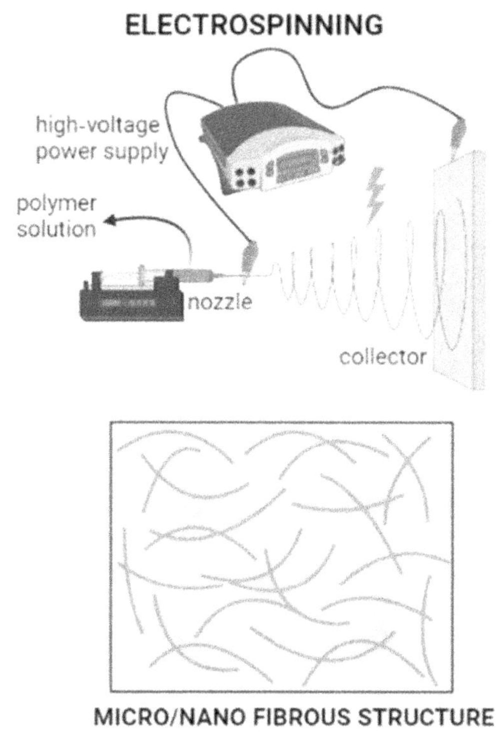

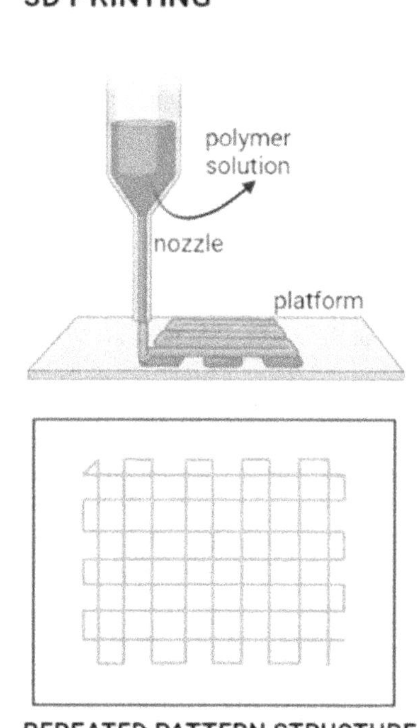

FIGURE 4.4 The basic setup of conventional electrospinning including power supply, syringe pump for the feeding polymer solution, and the collector plate and a basic 3D printer including the nozzle and platform.

TABLE 4.2
Recent Studies on Electropsun Scaffolds Produced for Bone Tissue Engineering

Polymer	Additive	Method	Advantages of Polymer	Advantages for BTE	Ref.
PHB	Keratin AL_2O3 nanowire	Conventional Electrospinning	Biodegradability with high mechanical properties	Alkaline phosphatase synthesis, increased calcium accumulation, cell growth, cell proliferation	Ghafari et al. (2023)
PCL	Lignin nanoparticle	Conventional electrospinning	Biocompatible polymer	A favorable physical and biological environment for the support and induction of preosteoblastic cell functions	Haider et al. (2023)
Silk fibroin-PCL	Ginsenosid	Co-electrospinning	Biodegradable, mechanical properties, biocompatible, and minimal inflammatory reaction	Upregulated ALP activity and osteogenic differentiation	Luo et al. (2021)
Gelatin Nylon 6 PU	-	Electrospinning with dual syringe pump setup	Cellular metabolism, morphogenesis during tissue regeneration, substantial mechanical stability and excellent spinnability	A wettable surface, promoted osteoblast cell attachment, migration, and proliferation throughout the scaffold porous structure	Ali et al. (2020)

*PHB: Polyhydroxybutyrate, PCL: polycaprolactone, PLGA: poly(lactic-*co*-glycolide), PU: polyurethane by combining the fibrous structure produced by electrospinning with other scaffold production techniques, researchers have aimed to improve the mechanical strength and form larger pore structures that can offer adequate sites for cell adhesion and better imitate the compact structure of the bone.

Additive manufacturing, also called 3D printing or rapid prototyping, can overcome many of the limitations of electrospinning and allows for fabricating scaffolds with precisely engineered morphologies that can assemble multimaterial structures (Huang et al., 2020). In general, we can define 3D printing as the process of creating 3D objects in a layer-by-layer structure using digital data (Tappa & Jammalamadaka, 2018). With this method, which has a feeder, extruder nozzle, and platform in its basic setup, the 2D-structured layer is printed on a rendering platform in the XY plane, then 3D objects formed from the repeated pattern structure combined by printing the subsequent layers in the z-axis (Shaik et al., 2021; Siripongpreda et al., 2023).

Various types of materials can be fabricated by 3D printing, including natural and synthetic polymers, metals, ceramics, and their composites, with customized shapes or macro/microporous architecture (Belgheisi et al., 2022). In tissue engineering, 3D printing has been presented as an effective method with many advantages, as the scaffolds produced in 3D-printed macro- and microstructures could morphologically simulate the heterogeneous structure of tissues and create patient-specific structures for irregular and nonuniform defects. The objects to be printed are organs and tissues, which already physically exist in the body, so developing tissue substitutes involves a reverse engineering approach that starts with collecting anatomical data.

Customized scaffold geometry is provided using computer-aided design (CAD) software and the specific parameters for the individual defect site. Before 3D printing a bone scaffold, computer modeling consists of essential data collection, image processing, and model creation. Significant differences in bone anatomy, types, and sizes of defects among patients make these steps important (Bahraminasab, 2020). To date, polymers with different features have been used as bioink to prepare 3D-printed scaffolds for bone tissue engineering. In Table 4.3, we have tabulated recent studies on applications related with 3D-printed tissues for bone regeneration.

TABLE 4.3
Recent Studies on 3D-Printed Scaffolds Produced for Bone Tissue Engineering

Polymer	Additive	Method	Advantages of Polymer	Advantages for BTE	Ref.
Polylactic acid	Lanthanum-doped octacalcium phosphate	Inkjet bioprinting	High mechanical properties	Promotes osteogenic differentiation and enhances bone defect regeneration	Xu et al. (2022)
Glycol chitosan	-	Visible light 3D printing	Suitable water solubility for printing	Cell proliferation and visible bone differentiation	Chang et al. (2022)
Silk fibroin	Bioactive glass	Extrusion bioprinting	Excellent biological compatibility	Superior compressive strength, biocompatibility, and stimulated bone formation ability	Du et al. (2019)
PCL	Nano hAp	Extrusion bioprinting	Easy to print due to its low melting temperature	Improved mechanical properties and enhanced bioactivity	Cestari et al. (2021)
Gelatin methacrylamide	hAp	Digital light processing	Similarity with tissue and cell environment	Significantly promotes the adhesion and proliferation of osteoblasts	Song et al. (2022)

Polymer	Additive	Method	Advantages of Polymer	Advantages for BTE	Ref.
Chitosan Alginate	hAp	Extrusion bioprinting	Osteoblast differentiation and mineralization	Biocompatible and did not have toxicity toward MSCs	Yousefiasl et al. (2023)
PP	Palm oil fuel ash	Fused deposition modeling	Easy workability	Bone repair potential	Darsani et al. (2021)
Alginatedialdehyde-gelatin	Silica-calcium nanoparticle	Pneumatic extrusion-based 3D printing	Abundant, inexpensive scaffold-forming features	Osteogenic drug release system, load-bearing capability, and provokes the activity of osteoblast cells	Monavari et al. (2021)

*BTE: bone tissue engineering, PCL: polycaprolactone, PP: polypropylene

Just like with electrospinning, scaffolds produced by 3D printing alone are not successful in imitating the complex structure of native bone. The main disadvantage encountered with 3D-printed scaffolds is that they can be reduced to only micrometer sizes. Reducing the pore size of the object printed in 3D printers is possible by changing three factors: pore design, scanning speed, and polymer injection temperature. However, commercial 3D printers have a resolution of around 250 μm, so it is difficult to have scaffolds with pores of less than 250 μm (Tylek et al., 2020). This feature produces very large pores and smooth strips in the micrometer range, but these structures cannot mimic the natural matrix and do not offer sufficient areas for cell adhesion. Therefore, such structures need nano-sized patterns (Belgheisi et al., 2022). To overcome these limitations, integrating electrospinning and additive manufacturing techniques has come to the fore for designing scaffolds combined by micro-sized filaments and nano-sized fibers.

4.4 INTEGRATING ELECTROSPINNING AND 3D PRINTING IN DESIGNING BONE TISSUE ENGINEERING SCAFFOLDS

In recent years, combining electrospinning and additive manufacturing to produce bone tissue engineering scaffolds has attracted considerable attention. The main purpose of this combination is to produce a single material with two different morphologies (nano and micro patterns) and to design the produced material according to the desired bone anatomy or defect morphology and size. Researchers combine the materials produced by these two methods in one of two combinations (Vaseashta et al., 2022).

In the first of these, the nanofibers are deposited directly on the 3D-printed patterns by electrospinning, either by electrospinning the coating for the outer surface of the final product or electrospinning coatings for each interlayer after each layer. The other approach is to homogeneously disperse premanufactured electrospun fibers in a polymer solution/melt and then scrape the fiber–polymer combination with 3D printing. Figure 4.5 summarizes how to integrate electrospinning and 3D printing. In addition, studies on the production of hybrid scaffolds for bone tissue engineering using these two methods together are presented in Table 4.4. Details of these combinations and case studies are explained in the following sections.

4.4.1 Surface Functionalization of 3D-Printed Scaffolds by Electrospinning

The most common approach to designing these hybrid scaffolds is to functionalize the outer surface of 3D-printed scaffolds using electrospun nanofibers. Here, fibrils produced by electrospinning

TABLE 4.4
Studies on Scaffolds Produced for Bone Tissue Engineering Using Both Electrospinning and Additive Manufacturing

Electrospun Polymer	3D-Printed Polymer	Integration Method	Advantages for BTE	Ref.
PCL Gelatin	PCL	Infusing dispersed nanofibers into the meshes of the PCL scaffold	Good mechanical stress, better for cell migration and proliferation than the 3D printing scaffold	Yu et al. (2016)
Gelatin–forsterite	PLA	Direct electrospinning on the top of the 3D-printed scaffold	An increase in elastic modulus, significant formation of bone-like apatite	Naghieh et al. (2017)
PCL Gelatin	PLA	3D printing of grids onto the electrospun mats	Increased mechanical strength while maintaining the ECM-like architecture	Pensa et al. (2019)
PCL	PCL PEGDA	3D printing on electrospun mats	Capable of simulating complex, functionally graded characteristics of the bone–ligament interface for tissue engineering scaffolds	Elghazali et al. (2019)
PCL PLGA, Gelatin, Collagen Bioactive glass	PCL	Melt electrowriting of PCL including short nanofibers	Improved cell adhesion and proliferation for rBMSCs and MC3T3-E1 cells	Elghazali et al. (2019)
PCL	PCL	Electrospinning on 3D-PCL	Faster degradation and high cell proliferation due to its porosity and composition	Rosales-Ibáñez et al. (2022)
Amoxicillin loaded PLGA	PLA	Wrapping nanofibers in 3D-printed cuboid frames	Capable of sustained release and of mimicking the morphology of the natural ECM of bone tissue	Chou et al. (2022)
PCL	PCL	Alignment of electrospun nanofiber using rotational electrospinning after printing two initial layers	Aligned double-scale anisotropic scaffolds that support cell attachment and proliferation, promote cell anisotropy, and an organized cytoskeleton with high expressions of osteogenic markers	Huang et al. (2020)
mPEG PCL mPEG-hAp	PCL PEG	Hybrid platform with thermal extrusion 3D printer and electrospinning	Suitable to support the adhesion and growth of MC3T3-E1 osteoblastic cells	Dong et al. (2019)
PLLA	PCL	Layer-by-layer deposition of fibers on the 3D-printed scaffold	Manipulates the osteoimmune environment to benefit bone regeneration with osteogenic differentiation, angiogenesis, and accelerated bone formation in vivo	Liu et al. (2021)
Gelatin	PLLA	Direct electrospinning on the surface of the 3D printed scaffold	Helps to entrap cells after cell seeding to distribute them well into the 3D-printed scaffold and suitable for nasal cartilage and subchondral bone reconstruction	Rajzer et al. (2018)

*PEGDA: polyethyleneglycol diacrylate, PLGA: poly(lactic-co-glycolic acid), PEG: polyethyleneglycol, PLLA: poly l-lactic acid

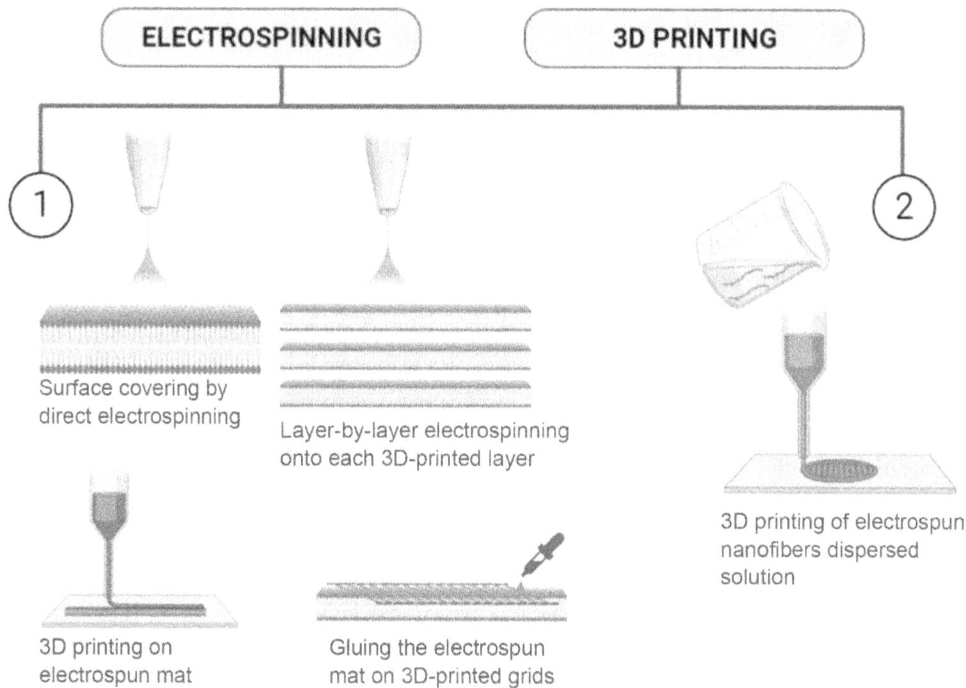

FIGURE 4.5 Classification of 3D-printed layer and electrospun nanofiber integration methods for bone tissue engineering: 1) electrospinning the surfaces of scaffolds and 2) developing bioinks reinforced with short electrospun fibers for use in 3D printing.

are utilized to imitate the structure of the natural bone matrix, while the additive manufacturing produces scaffolds with high precision, high resolution and repeatability through a layer-by-layer production. As an example, in a recent study, electrospinning and 3D printing techniques were integrated to formation of scaffolds having multiple gradual structures for bone tissue engineering.

Romero-Araya et al. (2021) selected PLA, which is easy to process, inexpensive, and has good mechanical properties, as a template polymer for both electrospun fibers and 3D-printed parts. To produce composite scaffolds, they placed rectangular-cut 3D-printed scaffolds on the collector in the electrospinning mechanism and collected the nanofibers on the 3D-printed layers. By repeating this process, they created a sandwich-like structure by combining PLA-based fibers as the middle layer with two layers of 3D-printed scaffolding. They observed that the 3D structure blended with the fibers exhibited a lower storage modulus than that of the bare 3D-printed parts, resulting in a softer composite. At the same time, the scaffold showed high cell viability as a result of good adherence and cells growing on both surfaces (Romero-Araya et al., 2021).

While nanofibers produced with electrospinning are coated on 3D-printed parts, there is another approach in which 3D-printed layers are created on fibrous mats. Wang et al. (2021) produced PCL/gelatin scaffolds hierarchically by melt electrospinning writing (MEW) and solution electrospinning for bone reconstruction applications. MEW is one of the emerging 3D printing techniques to fabricate 3D scaffolds with highly ordered microfibers.

After electrospinning, a conductive glass made by stacking alternating random nanofibers was placed on an XY moving platform coupled to a negative high voltage for MEW to obtain PCL grids on fibrous mats. For the scaffolds, the 3D-printed layer and electrospun nanofiber layer were stacked five times (Figure 4.6(A)), and the authors observed that the cells were able to penetrate through the spaces between nanofibers and evenly disperse throughout the multilayer composite scaffold after seven days of culture. Compared with conventional MEW scaffolds, composite scaffolds not only exhibited good mechanical properties and cell orientation effect but also appropriately mimicked the 3D ECM microenvironment (Wang et al., 2021).

Vyas and coworkers (2020) developed a double-scale scaffold by combining micro-sized 3D-printed fibers directly with electrospun nanofibers. A screw-assisted extrusion 3D printer and electrospinning system as shown in Figure 4.6(B) were employed to create PCL dual-scale scaffolds. The 3D-printed structures as scaffolds were created for bone tissue engineering applications with a pore size and fiber diameter (300 μm) suitable for achieving optimal cell proliferation, tissue growth, and progression of vascularization in vivo. Increased cell proliferation was observed on the double-scale scaffolds and the presence of aligned cells with a longitudinal morphology on the meshes in the pores of the printed microfibers (Vyas et al., 2020).

Another process is fabricating hybrid scaffolds by attaching electrospun nanofibers to the surface of 3D-printed layers. Belgheisi et al. (2022) studied this hybrid scaffold for bone tissue engineering applications by gluing electrospun nanofibers to 3D-printed grids. PCL, a biocompatible and

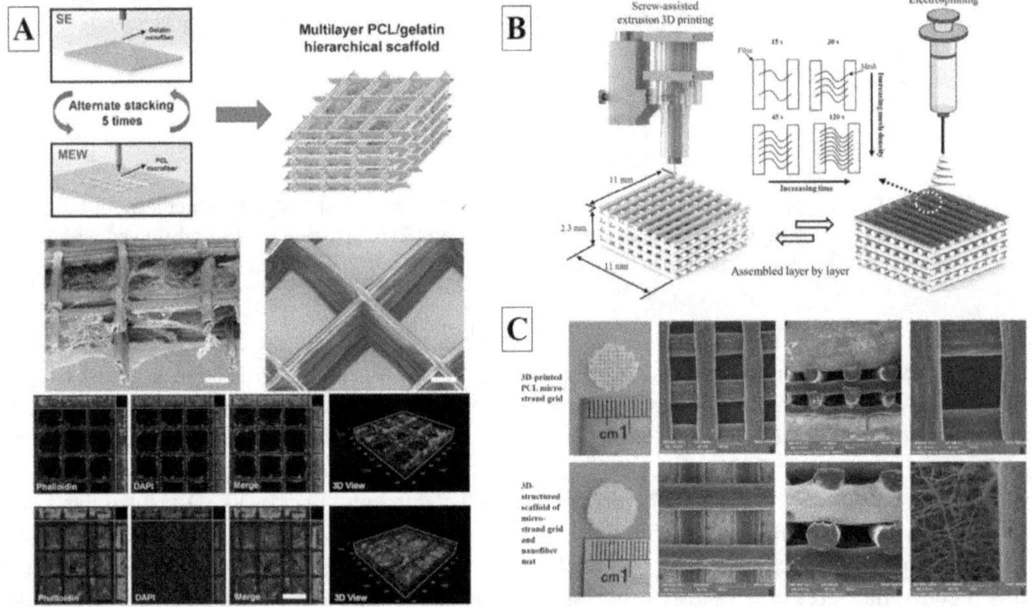

FIGURE 4.6 Scaffolds in multilayered structure designed for bone tissue engineering by using the integration of 3D printing and electrospinning: (A) schematic illustration and SEM image of the scaffold with multi-layer structure; after seven days of culture, images showing penetration and distribution of cells on scaffolds (reproduced with permission from Wang, Z., Wang, H., Xiong, J., Li, J., Miao, X., Lan, X., Liu, X., Wang, W., Cai, N., & Tang, Y.: Fabrication and In Vitro Evaluation of PCL/Gelatin Hierarchical Scaffolds Based on Melt Electrospinning Writing and Solution Electrospinning for Bone Regeneration. Mat. Sci. Eng. C. 2021. 128. 112287. Copyright 2021 Elsevier); (B) schematic display of the double-scale scaffold fabrication using both 3D printing and electrospinning (reproduced under the terms of CC-BY 4.0 (https://creativecommons.org/licenses/by/4.0/) International License from Vyas, C., Ates, G., Aslan, E., Hart, J., Huang, B., & Bartolo, P.: Three-Dimensional Printing and Electrospinning Dual-Scale Polycaprolactone Scaffolds with Low-Density and Oriented Fibers to Promote Cell Alignment. 3D Print. Add. Manuf. 2020. 7. 105–113. Copyright 2020 Vyas et al., published by Mary Ann Liebert, Inc.); (C) images of 3D-printed grid and 3D-structured scaffolds fabricated by nanofiber mats onto 3D-printed micro-strand layer grids (reproduced with permission from Belgheisi, G., Haghbin Nazarpak, M., & Solati-Hashjin, M.: Fabrication and Evaluation of Combined 3D Printed/Pamidronate-layered Double Hydroxides Enriched Electrospun Scaffolds for Bone Tissue Engineering Applications. Appl. Clay Sci. 2022. 225. Copyright 2022 Elsevier).

biodegradable polymer, was chosen for the preparation of both the fibers and the 3D-printed structure. Additionally, pamidronate-loaded layered double hydroxides were added to PCL nanofibers to improve the physicochemical and biological properties of the scaffolds and provide better cellular responses. Nanofibers and 3D-printed grids were prepared independently in separate assemblies. Then, with the help of glue (PCL 15% wt in DCM/DMF), the fibrous mats were attached to the surfaces of the two-layered grids. The physical and morphological images of the scaffolds produced are presented in Figure 4.I) (Belgheisi et al., 2022).

Another approach to hybrid scaffolds is fabricating scaffolds composed of micro/nanofibers by direct electrospinning onto each micro-patterned polymeric layer created during 3D printing. Studies show that this is an effective way of making porous scaffolds with interconnected macro channels that stimulate vasculogenesis and osteogenesis and connective micro channels that enhance osteochondral ossification and play important roles in bone regeneration (Diaz-Gomez et al., 2017). Gonzalez-Pujana et al. (2022) designed a hybrid scaffold consisting of electrospun nanofibers randomly distributed between 3D-printed layers to guide osteogenic differentiation.

Hybrid PCL scaffolds were fabricated using a 3D printer coupled with an electrospinning module, an extruder, and a heated platform. The scaffolds consisted of 10 consecutive 3D layers and electrospun fibers. The micro/nanoporous architecture exhibited imparted osteoinductive properties to the scaffolds supporting the expression of early and late osteogenic markers in MC3T3-E1 osteoblast cells, and these results showed that hybrid PCL scaffolds are a new platform that can guide osteogenic differentiation (Gonzalez-Pujana et al., 2022).

4.4.2 Short Electrospun Nanofiber-Reinforced Bioinks

It is well-known that printing materials (inks) are critically important for the preparation of 3D-printed scaffolds. Therefore, efforts have been made to create novel printing materials including synthetic and natural polymers, hydrogels prepared using them, cell-laden constructs, and composites prepared using nanomaterials and polymers. The materials to be used for the ink should have properties such as excellent cytocompatibility, good printability, high mechanical properties, and a fast/safe gelling process.

In bone tissue engineering applications, multiple structures with micro- and nanochannels that will support cell adhesion and growth and help osteogenic differentiation are possible by homogeneously dispersing the previously produced fibrous structures in the bioink and printing this combination as desired morphology. In addition, by dispersing the fibers in 3D-printed structures, the collagen fibers in the articular cartilage tissue are imitated, which enhances the mechanical features of the final scaffold (Shirazi et al., 2008). So far, few studies have been reported on bioinks that are both electrospun nanofiber-enhanced and suitable for 3D printing in bone tissue engineering applications such as cartilage regeneration.

In this concept, the nanofibers to be dispersed in the multi-composite bioink are first prepared by electrospinning. Then, the prepared fibrous structure is subjected to a series of processing techniques and chemical treatments including dehydration, homogenization, and evaporation drying to form small fibers (SFs). In one such study, hyaluronic acid and polyethylene oxide-based 3D-printed scaffolds were fabricated using bioink containing gelatin/PLGA electrospun nanofibers following those steps to make their composite bioink: dehydration of the fibrous mats, homogenization in a solvent, complete evaporation of the solvent, and dispersion of the short fibers (Chen et al., 2020). The formed fibers were dispersed in a viscous water solution consisting of hyaluronic acid and polyethylene oxide, and this composite mixture was 3D printed by extrusion.

As a continuation of this study, the bioactivity and regenerative potential of the hybrid scaffolds were further studied. Chen et al. (2020) prepared short electrospinning gelatin/PLGA fibers to improve mechanical features and increase their effectiveness in articular cartilage injuries in rabbits. A conventional electrospinning setup was used to prepare gelatin/PLGA fiber membranes. The membranes were dehydrated at high temperatures and then cut into small pieces and placed in tert-butanol.

Homogenized at 5000 rpm, fiber dispersions were obtained, and the dispersed gelatin/PLGA SFs were dried by evaporation of the solvent. As a final step, they combined these SFs with HAp and cartilage decellularized matrix powder as bioink to fabricate 3D scaffolds for complex tissue regeneration and provide mechanical support for cell growth. The final structure with 50% fiber content offers several advantages, including a fibrous network structure, flexibility, and biocompatibility, while in vivo studies have demonstrated the ability to significantly repair cartilage defects in rabbits (Figure 4.7) (Chen et al., 2020).

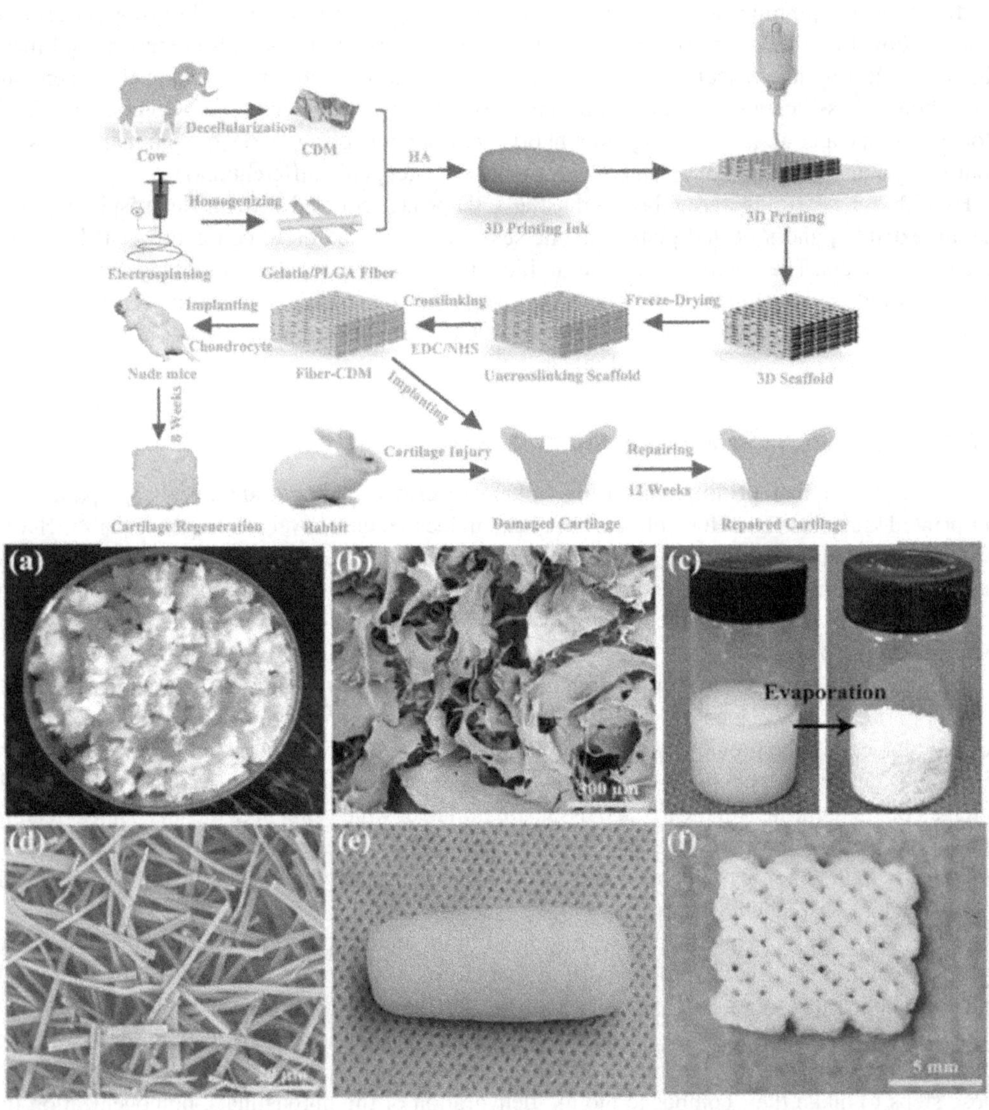

FIGURE 4.7 Schematic display of electrospinning fiber-reinforced cartilage decellularized matrix (CDM) based 3D-printed scaffold for cartilage regeneration and the morphology of products fabricated at each step: a: CDM powder, b: SEM image of CDM powder, c: dispersed gelatin/PLGA fibers in tert-butanol and after evaporation of tert-butanol, d: SEM image of dispersed gelatin/PLGA fibers, e: colloid consisting of CDM powder, gelatin/PLGA fibers, and HA solution as inks, f: 3D-printed fiber-reinforced CDM scaffold (reproduced with permission from Chen, W., Xu, Y., Li, Y., Jia, L., Mo, X., Jiang, G., & Zhou, G.: 3D Printing Electrospinning Fiber-Reinforced Decellularized Extracellular Matrix for Cartilage Regeneration. Chem. Eng. J. 2020. 382: 122986. Copyright 2020 Elsevier).

CONCLUSIONS AND FUTURE PERSPECTIVES

Electrospinning and 3D bioprinting show great potential for tissue engineering, showing promise for producing complex structures such as bone, cartilage, and osteochondral tissue. Many polymer types including natural and synthetic as well as composites of these polymers combined with different bioactive agents (drugs, essential oils, antibiotics) or functional materials (nanoparticles, bioceramics) have been successfully produced by using traditional production techniques or modified techniques alone or in combination, and the products have shown high potential in the field of clinical treatment. Electrospinning has powerful superiority in multifarious properties such as possible pilot-scale production, easy/simple production set-up, controlled fiber morphology, large surface area, easy functionalization, and the ability to provide nano-scale cues for cell orientation and maturation.

For bone tissue engineering, electrospun scaffolds mimic the topography of the fibrous nature of collagen fibers, the organic part of the bone matrix. However, a meticulous design is necessary for electrospun fibrous scaffolds to fabricate the suitable material and modify or functionalize the morphology for performing the bio-functions of osteogenesis. Additive manufacturing, also called 3D bioprinting, is a promising approach that allows using different polymers with controlled porosity and design, enhanced biological activity, improved mechanical properties, customization, and reproducibility and has many advantages, including the possibility of fabricating complex 3D structures.

Additionally, 3D printing has the problem of not being able to produce nano-sized patterns required for diffusion and vascularization. Combining electrospinning with 3D bioprinting provides a promising clinical platform for bone repair and regeneration that takes advantage of the positive features of both methods and is one of the biggest treatment steps for bone regeneration. Recent studies on the subject show that hybrid tissue scaffolds, which exhibit both micro and nanostructure, have high mechanical strength and can be designed according to the desired bone topography and bone defect shape; researchers have successfully imitated the composite structure of the bone consisting of spongy and hard parts. However, this combination is still in its infancy and some aspects need to be further investigated:

- Although bone tissue engineering with electrospinning and 3D printing has been explored, only a small fraction of this combination has been approved for clinical use so far. Studies are mostly on material characterization and determination of in vitro cell behavior, and a few are strategies on in vivo animal studies. For bone scaffolds produced by this combination to become a common clinical reality, studies that evaluate all components necessary for successful bone repair and regeneration are required.
- The research shows that easily printable synthetic polymers such as PCL and PLA are generally preferred for scaffold design experiments, but the final products exhibit poor mechanical and tensile properties. To overcome these limitations, fillers can be added to the polymeric matrix to act as reinforcing agents during manufacturing including inorganic and organic materials such as glass, carbon fibers, silicon, ceramics, or metals. Another approach is to use natural polymers (polysaccharides and proteins) from plants, biomass, or agricultural/industrial wastes as reinforcing agents. Thus, while improving the mechanical properties, antibacterial, biodegradability, and biocompatibility properties can be added to the final product with natural materials (such as chitosan), while mineralization can be contributed with inorganic or organic material additives (such as bioceramics).

LIST OF ABBREVIATIONS

ECM Extracellular matrix
HAp Hydroxyapatite crystals

MSCs Mesenchymal stem cells
PCL Polycaprolactone
PEG Polyethylene Glycol
PLGA Poly(lactic-co-glycolic acid)
PP Polypropylene
SFs Small fibers

REFERENCES

Abbasi, N., Hamlet, S., Love, R. M., & Nguyen, N. T. (2020). Porous scaffolds for bone regeneration. *J. Sci. Adv. Mater. Devices*. 5: 1–9.

Alcorta-Sevillano, N., Macías, I., Infante, A., & Rodríguez, C. I. (2020). Deciphering the relevance of bone ECM signaling. *Cells*. 9: 2630.

Ali, M. G., Mousa, H. M., Blaudez, F., Abd El-sadek, M. S., Mohamed, M. A., Abdel-Jaber, G. T., Abdal-hay, A., & Ivanovski, S. (2020). Dual nanofiber scaffolds composed of polyurethane- gelatin/nylon 6- gelatin for bone tissue engineering. *Colloids Surf.* 597: 124817.

Alonzo, M., Alvarez Primo, F., Anil Kumar, S., Mudloff, J. A., Dominguez, E., Fregoso, G., Ortiz, N., Weiss, W. M., & Joddar, B. (2021). Bone tissue engineering techniques, advances and scaffolds for treatment of bone defects. *Curr. Opin. Biomed.* 17: 100248.

Annamalai, R. T., Hong, X., Schott, N. G., Tiruchinapally, G., Levi, B., & Stegemann, J. P. (2019). Injectable osteogenic microtissues containing mesenchymal stromal cells conformally fill and repair critical-size defects. *Biomaterials*. 208: 32–44.

Bahraminasab, M. (2020). Challenges on optimization of 3D-printed bone scaffolds. *Biomed. Eng. Online*. 19: 1–33.

Belgheisi, G., Haghbin Nazarpak, M., & Solati-Hashjin, M. (2022). Fabrication and evaluation of combined 3D printed/pamidronate-layered double hydroxides enriched electrospun scaffolds for bone tissue engineering applications. *Appl. Clay Sci.* 225: 106538.

Bilgiç, E., Boyacıoğlu, Ö., Gizer, M., Korkusuz, P., & Korkusuz, F. (2020). Architecture of bone tissue and its adaptation to pathological conditions. In *Comparative Kinesiology of the Human Body: Normal and Pathological Conditions*. S. Angin, and I. E. Şimşek, Eds. Waltham, MA: Elsevier, pp. 71–90.

Bitar, K. N., & Zakhem, E. (2014). Design strategies of biodegradable scaffolds for tissue regeneration. *Biomed. Eng. Comput. Biol.* 6: BECB–S10961.

Bölgen, N., Demir, D., Aşık, M., Sakım, B., & Vaseashta, A. (2022). Introduction and fundamentals of electrospinning. In *Electrospun Nanofibers*. A. Vaseashta, and N. Bölgen, Eds. Cham: Springer, pp. 3–34.

Carvalho, M. S., Cabral, J. M. S., da Silva, C. L., & Vashishth, D. (2021). Bone matrix non-collagenous proteins in tissue engineering: Creating new bone by mimicking the extracellular matrix. *Polymers*. 13: 1095.

Cestari, F., Petretta, M., Yang, Y., Motta, A., Grigolo, B., & Sglavo, V. M. (2021). 3D printing of PCL/nano-hydroxyapatite scaffolds derived from biogenic sources for bone tissue engineering. *Sustainable Mater. Technol.* 29: e00318.

Chang, H. K., Yang, D. H., Ha, M. Y., Kim, H. J., Kim, C. H., Kim, S. H., Choi, J. W., & Chun, H. J. (2022). 3D printing of cell-laden visible light curable glycol chitosan bioink for bone tissue engineering. *Carbohydr. Polym.* 287: 119328.

Chen, S., John, J. V., McCarthy, A., & Xie, J. (2020). New forms of electrospun nanofiber materials for biomedical applications. *J. Mater. Chem. B*. 8: 3733.

Chen, W., Xu, Y., Li, Y., Jia, L., Mo, X., Jiang, G., & Zhou, G. (2020). 3D printing electrospinning fiber-reinforced decellularized extracellular matrix for cartilage regeneration. *Chem. Eng. J.* 382: 122986.

Chen, X., Fan, H., Deng, X., Wu, L., Yi, T., Gu, L., Zhou, C., Fan, Y., & Zhang, X. (2018). Scaffold structural microenvironmental cues to guide tissue regeneration in bone tissue applications. *Nanomaterials*. 8: 960.

Chou, P. Y., Lee, D., Chen, S. H., Liao, C. T., Lo, L. J., & Liu, S. J. (2022). 3D-printed/electrospun bioresorbable nanofibrous drug-eluting cuboid frames for repair of alveolar bone defects. *Int. J. Pharm.* 615: 121497.

Darsani, A., Marwah, O. M. F., Sa'ude, N., Adzila, S., Ibrahim, M., & Sharif, S. (2021). Capability behaviour of POFA composite filament for 3D printing user. *Lect. Notes Mech. Eng*. 46: 607–618.

Diaz-Gomez, L., García-González, C. A., Wang, J., Yang, F., Aznar-Cervantes, S., Cenis, J. L., Reyes, R., Delgado, A., Évora, C., Concheiro, A., & Alvarez-Lorenzo, C. (2017). Biodegradable PCL/fibroin/

hydroxyapatite porous scaffolds prepared by supercritical foaming for bone regeneration. *Int. J. Pharm.* 527: 115–125.

Dong, J., Jhu, R. J., Wang, L., Jiang, C. P., & Xian, C. J. (2019). A hybrid platform for three-dimensional printing of bone scaffold by combining thermal-extrusion and electrospinning methods. *Microsyst. Technol.* 1–15.

Du, X., Wei, D., Huang, L., Zhu, M., Zhang, Y., & Zhu, Y. (2019). 3D printing of mesoporous bioactive glass/silk fibroin composite scaffolds for bone tissue engineering. *Mater. Sci. Eng. C.* 103: 109731.

Elghazali, N., Rush, M., Garcia, E., Buksa, C., Perez, M., Trujillo, R., Lopez, S., & Salas, C. (2019). Bio-3D printing and near-field electrospinning of bone-ligament tissue engineering scaffolds. *Society of Biomaterials*. UNM Digital Repository.

Feng, X. (2009). Chemical and biochemical basis of cell-bone matrix interaction in health and disease. *Curr. Chem. Biol.* 3: 189.

Filipowska, J., Tomaszewski, K. A., Niedźwiedzki, Ł., Walocha, J. A., & Niedźwiedzki, T. (2017). The role of vasculature in bone development, regeneration and proper systemic functioning. *Angiogenesis*. 20: 291.

Florencio-Silva, R., Sasso, G. R. D. S., Sasso-Cerri, E., Simões, M. J., & Cerri, P. S. (2015). Biology of bone tissue: Structure, function, and factors that influence bone cells. *Biomed Res. Int.* 2015.

Ghafari, F., Karbasi, S., & Eslaminejad, M. B. (2023). Investigating of physical, mechanical, and biological properties of polyhydroxybutyrate-keratin/alumina electrospun scaffold utilized in bone tissue engineering. *Mater. Chem. Phys.* 297: 127340.

Gonzalez-Pujana, A., Carranza, T., Santos-Vizcaino, E., Igartua, M., Guerrero, P., Hernandez, R. M., & de la Caba, K. (2022). Hybrid 3D printed and electrospun multi-scale hierarchical polycaprolactone scaffolds to induce bone differentiation. *Pharmaceutics*. 14: 2843.

Haider, M. K., Kharaghani, D., Sun, L., Ullah, S., Sarwar, M. N., Ullah, A., Khatri, M., Yoshiko, Y., Gopiraman, M., & Kim, I. S. (2023). Synthesized bioactive lignin nanoparticles/polycaprolactone nanofibers: A novel nanobiocomposite for bone tissue engineering. *Biomat. Adv.* 144: 213203.

He, P., Sahoo, S., Ng, K. S., Chen, K., Toh, S. L., & Goh, J. C. H. (2013). Enhanced osteoinductivity and osteoconductivity through hydroxyapatite coating of silk-based tissue-engineered ligament scaffold. *J. Biomed. Mater. Res. A.* 101: 555–566.

Huang, B., Aslan, E., Jiang, Z., Daskalakis, E., Jiao, M., Aldalbahi, A., Vyas, C., & Bártolo, P. (2020). Engineered dual-scale poly (ε-caprolactone) scaffolds using 3D printing and rotational electrospinning for bone tissue regeneration. *Addit. Manuf.* 36: 101452.

Iglesias-Mejuto, A., & García-González, C. A. (2021). 3D-printed alginate-hydroxyapatite aerogel scaffolds for bone tissue engineering. *Mater. Sci. Eng. C.* 131: 112525.

Jeong, J., Kim, J. H., Shim, J. H., Hwang, N. S., & Heo, C. Y. (2019). Bioactive calcium phosphate materials and applications in bone regeneration. *Biomater. Res.* 23: 1–11.

Kemençe, N., & Bölgen, N. (2017). Gelatin- and hydroxyapatite-based cryogels for bone tissue engineering: Synthesis, characterization, in vitro and in vivo biocompatibility. *J. Tissue Eng. Regen. Med.* 11: 20–33.

Khorshidi, S., Solouk, A., Mirzadeh, H., Mazinani, S., Lagaron, J. M., Sharifi, S., & Ramakrishna, S. (2016). A review of key challenges of electrospun scaffolds for tissue-engineering applications. *J. Tissue Eng. Regen. Med.* 10: 715–738.

Kiernan, C., Knuth, C., & Farrell, E. (2018). Endochondral ossification: Recapitulating bone development for bone defect repair. In *Developmental Biology and Musculoskeletal Tissue Engineering: Principles and Applications*. M. J. Stoddart, A. M. Craft, G. Pattappa, and O. F. W. Gardner, Eds. Waltham, MA: Elsevier, pp. 125–148.

Kim, H. J., Park, I. K., Kim, J. H., Cho, C. S., & Kim, M. S. (2012). Gas foaming fabrication of porous biphasic calcium phosphate for bone regeneration. *Tissue Eng. Regen. Med.* 9: 63–68.

Kumar, P., Saini, M., Dehiya, B. S., Umar, A., Sindhu, A., Mohammed, H., Al-Hadeethi, Y., & Guo, Z. (2020). Fabrication and in-vitro biocompatibility of freeze-dried CTS-nHA and CTS-nBG scaffolds for bone regeneration applications. *Int. J. Biol. Macromol.* 149: 1–10.

Lee, S. S., Du, X., Kim, I., & Ferguson, S. J. (2022). Scaffolds for bone-tissue engineering. *Matter*. 5: 2722–2759.

Li, S., Dong, C., & Lv, Y. (2022). Magnetic liquid metal scaffold with dynamically tunable stiffness for bone tissue engineering. *Biomater. Adv.* 139: 212975.

Lin, X., Patil, S., Gao, Y. G., & Qian, A. (2020). The bone extracellular matrix in bone formation and regeneration. *Front. Pharmacol.* 11: 757.

Liu, X., Chen, M., Luo, J., Zhao, H., Zhou, X., Gu, Q., Yang, H., Zhu, X., Cui, W., & Shi, Q. (2021). Immunopolarization-regulated 3D printed-electrospun fibrous scaffolds for bone regeneration. *Biomaterials*. 276: 121037.

Lu, Y., Wang, J., Yang, Y., & Yin, Q. (2021). Bone defects are repaired by enhanced osteogenic activity of the induced membrane: A case report and literature review. *BMC Musculoskelet. Disord.* 22: 1–7.

Luo, J., Zhu, J., Wang, L., Kang, J., Wang, X., & Xiong, J. (2021). Co-electrospun nano-/microfibrous composite scaffolds with structural and chemical gradients for bone tissue engineering. *Mater. Sci. Eng. C*. 119: 111622.

Mantila Roosa, S. M., Kemppainen, J. M., Moffitt, E. N., Krebsbach, P. H., & Hollister, S. J. (2010). The pore size of polycaprolactone scaffolds has limited influence on bone regeneration in an in vivo model. *J. Biomed. Mater. Res. A*. 92A: 359–368.

Marques-Almeida, T., Cardoso, V. F., Gama, M., Lanceros-Mendez, S., & Ribeiro, C. (2020). Patterned piezoelectric scaffolds for osteogenic differentiation. *Int. J. Mol. Sci.* 21: 8352.

Miszuk, J., Liang, Z., Hu, J., Sanyour, H., Hong, Z., Fong, H., & Sun, H. (2021). Elastic mineralized 3D electrospun PCL nanofibrous scaffold for drug release and bone tissue engineering. *ACS Appl. Bio. Mater.* 4: 3639–3648.

Monavari, M., Homaeigohar, S., Fuentes-Chandía, M., Nawaz, Q., Monavari, M., Venkatraman, A., & Boccaccini, A. R. (2021). 3D printing of alginate dialdehyde-gelatin (ADA-GEL) hydrogels incorporating phytotherapeutic icariin loaded mesoporous SiO2-CaO nanoparticles for bone tissue engineering. *Mater. Sci. Eng. C*. 131: 112470.

Monier-Faugere, M. C., Chris Langub, M., & Malluche, H. H. (1998). Bone biopsies: A modern approach. In *Metabolic Bone Disease and Clinically Related Disorders*. L. V. Avioli, and S. M. Krane, Eds. Academic Press, Waltham, MA: Elsevier, pp. 237–280.

Murphy, C. M., & O'Brien, F. J. (2010). Understanding the effect of mean pore size on cell activity in collagen-glycosaminoglycan scaffolds. *Cell Adh. Migr*. 4: 377.

Naghieh, S., Foroozmehr, E., Badrossamay, M., & Kharaziha, M. (2017). Combinational processing of 3D printing and electrospinning of hierarchical poly(lactic acid)/gelatin-forsterite scaffolds as a biocomposite: Mechanical and biological assessment. *Mater. Des*. 133: 128–135.

Ng, J., Spiller, K., Bernhard, J., & Vunjak-Novakovic, G. (2017). Biomimetic approaches for bone tissue engineering. *Tissue Eng. Part B Rev*. 23(5): 480–493.

O'brien, F. J. (2011). Biomaterials & scaffolds for tissue engineering. *Mater. Today*. 14: 88–95.

Paiva, K. B. S., & Granjeiro, J. M. (2017). Matrix metalloproteinases in bone resorption, remodeling, and repair. *Prog. Mol. Biol. Transl. Sci.* 148: 203–303.

Paljevac, M., Gradišnik, L., Lipovšek, S., Maver, U., Kotek, J., Krajnc, P., Paljevac, M., Lipovšek, S., Krajnc, P., Gradišnik, L., Maver, U., & Kotek, J. (2018). Multiple-level porous polymer monoliths with interconnected cellular topology prepared by combining hard sphere and emulsion templating for use in bone tissue engineering. *Macromol. Biosci.* 18: 1700306.

Pensa, N. W., Curry, A. S., Bonvallet, P. P., Bellis, N. F., Rettig, K. M., Reddy, M. S., Eberhardt, A. W., & Bellis, S. L. (2019). 3D printed mesh reinforcements enhance the mechanical properties of electrospun scaffolds. *Biomater. Res*. 23: 1–7.

Qu, H., Fu, H., Han, Z., & Sun, Y. (2019). Biomaterials for bone tissue engineering scaffolds: A review. *RSC Adv*. 9: 26252–26262.

Rajzer, I., Kurowska, A., Jabłoński, A., Jatteau, S., Śliwka, M., Ziąbka, M., & Menaszek, E. (2018). Layered gelatin/PLLA scaffolds fabricated by electrospinning and 3D printing- for nasal cartilages and subchondral bone reconstruction. *Mater. Des*. 155: 297–306.

Reneker, D. H., & Yarin, A. L. (2008). Electrospinning jets and polymer nanofibers. *Polymer*. 49: 2387–2425.

Rezk, A. I., Rajan Unnithan, A., Hee Park, C., & Sang Kim, C. (2018). Rational design of bone extracellular matrix mimicking tri-layered composite nanofibers for bone tissue regeneration. *Chem. Eng. J*. 350: 812–823.

Romero-Araya, P., Pino, V., Nenen, A., Cárdenas, V., Pavicic, F., Ehrenfeld, P., Serandour, G., Lisoni, J. G., Moreno-Villoslada, I., & Flores, M. E. (2021). Combining materials obtained by 3D-printing and electrospinning from commercial polylactide filament to produce biocompatible composites. *Polymers*. 13: 1–19.

Rosales-Ibáñez, R., Viera-Ruiz, A. E., Cauich-Rodríguez, J. V., Carrillo-Escalante, H. J., González-González, A., Rodríguez-Martínez, J. J., & Hernández-Sánchez, F. (2022). Electrospun/3D-printed PCL bioactive scaffold for bone regeneration. *Polym. Bull.* 1–20.

Shaik, Y. P., Schuster, J., Shaik, A., Shaik, Y. P., Schuster, J., & Shaik, A. (2021). A scientific review on various pellet extruders used in 3D printing FDM processes. *OALib*. 8: 1–19.

Shirazi, R., Shirazi-Adl, A., & Hurtig, M. (2008). Role of cartilage collagen fibrils networks in knee joint biomechanics under compression. *J. Biomech.* 41: 3340–3348.

Siripongpreda, T., Hoven, V. P., Narupai, B., & Rodthongku, N. (2023). Emerging 3D printing based on polymers and nanomaterial additives: Enhancement of properties and potential applications. *Eur. Polym. J.* 184: 111806.

Smrke, D., Rožman, P., Veselko, M., Gubina, B., Smrke, D., Rožman, P., Veselko, M., & Gubina, B. (2013). Treatment of bone defects—Allogenic platelet gel and autologous bone technique. In *Regenerative Medicine and Tissue Engineering*. J. A. Andrades, Ed. London, UK: IntechOpen.

Song, P., Li, M., Zhang, B., Gui, X., Han, Y., Wang, L., Zhou, W., Guo, L., Zhang, Z., Li, Z., Zhou, C., Fan, Y., & Zhang, X. (2022). DLP fabricating of precision GelMA/HAp porous composite scaffold for bone tissue engineering application. *Compos. B. Eng.* 244: 110163.

Suamte, L., Tirkey, A., Barman, J., & Babu, P. J. (2023). Various manufacturing methods and ideal properties of scaffolds for tissue engineering applications. *Smart Mater. Manuf.* 1: 100011.

Tappa, K., & Jammalamadaka, U. (2018). Novel biomaterials used in medical 3D printing techniques. *J. Funct. Biomater.* 9: 17.

Thadavirul, N., Pavasant, P., & Supaphol, P. (2014). Improvement of dual-leached polycaprolactone porous scaffolds by incorporating with hydroxyapatite for bone tissue regeneration. *J. Biomater. Sci. Polym. Ed.* 25: 1986–2008.

Thavornyutikarn, B., Chantarapanich, N., Sitthiseripratip, K., Thouas, G. A., & Chen, Q. (2014). Bone tissue engineering scaffolding: Computer-aided scaffolding techniques. *Prog. Biomater.* 3: 61–102.

Tylek, T., Blum, C., Hrynevich, A., Schlegelmilch, K., Schilling, T., Dalton, P. D., & Groll, J. (2020). Precisely defined fiber scaffolds with 40 μm porosity induce elongation driven M2-like polarization of human macrophages. *Biofabrication*. 12: 025007.

Vaseashta, A., Demir, D., Sakım, B., Aşık, M., & Bölgen, N. (2022). Hierarchical integration of 3D printing and electrospinning of nanofibers for rapid prototyping. In *Electrospun Nanofibers*. A. Vaseashta, and N. Bölgen, Ed. Cham: Springer, pp. 631–655.

Vaseashta, A. (2007). Controlled formation of multiple Taylor cones in electrospinning process. *Appl. Phys. Lett.* 90: 093115.

Vyas, C., Ates, G., Aslan, E., Hart, J., Huang, B., & Bartolo, P. (2020). Three-dimensional printing and electrospinning dual-scale polycaprolactone scaffolds with low-density and oriented fibers to promote cell alignment. *3D Print Addit. Manuf.* 7: 105–113.

Wang, Z., Wang, H., Xiong, J., Li, J., Miao, X., Lan, X., Liu, X., Wang, W., Cai, N., & Tang, Y. (2021). Fabrication and in vitro evaluation of PCL/gelatin hierarchical scaffolds based on melt electrospinning writing and solution electrospinning for bone regeneration. *Mater. Sci. Eng. C.* 128: 112287.

Wu, S., Liu, X., Yeung, K. W. K., Liu, C., & Yang, X. (2014). Biomimetic porous scaffolds for bone tissue engineering. *Mater. Sci. Eng. R Rep.* 80: 1–36.

Xie, J., Shen, H., Yuan, G., Lin, K., & Su, J. (2021). The effects of alignment and diameter of electrospun fibers on the cellular behaviors and osteogenesis of BMSCs. *Mater. Sci. Eng. C.* 120: 111787.

Xu, Z., Lin, B., Zhao, C., Lu, Y., Huang, T., Chen, Y., Li, J., Wu, R., Liu, W., & Lin, J. (2022). Lanthanum doped octacalcium phosphate/polylactic acid scaffold fabricated by 3D printing for bone tissue engineering. *J. Mater. Sci. Technol.* 118: 229–242.

Xue, N., Ding, X., Huang, R., Jiang, R., Huang, H., Pan, X., Min, W., Chen, J., Duan, J. A., Liu, P., & Wang, Y. (2022). Bone tissue engineering in the treatment of bone defects. *Pharmaceuticals*. 15: 879.

Yousefiasl, S., Sharifi, E., Salahinejad, E., Makvandi, P., & Irani, S. (2023). Bioactive 3D-printed chitosan-based scaffolds for personalized craniofacial bone tissue engineering. *Eng. Reg.* 4: 1–11.

Yu, Y., Hua, S., Yang, M., Fu, Z., Teng, S., Niu, K., Zhao, Q., & Yi, C. (2016). Fabrication and characterization of electrospinning/3D printing bone tissue engineering scaffold. *RSC Adv.* 6: 110557–110565.

Zadpoor, A. A. (2015). Bone tissue regeneration: The role of scaffold geometry. *Biomat. Sci.* 3: 231–245.

Zhang, S., Zhang, M., Bai, R., Kong, L., Yang, H., Zhang, A., Dong, S., Chen, M., Ramakrishna, S., & Yang, F. (2022). Electrospun coaxial nanofibers loading with perovskite and icariin to enhance the bone scaffold-mediated osteogenesis. *Mater. Today Chem.* 26: 101246.

Zhao, C., Xia, L., Zhai, D., Zhang, N., Liu, J., Fang, B., Chang, J., & Lin, K. (2015). Designing ordered micropatterned hydroxyapatite bioceramics to promote the growth and osteogenic differentiation of bone marrow stromal cells. *J. Mater. Chem. B*. 3: 968–976.

Zhao, F., Xiong, Y., Ito, K., van Rietbergen, B., & Hofmann, S. (2021a). Porous geometry guided micro-mechanical environment within scaffolds for cell mechanobiology study in bone tissue engineering. *Front. Bioeng. Biotech*. 9: 819.

Zhao, R., Yang, R., Cooper, P. R., Khurshid, Z., Shavandi, A., & Ratnayake, J. (2021b). Bone grafts and substitutes in dentistry: A review of current trends and developments. *Molecules*. 26: 3007.

5 The 3D/4D Printing of Polymeric Scaffolds for Bone Tissue Engineering

Arkodip Mandal and Kaushik Chatterjee

5.1 INTRODUCTION

The endogenous self-repair/regeneration capacity of bone, especially in the younger population, ensures that minor fractures heal unaided without forming scar tissue and ultimately become indistinguishable and integrated with the adjacent healthy bone. However, in situations where the body lacks the template for orchestrated regeneration, such as in the skeletal reconstruction of critical-size bone defects caused by trauma, infection, congenital defects, tumor resections, or in conditions such as atrophic nonunions, osteonecrosis, and osteoporosis where the natural regeneration process is compromised, surgical interventions are warranted for the complete restoration of physiological function. Apart from sheltering the delicate internal organs, providing a structural framework, and aiding in locomotion, bone is responsible for the production and maturation of the cells of the immune system for immunoprotection, as well as functioning as a storage site for calcium, phosphate, and other ions (Sikavitsas et al., 2001). Hence, the restoration of damaged or lost bone is critical to avoid debilitating pain and negative impacts on the patient's mental well-being and quality of life.

5.1.1 Rationale for 3D Printing Bone Tissue Scaffolds

The prevalent approaches in reconstructive orthopedic or craniofacial surgery to treat defects and stimulate bone healing include the use of bone grafts, such as autografts, allografts, or xenografts. The 2021 valuation of the global market for bone grafts and substitutes was estimated at USD 2.91 billion, and it is anticipated to grow at a compound annual growth rate of 6.2% between 2022 and 2030, fueled by a steep upward incidence of bone and joint disorders, particularly in the aging population (Bone Grafts and Substitutes Market Report, 2022–2030). It is estimated that over four million procedures using bone grafts or bone substitute materials are being performed annually worldwide (Turnbull et al., 2018).

The current gold-standard treatment is bone autografts, in which the bone tissue is harvested from a non-load-bearing site (typically the iliac crest of the pelvis since it provides both cancellous and cortical bone and has the highest osteogenic potential) and transplanted to the defect site in the same individual. Autografts are universally preferred since they simultaneously provide optimal osteogenic (osteoprogenitor cells), osteoinductive (bone morphogenetic proteins [BMPs], matrix proteins, and growth factors), and osteoconductive (bone matrix scaffold) properties and are histocompatible and nonimmunogenic (Bauer & Muschler, 2000; Dimitriou et al., 2011). However, surgical complications associated with bone harvesting, multiple required surgeries, donor-site neurovascular injury, morphology mismatch, limited volume of autogenous bone, and high costs severely restrict their use in clinical settings (St John et al., 2003).

Allografts, which are procured from human cadavers or living donors, present a promising alternative to address the complications associated with bone harvesting and inadequate graft

DOI: 10.1201/9781003307310-6

material. Allogeneic bone is cleaned, processed (mainly by freezing and demineralizing), and sterilized to remove cells to minimize the risks of host-immune response and transmission of pathogens (Finkemeier, 2002). The lack of viable cells in allografts results in the loss of osteogenic properties, and the mechanical and biological properties vary in accordance with graft processing. Nevertheless, there remains the risk of immune reactions and of transferring viral (human immunodeficiency virus, hepatitis B and C) and bacterial infections, systemic diseases, or toxins (Giannoudis et al., 2005).

This pressing clinical need has spurred the search for alternative bone repair and regeneration therapies using synthetic material substitutes that outperform bone autografts and are closely comparable with the bone's physical, mechanical, and biological properties. In this context, bone tissue engineering (BTE) has gained immense popularity because it promises directly repairing bone at the defect site or synthesizing biofunctional bone-like tissue in vitro for transplantation through the synergistic combination of biomaterials and cell therapy (Stevens, 2008; Bose et al., 2013; Collins et al., 2021). The core component of BTE is the exogenous biomaterial scaffold, a 3D, porous biocompatible construct that mimics the extracellular matrix (ECM).

The scaffold provides spatiotemporal biophysical cues; a 3D matrix for cell attachment, differentiation, and proliferation; and mechanical support for the growing tissue; the scaffold also directs bone ingrowth and serves as a template for neo-tissue formation (Roseti et al., 2017). The scaffold is designed to undergo controlled biodegradation at a rate similar to mineralized tissue deposition and is ultimately replaced by newly synthesized biological tissue. Since the structure, property, and processing of the scaffolds largely dictate their biological activity, there has been considerable interest in bone tissue scaffold design and fabrication methodologies.

With rapid technological advances, increased accessibility, and reduced costs, 3D printing has emerged as the best-suited biofabrication tool for manufacturing bone tissue scaffolds due to its unprecedented capabilities in spatially positioning biomaterials in a predetermined, automated, and layer-by-layer fashion that enables the successful recapitulation of the complex multiscale structure, hierarchical architecture, distributions in porosity, and compositional gradients present in their natural counterparts. Given the vast differences in clinical requirements depending on the geometry and location of the defect site as well as patient-related factors such as health condition, age, and sex, 3D printing can be employed to fabricate on-demand, customized, and personalized bone tissue scaffolds based on 3D models derived from the patient's medical imaging data (computed tomography [CT] or magnetic resonance imaging [MRI] scans) using a computer-aided design (CAD) software. Such scaffolds are typically constructed by scanning the corresponding healthy anatomical region on the other half of the patient's body and mirroring it to serve as a CAD template (Ahn et al., 2018).

Biological components such as cells and growth factors can also be incorporated within the biomaterial formulation (bioink) to elicit a better cellular response, and this concurrent printing is referred to as 3D bioprinting. However, cell-based therapies face issues related to cell selection, viability, phenotypic stability, limited sources of cell types, stringent regulatory red tape, and high costs, making it challenging for human translation (Burdick et al., 2013). The scaffold can also act as a vehicle for the delivery of stem cells, genes, drugs, signaling molecules, and growth factors, which can further accelerate the bone regeneration process (Dang et al., 2018). This chapter will primarily focus on 3D-printed biodegradable polymeric scaffolds, their design considerations, and their fabrication strategies and discuss the latest innovations and state-of-the-art advances in this field.

5.1.2 Insights from the Natural Bone Tissue Structure

A basic understanding of the bone structure and its physiological environment will enable researchers to design bioinspired scaffolds for BTE (Lopes et al., 2018; Zhu et al., 2021). Bone is a highly dynamic, innervated, vascularized, mineralized connective tissue composed of organic (collagen, primary bone cells) and inorganic (hydroxyapatite, minerals) phases. It presents a hierarchical

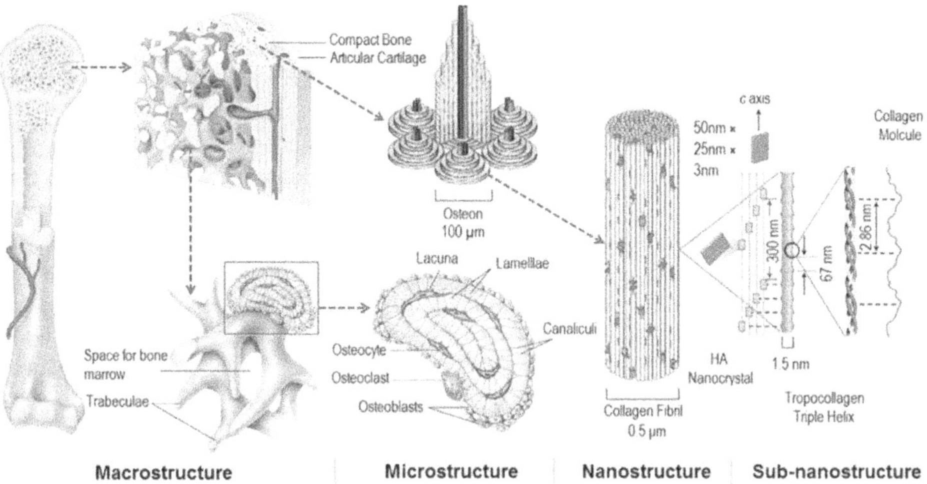

FIGURE 5.1 The multiscale hierarchical architecture of the human bone (reproduced with permission from Wang, X., Xu, S., Zhou, S., Xu, W., Leary, M., Choong, P., Qian, M., Brandt, M., & Xie, Y. M.: Topological design and additive manufacturing of porous metals for bone scaffolds and orthopedic implants: A review. Biomaterials. 2016. 83. 127–141. Copyright 2016 Elsevier).

architecture spanning multiple length scales that consists of macroscale (the outer cortical bone, also known as compact bone, and the inner cancellous bone, also referred to as trabecular bone), microscale, and sub-microscale (osteons, lamellae, Haversian systems) and nanoscale (nano-hydroxyapatite, fibrillar collagen) as shown in Figure 5.1 (Qu et al., 2019).

It is important to note that there exists a graded variation in density and porosity between the cortical and cancellous regions that forms the basis of many biomimetic scaffold designs (Di Luca et al., 2016; Shi et al., 2019; Bittner et al., 2019; Abbasi et al., 2020b). The proportions of cancellous and cortical bone vary depending on the anatomical location, with the cortical bone making up around 80% of the total skeletal mass (Clarke, 2008). As the name suggests, the compact bone is dense and solid (between 5 and 10% porosity) and consists of osteons (parallel cylinders of the matrix) arranged along the long axis of the bone (load-bearing direction). The osteon is the functional unit of the cortical bone and comprises osteocytes arranged in concentric layers called lamellae around central microscopic ducts referred to as the Haversian canals, which serve as conduits for nerve fibers and blood vessels. This characteristic arrangement of osteons imparts the cortical bone its characteristic mechanical strength.

On the contrary, the cancellous bone is light and much more porous (around 50–90%) with a higher bone-surface-area-to-bone-volume ratio and an elastic modulus and ultimate compressive strength 10 times lower than the cortical bone. The cancellous bone has a microarchitecture similar to cellular solids and comprises an interconnecting honeycomb-like network of anisotropically arranged trabeculae (rods, bars, and plates of bone matrix) with the cavities filled with bone marrow, blood vessels, and cells including hematopoietic stem cells and mesenchymal stem cells (MSCs) (Yin & Li, 2006). In addition to being the site of hematopoiesis, the cancellous bone facilitates the transmission and cushions against multidirectional stresses experienced during body movements.

5.2 SCAFFOLD REQUIREMENTS AND CONSIDERATIONS

The scaffold material should, first and foremost, be evaluated for its biocompatibility and toxicity (both local and systemic) and display no adverse effects such as local inflammation or immune-mediated reactions when implanted in the region of interest. Therefore, one must be aware of unreacted monomers or reactive functional groups on polymer chains, residual crosslinking agents, and/or degradation products, even for widely used polymers in tissue engineering. In addition to the material composition, the scaffold must be characterized for its pore size, total porosity, and mechanical properties.

Given its paramount importance in tissue engineering, Hollister stated by paraphrasing architect Robert le Ricolais, "The art of scaffolding is where to put the holes and the biofactors" (Hollister, 2005). The presence of an open and interconnected network of macropores is essential for maintaining high levels of cell viability as it facilitates efficient mass transport for delivering oxygen and nutrients to the cells and waste removal, allows cellular ingress (osteoconduction) and vascularization, and aids in osseointegration. While a minimum of 100–150 μm pore size is required for bone formation, larger pore sizes (> 300 μm) have been recommended as they favor direct osteogenesis (osteoinduction) and lead to the formation of blood capillaries (Karageorgiou & Kaplan, 2005; Jones et al., 2007; Bose et al., 2013).

While the porous architecture of the scaffold is critical for its biological performance, it has to be weighed against the mechanical requirements of the scaffold. The scaffold's elastic modulus and compressive and fatigue strength should be comparable with that of the native bone tissue to allow cell mechanoregulation and maintain the structural rigidity of the scaffold during bone regeneration (Turnbull et al., 2018). Therefore, *in silico* structure–function relationships of the scaffold can be performed as a preliminary step for scaffold design.

In the direct or forward design approach, the predesigned scaffold model serves as an input for the computation of effective elastic modulus and permeability properties. In general, the effective elastic modulus of the scaffold increases and the permeability decreases with increasing volume fraction (decreasing porosity). To solve these conflicting design requirements, topology optimization

TABLE 5.1
Porous Scaffold Characterization

Parameter	Definition	Scaffold property
Porosity	The total percentage of void space	Higher porosity decreases the effective elastic modulus but enhances the permeability of nutrients into the scaffold and facilitates waste removal.
Pore size	The diameter of an individual pore	A minimum pore size of 100 μm is recommended taking into consideration the cell size, transport, and migration requirements. Typically, a pore size of 100–300 μm is recommended, but larger pore sizes have also yielded favorable results.
Pore shape	The local curvatures at the pore boundary	The local curvatures can affect cell adhesion and focal adhesion and lead to differences in gene expression. High pore curvature is reported to enhance cell proliferation.
Pore interconnectivity	The percentage of pores that are interconnected	The presence of an interconnected porous network is critical for continuous bone ingrowth, as well as for vascularization and innervation of nascent tissue. It also impacts the transport properties of the scaffold.
Pore gradient	The difference in pore attributes in different scaffold regions	The presence of biomimetic gradient porosity can recapitulate the native bone architecture and can guide tissue ingrowth in vivo.
Surface area to volume ratio	The ratio of the total scaffold surface area to the total scaffold volume	A higher surface enhances cellular adhesion but leads to enhanced biodegradation.

(inverse method) can be employed to iteratively predict the material distribution that produces the desired elastic moduli while placing a constraint on the porosity (or vice versa) (Lin et al., 2004; Challis et al., 2010). For example, given a particular volume fraction, a unit cell microstructure with a cylindrical pore design is more permeable and less stiff than a spherical pore design (Hollister, 2005).

The direct approach, being a trial-and-error method to screen from a library of porous architectures, is computationally expensive but can accommodate the printing limitations such as producing the smallest feature sizes. While the inverse approach can generate porous scaffolds with the required properties, the scaffolds are not easily printable and therefore not manufacturable (Kelly et al., 2018). The increasing complexity and sophistication in scaffold designs call for a multifaceted approach to characterize the porous nature of the scaffold, which will enable better reproducibility and evaluation in animal studies (Table 5.1) (Salgado et al., 2004; Bose et al., 2013; Zhang et al., 2019; Cheng et al., 2019; Abbasi et al., 2020a; Kanwar & Vijayavenkataraman, 2021).

Since the scaffold is only intended to function as a temporary framework for host cells to deposit new mineralized tissue and, ultimately, designed to be entirely replaced by regenerated tissue, it should undergo controlled degradation by host enzymatic or biological processes. The scaffold's porosity also influences its degradation kinetics since higher porosity entails a greater surface area per unit volume and hence, faster degradation via chemical dissolution or enzymatic processes. Therefore, the biodegradation kinetics of the scaffold can also be tuned by varying the pore parameters to match those of bone regeneration to ensure optimal healing.

5.3 OVERVIEW OF 3D PRINTING TECHNIQUES

Traditional scaffold fabrication techniques such as chemical/gas foaming, particulate leaching, freeze drying, electrospinning, and thermally induced phase separation are limited in their ability to manufacture highly customizable, patient-specific scaffolds with tailored interconnected porous networks and hierarchical microarchitectures (Bose et al., 2013; Collins et al., 2021). Technological advances in 3D printing and advanced CAD methods have facilitated the production of highly reproducible scaffolds with greater control over the multiscale architecture, gradient porosity, pore size, microscale compositions, and tunable structural and mechanical properties in a cost-effective manner. This has opened new avenues for the design of sophisticated, biomimetic scaffold architectures that yield superior biological responses.

The 3D printing process relies on a CAD model derived from medical images of the patient. Medical imaging technologies such as MRI and CT generate cross-sectional 2D slices/images that are compiled on top of each other to create a 3D model of the target area. MRI scanners utilize strong magnetic fields and pulsating radio waves to map the location of water and adipose tissue in the body based on energy signals from hydrogen atoms in water and lipid molecules. CT, on the other hand, processes the X-ray attenuation data to produce images of the different tissues and organs. Because of the bone's low water and fat content and its high density, X-ray CT scans are generally preferred over MRI for generating better images of bone structures. Sometimes, computer modeling is required to construct the CAD model of the scaffold by comparing the medical images of the defect region and its analogous healthy counterpart.

While initially, 3D printing specifically referred to powder-based freeform fabrication in which an inkjet printhead was employed to deposit binders on a powder bed (Sachs et al., 1993), the definition has evolved to encompass a wide variety of processes that construct a 3D part in an additive manner, typically in a layer-by-layer fashion. Different 3D printing techniques operate via different mechanisms and pose some constraints on the properties of the material that can be printed (Figure 5.2). A detailed understanding of the process parameters and printing conditions, compatible material options, advantages, and limitations of these techniques can guide researchers in choosing the optimal 3D printing technique for BTE. Some of these techniques relevant to fabricating polymeric scaffolds are discussed in detail in Table 5.2 (Bose et al., 2013; Bedell et al., 2020; Qu et al., 2021).

TABLE 5.2
3D Printing Modalities

3D Printing Technique	Process Details	Materials	Pros	Cons
Fused deposition modeling (FDM) (also fused filament fabrication)	Heated polymer is extruded and hardens on cooling.	Thermoplastic polymers and their composites	No support structure is required.	Elevated temperatures are required to print the polymer in the molten phase.
Selective laser sintering (SLS)	A high-powered laser beam is used to fuse/bind powder particles into a solid construct.	Polymer powders and their composites	No support structure or post-processing is required. Process is fast.	Elevated temperatures are required. The resolution is dependent on the diameter of the laser beam.
Stereolithography (SLA)	A light beam is directed at specific spots based on computer design, which cures the polymer to form a solid construct.	Photocurable polymers and resins	Complex, high-resolution structures can be printed. Mild printing conditions enable the loading of cells, drugs, and other biological molecules.	Multimaterial structures are difficult to fabricate.
Digital light processing (DLP)	A digital light image of each layer of the 3D structure is projected, which leads to layer-by-layer photocrosslinking.	Photopolymerizable, low-viscous inks	Fast fabrication times Similar advantages as SLA	Limited multimaterial functionality
Inkjet	The ink droplets are ejected from the print head nozzle by applying thermal, piezoelectric, or electromagnetic forces.	Low-viscosity ink with rheopectic behavior	Low cost Ensures high viability of cells	Low printing accuracy
Extrusion	The ink is extruded from the nozzle and deposited on the print surface. Further crosslinking is required in some cases to ensure shape fidelity.	High-viscosity ink with shear-thinning behavior and thixotropic properties	Compatible with a wide variety of hydrogels Can support high cell densities and printing of cell spheroids	Process involves low resolution and slow printing speed. High shear forces may be detrimental to cell viability. Post-printing crosslinking steps are required.
Laser induced forward transfer (LIFT) (also laser assisted bioprinting	A laser pulse is projected on a shock-absorbing material that then dispenses the ink on the print bed. This is similar to inkjet printing, but the ink is not extruded through a nozzle in LIFT.	Low-viscosity ink	Supports high-density cell printing with high cell viability	Expensive Limited scope for multimaterial printing

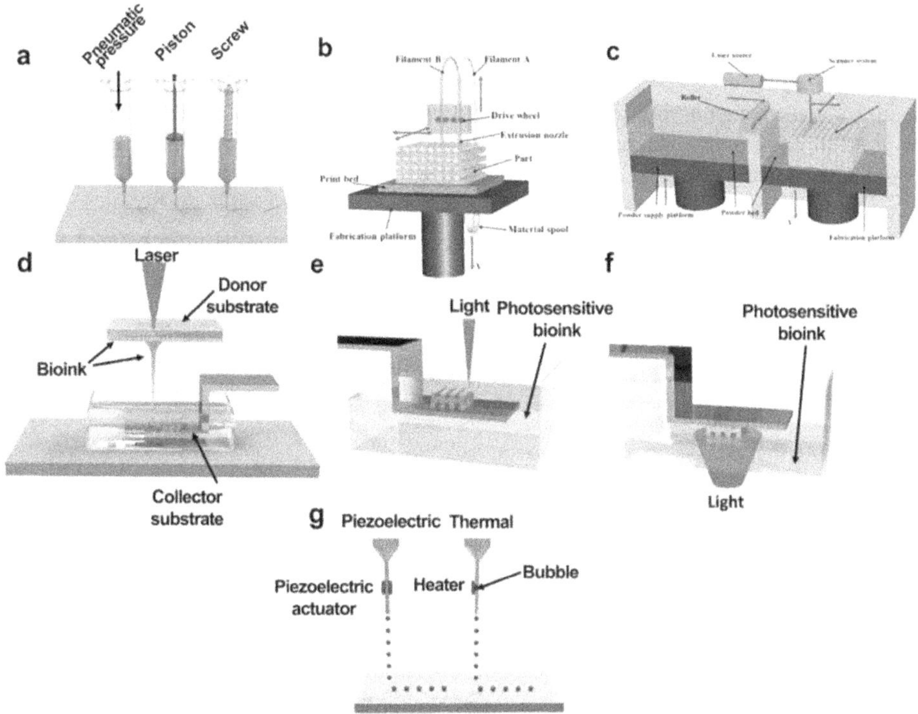

FIGURE 5.2 3D printing techniques: (a) extrusion, (b) FDM, (c) SLS, (d) LIFT, (e) SLA, (f) DLP, (g) ink-jet (reproduced under the terms of CC-BY 4.0 (https://creativecommons.org/licenses/by/4.0/) International License from Yi, H. G., Kim, H., Kwon, J., Choi, Y. J., Jang, J., & Cho, D. W.: Application of 3D bioprinting in the prevention and the therapy for human diseases. Sig. Transduct. Target Ther. 2021. 6. 177. Copyright 2021 The Authors, published by Springer Nature; Reproduced with permission from Wang, X., Jiang, M., Zhou, Z., Gou, J., & Hui, D.: 3D printing of polymer matrix composites: A review and prospective. Compos. B: Eng. 2017. 110. 442–458. Copyright 2017 Elsevier).

5.4 3D PRINTED/BIOPRINTED POLYMERIC BONE TISSUE SCAFFOLDS

Diverse material types and combinations including, but not limited to, natural/synthetic hydrogels, non-hydrogel-based polymers (polyesters, polyurethanes), bioceramics, biodegradable metals, composites, and hybrids have been explored as candidate materials to formulate ink compositions for 3D printing. In this section, we focus on 3D-printed/bioprinted polymeric scaffolds, which constitute the major category of materials used in BTE. Polymeric biomaterials used extensively in BTE can be classified as naturally derived materials (collagen, chitosan, cellulose, starch, alginate, gelatin, silk fibroin [SF], hyaluronic acid [HA]) or synthetic polymers (poly(ethylene glycol) [PEG], poly(vinyl alcohol) [PVA], poly(propylene fumarate), poly(ε-caprolactone) [PCL], poly(lactic acid) [PLA], poly(glycolic acid) [PGA], and their copolymers (poly(lactic-co-glycolic acid) [PLGA]) (Bedell et al., 2020).

Natural polymers have been extensively used in BTE owing to their low cost, chemical versatility, excellent biodegradability, and superior biological performance (low toxicity, presence of biofunctional molecules, and intrinsic osteogenic properties) (Guo et al., 2021). Owing to their hydrophilic character, these polymers are capable of forming hydrogels and support bioprinting.

However, the mechanical properties of natural polymers are typically low for load-bearing applications, and there remain concerns about potential immunogenicity and batch-to-batch variability (Koons et al., 2020).

To address these shortcomings, synthetic polymers have been formulated that can be appropriately tailored through a vast arsenal of chemical modifications in accordance with specific design requirements. However, synthetic polymers are often hydrophobic (water insoluble and cannot be used to encapsulate cells), lack cell-recognition sites, and must be extensively functionalized with cell-binding motifs such as RGD to achieve desired biological functions (Burdick & Anseth, 2002). In some cases, the bulk erosion of such polymer can cause the scaffold to fail in vivo, and the abrupt release and local accumulation of degradation products can trigger adverse inflammatory responses. This can be mitigated by manipulating the molecular weight, chemical composition (by copolymerization), and crystallinity to attain controlled biodegradation rates (Collins et al., 2021).

5.4.1 Natural Polymers

5.4.1.1 Alginate-Based Composite Scaffolds

Alginate is a linear polysaccharide that is predominantly derived from brown seaweed and has garnered significant attention for biomedical applications due to its exceptional biocompatibility, minimal toxicity, and propensity to undergo gelation in the presence of divalent cations like Ca^{2+}, Ba^{2+}, and Sr^{2+} (Alsberg et al., 2001; Augst et al., 2006; Venkatesan et al., 2015; Hernández-González et al., 2020). Ionically crosslinked hydrogels such as Ca-crosslinked alginates do not degrade but undergo dissolution of individual polymer chains, reducing mechanical strength mediated by loss of ions to the surrounding medium. However, alginate derivatives like oxidized alginate and poly(aldehyde guluronate) are known to undergo hydrolytic degradation (Drury & Mooney, 2003).

Park et al. (2018) synthesized a heparin-like alginate sulfate that exhibited a strong binding affinity for growth factors, thereby prolonging their biological activity. The authors prepared various alginate–sulfate/alginate bioinks to evaluate their feasibility in BTE. The addition of alginate–sulfate did not significantly affect the rheological properties or the printability of the bioinks. However, the alginate–sulfate-containing bioinks showed a greater and sustained release of bone morphogenetic protein-2 compared with the alginate-only ink. Furthermore, hydrogels that contained alginate-sulfate exhibited enhanced proliferation and differentiation of encapsulated MC3T3-E1 preosteoblasts and better cell growth and calcium deposition (Park et al., 2018). These findings highlight the potential of alginate-sulfate as a promising material for use in BTE.

Choe et al. (2019) investigated the potential of alginate/graphene oxide (GO) composite bioinks to enhance the rheological properties and osteoinductive abilities of alginate bioinks for use in BTE applications. The alginate/GO inks exhibited superior printability and structural stability compared with alginate-only inks. Notably, the presence of GO did not adversely affect the viability of human mesenchymal stem cells (hMSCs) encapsulated within the inks and, in fact, led to enhanced osteogenic induction of the hMSCs, as evidenced by higher alkaline phosphatase (ALP) activity, calcium deposition, and the expression of several osteogenic markers. These results suggest that incorporating GO into alginate bioinks holds great potential for improving the mechanical and biological performance of BTE constructs.

5.4.1.2 Chitosan-Based Composite Scaffolds

Chitosan is a linear polysaccharide derived from the deacetylation of chitin (found in the cell walls of fungi and crustacean exoskeletons) and bears a structural resemblance to naturally occurring glycosaminoglycans (GACs). Owing to its biodegradability, biocompatibility, and antimicrobial activity, chitosan has been widely used in the field of tissue engineering (Venkatesan & Kim, 2010; Lan Levengood & Zhang, 2014). Chitosan is insoluble at neutral pH but becomes soluble in dilute acids because of the protonation of the free amino groups. It has garnered significant attention for its positive impact on osteoblast activity and osteogenic differentiation in vitro (Klokkevold et al., 1996), as well as its efficacy in promoting bone repair in various animal models (Muzzarelli et al., 1993; Lee et al., 2000).

Zafeiris et al. (2021) fabricated chitosan/hydroxyapatite (HAp) scaffolds with customized shapes and a lattice-like microarchitecture via direct ink writing, matching the porosity and modulus of cancellous bone. Following 3D printing, the scaffolds were lyophilized to generate self-standing structures that imitate the microscale porosity and interconnectivity present in the natural bone. The biocompatibility of these scaffolds was assessed using MG63 human osteosarcoma cells. Preliminary results indicated that the scaffold's internal microarchitecture supported cell attachment and spreading and provided a conducive microenvironment for cell proliferation while maintaining high cell viability. Nonetheless, the osteoinductive capacity, gene expression, and mineralization of the chitosan/HAp scaffolds in long-term cell culture remain to be investigated for future applications.

Demirtaş et al. (2017) synthesized a bioprintable form of chitosan hydrogel (chitosan + glycerol phosphate + nano HAp + MC3T3-E1 preosteoblast cells) that is pH and thermosensitive in nature and allows extrusion printing at neutral pH. The printing process and hydrogel formulation were biocompatible and maintained high levels of cell viability. The inclusion of Hap further led to enhanced proliferation, and cytomorphological changes indicated the differentiation of preosteoblasts into mineralized and mature osteoblasts. The bioprinted hydrogels were also mechanically stable post-printing under simulated physiological conditions and outperformed similar alginate inks in terms of cell viability, proliferation, and osteogenic differentiation.

Chang et al. (2022) used a water-soluble glycol chitosan to synthesize photocurable methacrylated glycol chitosan (MeGC) by reacting with glycidyl methacrylate. The MeGC precursor solution, containing MG-63 cells, was crosslinked with visible light to generate a printable ink with optimal shape fidelity for extrusion-based bioprinting. The irradiation time was varied to achieve the optimal rheological properties, biocompatibility, and osteogenic differentiation of the bioink. This study proposes MeGC bioinks as an alternate chitosan-based bioprintable ink for fabricating applications in BTE.

5.4.1.3 HA-Based Composite Scaffolds

HA is a linear disaccharide and one of the simplest GACs and is generally extracted from genetically modified bacterial cultures. It constitutes a vital component of the human ECM, imparting elasticity and hydrophilicity to tissues and exhibiting inherent bioactivity (Collins & Birkinshaw, 2013; Xing et al., 2020). Additionally, HA can undergo degradation by hyaluronidase present in cells and serum (Patterson et al., 2010). The osteogenic efficacy of HA is contingent upon its molecular weight and concentration (Huang et al., 2003), although certain investigations suggest that the favorable osteogenic outcomes of HA stem from its degradation products that remain entrapped within the highly viscous high-molecular-weight HA (Sasaki & Watanabe, 1995).

Lee et al. (2018) developed a hybrid HA-based bioink (acrylated HA and tyramine-conjugated HA + hMSCs) with fast gelation kinetics (less than 200 sec) with an elastic modulus of ~ 1 kPa that had been previously reported to show higher MSC proliferation (Kim et al., 2008). The acrylated HA was also conjugated with different biofunctional peptides to induce angiogenesis and angiogenic differentiation of stem cells. The hydrogel scaffolds fabricated via bioprinting demonstrated high cell viability and retained their structural integrity. From gene expression results, it was concluded that hydrogels functionalized with BMP-7-derived peptide and substance P peptide could simultaneously support both bone regeneration and vascularization.

Poldervaart et al. (2017) modified HA by reaction with methacrylic anhydride to obtain photopolymerizable methacrylated hyaluronic acid (MeHA). The precursor hydrogel solution containing MeHA and photoinitiator was extrusion 3D printed and subsequently irradiated with ultraviolet (UV) light to enable photo-crosslinking. However, low-concentration solutions lacked shape fidelity and collapsed under their own weight before they could be crosslinked (Figure 5.3(f)). While the MeHA hydrogel scaffolds supported the survival of encapsulated human bone-marrow-derived MSCs and displayed intrinsic osteogenicity, the cell survival, morphology, and osteogenic differentiation were found to be highly dependent on polymer concentration. Taking into consideration printability and in vitro cell studies, an optimal polymer concentration of 2.5% was identified for the bioprinting of bone tissue scaffolds (Poldervaart et al., 2017).

Owing to the favorable osteoinductive ability of HA, Zhai et al. (2018) employed a high-concentration (20%) HA solution with encapsulated rat osteoblasts (ROBs) as a sacrificial bioink to improve the short-term viability, distribution uniformity, and deposition efficiency of osteoblasts within a nanocomposite hydrogel scaffold (polyethylene glycol diacrylate (PEGDA)/laponite XLG nanoclay). The ROBs released as a consequence of HA dissolution displayed better proliferation and differentiation than ROBs that were directly seeded onto the PEGDA-nanoclay scaffold, which was further confirmed by in vivo tibia repair and ectopic conduction experiments.

5.4.1.4 SF-Based Composite Scaffolds

SF is the fibrous protein part of silk that is produced by insects such as silkworms (e.g., *Bombyx mori*) and orb-weaving spiders (e.g., *Nephila clavipes*). SF is gaining traction for BTE because of its ease of processability, remarkable mechanical properties, excellent biocompatibility, minimal immunogenicity, and controlled proteolytic biodegradability (Vepari & Kaplan, 2007; Melke et al., 2016; Sun et al., 2021).

Fitzpatrick et al. (2021) printed porous SF/HAp bone cement scaffolds to facilitate vascularization and innervation of nascent bone following dental, oral, or maxillofacial surgery. The bioactive components, namely, bone morphogenetic protein-2 (for osteoinduction), vascular endothelial growth factor (VEGF, for angiogenesis), and neural growth factor (for innervation), were incorporated either by mixing with the bone cement prior to extrusion 3D printing or by soaking the scaffold in the morphogen solution post-printing. The synergistic effect of these morphogens enhanced the osteoblastic differentiation of human mesenchymal stem cells (hMSCs), increased proliferation of human umbilical vein endothelial cells (HUVECs), and neuronal differentiation of human-induced neural stem cells. Owing to their osteoconductivity and potential of osseointegration in vivo, the authors proposed the use of these SF/HAp bone cement scaffolds for non-load-bearing applications such as alveolar ridge augmentation (Fitzpatrick et al., 2021).

Zhou et al. (2021) incorporated tripeptide glycyl-l-histidyl-l-lysine (GHK)-copper (Cu) complex within 3D-printed silk scaffolds to accelerate bone repair and promote angiogenesis. The sustained release of GHK-Cu displayed therapeutic effects similar to those from free copper ions without the risk of toxicity and side effects associated with free copper Is (Figure 5.3(e)). The released GHK-Cu promoted osteogenic differentiation of bone marrow-derived stem cells (BMSCs) in the early stages of bone repair and HUVEC migration and tube formation via paracrine signaling by BMSCs. Implanting BMSC-seeded scaffolds in critical-sized calvarial bone defects in rats resulted in significantly enhanced vascularized bone regeneration compared with scaffolds without GHK-Cu, highlighting the potential of bioactive ion-based biomaterial strategies for BTE.

Rajput et al. (2022) synthesized a photo-crosslinkable derivative of SF, namely methacrylated-SF (SF-MA), by modifying SF with glycidyl methacrylate. MC3T3-E1 preosteoblast-laden SF-MA bioinks of varying polymer concentrations were investigated as a bioink for digital light processing (DLP) printing in terms of printing resolution and physical, rheological, and mechanical properties, as well as the potential for osteogenic differentiation. Various intricate bone-like architectures resembling the trabecular bone, Haversian systems, and vascular networks could be printed, highlighting the excellent printability of the bioink. An intermediate polymer concentration was identified to be the most efficient in driving the osteogenic differentiation of the encapsulated preosteoblasts even in the absence of soluble factors, thus making it a viable and promising candidate for bioprinting bone-mimetic structures (Figure 5.3(a–d)). Similar photopolymerizable polymers such as methacrylated-κ-carrageenancan (Kumari et al., 2022), methacrylated carboxymethyl cellulose (Melilli et al., 2020), and methacrylated chitosan (Shen et al., 2020) can also be explored for BTE applications using DLP printing.

5.4.1.5 Gelatin-Based Composite Scaffolds

Gelatin is a protein obtained from the irreversible denaturation of animal collagen and undergoes reversible thermal gelation, forming a triple-helix structure when the temperature is below 30 °C. In addition to its nontoxic and biocompatible nature, gelatin is rich in RGD (arginine-glycine-aspartic acid) motifs that enable excellent cell adhesion and spreading (Lukin et al., 2022). However, gelatin exhibits fast biodegradation under normal physiological conditions and has relatively low mechanical properties. Therefore, it is often blended with other biomaterials to enhance its suitability for use in BTE applications (C Echave et al., 2017).

Allen et al. (2022) developed a gelatin methacryloyl (GelMA)-gelatin-HAp bioink compatible with extrusion-based bioprinting for BTE applications. Adding gelatin facilitated the printing of GelMA at low concentrations, which is favorable for cell viability and proliferation. Furthermore, including HAp in the bioink slowed down enzymatic degradation, promoted osteoblastic proliferation and mineralization, and enhanced osteogenic gene expression without compromising cell viability and proliferation. Kara et al. (2022) incorporated decellularized bone particles (dbPTs) (rich in collagen and hydroxyapatite) as the bioactive reinforcing agent in a gelatin matrix to mimic the inorganic and organic components of the bone. Inks containing dbPTs of different concentrations were 3D printed, crosslinked with microbial transglutaminase, and lyophilized to obtain a highly porous scaffold with micro and macropores. This composite scaffold promoted the attachment, spreading, proliferation, and migration of MC3T3-E1 preosteoblast cells, indicating its potential for BTE.

To create functional vascularized bone tissue, Byambaa et al. (2017) fabricated a micro-architectured bone tissue scaffold with distinct vasculogenic and osteogenic niches using two GelMA bioinks with different degrees of methacryloyl substitution. Specifically, a central cylinder was bioprinted using VEGF-functionalized GelMA hydrogel with low methacryloyl substitution and was laden with HUVECs and hMSCs. In contrast, the outer cylinders were bioprinted using hMSC-laden GelMA hydrogel with high methacryloyl substitution and contained silica nanoplatelets with different concentrations of conjugated VEGF to generate a concentration gradient. The rapid degradation of the inner GelMA core led to the formation of a perfusable channel that was eventually lined by HUVECs and pericytes differentiated from hMSCs, forming a vessel-like lumen structure. Additionally, the presence of silica nanoplatelets and VEGF in the outer cylinders promoted osteogenic differentiation of the hMSCs.

5.4.2 Synthetic Polymers

5.4.2.1 PCL-Based Composite Scaffolds

PCL is a thermoplastic polyester with high mechanical strength and excellent blend compatibility and can be extruded at its glass transition temperature of 60 °C. The gradual in vivo hydrolytic degradation of PCL facilitates its utilization as a long-term load-bearing support during bone regeneration and the ossification of the scaffold (Yang et al., 2021). PCL is also popular as it is among the few synthetic polymers included in US Food and Drug Administration (FDA)-approved medical products. However, its lack of cell-adhesion properties necessitates surface functionalization or modification of surface characteristics for improved cell attachment (Koons et al., 2020).

Nyberg et al. (2017) employed FDM printing to fabricate porous PCL scaffolds functionalized with commercially and clinically used mineral additives such as tricalcium phosphate (TCP), HAp, Bio-Oss, and decellularized bone matrix (DCB). The presence of these mineral additives did not compromise the scaffold's mechanical properties, which ranged from 32 to 83 MPa for porous scaffolds. While the use of natural bone-derived matrix (PCL/Bio-Oss, PCL/DCB) resulted in a 10-fold increase in the expression of collagen I and osteocalcin genes (compared with only PCL) when adipose-derived stem cells were cultured on the scaffolds, synthetic additives (TCP and HAp) also led to enhanced osteoinductivity, although to a much lesser extent than Bio-Oss and DCB.

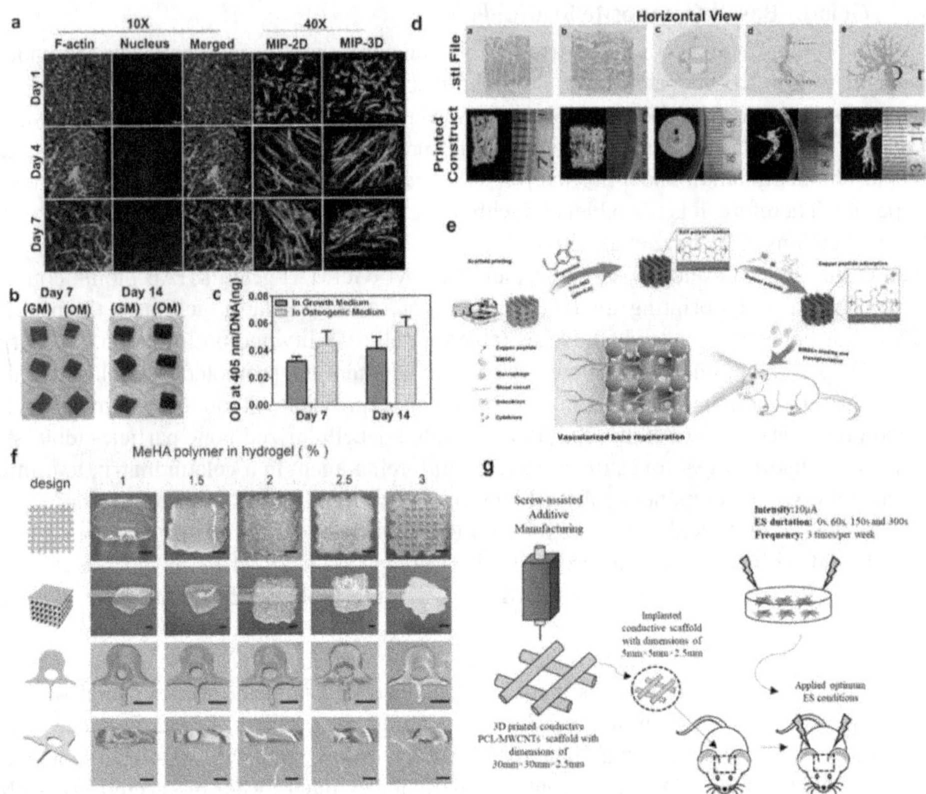

FIGURE 5.3 (a) The changes in the morphology of encapsulated MC3T3-E1 cells with time. (b) Digital photograph showing the calcium deposition in the SF-MA hydrogels stained with Alizarin Red dye; darker staining represents more calcium deposition (GM: growth medium, OM: osteogenic medium). (c) Plot of calcium deposition normalized to DNA content. (d) Fabrication of bone-mimetic architectures using SF-MA inks, demonstrating its excellent printability (reproduced with permission from Rajput, M., Mondal, P., Yadav, P., & Chatterjee, K.: Light-based 3D bioprinting of bone tissue scaffolds with tunable mechanical properties and architecture from photocurable silk fibroin. Int. J. Biol. Macromol. 2022. 202. 644–656. CopyrigI2022 Elsevier). (e) Schematic representation showing the fabrication of GHK-Cu-loaded 3D-printed silk scaffolds and its role in vascularized bone regeneration (reproduced with permission from Zhou, M., Wu, X., Luo, J., Yang, G., Lu, Y., Lin, S., Jiang, F., Zhang, W., & Jiang, X.: Copper peptide-incorporated 3D-printed silk-based scaffolds promote vascularized bone regeneration. Chem. Eng. J. 2021. 422. 130147. Copyright 2021 Elsevier). (f) Printability of Me-HA inks of different concentrations (reproduced under the terms of CC-BY 4.0 (https://creativecommons.org/licenses/by/4.0/) International License from Poldervaart, M. T., Goversen, B., Ruijter, M. de, Abbadessa, A., Melchels, F. P. W., Öner, F. C., Dhert, W. J. A., Vermonden, T., & Alblas, J.: 3D bioprinting of methacrylated hyaluronic acid (MeHA) hydrogel with intrinsic osteogenicity. PLOS ONE. 2017. 12. e0177628. Copyright 2017 Poldervaart et al., published by PLOS). (g) Schematic illustration of the experimental setup; the electroconductive PCL/MWCNT scaffolds are implanted in the rat calvarial defect and provided electrical stimulation for enhanced bone regeneration (reproduced under the terms of CC-BY 4.0 (https://creativecommons.org/licenses/by/4.0/) International License from e Silva, E. P., Huang, B., Helaehil, J. V., Nalesso, P. R. L., Bagne, L., de Oliveira, M. A., Albiazetti, G. C. C., Aldalbahi, A., El-Newehy, M., Santamaria-Jr, M., Mendonça, F. A. S., Bártolo, P., & Caetano, G. F.: In vivo study of conductive 3D printed PCL/MWCNTs scaffolds with electrical stimulation for bone tissue engineering. Bio-Des. Manuf. 2021. 4. 190–202. Copyright 2021 e Silva et al., published by Springer Nature).

Xu et al. (2014) evaluated the osteoconduction potential of PCL/HAp scaffolds for the in vivo repair of a partial segmental defect in the goat femur. Using CT-guided FDM, the authors 3D-printed porous PCL/HAp (pore diameter = 765 ± 83 µm, strand thickness = 280 ± 33 µm) and PCL (pore diameter = 746 ± 71 µm, strand thickness = 275 ± 28 µm) 3D artificial bones with both cortical and cancellous bone-like regions mimicking natural goat femurs. The PCL/HAp and PCL artificial bones were compared with BAM artificial bone and autologous bone (current primary options for repair of bone in load-bearing sites) on various parameters, including in vivo scaffold performance. The results indicated that PCL/HAp scaffolds possess osteoconductive abilities similar to those of autologous bone and mechanical properties closest to those of native bone, making them a compelling alternative to BAM artificial bones, which have limited shaping ability, excessive osteoconductivity, and poor mechanical strength and elastic modulus.

Xue et al. (2022) rationally designed a dexamethasone sodium phosphate-loaded CuS nanoparticle-PEG composite hydrogel coated 3D PCL scaffold as a multifunctional soft–hard scaffold to repair large bone defects. Incorporating CuS nanoparticles imparted excellent photothermal properties to the scaffold, and near infrared light-triggered local hyperthermia enhanced osteogenic differentiation in vitro and accelerated bone regeneration in vivo. While the 3D-printed (FDM) PCL component provided a rigid, structural framework, the hydrophilic PEG hydrogel served as a soft matrix for controlled and sustained drug release, cell adhesion, and interfacing with the surrounding bone tissues.

The release of active copper ions from the scaffold also conferred an antibacterial effect and augmented osteogenesis through the activation of VEGF and hypoxia-inducible factor-1α signaling pathways. This study highlights that the synergistic effect of photothermal therapy and osteogenesis-inducing drugs through multifunctional scaffolds may be a promising and efficient approach for the repair of bone defects. Electro-conductive composite scaffolds incorporating conductive polymers such as polypyrrole, polyaniline, and poly(3,4-ethylenedioxythiophene), as well as inorganic conductive materials, including graphene, carbon nanofibers, and carbon nanotubes are capable of transmitting electrical stimulation and promoting osteogenesis (Qu et al., 2021).

In another study, e Silva et al. (2021) investigated the effect of exogenous electrical stimulation on BTE by fabricating 3D-printed (extrusion-based) porous electro-conductive PCL/multiwall carbon nanotubes (MWCNTs) scaffolds. The PCL matrix reinforced with MWCNTs exhibited improved compressive modulus and surface hardness while preserving desirable pore characteristics. The combination of conductive PCL/MWCNT scaffolds and the electrical stimulation resulted in the formation of denser, more mineralized, and connective bone tissue as well as increased angiogenesis in animal bone defect models, providing yet another promising avenue for BTE (Figure 5.3(g)).

Lee et al. (2015) developed a coaxial extrusion 3D printing method to create multimaterial composite scaffolds with a core-shell architecture. The scaffold consisted of micro-sized struts with an inner polycaprolactone (PCL) core for mechanical support and an outer alginate shell loaded with bioactive phenamil methanesulfonate (PM) to induce osteoblastic differentiation and mineralization. By optimizing the PM concentration, the composite scaffolds exhibited higher MC3T3-E1 cell viability and ALP activity than PCL-only alginate scaffolds. The core-shell 3D printing technique demonstrated in this study can be used to impart bioactivity to scaffolds made of synthetic, hydrophobic polymers such as PCL and PLA.

5.4.2.2 PLA and Copolymer-Based Composite Scaffolds

PLA is another stiff, biocompatible, and low-cost thermoplastic polyester that is easily printable at its glass transition temperature of 65 °C. Its hydrolysis products are nontoxic (lactic acid), and it possesses adequate mechanical strength for load-bearing applications. The properties of PLA, including processability, mechanical strength, biodegradation rate, and biocompatibility, can be tuned by copolymerizing with various monomers, resulting in copolymers such as poly(lactic acid-co-glycolic acid) (PLGA), poly(lactic acid-co-caprolactone), poly(lactic acid-co-ethylene glycol), and poly(lactic acid-co-glutamic acid) (Narayanan et al., 2016). PLA is also approved by FDA for use in biomedical applications such as sutures and orthopedic and dental devices.

Zhang et al. (2022) fabricated a biomimetically hierarchical PLA/HAp scaffold with a porosity gradient that resembled the variations between cortical and cancellous bone regions using an FDM 3D printer. The scaffold was then infused with a soft gelatin methacryloyl hydrogel containing deferoxamine@poly(ε-caprolactone) nanoparticles (DFO@PCL NPs) and manganese carbonyl nanosheets to mimic the native extracellular milieu as well as to augment the local immune response of implantation. In vitro and in vivo analyses revealed the favorable osteo-immunomodulatory, osteoinductive, and angiogenic properties of this hybrid scaffold, making it well-suited for the repair of sizeable segmental bone defects.

A similar approach can increase the bioactivity of 3D-printed porous PLA scaffolds. Rajput et al. (2023) fabricated a porous PLA scaffold using an FDM printer and treated it with NaOH to increase the surface wettability. An hMSC-laden silk fibroin/alginate blend hydrogel was then introduced into the scaffold through the pores located between the PLA struts. The resulting hybrid scaffold exhibited a compressive modulus similar to that of cancellous bone and remained stable in an aqueous buffer solution for more than three weeks. Compared with a neat PLA scaffold, the hybrid scaffold showed significant enhancements in hMSC viability, proliferation, and osteogenic differentiation. The hybrid scaffold's optimum mechanical strength and bioactivity make it a promising strategy for bone repair and regeneration.

Surface engineering strategies can also be employed to enhance the bioactivity of neat PLA scaffolds. Jaidev and Chatterjee (2019) functionalized alkali-treated 3D-printed PLA scaffolds through covalent conjugation with polyethyleneimine (PEI) and citric acid (CA) via carbodiimide chemistry. The presence of CA on the PLA surface led to the precipitation of calcium and phosphate ions when immersed in simulated body fluid, resulting in the deposition of hydroxyapatite (HAp) crystals and surface mineralization of the scaffolds. The resulting PLA-HAp scaffolds exhibited significantly higher adhesion and proliferation of human mesenchymal stem cells (hMSCs) as well as improved osteogenic differentiation and mineralization than did PLA-only scaffolds. Using a similar approach, Nilawar and Chatterjee (2022) deposited ceria nanoparticles (instead of HAp) onto PEI and CA-grafted 3D-printed PLA scaffolds. The nanoceria-decorated scaffolds demonstrated reactive oxygen species scavenging and antibacterial properties, along with enhanced osteogenic differentiation, in contrast with alkali-treated PLA scaffolds. These works demonstrate a facile and versatile approach to augmenting the surface properties of neat PLA scaffolds for superior cell-material interactions and osteogenic activity.

Wei et al. (2022) introduced PVA-modified HAp microspheres into a PLGA matrix to fabricate (via extrusion-based printing) 3D scaffolds that possess superior mechanical properties and an inorganic composition similar to that of natural bone. Incorporating HAp microspheres led to a sixfold increase in compressive modulus compared with pure PLGA scaffolds and helped maintain the weak alkalinity of the degradation solution, even in the presence of acidic degradation products of PIGA. Moreover, the PLGA/HAp scaffolds exhibited improved cell adhesion, proliferation, and osteogenic differentiation of BMSCs and promoted osteogenesis and osseointegration in vivo.

Dou et al. (2021) fabricated a hierarchical bone-mimetic scaffold by infusing gelatin solution within a PLGA/nano HAp (PH) framework and subsequently lyophilizing it. While the extrusion-printed PH scaffold lends structural support, the gelatin network (G) is conducive for cell adhesion and protein adsorption. From in vivo rat femoral defect model data, it was concluded that the PHG scaffold presented denser and more continuous trabecular bone morphology and generated a better osteogenic response than the PH scaffold. The PHG scaffold also exhibited significant bone ingrowth at the defect site, resulting in a tight implant-natural tissue interface. The integration of different biofabrication techniques and the combination of natural and synthetic components, as demonstrated in this study, present a promising approach for the design of advanced 3D-printed scaffolds.

5.5 4D PRINTING

While 3D printing has made considerable advances in tissue engineering, it is not without its limitations. Tissues that are 3D printed are static and inanimate and cannot respond to physiochemical or biochemical cues, rendering them incapable of performing critical biological functions. Hence, there has been tremendous interest in developing 3D-printed scaffolds that can undergo dynamic changes in shape or configuration, transform their functionality, or alter properties in response to external (temperature, electric and magnetic fields, light, pH ions) or internal (cell traction forces) cues with the aid of smart materials or through built-in actuation mechanisms in the scaffold design. In a further advance, 4D printing refers to the inclusion of precise temporal control over the printed construct after leaving the print bed, in addition to the already present spatial command in the x, y, and z dimensions of the 3D printer.

Although 4D printing technology is hardly a decade old, it has witnessed rapid progress and widespread applications in biomedical engineering. The capabilities of 4D-printed scaffolds to undergo preprogrammed changes in shape and functionalities offers exciting avenues to design biomimetic tissue engineering constructs. In the context of BTE, 4D printing can be employed to engineer orthopedic scaffolds that can be first reshaped to facilitate its delivery into an irregular bone cavity in a minimally invasive manner through a small incision and subsequently stimulated to morph its shape to precisely fit the boundaries of the defect cavity.

This will be instrumental in reducing the risk of secondary trauma associated with surgical procedures and lead to better patient compliance. Strategies implementing 4D printing are also instrumental in creating complex shapes and constructs that are difficult to realize through conventional 3D printing technologies. For example, 4D printing can be adopted to impart complex curvatures mimicking the surface topology of the bone by encoding stresses in the print design, followed by structural evolution as a result of stimuli-triggered stress relaxation (Huang et al., 2017).

It can also be used to rapidly self-fold thin, flat sheets into microvessels with diameters matching those of blood capillaries and venules (as low as 50 μm) in a simple, fast, and facile manner. Such 4D-printed microvessels can be incorporated within the bone tissue scaffolds to facilitate the development of microvasculature and nervous networks, which is essential for large bone tissue scaffolds. A similar strategy can be beneficial for constructing long, hollow cylindrical constructs to recapitulate the functional units of the cortical bone, namely osteons (diameter between 150 to 350 μm) and Haversian systems (diameter between 60 to 90 μm) to mimic the hierarchical architecture of the bone tissue. The 4D printing technology also promises to create dynamic, phasic, or reconfigurable bone tissue scaffolds that self-remodel or functionally mature over time to better adapt to the physiological environment and dynamics of the healing tissue. For a comprehensive overview of recent developments in 4D-printed bone tissue scaffolds, the reader is directed to the supplementary file of this chapter.

5.6 INTRAOPERATIVE BIOPRINTING

Intraoperative bioprinting (IOB, also referred to as in situ bioprinting, in vivo bioprinting, or intravital bioprinting) is emerging as a promising technique for repairing and regenerating cutaneous tissue such as bone, cartilage, and skin (Li et al., 2023). In IOB, the bioink is directly positioned at the defect site in the living subject under surgical settings based on the information obtained from real-time processing of high-resolution digital images of the defect site (Figure 5.4(a)) (Moncal et al., 2022a; Wu et al., 2020). While IOB has yet to make its way into clinics, it offers several advantages in comparison with the conventional in vitro 3D printing/bioprinting of tissue scaffolds.

While prefabricated scaffolds may swell, contract, or deform in shape (as a consequence of ECM remodeling by the encapsulated cells) over time in the cell culture medium, direct printing into the defect site enables precisely fitting the printed material with the defect boundary (Ozbolat, 2015). Multi-axis robotic printheads capable of depositing bioinks on inclined/irregular surfaces can facilitate the in situ fabrication of scaffolds that conform to the complex, natural topographies of the defect site. By doing away with several key steps that are necessary in the conventional lab-to-clinic workflow (in vitro culture of bioprinted scaffolds for several weeks, implanting the irregularly shaped scaffolds during surgery, reshaping the scaffold to fit the defect geometry), IOB offers an efficient route for the rapid on-site management of tissue injuries and significantly reduces the risks of contamination during transportation or impairment of fragile hydrogel-based tissue scaffolds during implantation or suturing (Zhao et al., 2023).

More importantly, the neighboring native microenvironment can act as a natural bioreactor and direct the differentiation of stem cells or progenitor cells into tissue-specific lineages through endogenous biophysical or biochemical cues and thus bypass the extensive, time-consuming process of in vitro cell differentiation (Ozbolat, 2015; Wu et al., 2020). However, fundamental issues remain to be addressed, such as developing novel bioinks that can support bioprinting in the unique intracorporeal microenvironment (physiological temperature, wet surroundings, dynamic tissue interfaces, acidic pH condition), fast fabrication methods to reduce operating time, rapid in situ crosslinking mechanisms using mild agents to ensure high cell viability, customized and automated printers with precise motions that can adapt their print paths, and orientation of printheads following the dynamic wound environment so that there is minimum interference of the print tip/nozzle (extrusion) with the defect extremities.

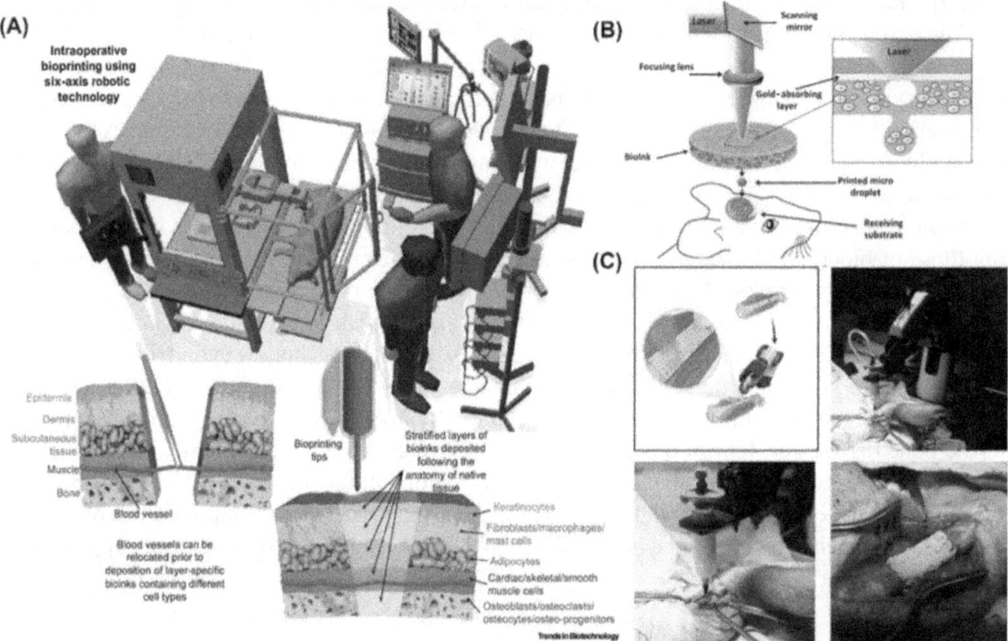

FIGURE 5.4 (a) Conceptual schematic illustration of intraoperative bioprinting in a surgical setting (reproduced with permission from Wu, Y., Ravnic, D. J., & Ozbolat, I. T.: Intraoperative Bioprinting: Repairing Tissues and Organs in a Surgical Setting. Trends. Biotechnol. 2020. 38. 594–605. Copyright 2020 Elsevier); (b) schematic illustration of intraoperative printing via LAB for the repair of mouse calvaria defect (reproduced under the terms of CC-BY 4.0 (https://creativecommons.org/licenses/by/4.0/) International License from Keriquel, V., Oliveira, H., Rémy, M., Ziane, S., Delmond, S., Rousseau, B., Rey, S., Catros, S., Amédée, J., Guillemot, F., & Fricain, J. C.: In situ printing of mesenchymal stromal cells, by laser-assisted bioprinting, for in vivo bone regeneration applications. Sci. Rep. 2017. 7. 1778. Copyright 2017 Keriquel et al., published by Springer Nature); (c) demonstration of intraoperative printing where a porous scaffold is directly printed at the defect site in a live subject with a robotic manipulator-based 3D printer (reproduced under the terms of CC-BY-NC-ND (https://creativecommons.org/licenses/by-nc-nd/4.0/) International License from Li, L., Shi, J., Ma, K., Jin, J., Wang, P., Liang, H., Cao, Y., Wang, X., & Jiang, Q.: Robotic in situ 3D bio-printing technology for repairing large segmental bone defects. J. Adv. Res. 2021. 30. 75–84. Copyright 2021 Li et al., published by Elsevier).

When Campbell and Weiss (2007) first proposed the concept of in situ bioprinting using inkjet technology in 2007, they argued that clinicians are more likely to opt for more straightforward off-the-shelf solutions rather than custom-printing tissue constructs on the operating table. Since then, there have been limited reports on IOB because of the elaborate requirements in terms of bioprinting modalities and the complexity involved with bioprinting within a live patient. However, this is poised to change in the coming years with the burgeoning advances in computer vision, sensing technologies, robot-assisted bioprinting modalities, and bioink formulations compatible with the demanding intracorporeal printing conditions.

Based on a previous study (Keriquel et al., 2010), Keriquel et al. (2017) developed an in situ laser-assisted bioprinting (LAB, or laser-induced forward transfer) approach to repair mice calvarial bone defect using a cellularized bioink comprising high-density (1.2×10^8 cells/mL) D1 cells (multipotent mouse bone marrow stromal precursor cells) and a nano-hydroxyapatite (nHA)n-collagen ink and tested the effect of two different morphologies (ring and disk) of cellular ink printing (Figure 5.4(b)). Two nHA-collagen disks were printed before and after cellular ink deposition to confine the cells in their morphology (disk or ring) as well as provide an osteoinductive matrix for the printed cells. Results from micro-CT indicated that there was marginal bone formation, restricted to the periphery of the defect in case of nHA-collagen material with D1 cells in a ring geometry even after two months. In contrast, the nHA-collagen with D1 cells in a disk geometry displayed homogeneous distribution of new osseous bone throughout the defect site; fully matured bone tissue formed even at the center of the defect.

Building on that study, Kérourédan et al. (2019) investigated the ability of LAB to guide the in vivo neovascularization of bone defects in a defined architecture and in turn, promote bone regeneration. To this end, a HUVEC bioink was printed on top of a collagen substrate containing VEGF and SCAPs (stem cells from apical papilla) that was deposited directly over the mouse dura mater. Post-printing, an additional layer of the collagen substrate was applied for the same purposes as in the previous study.

While random seeding of the cells led to interconnected but weakly organized vascular structures, primarily outside of the defect region, a vascularized area was observed for the ring geometry at two months, consistent with the initial printed pattern. The initial pattern was distorted for the cases of disk and closed circle geometries, but endothelial networks covered the entire region. While none of these conditions led to *ad integrum* bone regeneration, the disk and close-circle geometries showed a significant increase in bone regeneration compared to control groups (no implant, only collagen) (Kérourédan et al., 2019).

Li et al. (2017) explored the feasibility of treating segmental bone defects through in situ 3D printing utilizing high-resolution 3D scanning and robotic bioprinters. To create a model of the bone defect that needed to be 3D printed, the 3D scans of the damaged humeral bone (of a deceased New Zealand rabbit) and its corresponding healthy counterpart were processed and subtracted to generate the defect model. Alginate (partially crosslinked with $CaCl_2$)-PEGDA (poly(ethylene glycol) diacrylate) ink was directly printed into the defect and simultaneously UV-crosslinked to impart stability to thelinted part (Figure 5.4(c)). The authors hypothesized that the interpenetrating polymer network of alginate and PEGDA would lend sufficient mechanical strength and stiffness while it underwent regeneration and remodeling. Prompted by the successful implementation of this approach, the authors proceeded to employ this technique for fixing bone defects in large, living animals (pigs) in vivo (Li et al., 2021).

A similar biocompatible ink comprising partially-crosslinked alginate, PEGDA, and GelMA was extrusion-printed in a long segmental defect in the tibia (as well as internal fixation by a titanium plate to preserve tibial strength), with the help of a robotically assisted 3D bioprinter and photopolymerized after the printing of each layer. After three months, this experimental group presented a continuous cortical bone structure and an improved morphology with osteoblasts arranged regularly and in a compact fashion, indicating more active osteogenesis than in the blank control group (only internal fixation by titanium plate with no printed implant in the defect).

Moncal et al. (2021) developed a paste-like, shear-thinning, hard-tissue ink (HT ink) consisting of high-concentration collagen, chitosan (CS), nano-hydroxyapatite particles, and β-glycerophosphate disodium salt hydrate (βGP, as an osteogenesis induction reagent) for extrusion-based IOB. At body temperature, CS and βGP undergo temperature-induced physical crosslinking and a sol-gel phase transformation, which lends printability and shape fidelity to collagen. The HT ink encapsulated with primary rat bone marrow stem cells (rBMSCs) displayed favorable osteogenic properties without requiring any external osteogenic induction.

The defect created in the parietal bone was first scanned to generate the bioprinting path plan and subsequently filled through IOB using the HT ink with or without the inclusion of recombinant human bone morphogenetic protein-2 (rhBMP-2). After six weeks, the HT ink only and HT ink + rhBMP-2 groups exhibited greater bone volume to total bone volume, normalized bone mineral density, bone coverage area, and vascularization than the empty defect (control) group. Given that cell-based scaffolds tend to reduce hydrogel stiffness, accelerate degradation, and lead to instability, acellular forms of intraoperatively bioprinted constructs can also be explored as an effective and practical strategy for enhanced bone regeneration through the controlled in situ delivery of gene-based growth factors using nonviral gene vectors (Moncal et al., 2022a, 2022b).

CONCLUSION

The growing demand for customized, patient-specific bone tissue implants necessitates the development of new and innovative biofabrication techniques. Emerging technologies such as 4D printing and IOB show promise in mitigating some of the challenges associated with bioprinting and implanting these scaffolds at the defect site. However, regenerating vascularized and innervated bone tissue remains a formidable challenge in the field, owing to the complex, hierarchical architecture and multiscale porosity present in the native bone. To address this challenge, integrating biology-based approaches and engineering design principles is essential for developing effective therapies that can be translated to the clinic.

Toward this end, various hybrid and composite scaffold designs have been proposed that incorporate different components to serve specific functions. Generally, a synthetic hydrophobic polymer backbone is used to provide structural support, while a softer hydrogel network is employed to house cells, drugs, and bioactive factors, providing bio-instructive cues for cell proliferation and differentiation. This approach offers an opportunity for the orthogonal optimization of the mechanical properties and biological efficacy of the scaffolds.

The porosity, pore size, distribution, and interconnectivity are key parameters that dictate the mechanical properties and can be further reinforced with osteoinductive, inorganic components to match the mechanical properties of the native bone niche. On the other hand, the hydrogel stiffness, presence of cell-adhesive ligands, bioactive soluble factors, and biodegradability are the primary factors that determine long-term cell viability, proliferation, and differentiation into multiple lineages. Therefore, cutting-edge synthesis techniques are also being explored for designing and developing innovative hydrogel formulations that possess superior osteoinductive and osteoconductive properties.

ACKNOWLEDGEMENTS

The authors acknowledge support from the Science and Engineering Research Board, Government of India (IPA/2020/000025).

LIST OF ABBREVIATIONS

3D	Three-dimensional
4D	Four-dimensional

ALP	Alkaline phosphatase
BMP	Bone morphogenetic protein
BMSC	Bone marrow-derived stem cell
BTE	Bone tissue engineering
CAD	Computer-aided design
CT	Computed tomography
DLP	Digital light processing
DNA	Deoxyribonucleic acid
ECM	Extracellular matrix
FDM	Fused deposition modeling
GelMA	Gelatin methacryloyl
GHK	Glycyl-l-histidyl-l-lysine
HA	Hyaluronic acid
HAp	Hydroxyapatite
hMSC	Human mesenchymal stem cell
HSC	Hematopoietic stem cell
HUVEC	Human umbilical vein endothelial cell
IOB	Intraoperative bioprinting
LAB	Laser assisted bioprinting
MRI	Magnetic resonance imaging
MSC	Mesenchymal stem cell
MWCNT	Multiwall carbon nanotube
PCL	poly(ε-caprolactone)
PEG	poly(ethylene glycol)
PEGDA	poly(ethylene glycol) diacrylate
PEI	polyethyleneimine
PLA	poly(lactic acid)
PLGA	poly(lactic-co-glycolic acid)
PM	Phenamil methanesulfonate
Ppy	polypyrrole
ROB	Rat osteoblast
SF-MA	Methacrylated silk fibroin
SMP	Shape memory polymer
VEGF	Vascular endothelial growth factor

REFERENCES

Abbasi, N., Hamlet, S., Love, R. M., & Nguyen, N. T. (2020a). Porous scaffolds for bone regeneration. *J. Sci.: Adv. Mater. Devices*. 5: 1–9.

Abbasi, N., Ivanovski, S., Gulati, K., Love, R. M., & Hamlet, S. (2020b). Role of offset and gradient architectures of 3-D melt electrowritten scaffold on differentiation and mineralization of osteoblasts. *Biomater. Res*. 24: 2.

Ahn, G., Lee, J. S., Yun, W. S., Shim, J. H., & Lee, U. L. (2018). Cleft alveolus reconstruction using a three-dimensional printed bioresorbable scaffold with human bone marrow cells. *J. Craniofac. Surg*. 29: 1880.

Allen, N. B., Abar, B., Johnson, L., Burbano, J., Danilkowicz, R. M., & Adams, S. B. (2022). 3D-bioprinted GelMA-gelatin-hydroxyapatite osteoblast-laden composite hydrogels for bone tissue engineering. *Bioprinting*. 26: e00196.

Alsberg, E., Anderson, K. W., Albeiruti, A., Franceschi, R. T., & Mooney, D. J. (2001). Cell-interactive alginate hydrogels for bone tissue engineering. *J. Dent. Res*. 80: 2025–2029.

Augst, A. D., Kong, H. J., & Mooney, D. J. (2006). Alginate hydrogels as biomaterials. *Macromol. Biosci*. 6: 623–633.

Bauer, T. W., & Muschler, G. F. (2000). Bone graft materials: An overview of the basic science. *Clin. Orthop. Relat. Res*. 371: 10.

Bedell, M. L., Navara, A. M., Du, Y., Zhang, S., & Mikos, A. G. (2020). Polymeric systems for bioprinting. *Chem. Rev.* 120: 10744–10792.

Bittner, S. M., Smith, B. T., Diaz-Gomez, L., Hudgins, C. D., Melchiorri, A. J., Scott, D. W., Fisher, J. P., & Mikos, A. G. (2019). Fabrication and mechanical characterization of 3D printed vertical uniform and gradient scaffolds for bone and osteochondral tissue engineering. *Acta Biomater.* 90: 37–48.

Bone Grafts and Substitutes Market Report, 2022–2030. www.fortunebusinessinsights.com/bone-graft-substitutes-market-103106

Bose, S., Vahabzadeh, S., & Bandyopadhyay, A. (2013). Bone tissue engineering using 3D printing. *Mater. Today.* 16: 496–504.

Burdick, J. A., & Anseth, K. S. (2002). Photoencapsulation of osteoblasts in injectable RGD-modified PEG hydrogels for bone tissue engineering. *Biomaterials.* 23: 4315–4323.

Burdick, J. A., Mauck, R. L., Gorman, J. H., & Gorman, R. C. (2013). Acellular biomaterials: An evolving alternative to cell-based therapies. *Sci. Transl. Med.* 5: 176ps4.

Byambaa, B., Annabi, N., Yue, K., Trujillo-de Santiago, G., Alvarez, M. M., Jia, W., Kazemzadeh-Narbat, M., Shin, S. R., Tamayol, A., & Khademhosseini, A. (2017). Bioprinted osteogenic and vasculogenic patterns for engineering 3D bone tissue. *Adv. Healthc. Mater.* 6: 1700015.

Campbell, P. G., & Weiss, L. E. (2007). Tissue engineering with the aid of inkjet printers. *Expert Opin. Biol. Ther.* 7: 1123–1127.

C Echave, M., S. Burgo, L., L. Pedraz, J., & Orive, G. (2017). Gelatin as biomaterial for tissue engineering. *Curr. Pharm. Des.* 23: 3567–3584.

Challis, V. J., Roberts, A. P., Grotowski, J. F., Zhang, L. C., & Sercombe, T. B. (2010). Prototypes for bone implant scaffolds designed via topology optimization and manufactured by solid freeform fabrication. *Adv. Eng. Mater.* 12: 1106–1110.

Chang, H. K., Yang, D. H., Ha, M. Y., Kim, H. J., Kim, C. H., Kim, S. H., Choi, J. W., & Chun, H. J. (2022). 3D printing of cell-laden visible light curable glycol chitosan bioink for bone tissue engineering. *Carbohydr. Polym.* 287: 119328.

Cheng, A., Schwartz, Z., Kahn, A., Li, X., Shao, Z., Sun, M., Ao, Y., Boyan, B. D., & Chen, H. (2019). Advances in porous scaffold design for bone and cartilage tissue engineering and regeneration. *Tissue Eng. Part B Rev.* 25: 14–29.

Choe, G., Oh, S., Min Seok, J., A Park, S., & Young Lee, J. (2019). Graphene oxide/alginate composites as novel bioinks for three-dimensional mesenchymal stem cell printing and bone regeneration applications. *Nanoscale.* 11: 23275–23285.

Clarke, B. (2008). Normal bone anatomy and physiology. *Clin. J. Am. Soc. Nephrol.* 3: S131–S139.

Collins, M. N., & Birkinshaw, C. (2013). Hyaluronic acid based scaffolds for tissue engineering—A review. *Carbohydr. Polym.* 92: 1262–1279.

Collins, M. N., Ren, G., Young, K., Pina, S., Reis, R. L., & Oliveira, J. M. (2021). Scaffold fabrication technologies and structure/function properties in bone tissue engineering. *Adv. Funct. Mater.* 31: 2010609.

Dang, M., Saunders, L., Niu, X., Fan, Y., & Ma, P. X. (2018). Biomimetic delivery of signals for bone tissue engineering. *Bone Res.* 6: 25.

Demirtaş, T. T., Irmak, G., & Gümüşderelioğlu, M. (2017). A bioprintable form of chitosan hydrogel for bone tissue engineering. *Biofabrication.* 9: 035003.

Di Luca, A., Ostrowska, B., Lorenzo-Moldero, I., Lepedda, A., Swieszkowski, W., Van Blitterswijk, C., & Moroni, L. (2016). Gradients in pore size enhance the osteogenic differentiation of human mesenchymal stromal cells in three-dimensional scaffolds. *Sci. Rep.* 6: 1–13.

Dimitriou, R., Jones, E., McGonagle, D., & Giannoudis, P. V. (2011). Bone regeneration: Current concepts and future directions. *BMC Med.* 9: 66.

Dou, Y., Huang, J., Xia, X., Wei, J., Zou, Q., Zuo, Y., Li, J., & Li, Y. (2021). A hierarchical scaffold with a highly pore-interconnective 3D printed PLGA/n-HA framework and an extracellular matrix like gelatin network filler for bone regeneration. *J. Mater. Chem. B.* 9: 4488–4501.

Drury, J. L., & Mooney, D. J. (2003). Hydrogels for tissue engineering: Scaffold design variables and applications. *Biomaterials.* 24: 4337–4351.

e Silva, E. P., Huang, B., Helaehil, J. V., Nalesso, P. R. L., Bagne, L., de Oliveira, M. A., Albiazetti, G. C. C., Aldalbahi, A., El-Newehy, M., Santamaria-Jr, M., Mendonça, F. A. S., Bártolo, P., & Caetano, G. F. (2021). In vivo study of conductive 3D printed PCL/MWCNTs scaffolds with electrical stimulation for bone tissue engineering. *Bio-Des. Manuf.* 4: 190–202.

Finkemeier, C. G. (2002). Bone-grafting and bone-graft substitutes. *J. Bone Joint Surg*. 84: 454.

Fitzpatrick, V., Martín-Moldes, Z., Deck, A., Torres-Sanchez, R., Valat, A., Cairns, D., Li, C., & Kaplan, D. L. (2021). Functionalized 3D-printed silk-hydroxyapatite scaffolds for enhanced bone regeneration with innervation and vascularization. *Biomaterials*. 276: 120995.

Giannoudis, P. V., Dinopoulos, H., & Tsiridis, E. (2005). Bone substitutes: An update. *Injury*. 36: S20–S27.

Guo, L., Liang, Z., Yang, L., Du, W., Yu, T., Tang, H., Li, C., & Qiu, H. (2021). The role of natural polymers in bone tissue engineering. *J. Control. Release*. 338: 571–582.

Hernández-González, A. C., Téllez-Jurado, L., & Rodríguez-Lorenzo, L. M. (2020). Alginate hydrogels for bone tissue engineering, from injectables to bioprinting: A review. *Carbohydr. Polym*. 229: 115514.

Hollister, S. J. (2005). Porous scaffold design for tissue engineering. *Nat. Mater*. 4: 518–524.

Huang, L., Cheng, Y. Y., Koo, P. L., Lee, K. M., Qin, L., Cheng, J. C. Y., & Kumta, S. M. (2003). The effect of hyaluronan on osteoblast proliferation and differentiation in rat calvarial-derived cell cultures. *J. Biomed. Mater. Res. A*. 66A: 880–884.

Huang, L., Jiang, R., Wu, J., Song, J., Bai, H., Li, B., Zhao, Q., & Xie, T. (2017). Ultrafast digital printing toward 4D shape changing materials. *Adv. Mater*. 29: 1605390.

Jaidev, L. R., & Chatterjee, K. (2019). Surface functionalization of 3D printed polymer scaffolds to augment stem cell response. *Mater. Des*. 161: 44–54.

Jones, A. C., Arns, C. H., Sheppard, A. P., Hutmacher, D. W., Milthorpe, B. K., & Knackstedt, M. A. (2007). Assessment of bone ingrowth into porous biomaterials using MICRO-CT. *Biomaterials*. 28: 2491–2504.

Kanwar, S., & Vijayavenkataraman, S. (2021). Design of 3D printed scaffolds for bone tissue engineering: A review. *Bioprinting*. 24: e00167.

Kara, A., Distler, T., Polley, C., Schneidereit, D., Seitz, H., Friedrich, O., Tihminlioglu, F., & Boccaccini, A. R. (2022). 3D printed gelatin/decellularized bone composite scaffolds for bone tissue engineering: Fabrication, characterization and cytocompatibility study. *Mater. Today Bio*. 15: 100309.

Karageorgiou, V., & Kaplan, D. (2005). Porosity of 3D biomaterial scaffolds and osteogenesis. *Biomaterials*. 26: 5474–5491.

Kelly, C. N., Miller, A. T., Hollister, S. J., Guldberg, R. E., & Gall, K. (2018). Design and structure—Function characterization of 3D printed synthetic porous biomaterials for tissue engineering. *Adv. Healthc. Mater*. 7: 1701095.

Keriquel, V., Guillemot, F., Arnault, I., Guillotin, B., Miraux, S., Amédée, J., Fricain, J. C., & Catros, S. (2010). In vivo bioprinting for computer- and robotic-assisted medical intervention: Preliminary stud y in mice. *Biofabrication*. 2: 014101.

Keriquel, V., Oliveira, H., Rémy, M., Ziane, S., Delmond, S., Rousseau, B., Rey, S., Catros, S., Amédée, J., Guillemot, F., & Fricain, J. C. (2017). In situ printing of mesenchymal stromal cells, by laser-assisted bioprinting, for in vivo bone regenerati on applications. *Sci. Rep*. 7: 1778.

Kérourédan, O., Hakobyan, D., Rémy, M., Ziane, S., Dusserre, N., Fricain, J. C., Delmond, S., Thébaud, N. B., & Devillard, R. (2019). In situ prevascularization designed by laser-assisted bioprinting: Effect on bone regeneration. *Biofabrication*. 11: 045002.

Kim, J., Park, Y., Tae, G., Lee, K. B., Hwang, S. J., Kim, I. S., Noh, I., & Sun, K. (2008). Synthesis and characterization of matrix metalloprotease sensitive-low molecular weight hyaluronic acid based hydrogels. *J. Mater. Sci.: Mater. Med*. 19: 3311–3318.

Klokkevold, P. R., Vandemark, L., Kenney, E. B., & Bernard, G. W. (1996). Osteogenesis enhanced by chitosan (Poly-N-Acetyl glucosaminoglycan) in vitro. *J. Periodontol*. 67: 1170–1175.

Koons, G. L., Diba, M., & Mikos, A. G. (2020). Materials design for bone-tissue engineering. *Nat. Rev. Mater*. 5: 584–603.

Kumari, S., Mondal, P., & Chatterjee, K. (2022). Digital light processing-based 3D bioprinting of κ-carrageenan hydrogels for engineering cell-loaded tissue scaffolds. *Carbohydr. Polym*. 290: 119508.

Lan Levengood, S. K., & Zhang, M. (2014). Chitosan-based scaffolds for bone tissue engineering. *J. Mater. Chem. B*. 2: 3161–3184.

Lee, J., Lee, S. H., Kim, B. S., Cho, Y. S., & Park, Y. (2018). Development and evaluation of hyaluronic acid-based hybrid bio-ink for tissue regeneration. *Tissue Eng. Regen. Med*. 15: 761–769.

Lee, K., Seo, C. R., Ku, J. M., Lee, H., Yoon, H., Lee, J., Chun, W., Park, K. W., & Kim, G. (2015). 3D-printed alginate/phenamil composite scaffolds constituted with microsized core—Shell struts for hard tissue regeneration. *RSC Adv*. 5: 29335–29345.

Lee, Y. M., Park, Y. J., Lee, S. J., Ku, Y., Han, S. B., Klokkevold, P. R., Choi, S. M., & Chung, C. P. (2000). Tissue engineered bone formation using chitosan/tricalcium phosphate sponges. *J. Periodontol.* 71: 410–417.

Li, L., Shi, J., Ma, K., Jin, J., Wang, P., Liang, H., Cao, Y., Wang, X., & Jiang, Q. (2021). Robotic in situ 3D bio-printing technology for repairing large segmental bone defects. *J. Adv. Res.* 30: 75–84.

Li, L., Yu, F., Shi, J., Shen, S., Teng, H., Yang, J., Wang, X., & Jiang, Q. (2017). In situ repair of bone and cartilage defects using 3D scanning and 3D printing. *Sci. Rep.* 7: 9416.

Li, W., Wang, M., Wang, S., Wang, X., Avila, A., Kuang, X., Mu, X., Garciamendez, C. E., Jiang, Z., Manríquez, J., Tang, G., Guo, J., Mille, L. S., Robledo, J. A., Wang, D., Cheng, F., Li, H., Flores, R. S., Zhao, Z., Delavaux, C., Wang, Z., López, A., Yi, S., Zhou, C., Gómez, A., Schuurmans, C., Yang, G., Wang, Y., Zhang, X., Zhang, X., & Tang, G. (2023). An adhesive bioink toward biofabrication under wet conditions. *Small.* 1: 2205078.

Lin, C. Y., Kikuchi, N., & Hollister, S. J. (2004). A novel method for biomaterial scaffold internal architecture design to match bone elastic properties with desired porosity. *J. Biomech.* 37: 623–636.

Lopes, D., Martins-Cruz, C., Oliveira, M. B., & Mano, J. F. (2018). Bone physiology as inspiration for tissue regenerative therapies. *Biomaterials.* 185: 240–275.

Lukin, I., Erezuma, I., Maeso, L., Zarate, J., Desimone, M. F., Al-Tel, T. H., Dolatshahi-Pirouz, A., & Orive, G. (2022). Progress in gelatin as biomaterial for tissue engineering. *Pharmaceutics.* 14: 1177.

Melilli, G., Carmagnola, I., Tonda-Turo, C., Pirri, F., Ciardelli, G., Sangermano, M., Hakkarainen, M., & Chiappone, A. (2020). DLP 3D printing meets lignocellulosic biopolymers: Carboxymethyl cellulose inks for 3D biocompatible hydrogels. *Polymers.* 12: 1655.

Melke, J., Midha, S., Ghosh, S., Ito, K., & Hofmann, S. (2016). Silk fibroin as biomaterial for bone tissue engineering. *Acta Biomater.* 31: 1–16.

Moncal, K. K., Gudapati, H., Godzik, K. P., Heo, D. N., Kang, Y., Rizk, E., Ravnic, D. J., Wee, H., Pepley, D. F., Ozbolat, V., Lewis, G. S., Moore, J. Z., Driskell, R. R., Samson, T. D., & Ozbolat, I. T. (2021). Intraoperative bioprinting of hard, soft, and hard/soft composite tissues for craniomaxillofacial reconstruction. *Adv. Funct. Mater.* 31: 2010858.

Moncal, K. K., Tigli Aydın, R. S., Godzik, K. P., Acri, T. M., Heo, D. N., Rizk, E., Wee, H., Lewis, G. S., Salem, A. K., & Ozbolat, I. T. (2022a). Controlled co-delivery of pPDGF-B and pBMP-2 from intraoperatively bioprinted bone constructs improves the repair of calvarial defects in rats. *Biomaterials.* 281: 121333.

Moncal, K. K., Yeo, M., Celik, N., Acri, T. M., Rizk, E., Wee, H., Lewis, G. S., Salem, A. K., & Ozbolat, I. T. (2022b). Comparison of in-situ versus ex-situ delivery of polyethylenimine-BMP-2 polyplexes for rat calvarial defect repair via intraoperative bio printing. *Biofabrication.* 15: 015011.

Muzzarelli, R. A. A., Zucchini, C., Ilari, P., Pugnaloni, A., Mattioli Belmonte, M., Biagini, G., & Castaldini, C. (1993). Osteoconductive properties of methylpyrrolidinone chitosan in an animal model. *Biomaterials.* 14: 925–929.

Narayanan, G., Vernekar, V. N., Kuyinu, E. L., & Laurencin, C. T. (2016). Poly (lactic acid)-based biomaterials for orthopaedic regenerative engineering. *Adv. Drug Deliv. Rev.* 107: 247–276.

Nilawar, S., & Chatterjee, K. (2022). Surface decoration of redox-modulating nanoceria on 3D-printed tissue scaffolds promotes stem cell osteogenesis and attenuates bacterial colonization. *Biomacromolecules.* 23: 226–239.

Nyberg, E., Rindone, A., Dorafshar, A., & Grayson, W. L. (2017). Comparison of 3D-printed poly-ε-caprolactone scaffolds functionalized with tricalcium phosphate, hydroxyapatite, bio-oss, or decellularized bone matrix. *Tissue Eng.—A.* 23: 503–514.

Ozbolat, I. T. (2015). Bioprinting scale-up tissue and organ constructs for transplantation. *Trends Biotechnol.* 33: 395–400.

Park, J., Lee, S. J., Lee, H., Park, S. A., & Lee, J. Y. (2018). Three dimensional cell printing with sulfated alginate for improved bone morphogenetic protein-2 delivery and osteogenesis in bone tissue engineering. *Carbohydr. Polym.* 196: 217–224.

Patterson, J., Siew, R., Herring, S. W., Lin, A. S. P., Guldberg, R., & Stayton, P. S. (2010). Hyaluronic acid hydrogels with controlled degradation properties for oriented bone regeneration. *Biomaterials.* 31: 6772–6781.

Poldervaart, M. T., Goversen, B., de Ruijter, M., Abbadessa, A., Melchels, F. P. W., Öner, F. C., Dhert, W. J. A., Vermonden, T., & Alblas, J. (2017). 3D bioprinting of Methacrylated Hyaluronic Acid (MeHA) hydrogel with intrinsic osteogenicity. *PLoS One.* 12: e0177628.

Qu, H., Fu, H., Han, Z., & Sun, Y. (2019). Biomaterials for bone tissue engineering scaffolds: A review. *RSC Adv.* 9: 26252–26262.

Qu, M., Wang, C., Zhou, X., Libanori, A., Jiang, X., Xu, W., Zhu, S., Chen, Q., Sun, W., & Khademhosseini, A. (2021). Multi-dimensional printing for bone tissue engineering. *Adv. Healthc. Mater.* 10: 2001986.

Rajput, M., Mondal, P., Yadav, P., & Chatterjee, K. (2022). Light-based 3D bioprinting of bone tissue scaffolds with tunable mechanical properties and architecture from photocurable silk fibroin. *Int. J. Biol. Macromol.* 202: 644–656.

Rajput, M., Nilawar, S., & Chatterjee, K. (2023). Embedding silk fibroin-alginate hydrogel in a 3D-printed porous poly(Lactic acid) bone tissue scaffold augments stem cell function. *Regen. Eng. Transl. Med.* 1: 1–13.

Roseti, L., Parisi, V., Petretta, M., Cavallo, C., Desando, G., Bartolotti, I., & Grigolo, B. (2017). Scaffolds for bone tissue engineering: State of the art and new perspectives. *Mater. Sci. Eng. C.* 78: 1246–1262.

Sachs, E. M., Haggerty, J. S., Cima, M. J., & Williams, P. A. (1993). *Three-Dimensional Printing Techniques* (United States Patent No. US5204055A).

Salgado, A. J., Coutinho, O. P., & Reis, R. L. (2004). Bone tissue engineering: State of the art and future trends. *Macromol. Biosci.* 4: 743–765.

Sasaki, T., & Watanabe, C. (1995). Stimulation of osteoinduction in bone wound healing by high-molecular hyaluronic acid. *Bone.* 16: 9–15.

Shen, Y., Tang, H., Huang, X., Hang, R., Zhang, X., Wang, Y., & Yao, X. (2020). DLP printing photocurable chitosan to build bio-constructs for tissue engineering. *Carbohydr. Polym.* 235: 115970.

Shi, D., Shen, J., Zhang, Z., Shi, C., Chen, M., Gu, Y., & Liu, Y. (2019). Preparation and properties of dopamine-modified alginate/chitosan—Hydroxyapatite scaffolds with gradient structure for bone tissue engineering. *J. Biomed. Mater. Res. A.* 107: 1615–1627.

Sikavitsas, V. I., Temenoff, J. S., & Mikos, A. G. (2001). Biomaterials and bone mechanotransduction. *Biomaterials.* 22: 2581–2593.

Stevens, M. M. (2008). Biomaterials for bone tissue engineering. *Mater. Today.* 11: 18–25.

St John, T. A., Vaccaro, A. R., Sah, A. P., Schaefer, M., Berta, S. C., Albert, T., & Hilibrand, A. (2003). Physical and monetary costs associated with autogenous bone graft harvesting. *Am. J. Orthop. (Belle Mead NJ).* 32: 18–23.

Sun, W., Gregory, D. A., Tomeh, M. A., & Zhao, X. (2021). Silk fibroin as a functional biomaterial for tissue engineering. *Int. J. Mol. Sci.* 22: 1499.

Turnbull, G., Clarke, J., Picard, F., Riches, P., Jia, L., Han, F., Li, B., & Shu, W. (2018). 3D bioactive composite scaffolds for bone tissue engineering. *Bioact. Mater.* 3: 278–314.

Venkatesan, J., Bhatnagar, I., Manivasagan, P., Kang, K. H., & Kim, S. K. (2015). Alginate composites for bone tissue engineering: A review. *Int. J. Biol. Macromol.* 72: 269–281.

Venkatesan, J., & Kim, S. K. (2010). Chitosan composites for bone tissue engineering—An overview. *Mar. Drugs.* 8: 2252–2266.

Vepari, C., & Kaplan, D. L. (2007). Silk as a biomaterial. *Prog. Polym. Sci.* 32: 991–1007.

Wang, X., Jiang, M., Zhou, Z., Gou, J., & Hui, D. (2017). 3D printing of polymer matrix composites: A review and prospective. *Compos. B: Eng.* 110: 442–458.

Wang, X., Xu, S., Zhou, S., Xu, W., Leary, M., Choong, P., Qian, M., Brandt, M., & Xie, Y. M. (2016). Topological design and additive manufacturing of porous metals for bone scaffolds and orthopaedic implants: A review. *Biomaterials.* 83: 127–141.

Wei, J., Yan, Y., Gao, J., Li, Y., Wang, R., Wang, J., Zou, Q., Zuo, Y., Zhu, M., & Li, J. (2022). 3D-printed hydroxyapatite microspheres reinforced PLGA scaffolds for bone regeneration. *Biomater. Adv.* 133: 112618.

Wu, Y., Ravnic, D. J., & Ozbolat, I. T. (2020). Intraoperative bioprinting: Repairing tissues and organs in a surgical set ting. *Trends. Biotechnol.* 38: 594–605.

Xing, F., Zhou, C., Hui, D., Du, C., Wu, L., Wang, L., Wang, W., Pu, X., Gu, L., Liu, L., Xiang, Z., & Zhang, X. (2020). Hyaluronic acid as a bioactive component for bone tissue regeneration: Fabrication, modification, properties, and biological functions. *Nanotechnol. Rev.* 9: 1059–1079.

Xu, N., Ye, X., Wei, D., Zhong, J., Chen, Y., Xu, G., & He, D. (2014). 3D artificial bones for bone repair prepared by computed tomography-guided fused deposition modeling for bone repair. *ACS Appl. Mater. Interfaces.* 6: 14952–14963.

Xue, X., Zhang, H., Liu, H., Wang, S., Li, J., Zhou, Q., Chen, X., Ren, X., Jing, Y., Deng, Y., Geng, Z., Wang, X., & Su, J. (2022). Rational design of multifunctional CuS nanoparticle-PEG composite soft hydrogel-coated 3D hard polycaprolactone scaffolds for efficient bone regeneration. *Adv. Funct. Mater.* 32: 2202470.

Yang, X., Wang, Y., Zhou, Y., Chen, J., & Wan, Q. (2021). The application of polycaprolactone in three-dimensional printing scaffolds for bone tissue engineering. *Polymers.* 13: 2754.

Yi, H. G., Kim, H., Kwon, J., Choi, Y. J., Jang, J., & Cho, D. W. (2021). Application of 3D bioprinting in the prevention and the therapy for human diseases. *Sig. Transduct. Target Ther.* 6: 177.

Yin, T., & Li, L. (2006). The stem cell niches in bone. *J. Clin. Invest.* 116: 1195–1201.

Zafeiris, K., Brasinika, D., Karatza, A., Koumoulos, E., Karoussis, I. K., Kyriakidou, K., & Charitidis, C. A. (2021). Additive manufacturing of hydroxyapatite—Chitosan—Genipin composite scaffolds for bone tissue engineering applicatio ns. *Mater. Sci. Eng. C.* 119: 111639.

Zhai, X., Ruan, C., Ma, Y., Cheng, D., Wu, M., Liu, W., Zhao, X., Pan, H., & Lu, W. W. (2018). 3D-bioprinted osteoblast-laden nanocomposite hydrogel constructs with induced microenvironments promote cell viability, differentiation, and osteogenesis both in vitro and in vivo. *Adv. Sci.* 5: 1700550.

Zhang, J., Tong, D., Song, H., Ruan, R., Sun, Y., Lin, Y., Wang, J., Hou, L., Dai, J., Ding, J., & Yang, H. (2022). Osteoimmunity-regulating biomimetically hierarchical scaffold for augmented bone regeneration. *Adv. Mater.* 34: 2202044.

Zhang, L., Yang, G., Johnson, B. N., & Jia, X. (2019). Three-Dimensional (3D) printed scaffold and material selection for bone repair. *Acta Biomater.* 84: 16–33.

Zhao, W., Hu, C., & Xu, T. (2023). In vivo bioprinting: Broadening the therapeutic horizon for tissue injuries. *Bioact. Mater.* 25: 201–222.

Zhou, M., Wu, X., Luo, J., Yang, G., Lu, Y., Lin, S., Jiang, F., Zhang, W., & Jiang, X. (2021). Copper peptide-incorporated 3D-printed silk-based scaffolds promote vascularized bone regeneration. *Chem. Eng. J.* 422: 130147.

Zhu, G., Zhang, T., Chen, M., Yao, K., Huang, X., Zhang, B., Li, Y., Liu, J., Wang, Y., & Zhao, Z. (2021). Bone physiological microenvironment and healing mechanism: Basis for future bone-tissue engineering scaffolds. *Bioact. Mater.* 6: 4110.

6 Recent Advances in Biodegradable Implants in Bone Tissue Engineering

Shazia Shaikh, Rupita Ghosh, Ashiq Hussain Pandit, Shreya Mehrotra, and Ashok Kumar

6.1 INTRODUCTION

Bone defects/injuries occurring for various reasons such as trauma, accidents, inflammation, tumors, sports, and exercise demands orthopedic implants (Burny et al., 2000; Jin & Chu, 2019; Kim et al., 2020; Taddei et al., 2004). These orthopedic implants can be for both high and low load-bearing bone fractures. For high load-bearing fractures along with biocompatibility, implants need to have high mechanical properties to support the fractured bone structure and its functionality. These orthopedic implants are classified into two categories such as permanent and temporary implants (Palani, 2020).

Permanent bone implants (knee, hip, shoulder, elbow, ankle, wrist, and finger joints) cater to the human body throughout the lifespan, while temporary bone implants (plates, nails, screws, pins, wires, and intramedullary nails) are needed to fix the fractured bones until complete bone healing is achieved (Khodaei et al., 2023). Further, at present, temporary bone implants for high load-bearing fractures are primarily made up of nondegradable traditionally available metals such as titanium alloys and stainless steel. These metallic implants offer the advantages of high mechanical strength, durability, ductility, and biocompatibility. However, some of the major limitations associated with these implants are nondegradability, release of toxic ions in the surroundings, and higher mechanical properties than those of bone, resulting in stress shielding and subsequent implant failure (Bandyopadhyay et al., 2022).

Once the bone heals sufficiently, the major concern is performing revision surgery to remove these nondegradable implants placed as temporary bone supports in the form of screws, plates and pins (Han et al., 2019; Johnson et al., 2017). With the advent of technological advancement, third-generation biodegradable implants are constantly being explored that have bio-mimicking mechanical and physicochemical properties. Biodegradable polymers, ceramics, and metals are the three kinds of biomaterials widely studied as orthopedic implants (Tan et al., 2013). This chapter highlights the various recent biodegradable materials for bone tissue engineering and their clinical trials for commercialization are discussed.

6.2 INTERNAL BONE FIXATION DEVICES (BONE IMPLANTS)

Mechanical stimuli including stress, strain, topography, elasticity, and stiffness play vital roles in bone fracture healing process (Phillips, 2005). At present, the biomechanics of internal bone fixation devices (IBFDs) in the bone healing process is a cutting edge research topic. IBFDs not only provide stabilization but also help in creating biomimicking mechanical environment at the fracture site that promotes cellular bioactivity such as that of osteoblasts, chondrocytes, endothelial cells, fibroblasts, and mesenchymal stem cells (MSCs) (Ono et al., 2016).

DOI: 10.1201/9781003307310-7

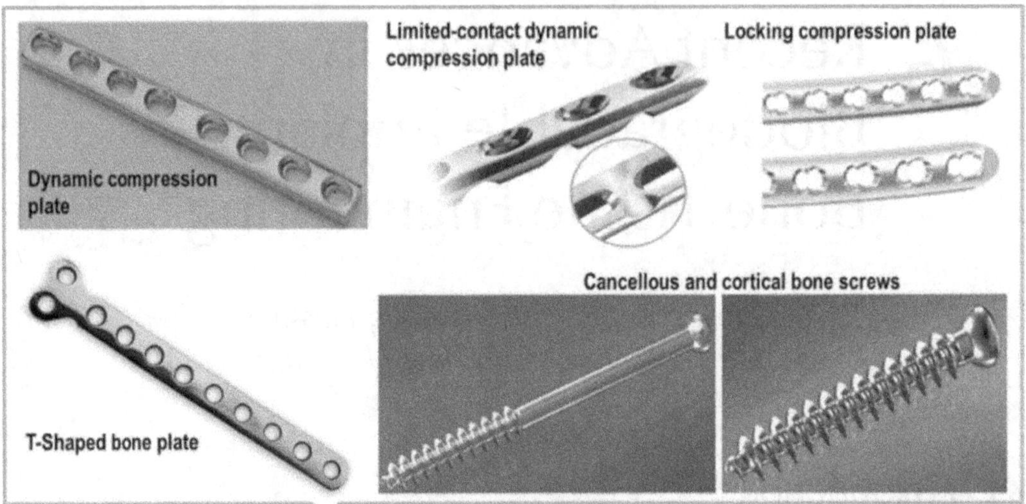

FIGURE 6.1 Successful IBFD designs. Bone fixation devices such as plates and screws are shown with different designs suitable for various types of bone fractures. Authors acknowledge all sources (online) from which images/photographs have been taken.

Moreover, fracture healing at various locations provides different microenvironments, and therefore, location-specific IBFD needs to be developed to provide desirable healing. When bone breaks sufficiently to disturb alignment, internal fixation devices are used for stabilization and proper natural remodeling/healing. Figure 6.1 shows various successful, medically certified IBFD designs including bone plates and screws that are already available in the implant market.

Meanwhile, the research on improving IBFD design is still in progress for both specific and nonspecific fractures. These internal fixation devices are made up of traditionally available nondegradable metals such as titanium alloys and stainless steel. Removing these IBFDs post healing is difficult and a financial burden to patients as well as society (Chaya et al., 2015; Hanson et al., 2008).

Bone plates and screws with different designs as shown in Figure 6.1 are the most commonly used IBFDs, providing compression resistance, stability, bending resistance, and so on. Both the plate and screw together bridge the gap between fractured and healthy bone and supports healing by biomechanical signaling. In addition, these IBFDs help in the normal functioning of fractured bones in day-to-day life.

6.3 BONE FRACTURE AND HEALING

Bone injuries can be produced by accidental load, cyclic load, or a constant over-ranged load over a long duration that involves both biological and mechanical aspects. In humans with habitual loads, the mechanical stability of bones is more than 50 years without failure. However, cyclic mechanical loading over prolonged durations beyond the mechanical range of bones leads to fractures, and these loads generate significant micro-damages that lead to fatigue failure. Further, bone is a tissue with intrinsic self-regeneration properties, but this self-regeneration property is limited by size; as fracture size exceeds the limit, implants are used to stabilize the fractured site and bone regeneration.

Additionally, bone self-regeneration is also age dependent, faster in children and slower in elderly people (Isaksson et al., 2007). Healing is also categorized as primary or secondary based on fracture size. In primary healing, the small voids are filled directly with bone tissues without forming any intermediate tissues, while secondary healing involves various steps including inflammation, repairing, and remodeling (Claes et al., 2012; Marsell & Einhorn, 2011). Moreover, fractured bone takes approximately three to six months to start working as normal bone and attains mechanical stability gradually (Busch et al., 2021; Sarian et al., 2022).

6.4 BIODEGRADABLE INTERNAL BONE FIXATION DEVICES

Biodegradable materials are degradable inside the human body environment and are eventually metabolized or replaced with cells and tissues (Zheng et al., 2014). For high load-bearing bone fractures, these materials are intended to provide mechanical support until the defect heals and is eventually replaced by bone tissue; the biodegradable material should maintain its mechanical integrity ideally for the three to six months of the bone-healing period. Table 6.1 shows some available biomaterials currently used as bone supports based on polymers, ceramics, composites, and metals.

6.4.1 Biodegradable Polymer for Orthopedic Applications

Over the last few decades, biodegradable polymers have attracted considerable attention from the scientific community due to their outstanding chemical, physical, physiological, and mechanical properties. They have been widely utilized in several biomedical applications, particularly in bone regeneration as an efficient biomaterial that mimics the 3D microenvironment of cells and tissues in vivo. Consequently, these biodegradable polymeric scaffolds enhance cell adhesion, their proliferation and differentiation (Rai et al., 2021). Thus, these bioscaffolds help in replacing damaged parts of the body without inducing any kind of immune response or inflammation.

Moreover, due to good biodegradability, these polymers can be employed as promising material for short- and long-term bone implants (Song et al., 2018). The synthetic biodegradable polymers present superior advantages over natural biopolymers, as they can be designed to offer numerous properties and have more uniformity than natural biopolymers. Moreover, a very reliable and safe source of raw material is obtained with these polymers that do not induce any sort of immunogenicity (Samir et al., 2022).

Several factors that largely influence the mechanical properties of biodegradable polymers are the monomer, initiator, and additives used. These factors in turn affect the hydrophilicity of polymers and their crystallinity, glass transition, melt temperatures, and molecular weight. Currently, synthetic biodegradable polymers are widely employed as orthopedic fixation devices (rods, screws, pins, ligaments).

Most of the synthetic biodegradable materials that are commercially available are either homopolymers of polyesters or copolymers of lactide or glycolide. There are also devices that are composed of copolymers of trimethylene carbonate, poly- dioxanone, and caprolactone (Middleton & Tipton, 2000). Next, we discuss some of the polymers and copolymers that are commonly used for developing bone fixation devices.

TABLE 6.1
Mechanical Properties of Bone, Nondegradable, and Biodegradable Materials

Materials	Density (g/cm^3)	Modulus (GPa)	Compressive Yield Strength (MPa)	Fracture Toughness (MPa m$^{1/2}$)
Cortical bone	1.8–2.1	7–20	130–180	3–6
Cancellous bone	1–1.4	0.01–3	2–12	NA
Ti alloys	4.2–4.5	110–120	750–1110	55–115
Co alloys	8.3–9.2	230	450–1000	NA
316 L steel	8.0	193	190	50–200
HAp	3.1	80–110	0.03–0.3	0.6–1.0
TCP	NA	24–39	2–3.5	0.3–1.0
Mg alloys	1.79–2.0	35–45	100–200	15–35

Ti: titanium, Co: cobalt, HAp: hydroxyapatite, TCP: tricalcium phosphate, Mg: magnesium (sourced from Haghshenas, 2017; Xing et al., 2022; Luthringer et al., 2014).

6.4.1.1 Polyglycolic Acid

Polyglycolic acid (PGA) is the first biodegradable polymer that has been extensively utilized as reinforcing material for pins, plates, and screws for bone surgery (Pina & Ferreira, 2012). It is a crystalline polymer with an average molecular weight in the range of 20,000 to 145,000 and melting point of about 220–230 °C (Singh & Tiwari, 2010). The ring opening polymerization of glycolide forms PGA with high molecular weight and 1 to 3% concentration of residual monomers (Figure 6.2).

PGA undergoes degradation via hydrolysis and with the help of certain nonspecific carboxypeptidases and esterases. It loses its mechanical properties within six weeks and degrades completely within a few months depending upon its purity, molecular weight, crystallinity, and size of the implant (On et al., 2020; Visan et al., 2021). However, some unfavorable tissue responses have been reported with PGA-based fixation implants with 2.0 to 46.7% incidence rate (Kontakis et al., 2007; Mavrogenis et al., 2009).

The maximum incidence has been reported in fractures of scaphoid bone and distal radius (Pelto-Vasenius et al., 1995), although the rate of foreign body reactions largely decreases after the dye is removed from the PGA-based implants (Böstman & Pihlajamäki, 2000). PGA has been used mainly in screws and rods as fracture-fixating material in cancellous bone due to its biodegradable nature. Some of the commercially available PGA-based devices for orthopedic application are shown in Table 6.2.

6.4.1.2 Polylactic Acid

Polylactic acid (PLA) is a synthetic semicrystalline biodegradable polymer with average molecular weight in the range of 180,000 to 530,000 with melting point of 174 °C (Chandra & Rustgi, 1998). It has two isomeric forms, L and D, and exists as poly-L-lactide (PLLA) and poly-D-lactide (PDLA) (de França et al., 2022). PLA usually degrades through hydrolysis. It forms by the ring opening polymerization of lactides (Figure 6.3).

The additional polymerization of PDLA with PLLA widens polymer chains, which results in more rapid degradation of the material (Balla et al., 2021). PLA-based plates and screws have been successfully employed as bone-fixation implants and treating various bone-related injuries such as ligament damage and various skeletal fractures (Narayanan et al., 2016). PLLA is considered a choice material for bone-fixation implants due to its higher mechanical strength in comparison with PDLLA (Capuana et al., 2022).

PLA-based bone implants show a good degree of biocompatibility with the host tissues (Castro et al., 2022). PLLA and PDLA show stainless steel-like tissue response inside muscles, although some complications like foreign body reactions were observed; however, these are not common to all PLLA-based materials (Hajebi et al., 2021). For instance, Eitenmüller et al. (1996) developed

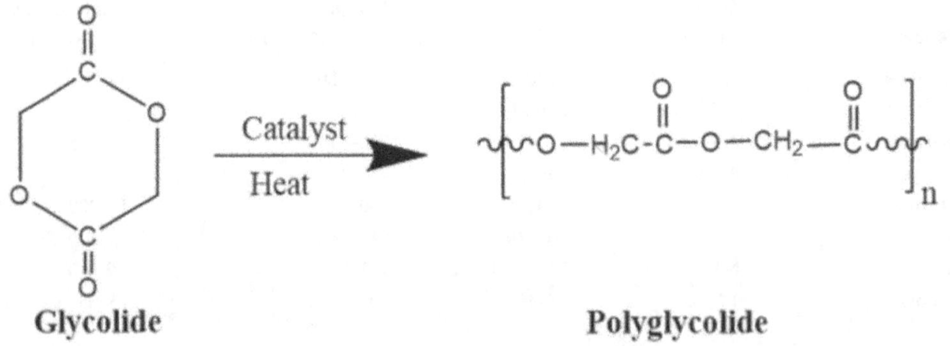

FIGURE 6.2 Synthesis of polyglycolic acid via ring opening polymerization of glycolide (drawn in ChemDraw).

TABLE 6.2
Commercially Available Biodegradable Polymer-Based Devices

Material	Commercial Name	Application	Manufacturer
SR-LPLA	Smart pins	Fracture fixation	Bionx Implants
SR-PGA	Smart pins	Fracture fixation	Bionx Implants
SR-LPLA	Smart screw	Fracture fixation	Bionx Implants
SR-LPLA	Smart tack	Fracture fixation	Bionx Implants
PDO	Orthosorb pin	Fracture fixation	J & J Orthopaedics
LPLA	Full-thread biointerference screw	Interference screws	Arthrex
LPLA	Bio screw	Interference screws	Linvatec
LLPLA	Sysorb	Interference screws	Sulzer Orthopedics
PGA	Lacto Sorbr SE	CMF Fixation	Biomet
PLLA/HA	Fixsorb	Fracture Fixation	Takiron
PGA-TMC	Suretak 6.0	Suture anchors	Smith and Nephew
LPLA	Bio Statak	Suture anchors	Zimmer

Reproduced with modification and permission from Middleton, J. C., & Tipton, A. J.: Synthetic biodegradable polymers as orthopedic devices. *Biomaterials*. 2000. 21(23). 2335–2346. Copyright 2000 Elsevier.; Reproduced under the terms of CC-BY 3.0 (https://creativecommons.org/licenses/by/3.0) International License from Pina, S., & Ferreira, J. M.: Bioresorbable plates and screws for clinical applications: a review. *J Healthc Eng*. 2012. 3. 243–260. Copyright 2012 Hindawi Publishing Corporation.

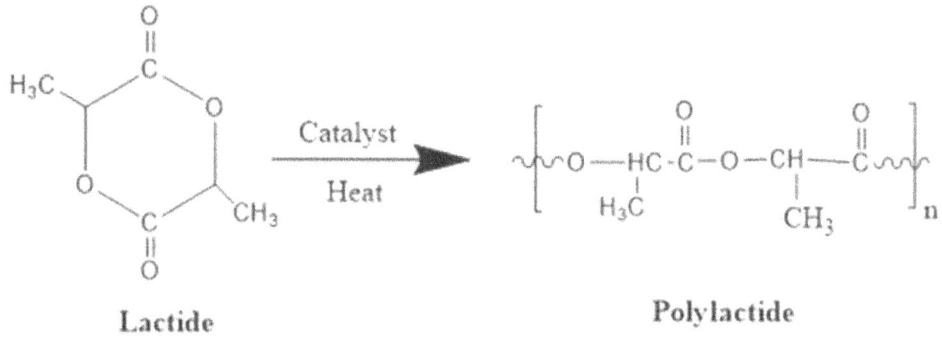

FIGURE 6.3 Ring-opening synthesis of polylactic acid from Lactides (drawn in ChemDraw).

PLLA-based plates for ankle fracture fixation and observed that more than 50% of the patients showed soft tissue complications due to slow clearance of the degraded PLA particles.

In another study, smaller PLLA-based plates and screws did not induce any kind of soft tissue reaction. Intraosseally implanted PLLA-based pins and screws have been shown to induce mild foreign body reactions, in contract with metallic materials, without showing any signs of inflammatory response during 48 weeks of follow-up (Pina & Ferreira, 2012). PLLA is known to persist in animal tissues for longer durations up to five years of post-implantation (Ngo et al., 2021).

Several resorbable orthopedic devices are produced from PLLA, and they result in fewer undesirable tissue reactions than do other biodegradable polymers (DeStefano et al., 2020). PLA behaves as a weaker acid and is more hydrophobic in nature due to the presence of methyl groups. The lower pH in body tissues close to these polymers may induce harmful effects. However, this issue can be addressed by incorporating some simple salts inside the polymer network (Agrawal & Athanasiou, 1997). Some of the commercially available PLA-based devices are shown in Table 6.2.

6.4.1.3 Poly(Dioxanone)

The first clinically tested monofilament synthetic suture was developed by the ring-opening polymerization of poly(p-dioxanone) which is commercially available in the market under the name PDS Ethicon (Figure 6.4). This material shows about 55% crystallinity and has a glass transition temperature of about −10 to 0 °C. Poly(dioxanone) exhibits no severe toxicity on implantation. Poly(dioxanone)-based absorbable pins used for fracture fixation are commercially available marketed by Johnson and Johnson Orthopedics (Middleton & Tipton, 2000).

6.4.1.4 Copolymers

The copolymerization of PLA and PGA together produces a full variety of PLGA polymers that includes both DL and L-lactides (Figure 6.5). The various properties of PLA and PGA copolymers can be easily regulated by varying the lactide-to-glycolide ratio (Pina & Ferreira, 2012). The rate of copolymer degradation largely depends on the ratio of monomers used. Generally, the higher concentration of PGA enhances the rate of degradation.

It is essential to mention that there is no linear correlation between the copolymer concentration and polymer degradation. For instance, a copolymer of 50% DL-lactide and 50% glycolide shows faster degradation than the homopolymer. Copolymers of 25–70% glycolide with L-lactide have amorphous nature because of disruption in the polymer chain regularity caused by the incorporation of another monomer (Makadia & Siegel, 2011).

The commercially available Biologically Quiet™ line developed by Instrument Makar is composed of an 85:15 ratio of poly (DL-lactide-*co*-glycolide). Biomet and surgical dynamics have developed PLA- and PGA-based copolymer screws and plates with an 82:18 poly(L-lactide-*co*-glycolide) ratio. Similarly, copolymerization of glycolide with trimethylene carbonate forms a polyglyconate that is used in sutures, pins, and screws. Usually these are prepared as A-B-A block copolymers with a glycolide-to-TMC (trimethylene carbonate) ratio of 2:1, glycolide-TMC at the center (B-block), and glycolide at end (A-block). These materials show better flexibility than pristine PGA and degrade within seven months. The tetra polymer of glycolide with TMC and p-dioxanone have also been developed to form sutures with low stiffness in comparison to pure PGA and can be easily absorbed within three to four months (Guo & Ma, 2014).

PGA on polymerization with TMC forms polyglyconate, which can be used as sutures, screws, and tacks (Hamza et al., 2022). Generally, these can be prepared by A-B-A block copolymers with a PGA:TMC ratio of 2:1, PGA-TMC in the center block, and PGA in the end blocks. These materials possess superior flexibility to that of pristine PGA and are completely absorbed within seven months. PGA can be also polymerized with p-dioxanone and TMC to form a terpolymer suture that shows less stiffness than pure PGA fibers and can be absorbed within two to four months (Nagarajan & Reddy, 2009). Currently, only a few biodegradable fixation devices based on copolymers of PGA, PLA, p-dioxanone, and trimethylene carbonate are available commercially in the market (Pina & Ferreira, 2012).

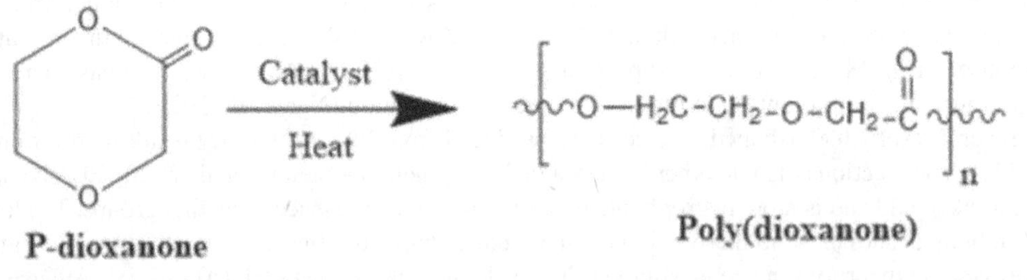

FIGURE 6.4 Synthesis of poly(dioxanone) through ring-opening polymerization (drawn in ChemDraw).

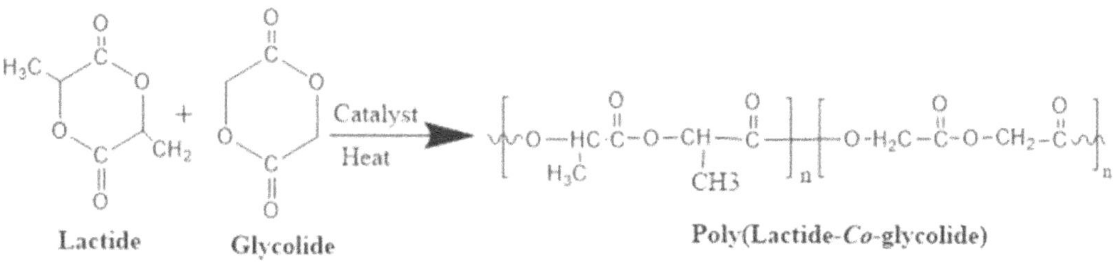

Lactide + Glycolide —Catalyst, Heat→ Poly(Lactide-*Co*-glycolide)

FIGURE 6.5 Copolymerization of PLA and PGA results in the synthesis of poly(lactide-co-glycolide) (drawn in ChemDraw).

6.4.2 Ceramics

Ceramics have been used by ancient civilizations for thousands of years in the form of pottery. It was discovered that clay could be hardened by mixing it with water and then shaping and drying it, finally followed by firing the product. However, the use of ceramics is not only restricted to firing naturally occurring substances for use in traditional household materials: Advances in the manufacture of ceramics over the past 100 years have led to their use in a variety of high-tech materials in applications as diverse as chemical, optical, magnetic, electrical, and biomedical (Ghosh, 2018).

Ceramics are inorganic compounds of metallic elements that are ionically and/or covalently bonded with nonmetallic elements (Mhadhbi & Sohani, 2022). They have the characteristic properties of high hardness, inherent brittleness, low tensile strength, very high elastic modulus, high compressive strength, durability, chemical stability, high corrosion resistance, and high melting temperatures. Ceramics are most commonly oxides, nitrides, and carbides (Turner, 2021).

6.4.2.1 Bioresorbable Ceramics

During the last few decades, revolutions have occurred in the use of ceramics to improve the quality of human life through reconstructive surgeries. This revolution led to the development of specially designed ceramics for the repair and reconstruction of damaged, diseased, or worn-out parts of the body. The ceramic-based materials within this medical implant class are called "bioceramics" (Hench, 1993). Among them, bioresorbable bioceramics are extensively used in bone tissue engineering applications for repairing and regenerating bone defects.

Bioresorbable ceramics can resorb with time when implanted in vivo and gradually replaced by new lamellar bone tissue (Tan et al., 2013). In general, natural bone tissue repairs itself and is gradually replaced by the constant turnover of cell populations throughout life (Hench, 1991). Therefore, in order for these implants to be successful, the dissolution rate must match the repair rates of the bone tissue (tunably resorbable). The dissolution rate of these ceramics also depends on the composition and structure of the material (Hench, 1993).

The use of bioresorbable ceramics was initially investigated as an alternative to metallic implants where revision surgery becomes necessary due to toxic ion release and stress-shielding effects (Dubok, 2000). As the bioresorbable ceramic implant degrades gradually, its mechanical property decreases, and the body's biological stress gradually shifts from the implant to the newly formed bone tissue, thus avoiding the stress-shielding effect while triggering tissue regeneration at the same time (Wei et al., 2020). Bioresorbable ceramics possess several other advantages such as biocompatibility, corrosion and wear resistance, and excellent biological activity. They do not disintegrate into the tissues, do not elicit an inflammatory response, and permit connective tissue and bone ingrowth into the pores (Wei et al., 2020). They are mainly used in the form of fillers, porous blocks, or sintered granules for filling bone defects, bone fracture repair or stabilization, and replacement of diseased tissue or as metallic implant coatings to increase their bioactivity and biocompatibility (Dorozhkin, 2010).

The primary bioresorbable ceramic material that is widely used in bone tissue engineering applications is calcium phosphate (CaP), mainly in the form of hydroxyapatite (HA) and β-tricalcium phosphate (β-TCP) ceramics. HA is a highly crystalline CaP ceramic with the empirical formula of $Ca_{10}(PO_4)_6(OH)_2$; it is the most extensively used CaP ceramic because of its chemical similarity with the inorganic phase of bone (Zhou & Lee, 2011). It has a Ca/P ratio of 1.67 and the most stable and least soluble CaP phase over the pH range of ~3.5 to ~9.7 (Samavedi et al., 2013).

HA is known to be osteoconductive in nature. Its resorption rate is slow, around 1–2% per year (Costantino & Friedman, 1994). Once implanted into the body, HA integrates into the regenerated bony tissue, promoting graft vascularization and the proliferation of stem cells and thereby guiding bone tissue regeneration. Doping with different ions can modify the HA crystalline structure and increase its dissolution rate. For example, doping with manganese and zinc increased HA degradation rates by modifying its crystallinity, microstructure, and solubility with the introduction of the cations (Kandasamy et al., 2020; Sheikh et al., 2015).

HA has received considerable recent attention as a bone substitute material. HA fabrication and processing have also developed with the growing importance of the biological applications of HA as artificial bone and teeth (Haider et al., 2017). HA has been used for repairing bone defects, spinal fusions, augmenting atrophic alveolar ridges, and craniofacial repair. It has also been used in dental surgery and as a vehicle for biomolecular and drug delivery. As a coating on orthopedic and dental implants, HA increases their bioactivity and biocompatibility (Murugan & Ramakrishna, 2005).

β-TCP is a biodegradable CaP ceramic with the empirical formula of $Ca_3(PO_4)_2$ and a Ca-to-P ratio of 1.5:1. β-TCP has been detected pathologically in calcified dental calculus and in renal and urinary stones, but it has not been identified in dentin, enamel, or bone (Dorozhkin & Epple, 2002). It promotes osteogenesis and new bone formation; specifically, when implanted in vivo, β-TCP resorbs completely and has a significantly faster degradation rate than HA, making it suitable for growth of new bone tissue (Fujita et al., 2003). However, HA has higher mechanical strength (Hing et al., 2007). To address this issue, researchers have combined HA with β-TCP to form biphasic calcium phosphate (BCP) with the optimized mechanical strength and biodegradation rate. BCP is therefore now widely used in bone tissue engineering applications (Ballouze et al., 2021; Sarkar et al., 2019).

The biodegradable ceramics have some shortcomings such as poor mechanical properties, low fatigue resistance, high stiffness and brittleness, and significantly less strength than metallic implants or nonresorbable ceramics (Hasan et al., 2013). Therefore, they are not widely used in load-bearing applications or as bone-fixation devices. Nevertheless, advantages are achieved by combining these bioresorbable ceramics with bioresorbable polymers to form bioresorbable polymer ceramic composites with optimized properties.

These composites are bioactive in nature and form chemical bonds with the host tissue and as a result fixation of these implants is accelerated (Elgendy et al., 1993; Ignjatović et al., 2006). Their application is successful when only low mechanical strength is required, and they are mainly used as biodegradable bone-fixation devices like interference screws and suture anchors to fix bone to soft tissues for treatment in arthroscopic surgeries and sports medicine. Bioresorbable interference screws are used to fix graft or tendon between the bone and the screw in biceps tenodesis and anterior cruciate ligament (ACL) reconstruction (Suchenski et al., 2010). The implantation of bioresorbable interference screws is associated with mechanical short-term stabilization that allows early movement while the bone tendon heals. This is followed by biological long-term stabilization through osteointegration while allowing effective load transmission and enhancing stability (Suchenski et al., 2010).

6.4.2.2 Bioresorbable Ceramic Bone-Fixation Devices

There are very few reports of bone-fixation devices made from pure ceramics in the literature, some of which will be discussed in this section, but the main reason is the low strength and brittleness of bioresorbable ceramics. However, considering the several advantages of these ceramics there is a high need for the development of bioresorbable pure ceramic bone fixation devices. Pure bioresorbable ceramic fixation devices are mainly used for the repair of ACL injuries where low mechanical strength is required.

Mayr et al. (2007) developed bioresorbable microporous pure β-TCP plugs to fix ACL grafts using patellar tendon by press fitting. It has comparable fixation strength with that of metallic interference screws. However, during the press fitting of the plug, the impaction on the graft by trocar can be a concern. To address this issue, Schumacher et al. (2017) developed a novel interference screw with a new screw geometry made of pure HA to allow insertion within the bone without applying any external torque, thereby preventing damage to the graft or surrounding tissue.

The screw had a large thread pitch, which helped in self-rotation during insertion without the need of any screwdriver. The screw had a significantly higher pullout force (486 ± 60 N) with rigid PU foam than that of the commercial BioComposite™ interference screw (435 ± 120 N). However, to insert the screw, compression is applied that causes chipping, mainly damaging the screw head (Schumacher et al., 2017). Therefore, to manufacture pure ceramic fixation devices, various critical factors need to be controlled: mainly the screw geometry such as shank diameter, thread diameter, screw length, thread pitch, thread geometry, and drive mechanism (Suchenski et al., 2010). Researchers are focusing on controlling these issues to be able to take them to the next level for clinical translation.

6.4.2.3 Bioresorbable Polymer Ceramic Composite Bone-Fixation Devices

PLA-, PGA-, and PLGA-based fixtures are available in the market and are preferred over the non-bioresorbable metallic bone fixation devices due to their resorbability, which avoids the need for a second surgery. Nevertheless, the poor mechanical properties and degradation of these implants results in the release of acidic monomers and oligomers, which sometimes results in a foreign body reaction called osteolysis (Bostman et al., 1990; Weiler et al., 1996), tunnel widening, and intra articular migration (Ramos et al., 2020). To minimize the undesired tissue reaction, composite screws made of bioresorbable polymer reinforced with ceramic-based biomaterials namely, β-TCP or HA have been developed (Akindoyo et al., 2017, 2018). Table 6.3 presents the commercially available bioresorbable composite bone-fixation screws.

In these composite ceramics, the ratio of polymer to ceramic should be optimized in such a way that the composite possesses maximum mechanical strength. The polymer component provides flexibility, while the ceramic component provides osteoconductivity, and altering the amount of polymer or ceramic greatly affects their strength at the interface; the composite materials can be either pliable or brittle. The elastic modulus of polymer ceramic composites can also be adjusted by controlling the ceramic content to be comparable with that of human bone, although their application is limited to the fixation of soft tissues.

Several researchers have observed that these composites have reduced or mild inflammatory response compared with that from pure polymers (Sheikh et al., 2015). The release of basic salts from the bioceramics buffers the acidic breakdown products of the polymers and reduces the rate of acidosis and causes less toxicity (Shikinami & Okuno, 1999). The introduction of ceramics in the polymer matrix also enhances their biocompatibility and osteoconductivity, providing good cell adhesion and replacement by newly formed bone tissue (Damien & Parsons, 1991).

6.4.3 Biodegradable Metals

As we have discussed, researchers have developed various types of biodegradable biomaterials such as biopolymers and bioceramics for temporary orthopedic implant applications. Between the two, biopolymers present good plasticity, biodegradability, and biocompatibility, but low strength and poor wettability limit their use as bone implants. On the other hand, bioceramics have high biocompatibility and osteoconductivity, but inert brittleness restricts their applicability as bone supports.

TABLE 6.3
Commercially Available Bioresorbable Polymer Ceramic Composite Interference Screws

Commercial Name	Composition	Manufacturer	Properties
ComposiTCP™ 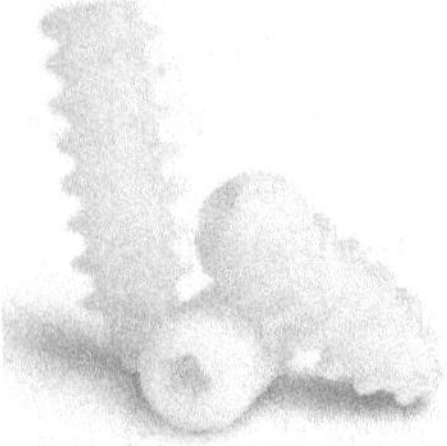	PLDLA/β-TCP	Zimmer Biomet, US	• Stimulates osteogenesis and ECM synthesis • Faster degradation kinetics and less inflammatory response than pure PLA (Aunoble et al., 2006)
CROSS lig® 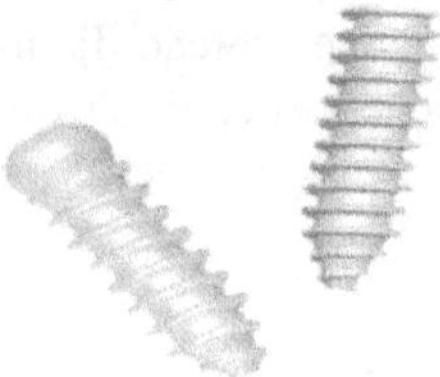	DL-PLA/β-TCP	FH ORTHO, US	• Use under high load conditions • Reduces inflammation and promotes human osteoblast proliferation, bone repair, and resorption (in contrast with pure lactic acid polymers) • Prevents tunnel enlargement and fibrous tissue formation (CROSS ling® interference screw, 2008)
Biotwin™ 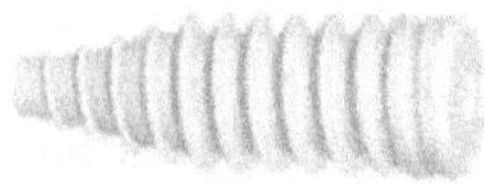 Osteotwin™ 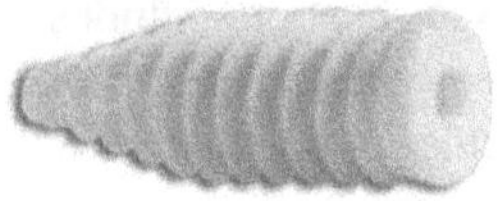	PLDLLA/BCP PLDLLA/MBCP	Biomatlante, France	• Provides the mechanical properties required for ligament reconstruction • Regulates resorption and osseointegration to form structural bone through hydrolysis (Barth et al., 2016; Biotwin™ Interference Screw)
FiberFIX™ 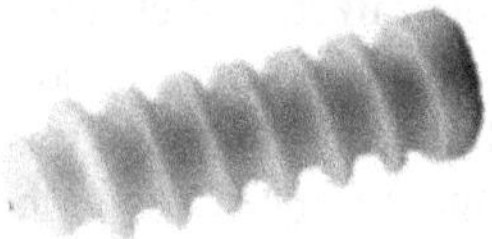	Patented bioresorbable polymer/HA nanofiber	Nanova, US	• Enhanced resistance to breakage or chipping during screw insertion • Reduced failure rates due to increased pull-out strength after insertion • Reduced acidic degradation of the composite and minimal inflammatory response (Vetalice, 2021)
Biosteon® 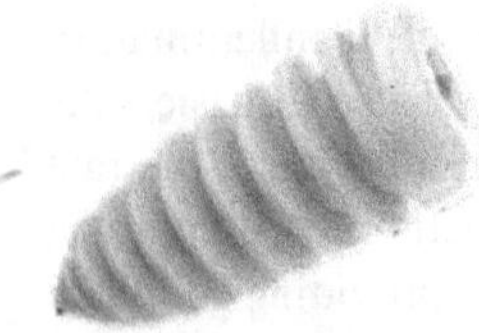	PLLA/HA	Biocomposites, UK	• Improved strength retention, osteointegration potential, and pH buffering during the graft healing period (Johnston et al., 2011) • Reduced tunnel widening (Lind et al., 2009)
Bilok® 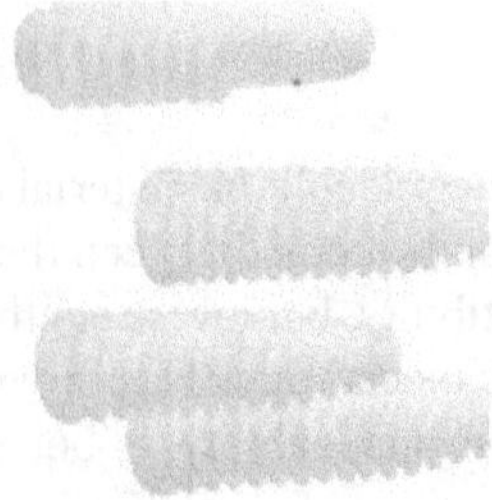	PLLA/β-TCP	Biocomposites, UK	• β-TCP particles distributed uniformly and well integrated into the PLLA matrix maximize the screw integrity (Barber & Dockery, 2008) • Improved degradation time and hydrophilicity due to low molecular weight and low crystalline PLLA (Barber & Boothby, 2007)

Commercial Name	Composition	Manufacturer	Properties
ActivaScrew™ Interference TCP	PLGA/β-TCP	Bioretek, Finland	• High strength • Easy insertion and safe medication use in the refixation of ligaments and tendons to bone • Enhanced fixation stability due to Self-Locking SL™ technology (ActivaScrew™ Interference)
BioComposite™	PLDLA/BCP	Anthrex, US	• Acidosis effect starts after significant tissue regeneration, reducing adverse reactions • The components act as a pH buffer, reducing the local acidosis effect (Arthrex 7 mm × 23 mm BioComposite Interference Screw vs. DePuy Mitek 7 mm × 23 mm Milagro Screw).
Bioact IF OSTEOTRANS	PLLA/unfired HA	Teijin Medical Technologies, Japan	• Strength higher than human cortical bone • Strength is retained for 4 ~ 6 months (Bioact IF OSTEOTRANS)
MILAGRO® Advanced Interference Screw	PLGA/β-TCP	Depuy Synthes, USA	• Microparticle dispersion technology enables uniform distribution of PLGA and β-TCP • Screw insertion rate is fast (Barber et al., 2011) • Osteoconductive, stable healing, no movement of graft • Tunnel enlargement • The rate of polymer degradation accounts for the high level of acidosis (Arthrex 7 mm × 23 mm BioComposite Interference Screw vs. DePuy Mitek 7 mm × 23 mm Milagro Screw)
GENESYS™ Matryx®	self-reinforced (SR) PLDA, ß-TCP	ConMed Linvatec, Finland	• Reliable fixation stability during the healing period • Promotes bone ingrowth (GENESYS™ Matryx® (β-TCP) Interference Screw).
BioRCI HA™	PLLA/HA	Smith & Nephew, US	• Additional fixation due to unique oversized head design • Reverse-threaded screws hold soft tissue grafts in the optimal position • Presence of HA reduces the pH as a result of combined HA and polymer resorption (Agrawal et al., 1996)

* β-TCP–β-tricalcium phosphate, HA–hydroxyapatite, BCP–biphasic calcium phosphate, ECM–extracellular matrix, MBCP–microporous biphasic calcium phosphate, PLLA–poly(L-lactic acid), PLDLA/DL-PLA–poly-L/D-lactide, PLDLLA–poly(L-lactide-co-D,L-lactide), PLGA–polylactic-co-glycolic scid, PGA–polyglycolic acid.

Note: Authors acknowledge all sources from which any information/image/photograph has been provided in this table.

When compared with biopolymers and bioceramics, biodegradable metals such as magnesium, zinc, and iron are recently capturing enormous research interest (Chandra & Pandey, 2020). Among them, Fe and Fe alloys have high mechanical properties with slow degradation rate, which does not match the requirement of bone regeneration. Moreover, Zn and Zn alloys have suitable degradation rate and low mechanical strength. In comparison, Mg and Mg alloys have similar mechanical properties (elastic moduli ~ 45 GPa, density ~ 1.75–1.85 g/cm^3) to those of natural bones (elastic moduli ~ 3–20 GPa, density ~ 1.75 g/cm^3), thereby lowering the stress-shielding effect between bone and Mg based implants (Tan et al., 2018). From a biological perspective, magnesium is an essential element in the human body, as Mg ions are needed in soft tissue healing and bone construction, and it acts as a cofactor for many enzymes; a healthy human contains 30 g of magnesium in total, and daily intake of 420 mg is recommended for good health (Jacobs et al., 2003). In case of bone healing, the release of Mg ions from Mg-based implants creates a localized alkaline environment that induces osteogenesis and increases bone mineralization (Galow et al., 2017; Yoshizawa et al., 2014).

However, the fast degradation profiles of Mg and Mg alloys in the human body environment result in premature loss of strength and implant failure (Ahmadkhaniha et al., 2017; Vinogradov et al., 2019). In addition, Mg has a hexagonal close-packed crystal structure that provides limiting slip systems and presents low formability and ductility (Tekumalla et al., 2014). Moreover, Mg and its alloys are highly biocompatible if alloying elements are below their toxic levels and are bioelements. The degradation of biodegradable magnesium-based metal alloys is driven by electrochemical reactions individually. The degradation products of Mg and its alloys are hydrogen gas and a porous magnesium hydroxide layer that forms on the surface and accelerates the corrosion in chlorine-containing physiological environments (Patil et al., 2019).

A tremendous amount of research has been focused on controlling the degradation rate of Mg and its alloys. Intrinsic impurity elements (Fe, Cu, Ni, and Co) in Mg form secondary phases with the alpha-Mg phase and cause micro-galvanic corrosion due to their higher corrosion potential than that of Mg, which is mostly responsible for the rapid Mg corrosion rate (Ho et al., 2020; Jaiswal et al., 2020; Pan et al., 2016; Zeng et al., 2006). Hence, it is crucial to create Mg-based biomaterials that have acceptable impurity levels to mitigate intrinsic corrosion.

To date, no pure magnesium has a long-term corrosion rate lower than that of commercially available ultra-high purity (UHP) magnesium, 0.25 mm/year as assessed by mass loss measurements in a 3.5% wt NaCl solution (Pan et al., 2016; Wu et al., 2021); however, UHP Mg is expensive. As a result, a variety of techniques were examined such as filtering, vacuum distillation, and fluxes, for lowering the cost of controlling the impurities in pure Mg and its alloys (Shaikh et al., 2022; Wu et al., 2021). It has also been demonstrated that alloying Mg can retard the biodegradation process, although there are few elements that are suitable for magnesium alloying from a medical standpoint.

There is a wealth of literature on alloying Mg to reduce its corrosion resistance for a variety of industrial and medical applications. Furthermore, all alloying elements form secondary phases with Mg, which causes corrosion (Ho et al., 2020; Zeng et al., 2006). Clinical approval has recently been granted for a few of the Mg and its alloys for use in bone implants, particularly high-purity (99.99%) Mg, Mg-Ca-Zn, and Mg-Y-RE-Zr (Hermawan, 2018).

Early attempts to use Mg as bone implants date to the early 1900s (Witte et al., 2008), but additional research wasn't possible until recent decades due to the material's rapid disintegration rate and inadequate refinement technologies at the time. The more modern Mg alloys demonstrated excellent osteointegration and osteogenesis capabilities after their extensive characterization using in vivo and animal experiments. Figure 6.6 presents the commercially available absorbable Mg- and Mg-alloy-based bone implants. Clinical trials of these implants are summarized in Table 6.4.

These trials were performed in Germany, China, Korea, Singapore, and Austria (Choo et al., 2019; Lee et al., 2016; Plaass et al., 2020; Wendelstein et al., 2021; Windhagen et al., 2013; Yu et al., 2015). The first clinical report was proposed in 2013 in Germany, where Mg-Y-RE-Zr alloy (MAGNEZIX®) screws were implanted in hallux valgus abnormalities. After this, the same screw

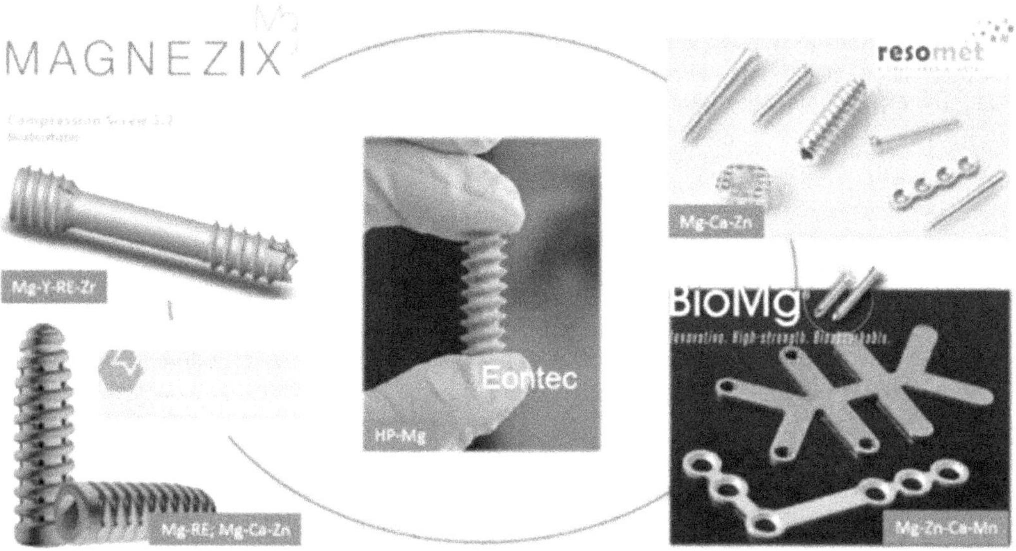

FIGURE 6.6 Commercially available magnesium-based absorbable bone implants (Reproduced under the terms of CC-BY 4.0 (https://creativecommons.org/licenses/by/4.0) International License from Sarian, M. N., Iqbal, N., Sotoudehbagha, P., Razavi, M., Ahmed, Q. U., Sukotjo, C., & Hermawan, H.: Potential bioactive coating system for high performance absorbable magnesium bone implants. Bioact. Mater., 2022. 12. 42–63. Copyright 2022 Sarian et al., published by Elsevier).

TABLE 6.4
Clinical Trials of Magnesium and Its Alloys and Implants Performed

Year	No. of Patients	Material	Location of Implantation	Duration
2013 (Windhagen et al., 2013)	26	MAGNEZIX vs. titanium implant	Foot	1–3 d, 4–8 d, 2 wk, 6 wk, 3 mo, 6 mo
2015 (Yu et al., 2015)	19	Pure Mg screw	Femoral Neck	3 mo, 6 mo, 12 mo
2016 (Zhao et al., 2016)	48	Pure Mg screw vs. without fixation	Femoral head	3 mo, 6 mo, 12 mo
2016 (Lee et al., 2016)	53	Mg (5wt%)-Ca (1wt%)-Zn screw	Hand	1 wk, 2 wk, 1 mo, 2 mo, 3 mo, 6 mo, 12 mo
2017 (Plaass et al., 2018)	26	MAGNEZIX vs titanium implant	Distal metatarsal	3y postoperative
2018 (Choo et al., 2019)	93	MAGNEZIX vs titanium implant	Distal metatarsal	Preoperative, 3 mo, 12 mo postoperative
2020 (Plaass et al., 2020)	70	MAGNEZIX vs titanium implant	Foot	6 wk, 12 wk, and 1 year
2020 (May et al., 2020)	48	Mg screw vs Ti screw	Ankle	12–53 months
2021 (Wendelstein et al., 2021)	44	Mg screw vs Ti screw vs K wire	Foot	Minimum of 12 months

d: day, wk: week, mo: month

was used in many clinical studies to treat various bone fractures. These studies were conducted for different durations (1 week to 1 year) and analyzed using various techniques including X-ray and low dose radiation computed tomography scans for understanding the bone healing and hydrogen evolution. Overall, clinical findings have shown promising results and confirmed magnesium and its alloys as safe bone fixtures. However, more clinical results with longer duration and load-bearing sites are required for future applications.

CONCLUSIONS AND FUTURE PERSPECTIVES

High incidences of bone fractures warrant the need for bone implants that can not only support the fractured native bone tissue but also promote bone healing. Bone healing is a slow process that usually takes three to six months depending on the site of injury/defect. Therefore, there is a high demand for biodegradable orthopedic supports and implant materials such as bone screws, plates, nails and rods.

Through this chapter, we have tried to focus on the development of biodegradable orthopedic implants for bone tissue engineering while highlighting the vital approaches adopted with clinical trials for commercialization. Ceramics, polymers, and their composites have shown potential, and commercial products are available in the implant market. However, many challenges remain to achieving good mechanical properties, tunable degradability, and osteoconductivity in bioactive composite materials to be used for osteologic repair and load-bearing implant applications.

On the other hand, biodegradable metal-based orthopedic implants, especially those fabricated using magnesium-based alloys, are attracting a great deal of attention due to enhanced properties. The major drawback of magnesium is high degradation in the human physiological environment. To overcome this high degradation, many steps are being adopted including purification, alloying, mechanical forging, and surface modifications. Researchers are now focusing on a combinatorial approach for fabricating tunably degradable magnesium-alloy based implants that can meet the desired outcomes in terms of load-bearing implants. Furthermore, it is expected that the next generation of biodegradable materials will demonstrate vast improvements in implant fabrication procedures as well as on their interface with the biological tissue. Materials scientists and physicians must constantly collaborate to develop innovative, bioactive, high-performance absorbable bone implants that accelerate bone fracture repair.

ACKNOWLEDGMENTS

The authors would like to acknowledge the funding received from the Indian Council of Medical Research (IMPRINT-6714; UAY/MHRD_IITK_006), India's Ministry of Human Resource Development (SPARC/2018–2019/P612/S), the Science and Engineering Research Board (IPA/2020/000026; CRG/2021/002179), the Government of India Department of Science and Technology (DST/NM/NT-2018/48) and Department of Biotechnology (DBT/IN/SWEDEN/08/AK/2017–18; BT/PR46254/AAQ/1/861/2022), and the Gangwal School of Medical Sciences and Technology, Indian Institute of Technology, Kanpur (initiation grant). Shazia Shaikh would like to acknowledge DBT-BioCARe for financial support (DBT/BSBE/2023606). Rupita Ghosh would like to acknowledge financial support from the DBT-RA program in Biotechnology and Life Sciences. Shreya Mehrotra would like to acknowledge the Department of Science and Technology for the Inspire faculty financial support.

LIST OF ABBREVIATIONS

ACL Anterior cruciate ligament
BCP Biphasic calcium phosphate

CaP Calcium phosphate
HA Hydroxyapatite
IBFD Internal bone fixation devices
PDLA Poly-D-lactide
PGA Poly(glycolic acid)
PLA Polymer poly(lactic acid)
PLGA Poly(lactic- co-glycolic acid)
PLLA Poly-L-lactide
TMC Trimethylene carbonate
UHP Ultra-high purity
β-TCP Beta tricalcium phosphate

REFERENCES

Agrawal, C. M., & Athanasiou, K. A. (1997). Technique to control pH in vicinity of biodegrading PLA-PGA implants. *J. Biomed. Mater. Res.* 38: 105–114.

Agrawal, C. M., Fan, M., Zhu, C., & Athanasiou, K. (1996). New technique to control the pH in the vicinity of biodegradable implants. *Proceedings of the 1996 5th World Biomaterials Congress: Part 2 (of 2).* Toronto, Canada.

Ahmadkhaniha, D., Fedel, M., Heydarzadeh Sohi, M., & Deflorian, F. (2017). Corrosion behavior of severely plastic deformed magnesium based alloys: A review. *Surf. Eng. Appl. Electrochem.* 53: 439–448.

Akindoyo, J. O., Beg, M. D., Ghazali, S., Heim, H. P., & Feldmann, M. (2017). Effects of surface modification on dispersion, mechanical, thermal and dynamic mechanical properties of injection molded PLA-hydroxyapatite composites. *Compos. Part A Appl. Sci. Manuf.* 103: 96–105.

Akindoyo, J. O., Beg, M. D., Ghazali, S., Heim, H. P., & Feldmann, M. (2018). Impact modified PLA-hydroxyapatite composites—Thermo-mechanical properties. *Compos. Part A Appl. Sci. Manuf.* 107: 326–333.

Aunoble, S., Clément, D., Frayssinet, P., Harmand, M. F., & Le Huec, J. C. (2006). Biological performance of a new β-TCP/PLLA composite material for applications in spine surgery: In vitro and in vivo studies. *J. Biomed. Mater. Res. A.* 78: 416–422.

Balla, E., Daniilidis, V., Karlioti, G., Kalamas, T., Stefanidou, M., Bikiaris, N. D., Vlachopoulos, A., Koumentakou, I., & Bikiaris, D. N. (2021). Poly (Lactic acid): A versatile biobased polymer for the future with multifunctional properties—From monomer synthesis, polymerization techniques and molecular weight increase to PLA applications. *Polymers (Basel).* 13: 1822.

Ballouze, R., Marahat, M. H., Mohamad, S., Saidin, N. A., Kasim, S. R., & Ooi, J. P. (2021). Biocompatible magnesium-doped biphasic calcium phosphate for bone regeneration. *J. Biomed. Mater. Res. B Appl. Biomater.* 109: 1426–1435.

Bandyopadhyay, A., Mitra, I., Goodman, S. B., Kumar, M., & Bose, S. (2022). Improving biocompatibility for next generation of metallic implants. *Prog. Mater. Sci.* 133: 101053.

Barber, F. A., & Boothby, M. H. (2007). Bilok interference screws for anterior cruciate ligament reconstruction: Clinical and radiographic outcomes. *Arthroscopy.* 23: 476–481.

Barber, F. A., & Dockery, W. D. (2008). Long-term absorption of β—Tricalcium phosphate poly-l-lactic acid interference screws. *Arthroscopy.* 24: 441–447.

Barber, F. A., Dockery, W., & Hrnack, S. A. (2011). Long-term degradation of a poly-lactide co-glycolide/β-tricalcium phosphate biocomposite interference screw. *Arthroscopy.* 27: 637–643.

Barth, J., Akritopoulos, P., Graveleau, N., Barthelemy, R., Toanen, C., & Saffarini, M. (2016). Efficacy of osteoconductive ceramics in bioresorbable screws for anterior cruciate ligament reconstruction: A prospective intrapatient comparative study. *Orthop. J. Sports Med.* 4: 2325967116647724.

Bioact IF OSTEOTRANS. Teijin Medical Technologies Co., Ltd. https://teijin-medical.co.jp/en/products/bonefix/osteotrans/bioact/

Bostman, O., Hirvensalo, E., Makinen, J., & Rokkanen, P. (1990). Foreign-body reactions to fracture fixation implants of biodegradable synthetic polymers. *J. Bone Joint Surg. Br.* 72: 592–596.

Böstman, O. M., & Pihlajamäki, H. K. (2000). Adverse tissue reactions to bioabsorbable fixation devices. *Clin. Orthop. Relat. Res.* 371: 216–227.

Burny, F., Donkerwolcke, M., Moulart, F., Bourgois, R., Puers, R., Van Schuylenbergh, K., Barbosa, M., Paiva, O., Rodes, F., & Bégueret, J. B. (2000). Concept, design and fabrication of smart orthopedic implants. *Med. Eng. Phys*. 22: 469–479.

Busch, A., Wegner, A., Haversath, M., & Jäger, M. (2021). Bone substitutes in orthopaedic surgery: Current status and future perspectives. *Z Orthop. Unfall*. 159: 304–313.

Capuana, E., Lopresti, F., Ceraulo, M., & La Carrubba, V. (2022). Poly-L-Lactic Acid (PLLA)-based biomaterials for regenerative medicine: A review on processing and applications. *Polymers (Basel)*. 14: 1153.

Castro, J. I., Valencia Llano, C. H., Tenorio, D. L., Saavedra, M., Zapata, P., Navia-Porras, D. P., Delgado-Ospina, J., Chaur, M. N., Hernández, J. H. M., & Grande-Tovar, C. D. (2022). Biocompatibility assessment of Polylactic Acid (PLA) and nanobioglass (n-BG) nanocomposites for biomedical applications. *Molecules*. 27: 3640.

Chandra, G., & Pandey, A. (2020). Biodegradable bone implants in orthopedic applications: A review. *Biocybern. Biomed. Eng*. 40: 596–610.

Chandra, R., & Rustgi, R. (1998). Biodegradable polymers. *Prog. Polym. Sci*. 23: 1273–1335.

Chaya, A., Yoshizawa, S., Verdelis, K., Myers, N., Costello, B. J., Chou, D. T., Pal, S., Maiti, S., Kumta, P. N., & Sfeir, C. (2015). In vivo study of magnesium plate and screw degradation and bone fracture healing. *Acta Biomater*. 18: 262–269.

Choo, J. T., Lai, S. H. S., Tang, C. Q. Y., & Thevendran, G. (2019). Magnesium-based bioabsorbable screw fixation for hallux valgus surgery—A suitable alternative to metallic implants. *Foot Ankle Surg*. 25: 727–732.

Claes, L., Recknagel, S., & Ignatius, A. (2012). Fracture healing under healthy and inflammatory conditions. *Nat. Rev. Rheumatol*. 8: 133–143.

Costantino, P. D., & Friedman, C. D. (1994). Synthetic bone graft substitutes. *Otolaryngol. Clin. North Am*. 27: 1037–1074.

Damien, C. J., & Parsons, J. R. (1991). Bone graft and bone graft substitutes: A review of current technology and applications. *J. Appl. Biomater*. 2: 187–208.

de França, J. O. C., da Silva Valadares, D., Paiva, M. F., Dias, S. C. L., & Dias, J. A. (2022). Polymers based on PLA from synthesis using D, L-lactic acid (or racemic lactide) and some biomedical applications: A short review. *Polymers (Basel)*. 14: 2317.

DeStefano, V., Khan, S., & Tabada, A. (2020). Applications of PLA in modern medicine. *Eng. Reg*. 1: 76–87.

Dorozhkin, S. V. (2010). Bioceramics of calcium orthophosphates. *Biomaterials*. 31: 1465–1485.

Dorozhkin, S. V., & Epple, M. (2002). Biological and medical significance of calcium phosphates. *Angew. Chem. Int. Ed. Engl*. 41: 3130–3146.

Dubok, V. A. (2000). Bioceramics—Yesterday, today, tomorrow. *Powder Metall. Met. Ceram*. 39: 381–394.

Eitenmüller, J., David, A., Pommer, A., & Muhr, G. (1996). Surgical treatment of ankle joint fractures with biodegradable screws and plates of poly-l-lactide. *Chirurg*. 67: 413–418.

Elgendy, H. M., Norman, M. E., Keaton, A. R., & Laurencin, C. T. (1993). Osteoblast-like cell (MC3T3-E1) proliferation on bioerodible polymers: An approach towards the development of a bone-bioerodible polymer composite material. *Biomaterials*. 14: 263–269.

Fujita, R., Yokoyama, A., Kawasaki, T., & Kohgo, T. (2003). Bone augmentation osteogenesis using hydroxyapatite and β-tricalcium phosphate blocks. *J. Oral Maxillofac. Surg*. 61: 1045–1053.

Galow, A.-M., Rebl, A., Koczan, D., Bonk, S. M., Baumann, W., & Gimsa, J. (2017). Increased osteoblast viability at alkaline pH in vitro provides a new perspective on bone regeneration. *Biochem. Biophys. Rep*. 10: 17–25.

Ghosh, R. (2018). *Study on the Development of Calcium Phosphate Based Machinable Bioceramics*. (Doctoral Dessertation, NIT Rourkela, India).

Guo, B., & Ma, P. X. (2014). Synthetic biodegradable functional polymers for tissue engineering: A brief review. *Sci. China Chem*. 57: 490–500.

Haghshenas, M. (2017). Mechanical characteristics of biodegradable magnesium matrix composites: A review. *J. Magnes. Alloys*. 5: 189–201.

Haider, A., Haider, S., Han, S. S., & Kang, I. K. (2017). Recent advances in the synthesis, functionalization and biomedical applications of hydroxyapatite: A review. *RSC Adv*. 7: 7442–7458.

Hajebi, S., Mohammadi Nasr, S., Rabiee, N., Bagherzadeh, M., Ahmadi, S., Rabiee, M., Tahriri, M., Tayebi, L., & Hamblin, M. R. (2021). Bioresorbable composite polymeric materials for tissue engineering applications. *Int. J. Polym. Mater*. 70: 926–940.

Hamza, A. A., El-Bakary, M. A., Ibrahim, M. A., Elgamal, M. A., & El-Sayed, N. M. (2022). Investigate the degradable behavior of a poly (glycolide-co-trimethylene carbonate) suture material used in a vascular surgery. *Polym. Bull.* 79: 10783–10801.

Han, H. S., Loffredo, S., Jun, I., Edwards, J., Kim, Y. C., Seok, H. K., Witte, F., Mantovani, D., & Glyn-Jones, S. (2019). Current status and outlook on the clinical translation of biodegradable metals. *Mater. Today.* 23: 57–71.

Hanson, B., van der Werken, C., & Stengel, D. (2008). Surgeons' beliefs and perceptions about removal of orthopaedic implants. *BMC Musculoskelet. Disord.* 9: 1–8.

Hasan, M. S., Ahmed, I., Parsons, A. J., Rudd, C. D., Walker, G. S., & Scotchford, C. A. (2013). Investigating the use of coupling agents to improve the interfacial properties between a resorbable phosphate glass and polylactic acid matrix. *J. Biomater. Appl.* 28: 354–366.

Hench, L. L. (1991). Bioceramics: From concept to clinic. *J. Am. Ceram. Soc.* 74: 1487–1510.

Hench, L. L. (1993). *An Introduction to Bioceramics* (Vol. 1). Singapore: World Scientific.

Hermawan, H. (2018). Updates on the research and development of absorbable metals for biomedical applications. *Prog. Biomater.* 7: 93–110.

Hing, K. A., Wilson, L. F., & Buckland, T. (2007). Comparative performance of three ceramic bone graft substitutes. *Spine J.* 7: 475–490.

Ho, Y. H., Joshi, S. S., Wu, T. C., Hung, C. M., Ho, N. J., & Dahotre, N. B. (2020). In-vitro bio-corrosion behavior of friction stir additively manufactured AZ31B magnesium alloy-hydroxyapatite composites. *Mater. Sci. Eng. C. Mater. Biol. Appl.* 109: 110632.

Ignjatović, N., Ninkov, P., Kojić, V., Bokurov, M., Srdić, V., Krnojelac, D., Selaković, S., & Uskoković, D. (2006). Cytotoxicity and fibroblast properties during in vitro test of biphasic calcium phosphate/poly-dl-lactide-co-glycolide biocomposites and different phosphate materials. *Microsc. Res. Tech.* 69: 976–982.

Isaksson, H., Comas, O., van Donkelaar, C. C., Mediavilla, J., Wilson, W., Huiskes, R., & Ito, K. (2007). Bone regeneration during distraction osteogenesis: Mechano-regulation by shear strain and fluid velocity. *J. Biomech.* 40: 2002–2011.

Jacobs, J. J., Hallab, N. J., Skipor, A. K., & Urban, R. M. (2003). Metal degradation products: A cause for concern in metal-metal bearings? *Clin. Orthop. Relat. Res.* 417: 139–147.

Jaiswal, S., Dubey, A., & Lahiri, D. (2020). The influence of bioactive hydroxyapatite shape and size on the mechanical and biodegradation behaviour of magnesium based composite. *Ceram. Int.* 46: 27205–27218.

Jin, W., & Chu, P. K. (2019). Orthopedic implants. *Encyclo. Biomed. Eng.* 425–439.

Johnson, I., Lin, J., & Liu, H. (2017). Surface modification and coatings for controlling the degradation and bioactivity of magnesium alloys for medical applications. *Orthop. Biomaterials.* 331–363.

Johnston, M., Morse, A., Arrington, J., Pliner, M., & Gasser, S. (2011). Resorption and remodeling of hydroxyapatite—Poly-L-lactic acid composite anterior cruciate ligament interference screws. *Arthroscopy.* 27: 1671–1678.

Kandasamy, S., Narayanan, V., & Sumathi, S. (2020). Zinc and manganese substituted hydroxyapatite/CMC/PVP electrospun composite for bone repair applications. *Int. J. Biol. Macromol.* 145: 1018–1030.

Khodaei, T., Schmitzer, E., Suresh, A. P., & Acharya, A. P. (2023). Immune response differences in degradable and non-degradable alloy implants. *Bioact. Mater.* 24: 153–170.

Kim, T., See, C. W., Li, X., & Zhu, D. (2020). Orthopedic implants and devices for bone fractures and defects: Past, present and perspective. *Eng. Reg.* 1: 6–18.

Kontakis, G. M., Pagkalos, J. E., Tosounidis, T. I., Melissas, J., & Katonis, P. (2007). Bioabsorbable materials in orthopaedics. *Acta Orthop. Belg.* 73: 159–169.

Lee, J. W., Han, H. S., Han, K. J., Park, J., Jeon, H., Ok, M. R., Seok, H. K., Ahn, J. P., Lee, K. E., & Lee, D. H. (2016). Long-term clinical study and multiscale analysis of in vivo biodegradation mechanism of Mg alloy. *Proc. Natl. Acad. Sci. U. S. A.* 113: 716–721.

Lind, M., Feller, J., & Webster, K. E. (2009). Tibial bone tunnel widening is reduced by polylactate/hydroxyapatite interference screws compared to metal screws after ACL reconstruction with hamstring grafts. *Knee.* 16: 447–451.

Luthringer, B. J. C., Feyerabend, F., & Römer, R. W. (2014). Magnesium-based implants: A mini-review. *Magnes. Res.* 27: 142–154.

Makadia, H. K., & Siegel, S. J. (2011). Poly Lactic-Co-Glycolic Acid (PLGA) as biodegradable controlled drug delivery carrier. *Polymers (Basel).* 3: 1377–1397.

Marsell, R., & Einhorn, T. A. (2011). The biology of fracture healing. *Injury.* 42: 551–555.

Mavrogenis, A. F., Kanellopoulos, A. D., Nomikos, G. N., Papagelopoulos, P. J., & Soucacos, P. N. (2009). Early experience with biodegradable implants in pediatric patients. *Clin. Orthop. Relat. Res.* 467: 1591–1598.

May, H., Alper Kati, Y., Gumussuyu, G., Yunus Emre, T., Unal, M., & Kose, O. (2020). Bioabsorbable magnesium screw versus conventional titanium screw fixation for medial malleolar fractures. *J. Orthop. Trauma.* 21: 1–8.

Mayr, H. O., Hube, R., Bernstein, A., Seibt, A. B., Hein, W., & von Eisenhart-Rothe, R. (2007). Beta-tricalcium phosphate plugs for press-fit fixation in ACL reconstruction—A mechanical analysis in bovine bone. *Knee.* 14: 239–244.

Mhadhbi, M., & Sohani, A. (2022). Introductory chapter: Smart and advanced ceramics and applications. In *Smart and Advanced Ceramic Materials and Applications*. M. Mhadhbi, Ed. London: IntechOpen, p. 8.

Middleton, J. C., & Tipton, A. J. (2000). Synthetic biodegradable polymers as orthopedic devices. *Biomaterials.* 21: 2335–2346.

Murugan, R., & Ramakrishna, S. (2005). Development of nanocomposites for bone grafting. *Compos. Sci. Technol.* 65: 2385–2406.

Nagarajan, S., & Reddy, B. (2009). Bio-absorbable polymers in implantation-an overview. *J. Sci. Ind. Res.* 68: 993–1009.

Narayanan, G., Vernekar, V. N., Kuyinu, E. L., & Laurencin, C. T. (2016). Poly (Lactic acid)-based biomaterials for orthopaedic regenerative engineering. *Adv. Drug Deliv. Rev.* 107: 247–276.

Ngo, H. X., Bai, Y., Sha, J., Ishizuka, S., Toda, E., Osako, R., Kato, A., Morioka, R., Ramanathan, M., & Tatsumi, H. (2021). A narrative review of u-HA/PLLA, a bioactive resorbable reconstruction material: Applications in oral and maxillofacial surgery. *Materials (Basel).* 15: 150.

On, S. W., Cho, S. W., Byun, S. H., & Yang, B. E. (2020). Bioabsorbable osteofixation materials for maxillofacial bone surgery: A review on polymers and magnesium-based materials. *Biomedicines.* 8: 300.

Ono, T., Okamoto, K., Nakashima, T., Nitta, T., Hori, S., Iwakura, Y., & Takayanagi, H. (2016). IL-17-producing γδ T cells enhance bone regeneration. *Nat. Commun.* 7: 10928.

Palani, N. (2020). Introduction to medical implants. In *Toxicological Aspects of Medical Device Implants*. P. S. T. Shanmugam, L. Chokkalingam, and P. Bakthavachalam, Eds. Cambridge, MA: Academic Press, pp. 1–15

Pan, F., Chen, X., Yan, T., Liu, T., Mao, J., Luo, W., Wang, Q., Peng, J., Tang, A., & Jiang, B. (2016). A novel approach to melt purification of magnesium alloys. *J. Magnes. Alloys.* 4: 8–14.

Patil, S. S., Misra, R., Gao, M., Ma, Z., Tan, L., & Yang, K. (2019). Bioactive coating on a new Mg-2Zn-0.5 Nd alloy: Modulation of degradation rate and cellular response. *Mater. Technol.* 34: 394–402.

Pelto-Vasenius, K., Hirvensalo, E., Böstman, O., & Rokkanen, P. (1995). Fixation of scaphoid delayed union and non-union with absorbable polyglycolide pin or Herbert screw: Consolidation and functional results. *Arch. Orthop. Trauma Surg.* 114: 347–351.

Phillips, A. (2005). Overview of the fracture healing cascade. *Injury.* 36: S5–S7.

Pina, S., & Ferreira, J. M. (2012). Bioresorbable plates and screws for clinical applications: A review. *J. Healthc. Eng.* 3: 243–260.

Plaass, C., Karch, A., Koch, A., Wiederhoeft, V., Ettinger, S., Claassen, L., Daniilidis, K., Yao, D., & Stukenborg-Colsman, C. (2020). Short term results of dynamic splinting for hallux valgus—A prospective randomized study. *Foot Ankle Surg.* 26: 146–150.

Plaass, C., von Falck, C., Ettinger, S., Sonnow, L., Calderone, F., Weizbauer, A., Reifenrath, J., Claassen, L., Waizy, H., & Daniilidis, K. (2018). Bioabsorbable magnesium versus standard titanium compression screws for fixation of distal metatarsal osteotomies—3 year results of a randomized clinical trial. *J. Orthop. Sci.* 23: 321–327.

Rai, P., Mehrotra, S., Priya, S., Gnansounou, E., & Sharma, S. K. (2021). Recent advances in the sustainable design and applications of biodegradable polymers. *Bioresour. Technol.* 325: 124739.

Ramos, D. M., Dhandapani, R., Subramanian, A., Sethuraman, S., & Kumbar, S. G. (2020). Clinical complications of biodegradable screws for ligament injuries. *Mater. Sci. Eng. C. Mater. Biol. Appl.* 109: 110423.

Samavedi, S., Whittington, A. R., & Goldstein, A. S. (2013). Calcium phosphate ceramics in bone tissue engineering: A review of properties and their influence on cell behavior. *Acta Biomater.* 9: 8037–8045.

Samir, A., Ashour, F. H., Hakim, A. A., & Bassyouni, M. (2022). Recent advances in biodegradable polymers for sustainable applications. *NPJ Mater. Degrad.* 6: 68.

Sarian, M. N., Iqbal, N., Sotoudehbagha, P., Razavi, M., Ahmed, Q. U., Sukotjo, C., & Hermawan, H. (2022). Potential bioactive coating system for high-performance absorbable magnesium bone implants. *Bioact. Mater.* 12: 42–63.

Sarkar, R., Agrawal, A., & Ghosh, R. (2019). Preparation of ex-situ mixed sintered biphasic calcium phosphate ceramics from its co-precipitated precursors and their characterization. *Trans. Indian Ceram. Soc.* 78: 101–107.

Schumacher, T. C., Tushtev, K., Wagner, U., Becker, C., große Holthaus, M., Hein, S. B., Haack, J., Heiss, C., Engelhardt, M., & El Khassawna, T. (2017). A novel, hydroxyapatite-based screw-like device for Anterior Cruciate Ligament (ACL) reconstructions. *Knee.* 24: 933–939.

Shaikh, S., Qayoom, I., Sarvesha, R., & Kumar, A. (2022). Bioresorbable magnesium-based alloys containing strontium doped nanohydroxyapatite promotes bone healing in critical sized bone defect in rat femur shaft. *J. Magnes. Alloys.* 11: 270–286.

Sheikh, Z., Najeeb, S., Khurshid, Z., Verma, V., Rashid, H., & Glogauer, M. (2015). Biodegradable materials for bone repair and tissue engineering applications. *Materials (Basel).* 8: 5744–5794.

Shikinami, Y., & Okuno, M. (1999). Bioresorbable devices made of forged composites of Hydroxyapatite (HA) particles and Poly-L-Lactide (PLLA): Part I: Basic characteristics. *Biomaterials.* 20: 859–877.

Singh, V., & Tiwari, M. (2010). Structure-processing-property relationship of poly (glycolic acid) for drug delivery systems 1: Synthesis and catalysis. *Int. J. Polym. Sci.* 2010: 652719.

Song, R., Murphy, M., Li, C., Ting, K., Soo, C., & Zheng, Z. (2018). Current development of biodegradable polymeric materials for biomedical applications. *Drug Des. Devel. Ther.* 12: 3117–3145.

Suchenski, M., McCarthy, M. B., Chowaniec, D., Hansen, D., McKinnon, W., Apostolakos, J., Arciero, R., & Mazzocca, A. D. (2010). Material properties and composition of soft-tissue fixation. *Arthroscopy.* 26: 821–831.

Taddei, E., Henriques, V., Silva, C., & Cairo, C. (2004). Production of new titanium alloy for orthopedic implants. *Mater. Sci. Eng. C.* 24: 683–687.

Tan, L., Dong, J., Chen, J., & Yang, K. (2018). Development of magnesium alloys for biomedical applications: Structure, process to property relationship. *Mater. Technol.* 33: 235–243.

Tan, L., Yu, X., Wan, P., & Yang, K. (2013). Biodegradable materials for bone repairs: A review. *J. Mater. Sci. Technol.* 29: 503–513.

Tekumalla, S., Seetharaman, S., Almajid, A., & Gupta, M. (2014). Mechanical properties of magnesium-rare earth alloy systems: A review. *Metals.* 5: 1–39.

Turner, I. G. (2021). Ceramics and glasses. In *Biomedical Materials.* R. Narayan, Ed. Cham: Springer, pp. 101–137.

Vetalice, J. A. (2021). *Nanova Biomaterials Launches FiberFIX Bioresorbable Implants.* www.orthoworld.com/nanova-biomaterials-launches-fiberfix-bioresorbable-implants/

Vinogradov, A., Vasilev, E., Kopylov, V. I., Linderov, M., Brilevesky, A., & Merson, D. (2019). High performance fine-grained biodegradable Mg-Zn-Ca alloys processed by severe plastic deformation. *Metals.* 9: 186.

Visan, A. I., Popescu-Pelin, G., & Socol, G. (2021). Degradation behavior of polymers used as coating materials for drug delivery—A basic review. *Polymers.* 13: 1272.

Wei, S., Ma, J. X., Xu, L., Gu, X. S., & Ma, X. L. (2020). Biodegradable materials for bone defect repair. *Mil. Med. Res.* 7: 1–25.

Weiler, A., Helling, H. J., Kirch, U., Zirbes, T. K., & Rehm, K. E. (1996). Foreign-body reaction and the course of osteolysis after polyglycolide implants for fracture fixation: Experimental study in sheep. *J. Bone Joint Surg. Br.* 78: 369–376.

Wendelstein, J., Holzbauer, M., Neubauer, M., Steiner, G., Gruber, F., & Schneider, W. (2021). Matched retrospective analysis of three different fixation devices for chevron osteotomy. *The Foot.* 47: 101779.

Windhagen, H., Radtke, K., Weizbauer, A., Diekmann, J., Noll, Y., Kreimeyer, U., Schavan, R., Stukenborg-Colsman, C., & Waizy, H. (2013). Biodegradable magnesium-based screw clinically equivalent to titanium screw in hallux valgus surgery: Short term results of the first prospective, randomized, controlled clinical pilot study. *BioMed. Eng. Online.* 12: 1–10.

Witte, F., Hort, N., Vogt, C., Cohen, S., Kainer, K. U., Willumeit, R., & Feyerabend, F. (2008). Degradable biomaterials based on magnesium corrosion. *Curr. Opin. Solid State Mater. Sci.* 12: 63–72.

Wu, G., Wang, C., Sun, M., & Ding, W. (2021). Recent developments and applications on high-performance cast magnesium rare-earth alloys. *J. Magnes. Alloys.* 9: 1–20.

Xing, F., Li, S., Yin, D., Xie, J., Rommens, P. M., Xiang, Z., Liu, M., & Ritz, U. (2022). Recent progress in Mg-based alloys as a novel bioabsorbable biomaterials for orthopedic applications. *J. Magnes. Alloys*. 10: 1428–1456.

Yoshizawa, S., Brown, A., Barchowsky, A., & Sfeir, C. (2014). Magnesium ion stimulation of bone marrow stromal cells enhances osteogenic activity, simulating the effect of magnesium alloy degradation. *Acta Biomater*. 10: 2834–2842.

Yu, X., Zhao, D., Huang, S., Wang, B., Zhang, X., Wang, W., & Wei, X. (2015). Biodegradable magnesium screws and vascularized iliac grafting for displaced femoral neck fracture in young adults. *BMC Musculoskelet. Disord*. 16: 1–6.

Zeng, R. C., Zhang, J., Huang, W. J., Dietzel, W., Kainer, K. U., Blawert, C., & Wei, K. E. (2006). Review of studies on corrosion of magnesium alloys. *Trans. Nonferrous Met. Soc. China*. 16: 763–771.

Zhao, D., Huang, S., Lu, F., Wang, B., Yang, L., Qin, L., Yang, K., Li, Y., Li, W., & Wang, W. (2016). Vascularized bone grafting fixed by biodegradable magnesium screw for treating osteonecrosis of the femoral head. *Biomaterials*. 81: 84–92.

Zheng, Y. F., Gu, X. N., & Witte, F. (2014). Biodegradable metals. *Mater. Sci. Eng. R Rep*. 77: 1–34.

Zhou, H., & Lee, J. (2011). Nanoscale hydroxyapatite particles for bone tissue engineering. *Acta Biomater*. 7: 2769–2781.

7 Recent Advances in Characterization Techniques for Bone Substitutes

Aman Nikhil and Ashok Kumar

7.1 INTRODUCTION

Bone is a dynamic tissue that constantly remodels throughout life and has the intrinsic property of healing without forming fibrous scar tissue (Marsell & Einhorn, 2011). Micro-damage in bone can repair itself, but when injury is critical, external interventions in the form of bone grafts or bone substitutes are required. Bone is the second most implanted tissue after blood (Shegarfi & Reikeras, 2009), where autologous grafts are the gold standard because they pose no adverse immunological response. However, there are limitations associated with autografts, namely the requirement of additional surgery for harvesting samples, morbidity at the harvest site, and the limited availability of sufficient tissue.

Alternatively, allografts and xenografts pose no limitations on availability but are prone to graft rejection and disease transmission (Fishman et al., 2012). Hence, there is a requirement for synthetic bone substitutes that can be utilized for repairing damaged bone due to trauma or diseases. The properties and functions of the materials used to fabricate the bone substitutes must be extensively characterized to guarantee that they are appropriate for biological applications.

A variety of methodologies are used to characterize materials' physical, chemical, microarchitectural, and mechanical properties to validate their potential as a bone substitute. Critical data regarding the material's chemical composition and crystallinity can be obtained through preliminary characterization using infrared spectroscopy and X-ray diffraction. The particle size of the bone graft components in the solution phase can be determined using dynamic light scattering (Stetefeld et al., 2016), while Raman spectroscopy provides information about different phases present in the sample (Morris & Mandair, 2011). This technique is also applied for determining the effects of sintering over different phases in the bone substitutes (Boullosa-Eiras et al., 2011).

The thermal stability of bone substitute materials is studied using thermogravimetric assays in which change in weight is monitored over a range of temperatures. Advanced imaging techniques like scanning electron microscopy (Mohammed & Abdullah, 2018) and transmission electron microscopy can reveal intricate details of the microarchitectures of bone substitutes including materials' surface architecture, porosity, and size. It is important for bone substitutes to have good mechanical properties so that they can provide initial support at the defect site, especially at load-bearing regions.

After the physicochemical evaluation of a material, a three-dimensional construct called a scaffold is designed using the characterized materials that is eventually utilized for in vitro and then in vivo testing. The fabricated scaffold is tested for its potential to support cell growth and induce osteogenic differentiation, in addition to its biodegradability. The scaffolds are implanted in bone defect in an animal model and tested for their potential to induce bone remodeling. Micro-CT (computed tomography) is a versatile technique for visualizing the radiographic images of scaffold inside the implantation site in addition to providing reconstructed images, 3D models, and assessing different bone parameters (Bedini et al., 2020).

DOI: 10.1201/9781003307310-8

These techniques provide researchers with powerful tools to characterize bone substitute materials and design scaffolds with osteogenic properties. This chapter details recent characterization techniques that can be employed to successfully validate the physical, chemical, and biological properties of bone substitute materials and ultimately their potential as scaffolds in treating bone injuries. Appropriate characterization and testing in preclinical and clinical trials is crucial for developed bone substitutes to ultimately reach patients.

7.2 BONE SUBSTITUTES

Bone injuries and fractures are caused by multiple factors that include age-related complications, hormonal changes, bone infections (osteomyelitis), osteoporosis, imbalanced loading during physical activities (e.g., sports-related injuries), and severe trauma (Loi et al., 2016; Osipov et al., 2018). Trauma that leads to considerable bone loss is primarily treated using autologous bone grafts; however, their limited availability and donor site morbidity pose major limitations. The remaining options are allografts and xenografts, but their complications include the potential for disease transmission, immunogenic reactions, susceptibility to infection, and limited availability.

Bone substitutes provide feasible alternatives using mostly ceramic- and polymer-based treatment options. Ceramic-based bone substitutes include hydroxyapatite, tricalcium phosphate, calcium sulphate, phosphate-based cements, and bioactive glass (Demir-Oğuz et al., 2023; Hou et al., 2022). Polymer-based materials are also employed in combination with ceramics and factor-based substitutes (natural and recombinant growth factors and hormones). Figure 7.1 presents the most common composite bone substitute materials for fabrication.

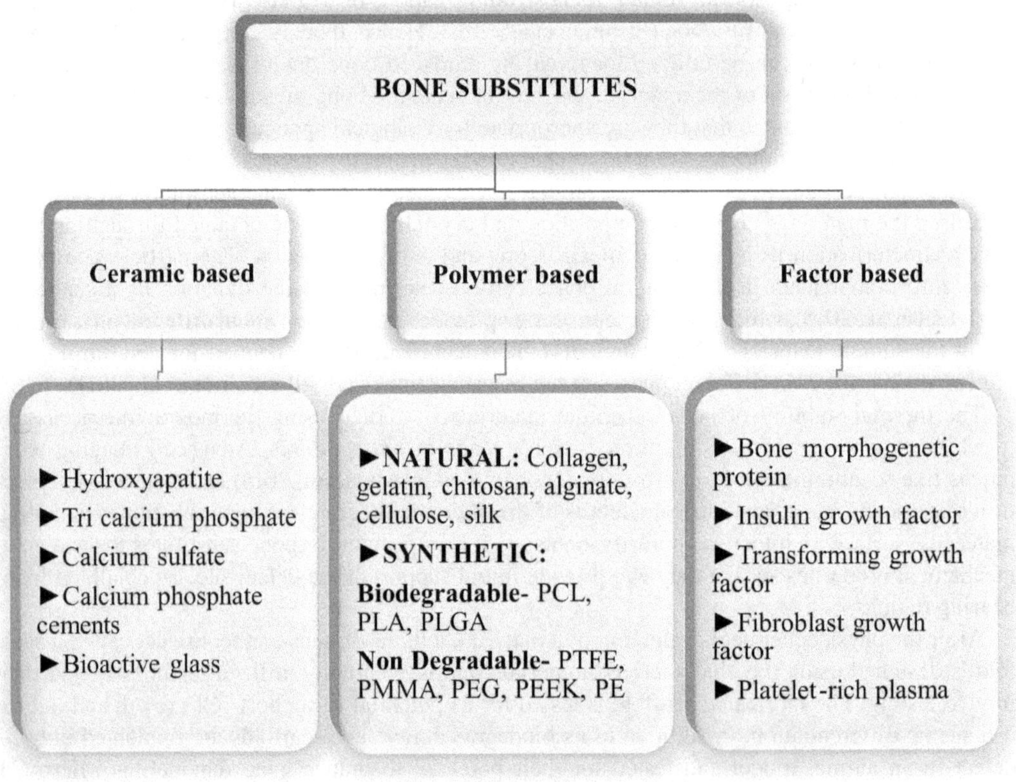

FIGURE 7.1 Different types of bone substitutes utilized for biomedical applications: PCL–polycaprolactone, PLA–polylactic acid, PLGA—polylactic-co-glycolic acid, PTFE–poly(tetrafluoroethylene), PMMA–poly(methyl methacrylate), PEG–polyethylene glycol, PEEK–poly(ether ketone), PE–polyethylene.

7.3 CHARACTERIZATION TECHNIQUES FOR BONE SUBSTITUTES

Advanced techniques are utilized to characterize the physicochemical properties of biomaterials for bone substitutes. Both material and scaffold have to be characterized so that the final bone substitute product can efficiently aid in bone remodeling. Here, we discuss the most recent physicochemical and biological techniques that are being utilized for detailed evaluation of the bone substitutes.

7.4 PHYSICOCHEMICAL CHARACTERIZATION TECHNIQUES

7.4.1 Infrared Spectroscopy

Fourier transform infrared spectroscopy (FTIR) is a technique utilized to characterize the bone matrix with which the absorbance of matrix components like hydroxyapatite (HAP) and collagen can be measured within a range of 500 cm^{-1} to 4000 cm^{-1}. To generate FTIR spectra, solid crushed samples are combined with infrared transparent alkali halides such as potassium bromide (KBr) salt to form pellets. The infrared radiation is passed through the pellet in the transmission mode; some radiation is absorbed by the sample, and the remainder is transmitted and recorded by the detector to make a transmittance spectrum (Figure 7.2(A)).

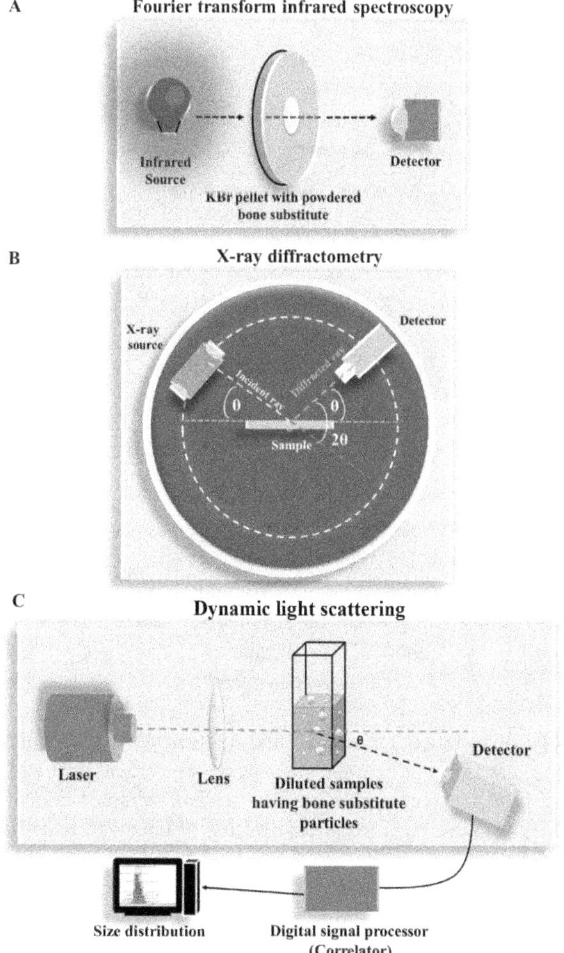

FIGURE 7.2 The working principle of A) Fourier transform infrared spectroscopy, B) X-ray diffractometry, and C) dynamic light scattering.

While in attenuated total reflection mode, powdered samples are directly analyzed without the addition of any other substance, which gives infrared spectrum interaction to about 2 μm from a sample's surface.

Bone matrix is a composite of HAP (mineral phase) and collagen (organic phase) that exhibits specific bands in the infrared spectrum. For HAP, the peaks are observed between 500 to 700 cm^{-1} and 900 to 1200 cm^{-1}, while for collagen, its range is between 1200 to 1799 cm^{-1} and between 2800 to 3700 cm^{-1} (Figueiredo et al., 2012). As the mineral phase is higher in composition in bone

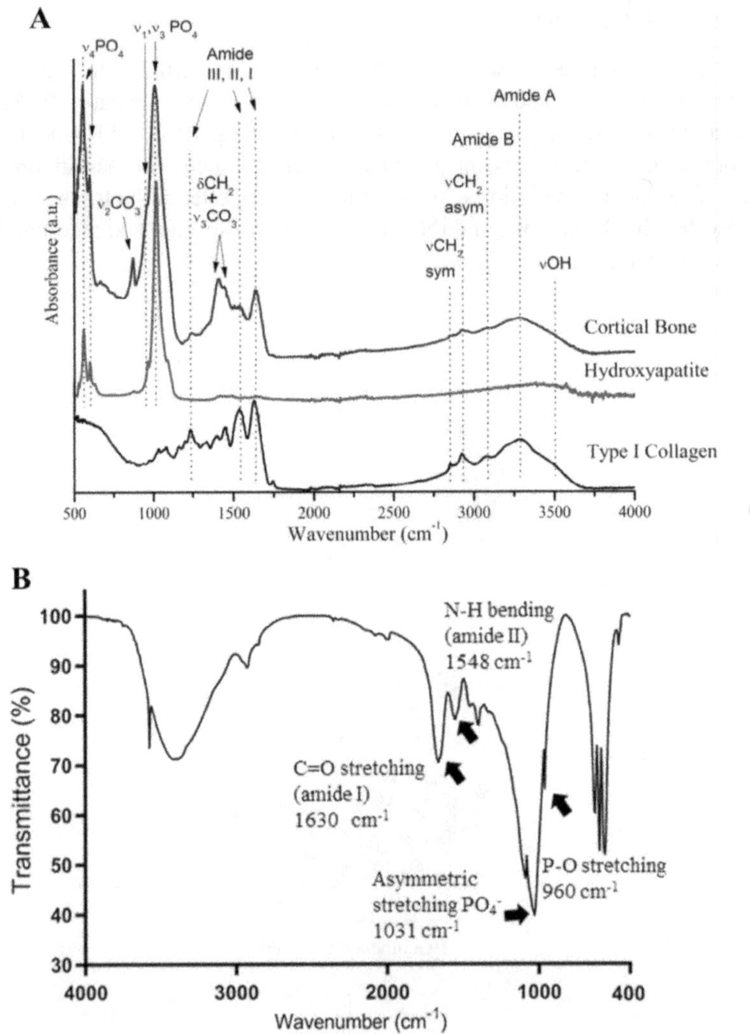

FIGURE 7.3 A) Typical FTIR spectra of bone, HAP, and collagen showing the vibrational assignments of the most significant bands. Different vibrations are shown using dotted vertical lines and arrows (reproduced under the terms of CC-BY 3.0 (https://creativecommons.org/licenses/by/3.0/) International License from Figueiredo, M. M., Gamelas, J. A. F., & Martins, A. G.: Characterization of bone and bone-based graft materials using FTIR spectroscopy. Infrared spectroscopy-life and biomedical sciences. 2012. 315–338. Copyright 2012 The authors, published by IntechOpen). B) FTIR spectrum of HAP-gelatin cryogel highlighting different vibrations typical of the components incorporated at the time of fabrication. The arrows indicate the major peaks utilized for characterizing the biomaterial present in the cryogel (reproduced with permission from Nikhil, A. & Kumar, A.: Evaluating potential of tissue-engineered cryogels and chondrocyte derived exosomes in articular cartilage repair. Biotechnol. Bioeng. 2022. 119. 605–625. Copyright 2022 John Wiley and Sons).

composite, major peaks originate from this phase; 557 and 600 cm^{-1} corresponds to bending vibration of v_4 PO_4^{3-} with some peaks due to amide bands of collagen as well. Further, absorptions obtained near 961 and 1012 cm^{-1} correspond to v_1 symmetric and v_3 asymmetric stretching vibration of phosphate. Typically, collagen shows peaks at 1634 and 1548 cm^{-1}, which correspond to amide I and amide II, respectively (Figure 7.3(A)). In short, the mineral and organic phases of bone contribute to infrared peaks that can be analyzed independent of each other and are beneficial for determining the relative ratio of the phases in bone samples.

Additionally, FTIR offers insights into incorporating nano-hydroxyapatite (nHAP) into scaffolds that prove the success of the fabrication process. In one study, the incorporation of nHAP into cryogels (scaffolds fabricated at sub-zero temperatures) designed for subchondral bone was evaluated using FTIR (Nikhil & Kumar, 2022). Scaffolds were fabricated using nHAP and gelatin with glutaraldehyde as crosslinking agent and using KBr pellet method, peaks were observed at 960 cm^{-1} corresponding to nondegenerate stretching of P–O bond present in PO_4^-. Further, the presence of nHAP was confirmed using a peak observed at 1031 cm^{-1}, which indicates PO_4^- asymmetric stretching. Peak at 1630 cm^{-1} corresponds to amide I (C=O stretching), and 1548 cm^{-1} for amide II (N–H bending) (Figure 7.3(B)).

7.4.2 X-Ray Diffractometry

X-ray diffractometry (XRD) is a robust analytical technique utilized to deduce the chemical composition, identify the phases of, and evaluate the crystallinity of powder-based bone substitute samples. X-rays with a wavelength of 1.54 angstroms are directed toward the sample and diffracted at different angles, and crystalline phases are recorded by the detector (Galia et al., 2011). The direction and intensity of diffracted rays depend on the crystal structure of the sample. One of the most common configurations is θ–2θ, where the X-ray source and detector are rotated while keeping the sample fixed and maintaining fixed angle θ (Figure 7.2(B)). The diffracted X-rays are continuously recorded by the detector and the data is plotted as X-ray counts with respect to 2θ (Schwartz, 2015).

XRD provides significant information on the phase transformation and nature of the material. In our earlier study (Teotia et al., 2017), we studied the phase transformation of nHAP in response to different temperature treatments to obtain a highly crystalline variant. Thermal treatment at 500 °C showed no phase transformation, while at 700 °C, we observed increased crystallinity after thermal treatment for a period of 4 h. We observed high nHAP (single phase) generation at 800 °C for 4 h (Figure 7.4(A)) with a diffractogram that was similar to the diffraction pattern of International Centre for Diffraction Data standard for HAP (card no. 09–432).

An investigation was conducted to assess the impact of iron addition on the structure of hydroxyapatite. The resulting nanocomposite exhibited no substantial alteration in the position of its XRD peak, indicating that the HAP structure underwent no significant changes (Predoi et al., 2021). Furthermore, this method may be applied to the comparison of various bone grafts.

Bio-Oss® is bovine-derived xenograft obtained from spinal bone, and Cerabone® is cattle femur condyle cancellous bone-derived xenograft for bone applications. Porcine-derived THE Graft was compared with Bio-Oss® and Cerabone®, and the XRD patterns showed low crystallinity for both THE Graft and Bio-Oss®, while Cerabone® showed narrower diffraction peaks pointing toward more crystallinity. The main peaks of all three grafts were nearly identical, showing that all grafts were composed of HAP. The XRD findings suggested that THE Graft and Bio-Oss® will be rapidly replaced by osteoblasts as less crystallinity makes a graft more degradable (Figure 7.4(B)) (Lee et al., 2017).

XRD has proved to be of importance where crystalline and amorphous nature of material needs to be deduced. A study demonstrated the amorphous nature of bioactive glass (58 S) that had dispersive peaks with no sharp diffraction peaks. At a 2θ angle of 23 °C, a broad peak appeared that was the characteristic peak of typical amorphous structure of silicate glass (Chen et al., 2018).

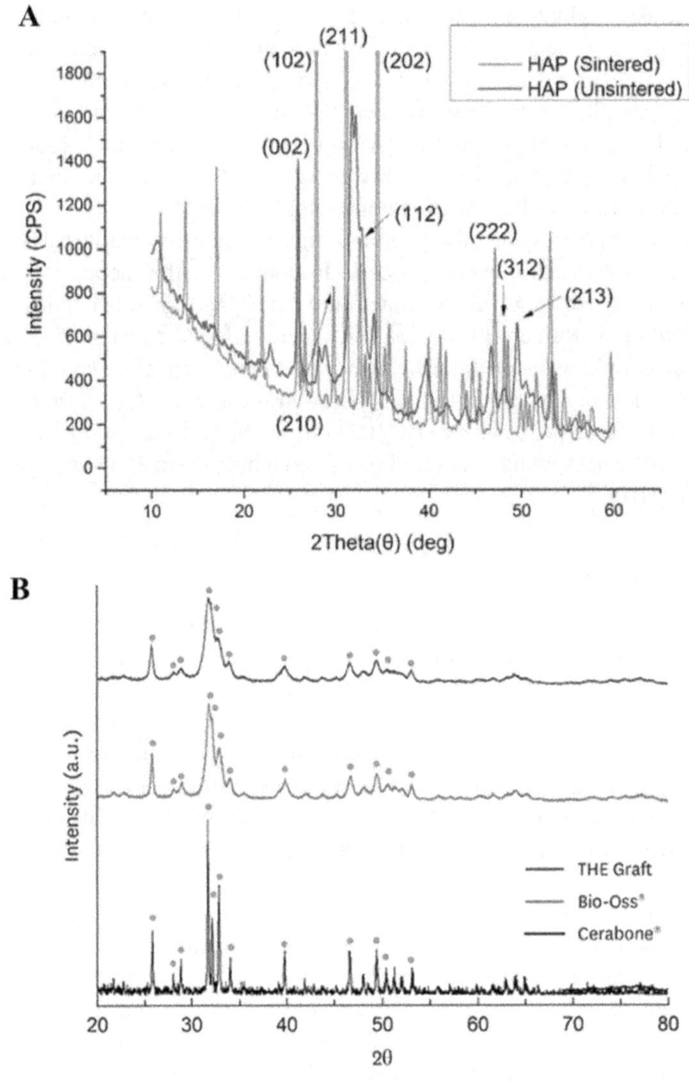

FIGURE 7.4 **A**) XRD of nHAP unsintered and post-sintering at 800 °C for 4 h; the numbers denote the miller indices from the International Centre for Diffraction Data standard for HAP (card no. 09–432) (Reproduced with permission from Teotia, A. K., Raina, D. B., Singh, C., Sinha, N., Isaksson, H., Tägil, M., Lidgren, L., & Kumar, A.: Nano-hydroxyapatite bone substitute functionalized with bone active molecules for enhanced cranial bone regeneration. ACS Appl. Mater. Interfaces. 2017. 9. 6816–6828. Copyright 2017 American Chemical Society). **B**) XRD patterns of THE Graft, Bio-Oss®, and Cerabone®. The blue dots mark the reference HAP peaks that were present in all three curves at respective 2θ values (reproduced under the terms of CC-BY 4.0 (https://creativecommons.org/licenses/by/4.0/) International License from Lee, J. H., Yi, G. S., Lee, J. W., & Kim, D. J.: Physicochemical characterization of porcine bone-derived grafting material and comparison with bovine xenografts for dental applications. J. Periodontal Implant Sci. 2017. 47. 388–401. Copyright 2017 Korean Academy of Periodontology).

7.4.3 Dynamic Light Scattering

The particle sizes of the components present in bone substitutes can be determined using dynamic light scattering (DLS), whereby the Brownian motion of the particles present in liquid samples occurs because of solvent molecule bombardment. The particle movement is monitored over a time range in the sample to deduce the size-related information as larger particles diffuse more slowly than smaller particles in a sample (Stetefeld et al., 2016). DLS has been extensively utilized for characterizing the particle sizes of the bone substitutes utilized for scaffold preparation or coating of bone-based implants (Figure 7.2(C)).

An iron-doped HAP coating was developed for bone applications (Predoi et al., 2021), and DLS provided average particle sizes of 57.09 nm (data weighed by number) and 64.62 nm (data weighed by volume). DLS provided a thorough distribution of the particles present in the sample as well as the number of particles in a specific range. Further, it was utilized for characterizing the calcium phosphate (CaP) present in gelatin/calcium phosphate electrospun composite scaffold fabricated for bone tissue engineering (Miguez et al., 2022). Different samples were tested to select the one with the most nano-sized particles, and CaP-12 had the highest percentage (31.9% had a mean diameter of 198.2 ± 44.2 nm, and 68.1% had a diameter 1073 ± 223.9 nm).

Biological entities like extracellular vesicles (ECVs) can be studied for their size distribution using DLS. ECVs isolated from MG63 osteosarcoma cell lines were characterized using a nanoparticle analyzer (SZ-100) with a 532 nm wavelength and power of 10 mW (Emami et al., 2020). Three independent measurements were carried out at room temperature, and results confirmed the heterogeneity in the size, which ranged from 28.8 nm to 1331.8 nm. The study showed a beneficial effect of ECVs on mineralization and mandibular bone regeneration when loaded on scaffold fabricated using a decellularized matrix and hydroxyapatite.

7.4.4 Thermogravimetric Assay

Thermogravimetric assay (TGA) is an analytical technique utilized for characterizing the thermal stability of bone substitute material. The TGA equipment consists of a sample pan supported by a precision balance. The pan is situated inside a furnace that undergoes a cycle of heating and cooling during the experiment with influx of an inert gas. The weight loss is continuously monitored as the sample is heated to high temperatures beyond 1000 °C (Figure 7.5(A)).

This technique was recently utilized to estimate the collagen and HAP content in archaeological bone samples (Durga et al., 2022). The thermal stability of the volatile components is determined by constantly monitoring the change in weight of the material when the sample is heated at a constant rate (Zafeiropoulos, 2011). TGA is advantageous as it requires much less material for analysis and does not require extensive preparation of samples.

TGA was utilized to confirm the crystallization temperature of phosphate glass bone substitute at temperatures ranging from room temperature to 900 °C heated at 20 °C/min in the air. The measured parameters included glass transition temperature (T_g), onset of crystallization ($T_{c(ON)}$), crystallization temperature (T_c), and melting temperature (T_m). The results showed that T_c was 660 °C and T_m was 740 °C, while $T_{c(ON)}$ started at 640 °C and T_g was 500 °C (Chauhan et al., 2021).

The stability of fabricated bone scaffolds can be tested using TGA as performed in a study to check percentage weight loss in collagen-nHAP composite scaffold (CS) and a collagen–gelatin–chitosan polymer scaffold (SC) (Teotia et al., 2018). Further, the authors studied incorporating nHAP in CS when the samples were heat treated till 600 °C. The results showed that CS showed 25.5% weight loss, while SC's weight loss was 70.9%, which implied that presence of HAP in CS was the reason for the difference observed in the weight loss.

TGA has also been used to quantify the incorporation of HAP and tricalcium phosphate (TCP) in 3D-printed poly (trimethylene carbonate) scaffolds (Teotia et al., 2020). Samples were heated to a final temperature of 600 °C at a heating rate of 20 °C/min, which resulted in polymer decomposition. The residual weight of the material gave insight into the percentage weight incorporation of ceramics in the printed scaffolds. The 3D-printed PTMC scaffold showed complete decomposition with residual mass of 0.4% at 300 °C degradation temperature. For composite 3D-printed scaffolds with both PTMC and HAP, residual mass was 54 ±1%, while for the PTMC and TCP scaffold, residual mass was 53 ±1%, corresponding to their ceramic content.

A new bone substitute was developed that introduced demineralized bone matrix (DBM) into a carrier with a polyvinyl alcohol (PVA)/glycerol network crosslinked using borax and reinforced with calcium carbonate ($CaCO_3$) (Medrano-David et al., 2021). To investigate the thermal behavior of this injectable formulation (weight percentage composition of 26% DBM, 2% $CaCO_3$, 2% PVA, 6.5% glycerol, 0.5% borax and 63% water), TGA was carried out. The sample was heated from 30 °C to 1200 °C at a heating rate of 5 °C/min under nitrogen atmosphere. The results showed that at around 100 °C, the first event occurred where weight loss of 5.5% occurred which was attributed to loss of moisture and various volatile functional groups (Medrano-David et al., 2021).

The PVA side chain degradation occurred at 225 °C with associated weight loss of 21.81%. Further, 26% of material degradation occurred at around 390 °C that was identified with PVA hydroxyl group dehydration. At 480 °C, 5.5% weight loss occurred that was attributed to carbonation (breaking the C-C bond of the main PVA chain). The thermal decomposition of $CaCO_3$ into calcium oxide (CaO) and carbon dioxide (CO_2) also occurred, and at the end of the thermal cycle, CaO did not degrade. The total weight loss was 84.5%, and the residual sample consisted of phosphates of DBM and CaO of $CaCO_3$ (Medrano-David et al., 2021).

7.4.5 Raman Spectroscopy

Raman spectroscopy is based on scattering (Raman effect), wherein the frequency of scattered radiation is different from monochromatic incident radiation frequency because of its interaction with vibrating molecules of the sample. For testing bone substitutes, the monochromatic radiation is

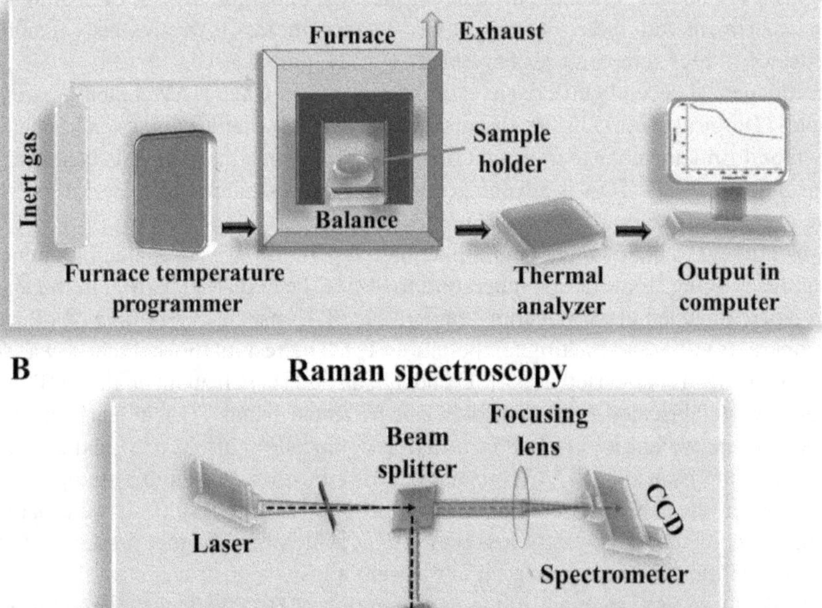

FIGURE 7.5 The working principle of A) thermogravimetric assay and B) Raman spectroscopy.

made to strike over the sample, where inelastic collisions occur between the molecules of substitute material and incident radiation, and the radiation is scattered in different directions. Most scattered radiation has the same frequency as that of incident radiation, which constitutes Rayleigh scattering, while a small fraction of scattered radiation has different frequencies that constitute Raman scattering (Figure 7.5(B)). When the scattered light frequency is lower than incident, stroke lines appear on Raman spectra, but when the frequency is higher, anti-stroke lines appear (Bumbrah & Sharma, 2016). Raman spectroscopy is a nondestructive characterization technique utilized for distinguishing different phases present in the material. It is a very specific and versatile technique that requires only minimal sample preparation, and it can be utilized for hydrated samples as well.

Raman spectra were obtained for HAP sintered at different temperatures for 4 h (Teotia et al., 2017), and the Raman shifts are shown in Figure 7.6(A). The spectra show that sintering at high temperature for extended periods improved the quality of the HAP powder. HAP formation from amorphous calcium phosphate phases was temporally studied using dynamic in situ Raman spectroscopy (Montes-Hernandez & Renard, 2020). The spectra showed the synchronous transformation of both octacalcium phosphate and amorphous tricalcium phosphate into HAP. The results show the time-lapse Raman spectroscopy monitoring of HAP formation where evolution of peaks were used for deconvolution fitting (Figure 7.6(B)).

Raman spectroscopy has also been used to study HAP samples produced from various types of bone tissues belonging to cow, ram, turkey, duck, goose (Timchenko et al., 2018). Timchenko et al. (2018) studied HAP powders obtained from cancellous bone with several degrees of demineralization and thermal processing regimes. The results showed that thermal treatment at 700 °C improved HAP powder quality as it led to decomposition of the organic components with increases in mineral concentration. This technique was utilized to assess ion substitution and has been widely applied for phosphate minerals.

Doping of nHAP with yttrium and fluoride ions was tested with sintering carried out at different temperatures (Yilmaz & Evis, 2014). In the case of pure HAP Raman spectra, the characteristic band at 963 cm^{-1} for v_1 (PO_4^-) was prominent, with two fluorescence bands observed at 770 cm^{-1} and 697 cm^{-1}. A shift in wavenumber was seen where bands shifted toward higher wavenumbers in the spectra when HAP was doped with iron or yttrium. Iron-doped HAP showed variations between 1000 cm^{-1} and 1100 cm^{-1}.

7.4.6 The Porosity of Bone Scaffolds

The porosity of the scaffolds fabricated using bone substitute material is an essential property that plays a key role in efficient bone remodeling. Typically, for a bone graft/scaffold, pore size less than 100 μm is not suitable because it directly impacts the bone ingrowth and vascularization, which are both crucial factors for bone remodeling. Contrarily, large pore sizes in the range of 300 to 500 μm are considered ideal for bone remodeling as reported previously (Hannink & Arts, 2011).

Bone substitute scaffolds are characterized using solvent-based cyclohexane method. In this technique, the pores present inside the scaffold are filled with cyclohexane, and porosity can be deduced with respect to the scaffold dry weight. Cryogels fabricated using nHAP and gelatin for subchondral bone of knee joint were assessed for porosity and pore volume using the cyclohexane method (Nikhil & Kumar, 2022). The dry weight of the cryogel was monitored, and then the cryogel immersed in cyclohexane at room temperature for 1 h. The weight of cryogel with cyclohexane was monitored, and percentage porosity (70%) was evaluated; the calculated pore volume was 2.5 mm^3/mg of cryogel. Such indirect assessments provide crucial information on the porosity of the entire 3D scaffold and its potential to support bone ingrowth.

7.4.7 Scanning Electron Microscopy

The microarchitecture of bone substitutes can be characterized by visualizing them using scanning electron microscopy (SEM). A dehydrated sample is affixed over a copper stub and then sputter

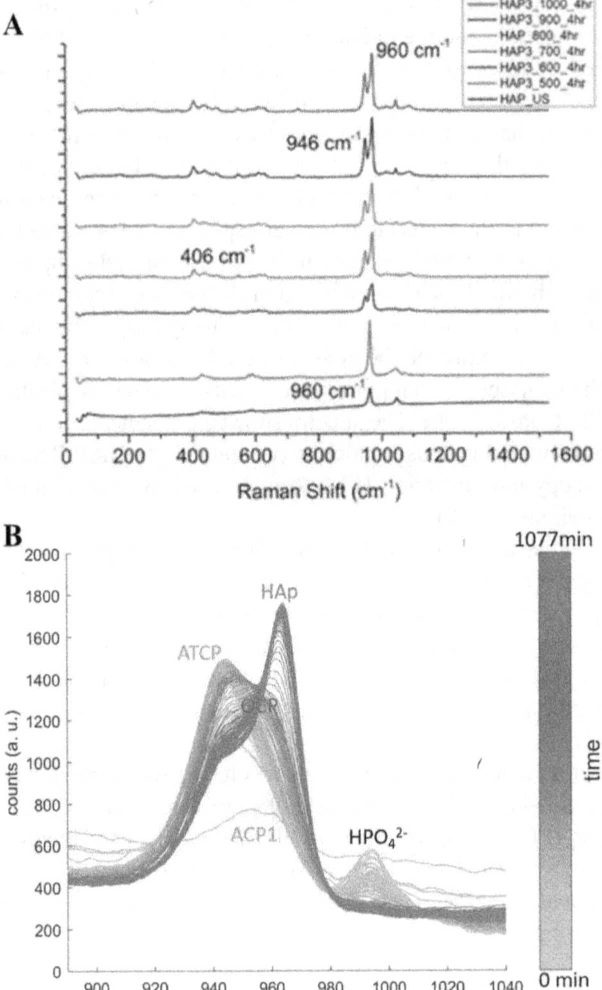

FIGURE 7.6 **A)** Raman spectra of nHAP after thermal treatment at different temperatures (ranging from 500 °C to 1000 °C) for a period of 4 h. The spectra were compared with the reference HAP spectra, and major peaks are mentioned (reproduced with permission from Teotia, A. K., Raina, D. B., Singh, C., Sinha, N., Isaksson, H., Tägil, M., Lidgren, L., & Kumar, A.: Nano-hydroxyapatite bone substitute functionalized with bone active molecules for enhanced cranial bone regeneration. ACS Appl. Mater. Interfaces. 2017. 9. 6816–6828. Copyright 2017 American Chemical Society). **B)** Time-lapse evolution of the main peaks used for deconvolution fitting in Raman spectroscopy monitoring of the formation of HAP. The spectra show the transformation of octacalcium phosphate into HAP and amorphous tricalcium phosphate (ATCP) into HAP (reproduced with permission from Montes-Hernandez, G., & Renard, F.: Nucleation of brushite and hydroxy-apatite from amorphous calcium phosphate phases revealed by dynamic in situ Raman spectroscopy. J. Phys. Chem. C. 2020. 124. 15302–15311. Copyright 2020 American Chemical Society).

coated with gold (Cruz et al., 2007) to make the sample surface conductive, prevent surface charging, and promote the emission of secondary electrons to be collected by detector. Samples are then subjected to an accelerating voltage to deduce the surface architecture (Figure 7.7(A)).

The microarchitecture provides details about physical properties of the material like particle size, porosity, and entities present in a scaffold. SEM was utilized to investigate the morphology of the iron-doped HAP bone substitute particles and coating, which was captured at 30 kV accelerating voltage. The average particle size obtained was 25 ± 2 nm having spherical morphology and coating was homogeneous, continuous, with no cracks (Predoi et al., 2021).

Our group optimized a nano-cement made up of a combination of nHAP and calcium sulphate hemihydrate to make an injectable formulation for bone defects and used SEM to observe the presence of nHAP particles in the fabricated cryogel with pore diameters in range of 40 to 50 µm (Figure 7.8(A)) (Teotia et al., 2018). Similarly, HAP-gelatin cryogel was characterized using SEM where samples were scanned at an accelerating voltage of 20 kV (Nikhil & Kumar, 2022). We observed an interconnected porous network and nHAP particles embedded in the pore walls of the cryogel with pore diameters from 40 nm to 110 nm (Figure 7.8(B)).

In orthopedics, infection of bone graft is a serious complication, and increasing resistance to antibiotics requires certain novel treatment strategies. Magnesium oxide (MgO) provides an alternative because of its broad-spectrum antibiotic activity. In this direction, spherical HAP and MgO granules were fabricated that showed cytocompatibility and antibacterial activity, and the researchers observed that higher sintering temperature caused HAP particles to coalesce (Coelho et al., 2020).

When sintering was carried out at a higher temperature like 1300 °C, granules possess bigger HAP crystals than those that form at lower sintering temperatures. MgO was enclosed in the middle

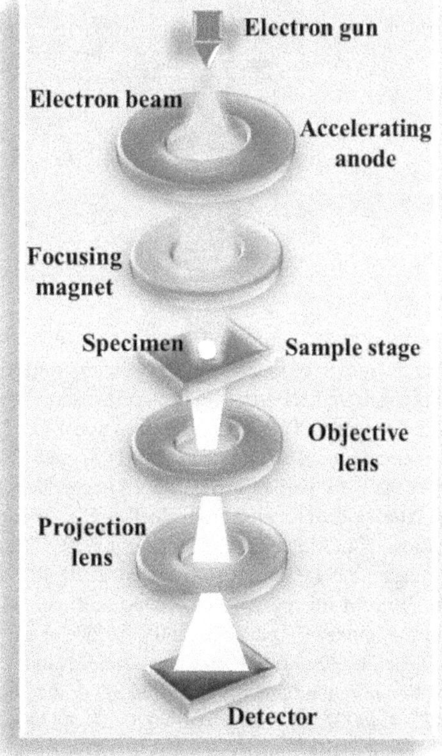

FIGURE 7.7 The working principle of A) scanning electron microscopy and B) transmission electron microscopy.

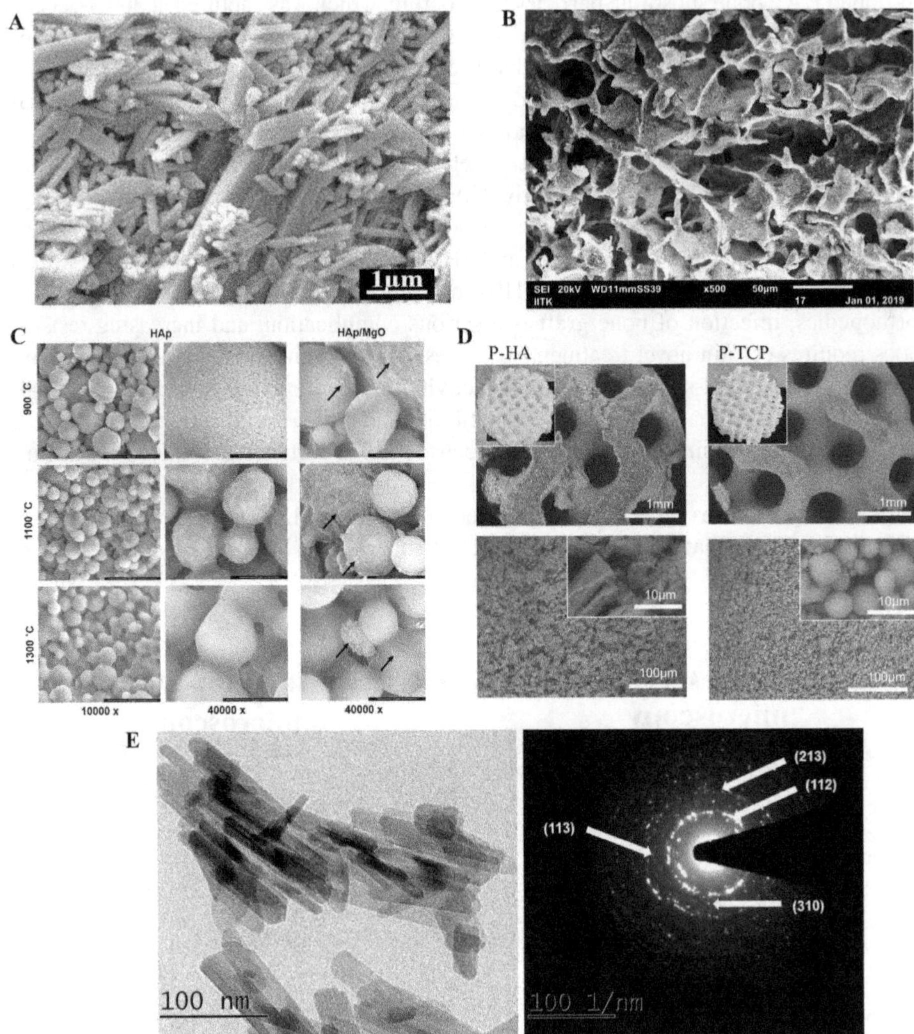

FIGURE 7.8 A) SEM image of nano-cement (scale bar: 1 µm). B) SEM image of hydroxyapatite-gelatin cryogel (scale bar: 50 µm) (reproduced with permission from Nikhil, A., & Kumar, A.: Evaluating potential of tissue-engineered cryogels and chondrocyte derived exosomes in articular cartilage repair. Biotechnol. Bioeng. 2022. 119. 605–625. Copyright 2022 John Wiley and Sons). C) SEM images showing the surface details of HAP and HAP/MgO spherical granules sintered at 900, 1100, and 1300 °C. Arrows point out the MgO particles enclosed in the middle of the HAP particles (reproduced under the terms of CC-BY 4.0 (https://creativecommons.org/licenses/by/4.0/) International License from Coelho, C. C., Padrão, T., Costa, L., Pinto, M. T., Costa, P. C., Domingues, V. F., Quadros, P. A., Monteiro, F. J., & Sousa, S. R.: The antibacterial and angiogenic effect of magnesium oxide in a hydroxyapatite bone substitute. Sci. Rep. 2020. 10. 19098. Copyright 2020 Coelho et al., published by Springer Nature). D) SEM micrographs of printed scaffolds with asymmetric HA particles on the surface of the P–HA scaffold and round TCP particles on the surface of the P–TCP scaffold (reproduced with permission from Teotia, A. K., Dienel, K., Qayoom, I., van Bochove, B., Gupta, S., Partanen, J., Seppälä, J., & Kumar, A.: Improved bone regeneration in rabbit bone defects using 3D printed composite scaffolds functionalized with osteoinductive factors. ACS Appl. Mater. Interfaces. 2020. 12. 48340–48356. Copyright 2020 American Chemical Society). E) TEM image of nHAP (unsintered) and SAED electron diffraction pattern of nHAP (unsintered) (reproduced with permission from Teotia, A. K., Raina, D. B., Singh, C., Sinha, N., Isaksson, H., Tägil, M., Lidgren, L., & Kumar, A.: Nano-hydroxyapatite bone substitute functionalized with bone active molecules for enhanced cranial bone regeneration. ACS Appl. Mater. Interfaces. 2017. 9. 6816–6828. Copyright 2017 American Chemical Society).

of HAP as bigger aggregates and was observed under SEM as small particles over the surface of HAP (Figure 7.8(C)). We used SEM to observe the surface topology of the 3D-printed bone scaffolds including the surface roughness and distribution of HAP and TCP ceramic in PTMC scaffold; we observed asymmetric HAP-based particles over the surface of PTMC-HAP but rounded TCP particles on the PTMC-TCP scaffold (Figure 7.8(D)) (Teotia et al., 2020).

Energy-dispersive X-ray spectroscopy (EDX) is utilized in combination with SEM that provides the micro-scale chemical composition of the sample using X-rays. Researchers analyzed the surface composition of bovine-derived xenogeneic bone substitute mixed with hydroxypropyl methylcellulose hydrogel to make bone graft material. They observed that this graft had a calcium-to-phosphate ratio of 1.434 (atomic percentages were 6.837 ± 6.433 for carbon, 34.78 ± 5.6999 for oxygen, 33.79 ± 7.053 for phosphorous, and 48.44 ± 8.954 for calcium) using EDX (Kim et al., 2021).

7.4.8 Transmission Electron Microscopy

For material characterization, transmission electron microscopy (TEM) is a very powerful tool. The electron source emitted from the top of the microscope travels through vacuum via electromagnetic lens to strike the bone substitutes or scaffolds. The electrons pass through the specimen and are captured by the detector (Figure 7.7(B)).

The principle of TEM is similar to that of light microscopy with the exception that electrons are utilized instead of light. As the wavelength of incident electrons is much smaller than light, resolution obtained with TEM is considerably high and provides the finest details of samples. TEM was utilized to analyze the size, shape, and architecture of HAP and showed that the crystals were in the nano-size range (Teotia et al., 2017). Selected area electron diffraction (SAED) was also carried out to obtain crystallographic data to analyze the crystallinity and crystal structure. The SAED showed that the diffraction rings obtained were characteristic of HAP, showing the successful fabrication of crystalline nHAP (Figure 7.8(E)).

7.4.9 Mechanical Characterization

In the case of bone-based applications, the scaffold must possess adequate mechanical strength to address bone damage during the earliest stages of implantation. In a mechanical testing system, the scaffold fabricated using the bone substitute is placed over the sample holder, and a load is applied using a load cell. The sample is then compressed at a fixed crosshead speed till the sample fractures. The stress vs. strain data is recorded and compressive strength can be deduced (Figure 7.9(A)).

Different commercially available bone graft substitute cements have been compared based on the compressive as well as the flexural strength (Drosos et al., 2012). Bone grafts included for testing were polymethymethacrylate (PMMA) (Genatafix 3 Mathys Ltd, Switzerland), calcium phosphate (Calcibon Biomet, Germany-CP1, Graftys HBS-CP2), nanocrystalline hydroxyapatite (OSTIM Biomaterials GmbH & CO, Germany-HA), calcium sulfate (MIIG-115 Wright Medical Technology Inc, USA-CS1, MIIG-X3 Wright Medical Technology Inc, USA-CS2). For compression testing, cylindrical samples were fabricated that were 6 mm in diameter and 12 mm in length and compressed at loading speed of 20 mm/min. Average compressive strength with standard deviation obtained was 88.5 ± 0.8 MPa for PMMA, 52.9 ± 3.6 MPa for CS2, 15.1 ± 2.5 MPa for CP1, 9.9 ± 1.6 MPa for CS1, 4.0 ± 0.4 MPa for CP2, and 3.8 ± 1.6 MPa for HA. For the bending test, sample dimensions were 75 mm × 10 mm × 3.3 mm (length × breadth × height) that was subjected to a loading speed of 5 mm/min between two parallel cylindrical supports. Average bending strength with standard deviation obtained was 54.8 ± 7.4 MPa for PMMA, 11.9 ± 3.4 MPa for CS2, 6.1 ± 1.1 MPa for CS1, 4.3 ± 0.5 MPa for CP1, and 2.1 ± 0.6 MPa for CP2.

Mechanical testing is utilized for analyzing the effect of changing the composition of bone substitutes over the strength of fabricated scaffolds. Several new combinations have been tested for enhancing the mechanical strength of the already available bone substitutes. The combination of

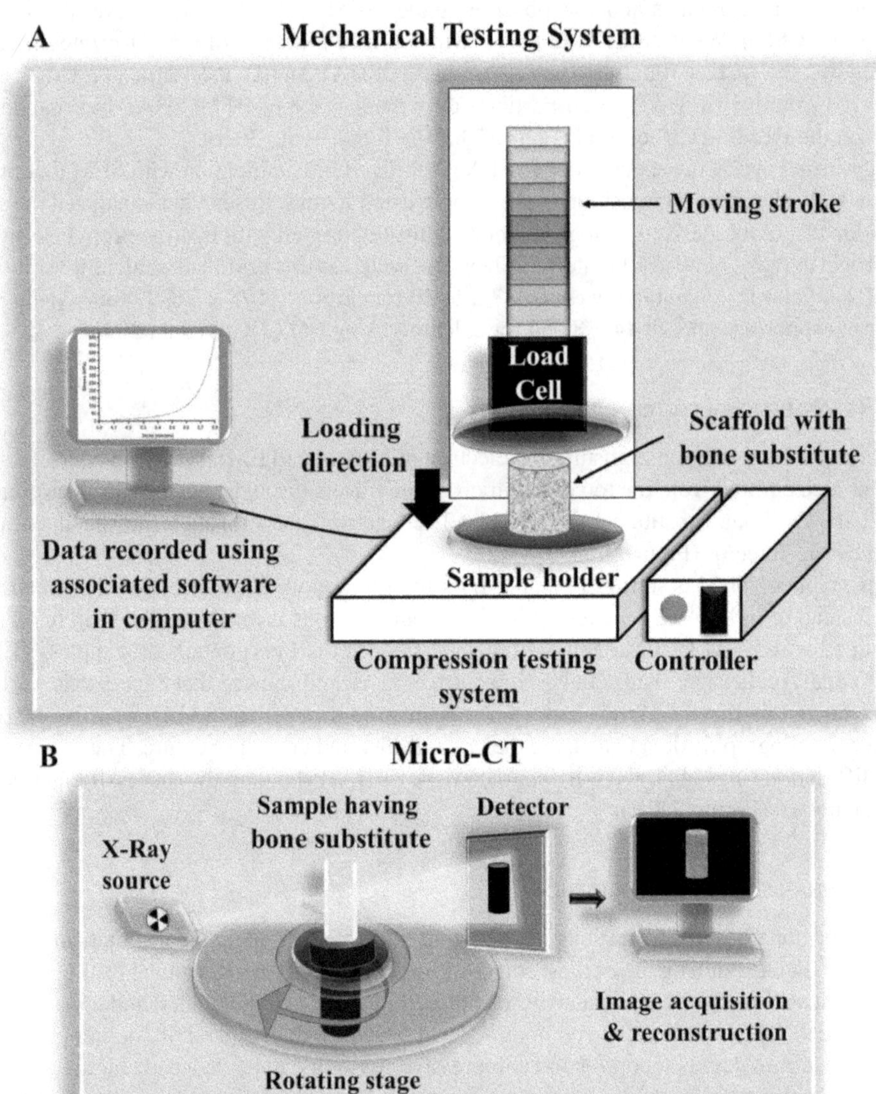

FIGURE 7.9 The working principle of A) mechanical testing system and B) micro-CT.

bioglass (BG; $60SiO_2\_35CaO\_5P_2O_5$) with different concentrations of graphene oxide (0.5%, 1%, 2%, 3%) was tested to improve the mechanical properties (El-khooly et al., 2022). It was observed that compressive strength increased from 55.06 ± 4.49 MPa for BG to 100.23 ± 2.93 MPa for the sample with 0.5% GO, but for 1%, 2%, and 3% GO, it was 74.53 ± 2.43 MPa, 70.48 ± 2.95 MPa, and 75.7 ± 2.42 MPa, respectively. The limited enhancement with 1%, 2%, and 3% GO was attributed to degradation in dispersion of GO at high concentration.

Similarly, researchers investigated mechanical characteristics of β-TCP and its doped variants with zinc, magnesium, and titanium as bone substitutes for biomedical applications (Samanta et al., 2019). Vikers hardness testing was carried out where the indenter was pitched inside the sample with accurately measured force. After 30 s, size of the indent was optically measured, and the average hardness of different compositions was calculated as a function of 300 mN indentation load.

The study revealed that the hardness of β-TCP can be improved to certain extent by incorporation of dopants. Pure β-TCP has hardness of 0.652 ± 0.03 GPa that increased to 0.704 ± 0.03 GPA with 5% zinc oxide doping, 0.687 ± 0.09 GPa with 5% magnesium chloride doping, and 0.672 ± 0.08 GPa with 5% titanium oxide doping.

We thoroughly studied the effects of different ratios of calcium sulphate hemihydrate and nano-hydroxyapatite (CSH:nHAP) on mechanical properties of nano-cement (Teotia et al., 2017). For this purpose, we fabricated nano-cement and calcium sulphate monoliths in dimensions of 1.6 × 1.6 × 1.6 cm and subjected them to load at a speed of 0.6 mm/min. The results showed that calcium sulphate material had a compressive modulus of 424 ± 51 MPa while the nano-cement with a 6:4 CSH:nHAP) ratio showed compressive modulus of 328 ± 63 MPa.

7.4.10 X-Ray

X-ray imaging is a powerful and crucial technique utilized in medical imaging and diagnosis. The beam of X-ray (electromagnetic radiation) is passed through the region of interest for visualizing internal structures like bone and implanted radiopaque bone substitute materials. The X-ray beam is absorbed or scattered by the internal organs, structures, and remaining radiation is transmitted, which is captured by the detector to obtain the X-ray radiograph.

A clinical study was carried out where calcibon (artificial bone graft substitute) was utilized for filling the bone cavities (Friesenbichler et al., 2017). Calcibon has osteoconductive properties, with a chemical composition of α-TCP (62.5%), dicalcium phosphate dihydrate (26.8%), calcium carbonate (8.9%), and hydroxyapatite (1.8%). The non-randomized study was carried out to deduce the calcibon's efficacy for resorption and healthy bone remodeling after bone tumor curettage. The bone substitute was provided in a minimally invasive percutaneous manner, and the calcibon showed rapid bone consolidation, durability, and incorporation with a low rate of complications. Although calcibon integrated well with bone, it requires a longer period for resorption as shown in follow-up X-ray imaging (Figure 7.10(A)).

The radiological changes can be monitored after filling the bone defect using ceramic bone graft substitute like Cerament bone void filler (Horstmann et al., 2018). Proximal humerus and distal tibia were treated by curettage and defect filling with cerament and analysed at different follow up time points of 6 weeks, 3 months, 6 months, and 12 months, respectively. Increasing product resorption and cortical thickening has been observed using radiographical imaging on treatment with this bone substitute (Figure 7.10(B)).

7.4.10.1 Dual-Energy X-Ray Absorptiometry

Another technique utilized in clinics for assessment of the bone mineral density is dual-energy X-ray absorptiometry (DEXA). It uses a small dose of radiation to easily image bones or bone substitutes, and it is the gold standard for measuring crucial information regarding changes in bone density, especially in osteoporotic patients; it can be further utilized to calculate fracture risk. It is a fast and noninvasive technique whereby two energy peaks are created to separate soft tissue from the bone (Litak et al., 2022).

In our recent study, DEXA technique was utilized for assessing the development of osteoporotic conditions in rats in response to ovariectomy (Nikhil et al., 2024). The sepsis-induced bone was treated using nano-cement-based functionalized bone substitute, and subsequent improvement in bone mineral density was deduced using DEXA.

7.4.10.2 Micro-CT

Micro-CT is an advanced imaging technique that captures high-resolution images at small scale for scaffold and bone substitute treated specimen. X-rays are made to fall over the sample, and then transmitted radiation is detected by the detector. The sample is placed over a rotating stage, and

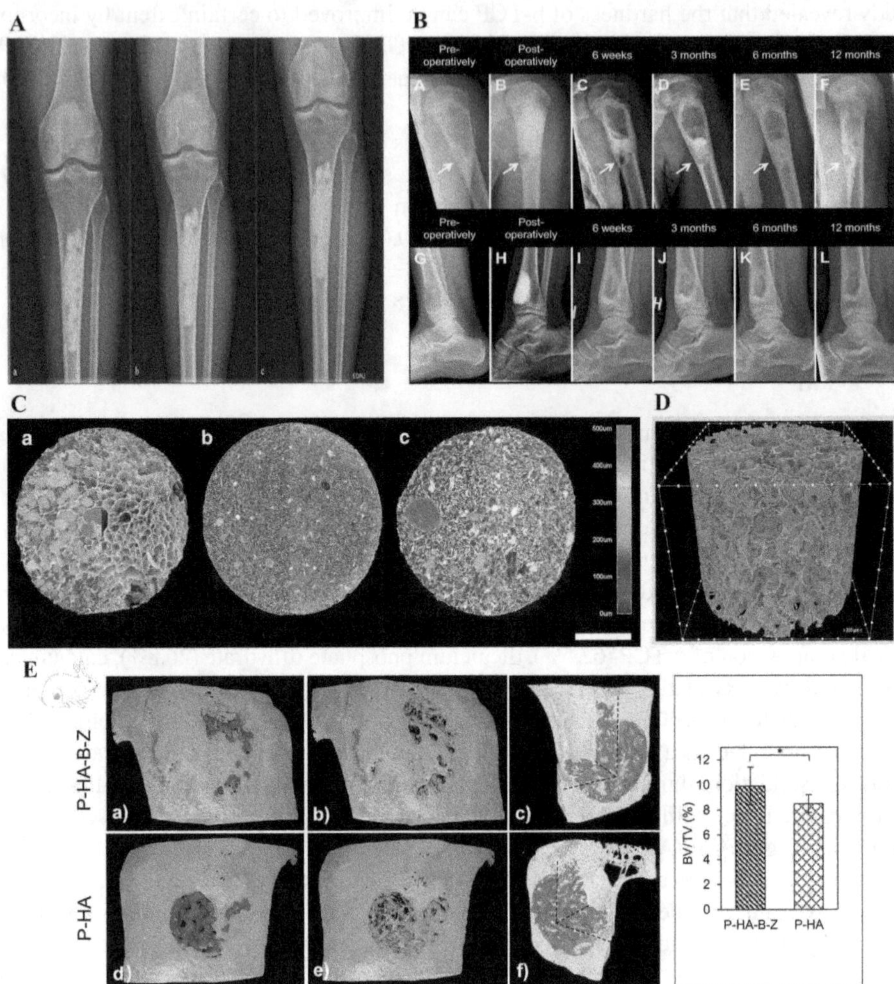

FIGURE 7.10 **A)** (a) X-ray of a 36-year-old male patient a few days following curettage of a low-grade chondrosarcoma of the left proximal tibia; (b and c) follow-up radiographs 7 and 13 months following index surgery showing integration but no resorption of the artificial bone graft substitute (reproduced under the terms of CC-BY 4.0 (https://creativecommons.org/licenses/by/4.0/) International License from Friesenbichler, J., Maurer-Ertl, W., Bergovec, M., Holzer, L. A., Ogris, K., Leitner, L., & Leithner, A.: Clinical experience with the artificial bone graft substitute Calcibon used following curettage of benign and low-grade malignant bone tumors. Sci. Rep. 2017. 7. 1–5. Copyright 2017 Friesenbichler et al., published by Springer Nature). **B)** Upper row: Simple cyst of the proximal humerus treated by curettage and defect-filling using CERAMENT|*BONE VOID FILLER*. (A,B) Pre- and postoperative X-rays showing decreased cortical thickness and an isolated chamber in the distal part of the affected bone (arrow), which is not accessed or filled during the operation. (C–E) X-rays taken after 6 weeks and 3 and 6 months, respectively, showing increased product resorption and cortical thickening. (F) X-ray taken after 12 months showing normal cortical thickness in the main part of the cyst and reduced cortical thickness in the non-treated distal chamber as a sign of possible local recurrence. Lower row: Aneurysmal bone cyst of the distal tibia treated by curettage and defect filling using CERAMENT|*BONE VOID FILLER*. (G,H) Pre- and post-operative X-rays showing decreased anterior cortical thickness and complete defect filling. (I–L) X-rays taken after 6 weeks and 3, 6, and 12 months, respectively, showing increased product resorption and cortical thickening. Note the increasing distance between the growth-plate and the distal aspect of the cyst (reproduced under the terms of CC-BY 4.0 (https://creativecommons.org/licenses/by/4.0/) International License from Horstmann, P. F., Hettwer, W. H., Kaltoft, N. S., & Petersen, M. M.: Early clinical and radiological experience with a ceramic bone graft substitute

in the treatment of benign and borderline bone lesions. Sci. Rep. 2018. 8. 1–8. Copyright 2018 Horstmann et al., published by Springer Nature). **C)** Micro-CT 3D visualization of selected specimens: a: RT MID, b: ORIG, c: 37 MIN. The right halves depict the scaffold matrix, and the left halves combine the scaffold matrix with color-coded pore sizes. In the ORIG (b) specimen, red pores seem to be much smaller than the red and green pores in RT MID and 37 MIN; scale bar (white) = 3 mm (reproduced under the terms of CC-BY 4.0 (https://creativecommons.org/licenses/by/4.0/) International License from Bartoš, M., Suchý, T., & Foltán, R.: Note on the use of different approaches to determine the pore sizes of tissue engineering scaffolds: what do we measure? Biomed. Eng. Online. 2018. 17. 1–15. Copyright 2018 Bartoš et al., published by Springer Nature). **D)** A 3D micro-CT image of the polycaprolactone–polyurethane scaffold. The distance between two adjacent white dots is 250 μm (reproduced under the terms of CC-BY 4.0 (https://creativecommons.org/licenses/by/4.0/) International License from Cengiz, I. F., Oliveira, J. M., & Reis, R. L.: Micro-CT—a digital 3D microstructural voyage into scaffolds: a systematic review of the reported methods and results. Biomater. Res. 2018. 22. 1–11. Copyright 2018 Cengiz et al., published by Springer Nature). **E)** Representative micro-CT 3D reconstructions of tibia defect with implanted scaffolds colored red in a) and d). The scaffold has been removed in b) and e), showing a bone infiltration pattern within the defect. The sectioned images of scaffolds display implantation within the defect with the bone (light brown) infiltrating within the scaffolds in c) and f). BV (bone volume) relative to the TV (tissue volume) within the scaffolds is shown for both study groups (mean ± SD, n = 5, two-tailed t test, $\alpha = 0.05$). (Reproduced with permission from Teotia, A. K., Dienel, K., Qayoom, I., van Bochove, B., Gupta, S., Partanen, J., Seppälä, J., & Kumar, A.: Improved bone regeneration in rabbit bone defects using 3D printed composite scaffolds functionalized with osteoinductive factors. ACS Appl. Mater. Interfaces. 2020. 12. 48340–48356. Copyright 2020 American Chemical Society).

a series of images are captured that are further reconstructed into a cross-sectional image of the sample (Figure 7.9(B)). It can be further processed into 3D models to obtain detailed information of the internal microarchitecture. It provides crucial data like bone volume, tissue volume, bone mineral density, porosity, trabecular thickness, and trabecular separation.

Researchers used micro-CT to evaluate a collagen-based composite scaffold structure (Bartoš et al., 2018). Different composite scaffolds were fabricated with varying genipin/collagen concentrations at different temperatures. RT MID was fabricated at 0.053 g/1 g of collagen at 20 °C, 37 min at 0.026 g/1 g at 37 °C, while ORIG was control non-crosslinked scaffold. Micro-CT of the scaffold matrix was carried out and combined with color-coded pore size values (Figure 7.10(C)) to obtain details of the pore size of fabricated scaffolds at different concentrations and temperatures. Micro-CT imaging can be utilized to observe microarchitecture of scaffolds like polycaprolactone-polyurethane (Figure 7.10(D)) (Cengiz et al., 2018). In several preclinical trials, bone formation at the defect site has been evaluated using micro-CT. In a rabbit tibia defect, we analyzed bone formation with a PTMC-HAP scaffold and PTMC-HAP with BMP and ZA (Teotia et al., 2020). We analyzed the reconstructed images of the defect site of the tibia (Figure 7.10(E)) and calculated the relative BV/TV (%) for the two groups and found that incorporating BMP and ZA significantly increased bone remodeling.

7.5 BIOLOGICAL CHARACTERIZATION

After thorough characterization of the bone substitute, it is utilized to make a suitable scaffold that can be further tested for in vitro cell–material interactions. A suitable bone substitute material should be osteoconductive, osteoinductive, and osteogenic (Khan et al., 2012). Scaffolds can be fabricated using different techniques like hydrogelation, cryogelation, lyophilization, electrospinning, or 3D printing and then assessed for their ability to support cell growth in laboratory conditions.

7.5.1 In Vitro Characterization

The cell growth over the bone substitute scaffold can be assessed in cell culture conditions in a carbon dioxide incubator at a steady temperature of 37 °C. The fabricated scaffold is sterilized using ethanol gradient and UV, and then cells are seeded over the scaffold. Cell growth assessment assays are performed using MTT reagent (3-(4,5-dimethylthiazol-2-yl)-2,5-diphenyltetrazolium bromide), which is a tetrazolium reduction assay to purple formazan crystals by metabolically active cells. The alkaline phosphatase (ALP) cell differentiation assay is also utilized to check the potential of the scaffold to drive cells toward osteogenic lineage.

Cryogels fabricated using nHAP and gelatin were assessed for cell proliferation and differentiation of the preosteoblasts (Nikhil & Kumar, 2022). The scaffold favored the adhesion of preosteoblasts and subsequently aided in their proliferation for a period of 18 days. Further, ALP showed increased expression from day 7 onwards, inclining toward its osteogenic differentiation potential. Further, imaging techniques like SEM are utilized for visualizing cell seeded scaffolds, where cells and their secreted extracellular matrix can be observed. Similarly, in confocal microscopy, cells are fluorescently labeled and imaged over the scaffold in all three planes using Z stacking. The procedure provides the flexibility to image the live cells, which provides very important information regarding cell-material interaction.

7.6 PRECLINICAL TRIALS

In vitro results are further confirmed in preclinical animal trials that utilize a suitable small animal model like mice, rat, or rabbit to test the bone substitute material in a critical- or sub-critical-size bone defect to assess its efficacy, cytocompatibility, and potential to enable bone remodeling (McGovern et al., 2018). In a typical animal surgery, the bone defect is created in a controlled manner, and then the defect is filled with scaffold fabricated using bone substitute material. By deducing parameters from micro-CT evaluations of the bone, the potential of the material is assessed to determine the efficacy of the treatment administered over the course of an experiment.

Histological staining like hematoxylin and eosin and Masson's trichrome are utilized to deduce the cell infiltration and collagen deposition at the defect site. Picrosirius red staining has been widely utilized to analyze the type of collagen deposition at the treatment site (Qayoom et al., 2022). Immunohistochemistry is a technique that employs antibodies to assess the presence of specific antigens or proteins within a tissue sample derived from a remodeling site, such as collagen I. After confirming the potential of bone-based substitute in small animals, higher animal models like pig, sheep, or goat are utilized for testing a material before its clinical evaluation. The animal experiments are carried out under strict ethical guidelines, and a national-level committee like the Committee for the Control and Supervision of Experiments on Animals strictly scrutinize the protocols of experimentation. A controlled clinical trial is then carried out to check the efficacy and dosage in humans, and finally, a bone substitute material can be approved for clinical use. After this rigorous chain of characterization, testing, and approvals, a bone substitute product reaches the orthopedic clinics.

CONCLUSION

Bone substitutes have a broad market, and there is an increasing demand for novel materials that can be employed in the clinics to treat injuries. There are several bone substitutes already available in the market, but research is continuously proceeding toward obtaining an ideal bone substitute. The characterization techniques play a vital role in elucidating the potential of new bone substitutes by determining their physicochemical properties.

Ceramic-based bone substitutes are widely being pursued in combination with polymer- and factor-based substitutes to get a combination of strong, biodegradable, and biocompatible material, and characterization is paving the way toward successful preclinical and clinical trials of bone substitute materials.

ACKNOWLEDGEMENTS

Aman Nikhil would like to thank the Department of Biotechnology for his PhD fellowship at Indian Institute of Technology Kanpur.

LIST OF ABBREVIATIONS

ALP	Alkaline Phosphatase
BMD	Bone Mineral Density
BMP	Bone Morphogenetic Protein
CaP	Calcium Phosphate
CT	Computed Tomography
DBM	Demineralized Bone Matrix
DLS	Dynamic Light Scattering
FTIR	Fourier Transform Infrared Spectroscopy
HAP	Hydroxyapatite
nHAP	Nanohydroxyapatite
PMMA	Polymethylmethacrylate
PTMC	Poly (trimethylene carbonate)
PVA	Polyvinyl Alcohol
SEM	Scanning Electron Microscopy
TCP	Tricalcium Phosphate
TEM	Transmission Electron Microscopy
TGA	Thermogravimetric Assay
XRD	X-Ray Diffractometry
ZA	Zoledronic Acid

REFERENCES

Bartoš, M., Suchý, T., & Foltán, R. (2018). Note on the use of different approaches to determine the pore sizes of tissue engineering scaffolds: What do we measure? *Biomed. Eng. Online*. 17: 1–15.

Bedini, R., Pecci, R., Meleo, D., & Campioni, I. (2020). Bone substitutes scaffold in human bone: Comparative evaluation by 3D micro-CT technique. *Appl. Sci.* 10: 3451.

Boullosa-Eiras, S., Vanhaecke, E., Zhao, T., Chen, D., & Holmen, A. (2011). Raman spectroscopy and X-ray diffraction study of the phase transformation of ZrO2—Al2O3 and CeO2—Al2O3 nanocomposites. *Catal. Today*. 166: 10–17.

Bumbrah, G. S., & Sharma, R. M. (2016). Raman spectroscopy—Basic principle, instrumentation and selected applications for the characterization of drugs of abuse. *Egypt. J. Forensic Sci.* 6: 209–215.

Cengiz, I. F., Oliveira, J. M., & Reis, R. L. (2018). Micro-CT—A digital 3D microstructural voyage into scaffolds: A systematic review of the reported methods and results. *Biomater. Res.* 22: 1–11.

Chauhan, N., Lakhkar, N., & Chaudhari, A. (2021). Development and physicochemical characterization of novel porous phosphate glass bone graft substitute and in vitro comparison with xenograft. *J. Mater. Sci.: Mater. Med.* 32: 60.

Chen, J., Zeng, L., Chen, X., Liao, T., & Zheng, J. (2018). Preparation and characterization of bioactive glass tablets and evaluation of bioactivity and cytotoxicity in vitro. *Bioact. Mater.* 3: 315–321.

Coelho, C. C., Padrão, T., Costa, L., Pinto, M. T., Costa, P. C., Domingues, V. F., Quadros, P. A., Monteiro, F. J., & Sousa, S. R. (2020). The antibacterial and angiogenic effect of magnesium oxide in a hydroxyapatite bone substitute. *Sci. Rep.* 10: 19098.

Cruz, G. A. da, Toledo, S. de, Sallum, E. A., & Lima, A. F. M. de. (2007). Morphological and chemical analysis of bone substitutes by scanning electron microscopy and microanalysis by spectroscopy of dispersion energy. *Braz. Dent. J.* 18: 129–133.

Demir-Oğuz, Ö., Boccaccini, A. R., & Loca, D. (2023). Injectable bone cements: What benefits the combination of calcium phosphates and bioactive glasses could bring? *Bioact. Mater.* 19: 217–236.

Drosos, G. I., Babourda, E., Magnissalis, E. A., Giatromanolaki, A., Kazakos, K., & Verettas, D. A. (2012). Mechanical characterization of bone graft substitute ceramic cements. *Injury*. 43: 266–271.

Durga, R., Jimenez, N., Ramanathan, S., Suraneni, P., & Pestle, W. J. (2022). Use of thermogravimetric analysis to estimate collagen and hydroxyapatite contents in archaeological bone. *J. Archaeol. Sci.* 145: 105644.

El-khooly, M. S., Abdraboh, A. S., Bakr, A. M., & Ereiba, K. H. T. (2022). Bioactivity and mechanical properties characterization of bioactive glass incorporated with graphene oxide. *Silicon*. 15: 1263–1271.

Emami, A., Talaei-Khozani, T., Tavanafar, S., Zareifard, N., Azarpira, N., & Vojdani, Z. (2020). Synergic effects of decellularized bone matrix, hydroxyapatite, and extracellular vesicles on repairing of the rabbit mandibular bone defect model. *J. Transl. Med.* 18: 1–18.

Figueiredo, M. M., Gamelas, J. A. F., & Martins, A. G. (2012). Characterization of bone and bone-based graft materials using FTIR spectroscopy. In *Infrared Spectroscopy-Life and Biomedical Sciences*. T. Theophile, Ed. Norderstedt: Books on Demand, pp. 315–338.

Fishman, J. A., Scobie, L., & Takeuchi, Y. (2012). Xenotransplantation-associated infectious risk: A WHO consultation. *Xenotransplantation*. 19: 72–81.

Friesenbichler, J., Maurer-Ertl, W., Bergovec, M., Holzer, L. A., Ogris, K., Leitner, L., & Leithner, A. (2017). Clinical experience with the artificial bone graft substitute calcibon used following curettage of benign and low-grade malignant bone tumors. *Sci. Rep.* 7: 1–5.

Galia, C. R., Lourenço, A. L., Rosito, R., Macedo, C. A. S., & Camargo, L. M. A. Q. (2011). Physicochemical characterization of lyophilized bovine bone grafts. *Rev. Bras. Ortop. (English Edition)*. 46: 444–451.

Hannink, G., & Arts, J. J. C. (2011). Bioresorbability, porosity and mechanical strength of bone substitutes: What is optimal for bone regeneration? *Injury*. 42: S22–S25.

Horstmann, P. F., Hettwer, W. H., Kaltoft, N. S., & Petersen, M. M. (2018). Early clinical and radiological experience with a ceramic bone graft substitute in the treatment of benign and borderline bone lesions. *Sci. Rep.* 8: 1–8.

Hou, X., Zhang, L., Zhou, Z., Luo, X., Wang, T., Zhao, X., Lu, B., Chen, F., & Zheng, L. (2022). Calcium phosphate-based biomaterials for bone repair. *J. Funct. Biomater.* 13: 187.

Khan, W. S., Rayan, F., Dhinsa, B. S., & Marsh, D. (2012). An osteoconductive, osteoinductive, and osteogenic tissue-engineered product for trauma and orthopaedic surgery: How far are we? *Stem Cells Int.* 2012: 1–7.

Kim, S. Y., Lee, Y. J., Cho, W. T., Hwang, S. H., Heo, S. C., Kim, H. J., & Huh, J. B. (2021). Preliminary animal study on bone formation ability of commercialized particle-type bone graft with increased operability by hydrogel. *Materials*. 14: 4464.

Lee, J. H., Yi, G. S., Lee, J. W., & Kim, D. J. (2017). Physicochemical characterization of porcine bone-derived grafting material and comparison with bovine xenografts for dental applications. *J. Periodontal Implant Sci*. 47: 388–401.

Litak, J., Grochowski, C., Rysak, A., Mazurek, M., Blicharski, T., Kamieniak, P., Wolszczak, P., Rahnama-Hezavah, M., & Litak, G. (2022). New horizons for hydroxyapatite supported by DXA assessment—A preliminary study. *Materials*. 15: 942.

Loi, F., Córdova, L. A., Pajarinen, J., Lin, T., Yao, Z., & Goodman, S. B. (2016). Inflammation, fracture and bone repair. *Bone*. 86: 119–130.

Marsell, R., & Einhorn, T. A. (2011). The biology of fracture healing. *Injury*. 42: 551–555.

McGovern, J. A., Griffin, M., & Hutmacher, D. W. (2018). Animal models for bone tissue engineering and modelling disease. *Dis. Models Mech.* 11: dmm033084.

Medrano-David, D., Lopera, A. M., Londoño, M. E., & Araque-Marín, P. (2021). Formulation and characterization of a new injectable bone substitute composed PVA/borax/CaCO3 and demineralized bone matrix. *J. Funct. Biomater.* 12: 46.

Miguez, M., Sabarots, M. G., Cid, M. P., Salvatierra, N. A., & Comín, R. (2022). Fabrication and characterization of gelatin/calcium phosphate electrospun composite scaffold for bone tissue engineering. *Fibers Polym.* 23: 1915–1923.

Mohammed, A., & Abdullah, A. (2018). Scanning Electron Microscopy (SEM): A review. *Proceedings of the 2018 International Conference on Hydraulics and Pneumatics—HERVEX*. Băile Govora, Romania, pp. 7–9.

Montes-Hernandez, G., & Renard, F. (2020). Nucleation of brushite and hydroxyapatite from amorphous calcium phosphate phases revealed by dynamic in situ raman spectroscopy. *J. Phys. Chem. C*. 124: 15302–15311.

Morris, M. D., & Mandair, G. S. (2011). Raman assessment of bone quality. *Clin. Orthop. Relat. Res.* 469: 2160–2169.

Nikhil, A., & Kumar, A. (2022). Evaluating potential of tissue-engineered cryogels and chondrocyte derived exosomes in articular cartilage repair. *Biotechnol. Bioeng.* 119: 605–625.

Nikhil, A., Qayoom, I., Das, A., & Kumar, A. (2024). Preventing septic implant failures in osteoporotic hip fractures using antibiotic-loaded functionalized nanocement. *Chem. Eng. J.* 486: 149908.

Osipov, B., Emami, A. J., & Christiansen, B. A. (2018). Systemic bone loss after fracture. *Clin. Rev. Bone Miner. Metab.* 16: 116–130.

Predoi, D., Iconaru, S. L., Ciobanu, S. C., Predoi, S.-A., Buton, N., Megier, C., & Beuran, M. (2021). Development of iron-doped hydroxyapatite coatings. *Coatings.* 11: 186.

Qayoom, I., Srivastava, E., & Kumar, A. (2022). Anti-infective composite cryogel scaffold treats osteomyelitis and augments bone healing in rat femoral condyle. *Biomat. Adv.* 142: 213133.

Samanta, S. K., Chanda, A., & Nandi, S. K. (2019). Physical and mechanical characterization of crystalline pure β-tri calcium phosphate & its dopants as bone substitutes. *IOP Conf. Ser. Mater. Sci. Eng.* 577: 12138.

Schwartz, D. (2015). *ITWG Guideline on Powder X-Ray Diffraction (XRD)-General Overview.* Lawrence Livermore, California, USA: Livermore National Laboratory.

Shegarfi, H., & Reikeras, O. (2009). Bone transplantation and immune response. *J. Orthop. Surg.* 17: 206–211.

Stetefeld, J., McKenna, S. A., & Patel, T. R. (2016). Dynamic light scattering: A practical guide and applications in biomedical sciences. *Biophys. Rev.* 8: 409–427.

Teotia, A. K., Dienel, K., Qayoom, I., van Bochove, B., Gupta, S., Partanen, J., Seppälä, J., & Kumar, A. (2020). Improved bone regeneration in rabbit bone defects using 3D printed composite scaffolds functionalized with osteoinductive factors. *ACS Appl. Mater. Interfaces.* 12: 48340–48356.

Teotia, A. K., Qayoom, I., & Kumar, A. (2018). Endogenous platelet-rich plasma supplements/augments growth factors delivered via porous collagen-nanohydroxyapatite bone substitute for enhanced bone formation. *ACS Biomater. Sci. Eng.* 5: 56–69.

Teotia, A. K., Raina, D. B., Singh, C., Sinha, N., Isaksson, H., Tägil, M., Lidgren, L., & Kumar, A. (2017). Nano-hydroxyapatite bone substitute functionalized with bone active molecules for enhanced cranial bone regeneration. *ACS Appl. Mater. Interfaces.* 9: 6816–6828.

Timchenko, P. E., Timchenko, E. V., Pisareva, E. V., Vlasov, M. Y., Volova, L. T., Frolov, O. O., & Kalimullina, A. R. (2018). Experimental studies of hydroxyapatite by Raman spectroscopy. *J. Opt. Technol.* 85: 130–135.

Yilmaz, B., & Evis, Z. (2014). Raman spectroscopy investigation of nano hydroxyapatite doped with yttrium and fluoride ions. *Spectrosc. Lett.* 47: 24–29.

Zafeiropoulos, N. E. (2011). *Interface Engineering of Natural Fibre Composites for Maximum Performance.* Cambridge: Elsevier.

II

Application of Nanotechnology and Phytomedicines for Bone Repair and Regeneration

8 Spatially Controlled Delivery of Bioactive Cues for Bone Tissue Engineering

From Nano to Macro Scale

Chandra Khatua, Eshita Mukherjee, and Debrupa Lahiri

8.1 INTRODUCTION

Bone tissue engineering has attracted much research and therapeutic attention recently. Researchers tried to learn how to take advantage of the self-healing ability of bone for repairing its minor defects. It became clear that it would be beneficial to have naturally produced biochemical signalling cues during bone self healing, either by providing them directly or by using other substances for stimulating bone regeneration (Zhu et al., 2022).

Bone tissue engineering involves delivering bioactive cues that are able to respond to biochemical signals and generate new, functional bone tissue that can integrate with neighbouring tissue. A variety of biomaterials can transmit biochemical signals to cells in both temporally and spatially controlled ways (Bittner et al., 2018; Chen et al., 2021; Subbiah et al., 2021). They include bioactive substances such as growth factors, small molecules and drugs.

For instance, collagen sponges that release bone morphogenetic proteins have been utilized in therapeutic studies to treat spinal fusions (McKay & Sandhu, 2002) and nonunions of the femur and tibia (Kanakaris et al., 2009). These systems provided limited spatially and temporally controlled release of growth factors. Therefore, these factors were required in significantly higher concentrations than that observed in the natural healing process (Smucker et al., 2006). As a result, when used on the anterior cervical spine, collagen sponges have led to major vertebral body bone resorption and swelling (McClellan et al., 2006).

These restrictions inspired the development of a system with improved temporally and spatially controlled delivery of bioactive cues. Numerous researchers have discussed the spatiotemporally controlled release profiles of bioactive cues for bone growth (Mehta et al., 2012; Vo et al., 2012). Some recent research has been focused on developing delivery systems that are able to not only temporally but also spatially control the release of desired bioactive cues (Bittner et al., 2018; He et al., 2022).

The majority of the previous work on the delivery of bioactive cues was carried out using homogeneous cues. However, recent studies have focused on functionalized spatial and temporal arrangements of these molecules (He et al., 2022). Temporal control is helpful because it enables the bioactive cues to be released for a certain time period to reach the desired cellular responses without requiring additional dosage. There have been some attempts to explain how the timing of signal presentation coincides with bone formation and healing time (Jantz, 1999). Gene expression as well as extracellular matrix (ECM) formation are closely modulated in time and space during these processes. Hence, there is a need to develop a scaffold with spatially controlled bioactive cues for bone regeneration applications. This book chapter explores different approaches for the spatially controlled delivery of bioactive cues for bone tissue engineering.

DOI: 10.1201/9781003307310-10

8.2 SPATIAL CONTROL OF BIOACTIVE CUES

The majority of growth factor proteins are unstable and have a short half-life in nature (Penheiter et al., 2002). High doses are needed for the conventional administration of these compounds, which is not physiologically appropriate or cost effective. Finally, high concentrations can have negative effects like poor immune responses, tumour formation and high cost. Therefore, it should be ensured that the bioactive cues have controlled local concentrations during application.

8.3 BIOACTIVE CUES FOR BONE TISSUE ENGINEERING

Different bioactive cues are crucial for controlling cellular processes and tissue growth for bone tissue engineering (Figure 8.1). The growth factor is a kind of protein or polypeptide that can aid in tissue regeneration. In addition to the traditional polypeptide or protein-based growth factors, other bioactive molecules, such as nucleic acids and hormones, have also shown significant potential for accelerating bone regrowth. Due to the exceptional physiochemical and biological properties of these molecules, specific design approaches for delivery systems are required.

8.3.1 Growth Factors

Growth factors refer to soluble signalling proteins or polypeptides that can be secreted by cells in order to regulate biological activities like cell proliferation, migration, differentiation and ECM synthesis (Cross & Dexter, 1991). They act by attaching to receptors on the cell surfaces and influence gene expression. After binding, phosphorylation of the receptor causes conformational changes in the receptor that trigger signalling cascades inside the cell (Schlessinger & Ullrich, 1992).

Growth factor receptors that have been internalized have the ability to produce phosphorylate intracellular signalling proteins like transcription factors. This can translocate to the nucleus and control gene activation. These factors work locally and diffuse in the short range through the ECM. For cellular activities, the half-life of the growth factor is in the order of hours, as they degrade through proteolysis (Penheiter et al., 2002).

There are various growth factors employed in bone tissue engineering, both individually and in different combinations: fibroblast growth factors-2 (FGF-2), bone morphogenetic protein (BMP-2, BMP-4, BMP-7), insulin-like growth factor (IGF-1), transforming growth factor-β (TGF-β1, TGF-β2, TGF-β3), vascular endothelial growth factor (VEGF), platelet-derived growth factor (PDGF) and stromal cell-derived factor 1 (De Witte et al., 2018) (Table 8.1).

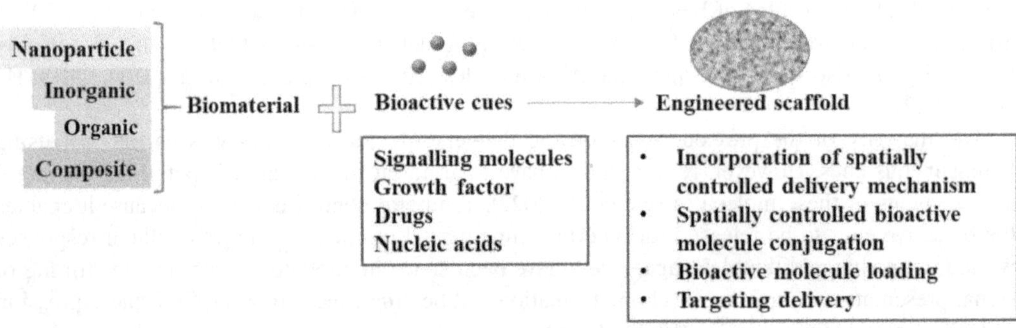

FIGURE 8.1 Schematic representation of a delivery system for bioactive cues.

TABLE 8.1
Growth Factors for Bone Tissue Engineering

Growth Factor	Function	Reference
Bone morphogenetic proteins	Promote differentiation	Park et al. (2015)
Vascular endothelial growth factor	Angiogenesis	Madrigal et al. (2018)
Platelet-derived growth factor	Vascularization, increase proliferation	Wang et al. (2021)
Fibroblast growth factor	Angiogenesis, increase proliferation and promote osteogenic differentiation	Novais et al. (2021)
Insulin-like growth factor	Promote osteogenic differentiation	He et al. (2020)
Transforming growth factor beta	Promote osteogenic, chondrogenic differentiation	Gonzalez-Fernandez et al. (2019)

BMP-2, BMP-7, VEGF and FGF-2 exhibited excellent potential for bone regeneration and are involved in various preclinical studies (Oliveira et al., 2021). However, the prospective outcomes shown in animal models have not yet been effectively translated to human trials because of adverse effects. For example, vascular permeability is considerably increased by VEGF, which could cause swelling and systemic hypotension. Most BMP-related side effects are associated with heterotopic bone development and BMP-2 also increases the possibility of developing cancer.

Most of the growth factors used for therapeutic applications are delivered at high doses, and side effects of growth factors are caused by improperly controlled release and dosages above physiological levels. At fracture sites, these growth factors are present in extremely low amounts (between pg/mL and a few ng/mL) (Glass et al., 2011). To promote new bone formation in current clinical therapies, growth factors are required in higher concentrations; for instance, although each vial of Osigraft® contains 3.5 mg of BMP-7, sometimes more than one vial is used for bone treatment (Friedlaender et al., 2001).

Patients have utilized these recombinant human growth factors for many years with no adverse effects (Guler et al., 1987). However, the production cost of sufficient growth factors for clinical uses is high. According to a 2008 report, the price of BMP-7 containing 3.5 mg, which was used for tibia fracture treatment, was GBP 3000 (about USD 3800) (Dahabreh et al., 2009). New production techniques help to decrease the price of growth factors and make possible more clinical applications (Von Einem et al., 2010).

Another option to mimic growth factors is synthetic peptides. The growth factor receptors are still activated by these shorter peptide sequences, but these small molecules can be easily modified with other chemical groups. Several peptide sequences that mimic BMP-2 promote osteogenic behaviour both in vitro (Lee et al., 2010) and in vivo (Lin et al., 2007). Additionally, peptide sequences that resemble other growth factors, such as VEGF (D'Andrea et al., 2005) and FGF-2 (Lin et al., 2006), have been identified and their biological activities described. Ultimately, it is crucial to make a delivery system that enables an efficient low-dose delivery of growth factor through controlled release profiles and specific in vivo localization.

The sustained in vivo release of BMP over four weeks resulted in considerably better bone growth than the same amount of BMP-2 released in a burst (Jeon et al., 2008). Osteoprogenitor cells increased BMP-2 expression at around 21 days at the area of bone fracture, and BMP-2 closely imitates the signalling cascade after injury (Dimitriou et al., 2005). Therefore, current studies have concentrated on the release timing of growth factors and their combinatorial effects. The combinational delivery of IGF-1 and BMP-2 did not show osteogenic differentiation of mouse pluripotent stem cells, while the initial dose of BMP-2 improves bone mineralization (Raiche & Puleo, 2004).

Additionally, controlled release of growth factor helps blood vessel formation (Shah et al., 2011). The early release of VEGF along with an osteogenic growth factor enhanced bone formation in vivo (Shah et al., 2011). In contrast, some researchers claimed that the timing of vasculogenic growth factor was not essential for bone formation and that the release kinetics of osteogenic growth factor were more important (Geuze et al., 2012). Several studies have been carried out to determine the release sequence of these growth factors for bone formation (Dang et al., 2018; Nurkesh et al., 2020; Vo et al., 2012).

8.3.2 Genetic Material

Nucleic acids such as RNA and DNA can modify gene expression at the transcriptional or posttranscriptional stages. They can be used as genetic material as an alternative to growth factors. These are responsible for enhancing bone formation or inhibiting antagonistic pathways (Evans et al., 2012). Extensive research has been done on the effects of genetic material both individually and incorporated into scaffolds (Krebs & Alsberg, 2011).

At the genetic level, nucleic acids can modify cellular activity and regulate the process of bone formation. Prolonged protein expression can be enabled by DNAs and mRNAs that can code for differentiation and growth factors (Franceschi, 2005). For instance, genes encoding BMPs, FGF-2, IGFs, TGF-β, PDGF, VEGF and IGFs can promote bone regeneration (Chang et al., 2010; Gonzalez-Fernandez et al., 2016; McMillan et al., 2018).

Noncoding genes that control cell activity and gene expression such as miRNA (Zhang et al., 2016) and siRNA (Ghadakzadeh et al., 2016) also have promising use as innovative therapeutic agents and have significant roles in bone repair. It is difficult to cross the same charged cell membrane with negatively charged nucleic acids due to electrostatic repulsion (Nitta & Numata, 2013). Another challenge is the fast degradation of certain RNAs in vivo (Guo et al., 2010). Spatiotemporal controlled delivery systems of RNA may be helpful for promoting bone growth when more miRNA and siRNA sites are identified for osteogenesis.

8.3.3 Drugs

A variety of anti-inflammatory drugs or antibiotics, individually or in combination with other biomaterials, have been widely used for bone tissue applications (Feng et al., 2010) to treat bacterial inflammation that could develop during and after the implantation of scaffolds. A wound's inflammation needs to be lessened so that the healing process can begin (Snoddy & Jayasuriya, 2016). The sustained release of antibiotics helps to prevent infection at a bone fracture site produced by debridement and promotes bone regeneration.

Antibiotic drugs such as gentamicin, vancomycin, tetracycline and silver nanoparticles are usually used in bone tissue engineering (Mouriño & Boccaccini, 2010). To inhibit infection in a rabbit bone injury model, polycaprolactone membranes loaded with vancomycin have been used as a delivery system (Wei et al., 2018). This controlled antibiotic-delivery membrane decreases bone infection and enhances bone regeneration.

Several orthopedic implants and scaffolds contain minerals like calcium phosphonate (CaP) and hydroxyapatite, and both these minerals and the ions they release can promote preosteoblast proliferation and differentiation (Lin et al., 2018; Liu et al., 2009; Yang et al., 2008). There are many ways to produce controlled and uniform mineral deposition throughout the implants. Initially, mineral deposition onto scaffolds was accomplished by simulated body fluid (SBF) incubation, but it had been a time consuming process, requiring several weeks to complete (Wei & Ma, 2006). Electrodeposition was afterward established and was capable of producing rapid mineralized coating (CaP) on the surface of scaffolds. A superior-quality mineral coating can be produced rapidly (0.5–3 h), and after deposition, the surface topography can be adjusted according to the parameters of the electrochemical process (He et al., 2010). Antibiotics and anti-inflammatory medications should be used locally to the defect site to prevent side effects related to systemic delivery.

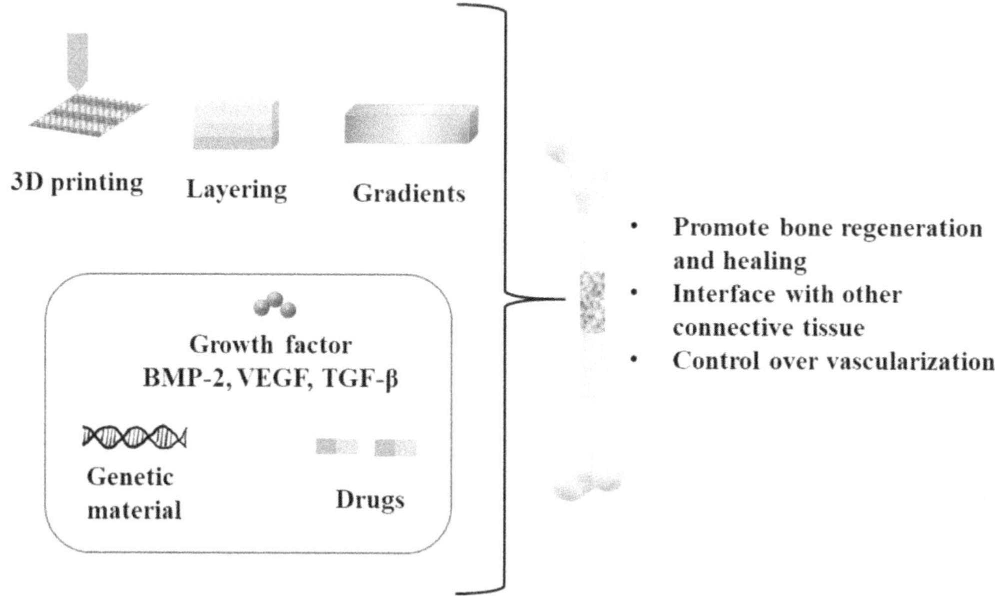

FIGURE 8.2 Different techniques of delivery systems for bioactive cues.

8.4 DELIVERY SYSTEMS

The biochemical environment of bone is composed of a range of bioactive molecules. To re-create this milieu and promote bone regeneration, several strategies for delivering bioactive cues have been suggested (Figure 8.2). The crosslinking or direct adsorption of bioactive molecules to the implant usually produced less-than-ideal results because of burst release and molecular denaturation. Delivery methods should be improved for more accurate and efficient control over release. The nanostructured delivery methods are promising because they are precisely tailored to offer better loading efficiency and controlled release over time.

Osteogenic growth factors like BMP-2, BMP-7 and TGF-β are essential for cell proliferation, differentiation and eventually osteogenesis. An absorbable collagen sponge (INFUSE™) is used to deliver BMP-2 for therapeutic applications that was US Food and Drug Administration (FDA) approved in 2002 (McKay et al., 2007). Despite its being effective, the sponge requires supraphysiologic levels of the growth factor, and these are related to many negative side effects, as discussed earlier. Therefore, innovative delivery systems that can allow the controlled release of lower dosages of bioactive cues for improving bone growth have drawn a great deal of research attention.

8.4.1 Inorganic Delivery Systems

The benefits of using ceramic materials in the area of bone regeneration are its inherent osteoconductive properties. Ceramics that are frequently used are calcium phosphate (CaP) based, for instance tricalcium phosphate (TCP) and hydroxyapatite (HA). When HA-based delivery methods were first being studied, bioactive molecules like BMP-2 were directly coated on HA, which got adsorbed (Xie et al., 2010). However, these adsorbed molecules are released rapidly.

Thus, alternate approaches were required for sustained release such as chemically bonding bioactive factors to the surface of inorganic material to enable more controlled release over time. For the binding of bioactive molecules, the surface of CaP can be functionalized in various ways. For instance, functionalized nano-HA particles can bind to BMP-2 and offer controlled release over time to promote osteogenesis (Zhou et al., 2018).

Metal oxide nanoparticles such as titanium oxide (TiO_2) and silica (SiO_2) have been functionalized as nano-structured vehicles for delivering various bioactive compounds used for bone regeneration (Shadjou & Hasanzadeh, 2015; Zhou et al., 2015). Mesoporous silica is one example of a silica-based nanomaterial that has been designed to offer a controlled release of various bioactive molecules (Eivazzadeh-Keihan et al., 2020). These are biocompatible and can be functionalized with different types of linkers (Yao et al., 2018). They have been used to carry BMP-2 and dexamethasone and regulate the release of BMP-2 both in vitro and in vivo. These silica-based materials have certain remarkable benefits, including their adjustable mesoporous structure and capability to bind with various molecules. Furthermore, the design and architecture of these nanomaterials can be modified to improve bone tissue regeneration (Zhu et al., 2021).

TiO_2 nanotubes can be used to deliver drugs and other biomolecules for bone development (Kwon et al., 2017). They can be functionalized to impregnate the target molecule on the material surface as well as to encapsulate it. The surface-impregnated BMP-2 on TiO_2 nanotubes was used for in vitro bone regeneration. In addition to being used to deliver bioactive cues, CaP and HA coatings have been applied to the surfaces of TiO_2 nanotubes. The toxic effect of TiO_2-based nanomaterials, however, has been a concern, as some studies have described that strong osteoblast adhesion to the metallic substance may cause apoptosis (Liu et al., 2017). The cytotoxicity of TiO_2 monofilaments has also been discussed elsewhere (Magrez et al., 2009).

8.4.2 Organic Delivery Systems

Both natural and synthetic components are used to develop polymer-based delivery systems as alternatives to inorganic delivery systems (Jacob et al., 2018). Polycaprolactone (PCL), polyethylene glycol (PEG), poly (L-lactic acid) (PLA) and poly (lactic-co-glycolic acid) (PLGA) are synthetic polymers that are generally employed as bioactive molecule delivery systems. PLGA is used as copolymers, whereas PEG, PCL and PLA are made from single monomers.

Synthetic polymers have been widely used as delivery systems for BMP-2, dexamethasone, and other bioactive cues for promoting bone growth. Micro-encapsulation has allowed for the accurate and regulated delivery of bioactive cues, increasing the sustained administration of therapeutic dosage while minimizing negative effects at the same time. Polymeric encapsulation, as nano- or microspheres, is frequently used in formulations.

PCL, PLGA and PEG are biocompatible, and PLGA is preferred because it is FDA approved and has shown anti-inflammatory efficacy (Makadia & Siegel, 2011). Furthermore, the molecular weight, L/G ratio and stereochemistry of PLGA can be changed alter the polymer's characteristics and degradation (Habraken et al., 2007). However, PLA and PLGA can produce toxic acidic substances during degradation. To reduce toxicity and burst release of bioactive molecules, controlled degradation of the polymer delivery system is crucial.

Alginate, collagen, chitosan, hyaluronic acid (HA), gelatin, silk fibroin and fibrin are some examples of natural polymers that are employed for the controlled delivery of bioactive cues for bone tissue application (Jacob et al., 2018). These materials have the advantages of biocompatibility and biomimetic properties because they are very similar to natural ECM and they are also completely degradable. Natural polymer-based delivery systems have been used to deliver VEGF (Farokhi et al., 2014), BMP-2 (Shen et al., 2016), antibiotics (Cai et al., 2016) and immunomodulators (Amjadian et al., 2016).

However, employing natural polymers as a delivery system has some limitations. It is difficult to regulate the release of bioactive cues from these degradable polymers. Collagen degrades rapidly due to its protease action (Li et al., 2021a), although the degradation rates of natural polymers can be reduced significantly by employing various chemical modifications such as crosslinking or combining them with other substances (Ding et al., 2016; Oliveira et al., 2019). Natural polymers also have limitations associated with their production cost and reproducibility in different batches (Vo et al., 2012).

8.4.3 Composite Delivery Systems

Composite materials have been developed that aim to overcome the limitations of the synthetic and natural polymers we have discussed so far. Combining multiple materials can synergize their individual properties into one delivery system. Composite materials allow the precise control of the release profile of a particular molecule, for instance the osteogenic growth factors that are essential for in vivo application.

Polymer blends, polymer/silica composites and polymer/ceramic composites are examples of composite delivery systems (Kim et al., 2018; Liu et al., 2022; Oliveira et al., 2021). Polymer and HA composite materials such as poly(ethylene oxide)/silk fibroin/nano-HA (Liu et al., 2022; Shen et al., 2016), gelatin/nano-HA (Udomluck et al., 2020), PLA/collagen/nano-HA (Liu et al., 2022), PCL/HA (Rittipakorn et al., 2021) and chitosan/nano-HA (Liu et al., 2022) have been developed for regulated BMP-2 delivery. In composite systems, the ceramic components give osteoconductive benefits, while the polymer constituents can be used for crosslinking and functionalization.

Polymer blends have also been developed for regulating degradation rates (Wang et al., 2018). In bone tissue engineering research, metal and polymer composites as bioactive molecule delivery systems have attracted great interest. Although biomolecules can be quickly released from functionalized metal oxides like silica, conjugation with polymers can also lead to sustained release over time. Mesoporous silica combined with PLGA has been developed as a delivery system to deliver therapies such as BMP-2 (Minardi et al., 2020) as well as other growth factors (Minardi et al., 2015). It has exhibited interesting release studies, cytotoxicity and osteogenicity both in vitro and in vivo.

Similar composite materials have been used by others for bone formation (Zhang et al., 2018). Coated mesoporous silica-incorporated PCL nanofibers were developed that can bind several bioactive compounds and sustained release over time, which enhanced osteogenic differentiation in vitro (Singh et al., 2015). Researchers are involved in making spatiotemporally regulated biomaterials that can distribute rhBMP-2 to the bone defect site because of the exceptionally pro-osteogenic properties of this growth factor (El Bialy et al., 2017). More broadly, various types of ceramic scaffolds and polymeric and hydrogel-based materials have been investigated in the last decade, which exhibited very promising results (Quinlan et al., 2015a).

By conjugating synthetic or natural BMP-2-binding ligands with the polymer matrix, it is possible to control BMP-2 delivery more precisely. An alginate/PCL scaffold-based BMP-2 delivery system showed strong interactions between bone morphogenic proteins and heparin microparticles (HMPs) (Hettiaratchi et al., 2020). The diffusion of BMP-2 was slowed by interacting with HMPs, which produced a persistent gradient and spatially regulated localization. The osteogenic gene expression was spatially controlled by the BMP-2 concentration, which helps to form a graded microstructure from low-stiffness cartilage to high-stiffness mineralized bone. A magnetically induced biochemical gradient of BMP-2 was produced using heparin-conjugated superparamagnetic iron oxide nanoparticles in agarose hydrogel. This conjugate provides new potential for complex tissue engineering systems (Li et al., 2018).

Advanced technology has made it possible to fabricate scaffolds with gradients of growth factors that are differentially arranged. The cutting-edge techniques that can be used to incorporate biomolecules within scaffolds include layer-by-layer, microfluidics and 3D bioprinting (Li et al., 2018, 2021b). Alginate-based hydrogels with a spatial gradient of bioactive cues were incorporated in 3D-printed PCL scaffolds. The growth factor was combined with VEGF and BMP-2 combination and applied at peripheral and central locations for the regeneration of bone (Freeman et al., 2020); alginate and laponite slowed the release rate compared with that with pure alginate, leading to the controlled release of the signaling biomolecule. In a different study, researchers used mesoporous bioactive glass nanospheres that incorporated electrospun PCL nanofibers to deliver FGF2 and FGF18 (Kang et al., 2015).

Researchers have also used 3D-printed scaffolds to deliver bioactive cues for tissue regeneration. For example, 3D-printed composite of PCL/PLGA/β-TCP was made in membrane form, and BMP-2 in collagen gel was incorporated into the pores of the membrane (Park et al., 2017). TGF-β1 encapsulated in PLGA microspheres and n-HA composite were used to make osteochondral scaffolds using stereolithography (SLA). A micro-precise spatiotemporal delivery system was developed by incorporating PLGA microspheres encapsulating growth factors in 3D-printed polymeric microstrands (Tarafder et al., 2016).

8.5 FUNCTIONALIZED DELIVERY SYSTEMS

Functionalized scaffolds (Figure 8.3) can be developed to offer both the spatiotemporally controlled release of bioactive molecules that promote bone growth (Minardi et al., 2016a). For clinical applications, the spatially controlled release of bioactive molecules ensures that they are released into the fracture or target area of interest (Minardi et al., 2016a). On the other hand, to coordinate the cascade of molecular and cellular activities required for bone repair, temporally controlled release is crucial. Scaffold is combined with nanostructured delivery systems in various forms such as hydrogels, fibers and 3D-printed materials (Yi et al., 2016). These scaffolds can be functionalized with growth factors, peptides, antibiotics and even cells (Minardi et al., 2016a).

Angiogenic factors including PDGF, VEGF and FGF are crucial for bone regeneration (David Roodman, 2003; De la Riva et al., 2010). Inflammatory reaction of the host is a key factor in osteogenesis and regrowth of bone. Incorporating immunomodulatory bioactive molecules into scaffolds is another way to improve bone healing (Corradetti et al., 2015; Guihard et al., 2015). Implanted biomaterials offer the significant advantage of the controlled release of antibiotics to minimize the risk of infection during implantation (Adams et al., 2009). For instance, several types of scaffolds including PLA/HA composite (Amjadian et al., 2016) and electrospun fiber discs (Li et al., 2015a) have been modified to deliver dexamethasone to enhance bone regeneration.

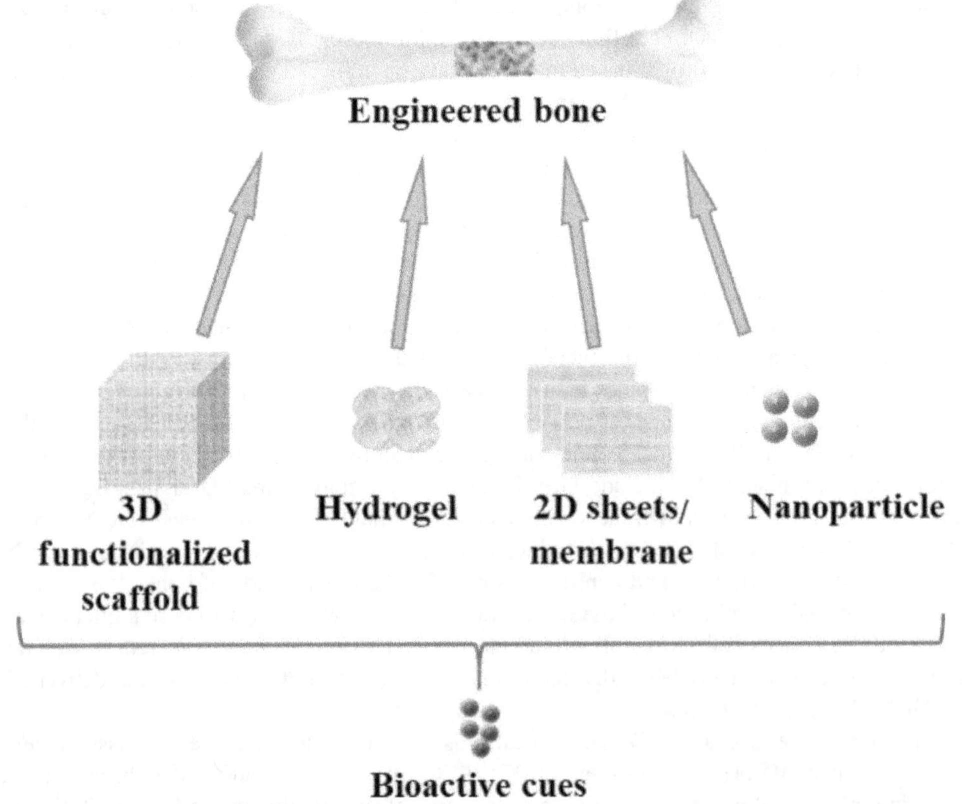

FIGURE 8.3 Different systems to deliver bioactive cues.

8.5.1 Incorporating Nanocarriers in 3D Delivery Systems

There have been numerous methods for directly incorporating bioactive cues and nanostructured carriers into 3D scaffolds. Among them, hydrogels are widely used (Hoare & Kohane, 2008). Hydrogels can be tailored to regulate the release of bioactive molecules (Gibbs et al., 2016) as well as improve the adhesion and proliferation of cells (Tibbitt & Anseth, 2009). Therefore, different types of polymeric hydrogels have been developed that are biocompatible. By altering their surface with different ligands, they can be easily functionalized (Hoffman, 2012).

There are a few limitations to fabricating these hydrogels and to their therapeutic applications (Hoare & Kohane, 2008). They are difficult to handle because they are inherently weak. Additionally, the clinical utilization of hydrogels is constrained by their sterilization difficulties (Hoffman, 2012). However, in vitro studies have revealed that alginate hydrogels conjugated with peptide mimicking BMP-2 improve osteogenic differentiation markers and enhance mineralization (Madl et al., 2014). Polymeric hydrogel scaffolds have also been used as delivery systems for angiogenic agents like VEGF (Kempen et al., 2009).

8.5.2 Surface Modification and Crosslinking of Nanocarriers in 3D Delivery Systems

There are other ways to functionalize biomaterials including surface modification and crosslinking. Surface chemistries have the ability to provide controlled release by facilitating the stable, covalent attachment of molecules (Nie et al., 2007). For example, heparin-based linkers are frequently used for the surface adhesion of growth factors (Liang & Kiick, 2014). They are used for the local delivery of angiogenic factors like VEGF and PDGF as well as BMP-2 (Yun et al., 2013).

Additionally, BMP-2 delivery systems have been integrated directly into the surfaces of 3D-printed ceramic based scaffolds utilizing polymeric emulsion (Kim et al., 2018). Additionally, immunomodulatory molecules can modify surfaces. To facilitate the quick release of interferon gamma (IFN-γ), decellularized scaffolds were functionalized with IFN-γ via adsorption and/or IL-4 via biotin-streptavidin binding and regulated the sustained release of IL-4 for promoting M2 macrophages polarization (Spiller et al., 2015).

IFN-γ functionalized scaffolds showed enhanced vascularization in comparison with a control group (Spiller et al., 2015). Other immunomodulatory molecules such as IL-4 (Minardi et al., 2016b), IL-10 (Rodell et al., 2015) and IL33 (Liu et al., 2018) are used to functionalize scaffolds, for instance to offer the controlled release of conjugated BMP-2, (Gan et al., 2015; Kim et al., 2018; Mohammadi et al., 2018). In a cranial lesion rat model, porous scaffolds made of sintered nano-HA were designed with either BMP-2 or BMP-2-related peptide with efficient osteogenic potential (Sun et al., 2018). TiO_2 nanotubes were developed by anodizing a titanium substrate and loaded with BMP-2 for sustained release (Hu et al., 2012); these nanotubes demonstrated promise in the in vitro stimulation of osteogenic differentiation.

8.5.3 Multifunctional Scaffolds as Delivery Systems

Multifunctional materials can be used to construct 3D scaffolds loaded with bioactive compounds, such as peptide amphiphiles (PA); the nanogel of heparin-binding PA can bind and mimic native BMP-2 signaling (Lee et al., 2013). PA binding with BMP-2 can stimulate bone regrowth in rat femoral defect using 10-fold lower doses of BMP-2 than are generally needed (Lee et al., 2013). Another research group demonstrated that the nanogel of BMP-2-binding PA also increased bone healing in a preclinical posterolateral lumbar fusion model using 10 times lower doses of BMP-2 than are generally needed (Lee et al., 2015).

BMP-2-mimicking peptides were used to make hydrogels that could induce MSCs to differentiate into osteoblasts (Liang et al., 2019). Binding many osteogenic growth factors with heparin in the physiological condition is difficult, as heparin sulfate chains have a complex motif; therefore, nanostructures of supramolecular glycopeptide comprising sulfated monosaccharides were used to functionalize PAs (Lee et al., 2017). The PA nanostructures with 100-fold lower doses of BMP-2 than are generally needed (100 ng of BMP-2 per animal) produced 100% fusion in a rat model (Lee et al., 2017).

The preclinical evidence is promising for the use of PA-based controlled delivery systems in bone regeneration, although controlling the nano-scale characteristics of PAs and functionalization by various binding motifs, as well as gelling substances into macrostructures for clinical applications, are all challenging undertakings. The future challenges for these materials include their large-scale production, batch-to-batch inconsistency and optimizations of therapeutic applications. The potential for spatially controlled delivery for bone regeneration applications is constantly growing with a wide range of variables that can be modified.

8.6 DELIVERY TECHNIQUES

Cells are naturally sensitive to regional micro- and nanoscale patterns of chemistry and topography, which causes a variety of changes in cell behavior. This includes changes in cell orientation and adhesion and in intracellular signalling pathways that control gene expression and transcriptional activity (Stevens & George, 2005). A highly interconnected porous architecture creates an optimal in vivo milieu to accommodate a variety of signalling cues that affect cell destiny.

Current biomaterial scaffolds for bone repair are made to mimic such milieus to support osteogenesis by promoting cell ingrowth, differentiation and vascularization. The most promising bone substitutes are scaffolds with 3D hierarchical architectures and porous nanostructures (Zhou et al., 2019). The bone scaffold materials' functionality can be improved by incorporating bioactive cues (such as drugs or growth factors) to promote bone regeneration or treat bone disorders by enhancing cell proliferation, differentiation and adhesion (Lynn & Langer, 2000; Romagnoli et al., 2013; Wohl & Engbersen, 2012). Hence, spatially controlled delivery of bioactive cues is needed (Mouriño & Boccaccini, 2010) for bone tissue engineering applications.

As a bone substitute, 3D porous biomaterial scaffolds have been developed using a variety of techniques. The conventional techniques include gas forming, solvent casting particulate leaching, powder foaming, thermally induced phase separation, lyophilization and sol-gel (Kim et al., 2017), while the recent fabrication methods include self-assembly (Chen et al., 2013), bioprinting or additive manufacturing (Inzana et al., 2014; Peltola et al., 2008), layer by layer (LBL) (Chung et al., 2007) and electrospinning (Xue et al., 2017). In many instances, rather than relying just on one technology, fabricating hierarchical scaffolds relies on the combination of various techniques (Wubneh et al., 2018). Herein, we mostly emphasize the advanced methods for fabricating scaffolds to spatially control the delivery of bioactive cues from nano to micro range for bone tissue engineering applications.

8.6.1 Self-Assembly

Self-assembly is the method by which molecules spontaneously combine to create a well-defined, stable entity via noncovalent bonding (Whitesides et al., 1991). In biological systems, self-assembly is common and is thought to be the key to creating complex biological structures (Whitesides et al., 1991). For example, natural ECM is formed by the self-assembly of many nanofibrillar proteins released by cells, namely, collagen fibrils.

Biomaterials that mimic bone biomineralization offer a bone-like milieu for osteoblast proliferation and differentiation, giving the substitute bone required stiffness and mechanical strength (Liu et al., 2016). One of the most difficult parts of biomaterial self-assembly is the compatibility of the scaffolds' structural and biological activities with the native bone (Li et al., 2015b). Some natural polymers such as silk and collagen and synthetic polymers including PLA, PLGA and PGA are of particular interest because of their unique biodegradability and biocompatibility (Farokhi et al., 2018). Because of its affinity for hard tissues and mechanical qualities, bioactive glasses are frequently employed for bone repair.

For instance, a porous biomaterial scaffold was developed by combining collagen-glycosaminoglycan (CG) and bioactive glass, using freeze-drying and self-assembly (O'Brien et al., 2004; Quinlan et al., 2015b). A hydroxyl carbonate apatite layer was created on the particle's surface when the bioactive glass particles were added to the CG slurry via ion exchange reactions of Na^+ and Ca^{2+} with H^+ or H_3O^+. Enhanced VEGF production in endothelial cells and the compressive modulus of the assembled composites was observed because of bioactive glass addition (Quinlan et al., 2015b).

In another study, a novel scaffold system was prepared in which nanospheres were encapsulated into microspheres. Here, BMP-2-bound heparin-conjugated gelatin nanospheres encapsulated into nanofibrous microspheres of poly (l-lactic acid) (PLLA) result in the release of BMP-2 in a controlled manner. This nanofibrous microsphere is a self-assembled carrier made of synthetic nanofibers that supports tissue ingrowth and cell attachment. It is also a scaffold that has osteoinductive properties for accelerated repairing of bone, according to an in vivo calvarial defect model (Ma et al., 2015).

8.6.2 Bioprinting

Bioprinting (Figure 8.4) is the application of computer-based transfer methods for the assembly and patterning of nonliving and living materials with a predetermined 3D or 2D organization for constructing bioengineered model structures useful in basic cell biology studies, pharmacokinetics and regenerative medicine (Moroni et al., 2018). Printed biomaterials, bioactive cues and living cells are all feasible with this method (Dalton et al., 2016), but like all printing processes, ink is required.

A bioink is a formulation of materials and cells or biological molecules produced utilizing the technology of bioprinting (Moroni et al., 2018). If the formulation does not contain any cells, it is called ink. When promoting cell development into tissues, additive manufacturing, which is mainly cell seeding after developing a 3D scaffold, is considered bioprinting (Dalton et al., 2016; Moroni

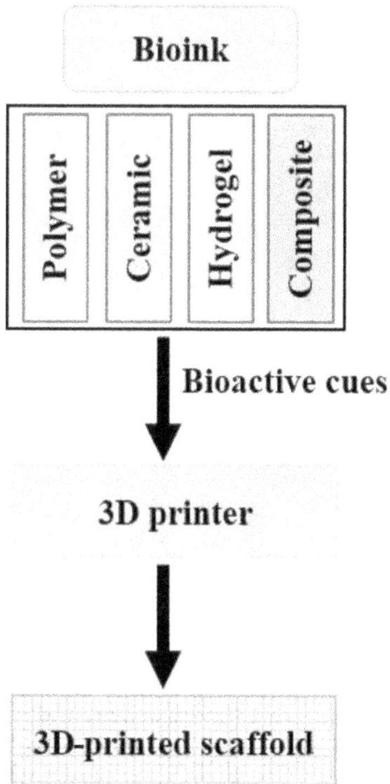

FIGURE 8.4 Schematic of 3D-printed scaffold formation via bioprinting.

et al., 2018). Despite being a subset of bioprinting, additive manufacturing employs inks (rather than bioinks), with cells seeded subsequently.

Micro- and nanoscale surface patterns are beneficial for delivering bioactive cues, like drugs, growth factors, nucleic acids or genes. In regenerative medicine, these bioactive cues should be delivered in a spatially controlled manner for optimal tissue regeneration. Effective cell differentiation, proliferation and function rely heavily on the spatially controlled delivery of the bioactive cues.

In one study, gelatin microparticles were loaded with BMP-2 incorporated into an alginate-containing bioink. This system containing goat-derived multipotent stromal cells permitted the continuous release of BMP-2 for three weeks, which helped in bone regeneration and significant osteogenic differentiation in rats and mice (Poldervaart et al., 2013). When VEGF was loaded into microspheres, due to their spatially controlled bioprinting and depending on the release of VEGF, regional differences in vascularization of scaffolds were observed in vivo. Bioprinting was also utilized for printed constructs of various types of cells to spatially control the release of growth factor, which was modified regionally for each type of cell (Poldervaart et al., 2014).

For osteochondral regeneration, a 3D nanocomposite was designed consisting of growth factors BMP-2 and TGF-β1 for, respectively, osteogenic and chondrogenic differentiation. For optimal growth factor encapsulation and prolonged delivery, nanospheres were functionalized to the cartilage and bone layers. Adhesion and differentiation of stem cells in cartilage and bone layers were markedly improved (Castro et al., 2014).

In a bioprinted model, TGF-β1 was delivered to human bone marrow MSCs using a similar approach. The strategy makes use of the core-shell nanospheres' sustained release capabilities (Zhu et al., 2018). Properly placed nanospheres inside the bioprinted cartilage model allowed for a TGF-β delivery up to 21 days that boosted the encapsulated MSCs' chondrogenic differentiation.

A 3D bioprinted scaffold containing sodium alginate, polyethylenimine (PEI) and silica gel (inorganic filler) was developed for a release study of BMP-7 growth factor in bone tissue regeneration (Sithole et al., 2023). BMP-7 was loaded onto the surface of the 3D-printed scaffold and showed sustained release. After eight weeks, BMP-7 containing 3D-printed scaffolds exhibited more osteogenesis than the scaffolds without BMP-7 (Figure 8.5).

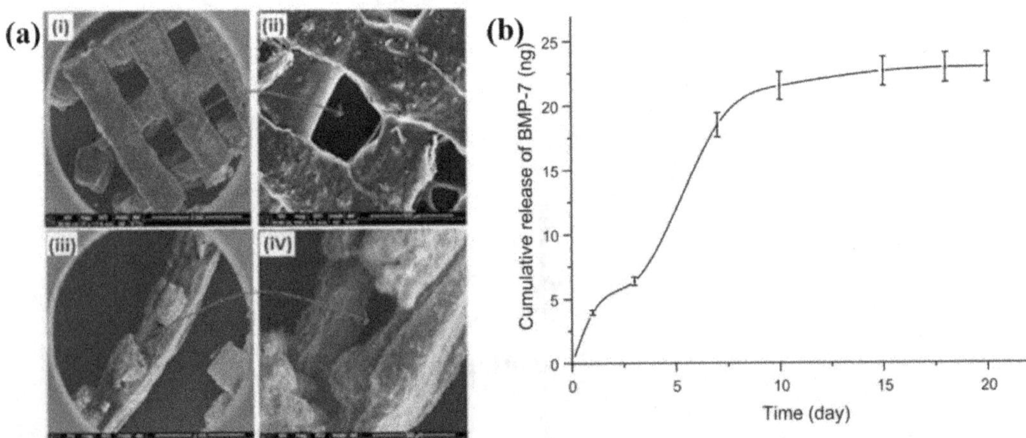

FIGURE 8.5 Surface morphology and release profile of a 3D-printed biomaterial scaffold: (a) cross-section and biomineralization of the scaffold: (i) surface of scaffold, (ii) magnified surface of scaffold, (iii) cross-section of scaffold, and (iv) magnified cross-section of scaffold; (b) in vitro BMP-7 release from the 3D-printed scaffold (reproduced under the terms of CC-BY 4.0 (https://creativecommons.org/licenses/by/4.0/) International License from Sithole, M. N., Kumar, P., Du Toit, L.C., Erlwanger, K.H., Ubanako, P.N., & Choonara, Y.E.: A 3D-Printed Biomaterial Scaffold Reinforced with Inorganic Fillers for Bone Tissue Engineering: In Vitro Assessment and In Vivo Animal Studies. Int. J. Mol. Sci. 2023. 24. 7611. Copyright 2023 Sithole et al., published by MDPI).

The spatial delivery of bioactive cues such as growth factors is possible by printing on ceramic matrices (Becker et al., 2012; Cornelsen et al., 2013), and magnetic particles are also sometimes used to bind growth factors that can effectively deliver growth factors in a spatially controlled manner using external magnetic stimulation (Lee et al., 2014). In addition to particles, fibers are highly useful for the spatially controlled release of growth factors. In comparison with microfibers without growth factor, bioprinted collagen microfibers incorporating BMP-2 effectively promoted bone MSC differentiation into osteocytes (Du et al., 2015).

Additionally, when aligned submicron fibers were functionalized with different printed growth factors, specific cell differentiation was seen in a spatially controlled way (Ker et al., 2011). Researchers studied the controlled release of bovine serum albumin (BSA) and VEGF by loading them into a bioink containing methyl cellulose and sodium alginate blended with laponite (a synthetic nanosilicate clay). The research group 3D printed the scaffold by extrusion (Ahlfeld et al., 2017). The findings we have discussed so far have shown that particles and fibers are highly effective for the delivery of growth factors, but bioprinting can influence the biological activity of loaded growth factors. For example, when bioceramic matrices with recombinant BMP-2 were printed using inkjet printing technology, the biological activity of the growth factor decreased by 10% compared with the nonprinted control solution (Vorndran et al., 2010).

Antibiotics and anti-inflammatory drugs are typical therapeutic strategies in regenerative medicine to reduce infections and inflammatory responses. Drugs can be released in a spatially controlled manner when they are included in scaffolds containing fibers or particles. Non-printed nanostructured materials were reviewed for tissue engineering and regenerative medicine purposes (Tang et al., 2016). Recently, drug-incorporated particles and fibers are being used as composite bioinks along with cells and biomaterials.

Antibiotic-loaded ceramic particles have been investigated for treating a number of infection-related bone diseases such as bone tuberculosis (Li et al., 2015c; Zhu et al., 2015) and osteomyelitis (Inzana et al., 2015). For instance, researchers coprinted rifampicin and isoniazid on mesoporous bioactive glass matrix which was used as a drug delivery system to treat osteoarticular tuberculosis. The method was highly appreciated due to its good osteogenic potential and spatial drug release in a defective bone model of a rabbit (Li et al., 2015c), and another composite scaffold containing mesoporous silica nanoparticles incorporated with two antibiotics, rifampicin and isoniazid, showed almost the same fruitful outcome (Zhu et al., 2015).

Antibiotics in the form of powder can be incorporated into calcium phosphate-containing bioceramic scaffolds before printing, but antibiotics in the form of solution can be included onto scaffolds by using another set of inkjets. These were coprinted with rifampicin and vancomycin to treat osteomyelitis after surgery (Inzana et al., 2015). In another study, drug release was delayed when microporous 3D-powder-printed bioceramic was loaded with tetracycline, ofloxacin and vancomycin. Additionally, when the drug was incorporated with a 50:50 mixture of polymer solutions containing polyglycolide and polylactide, it was released in a controlled manner (Gbureck et al., 2007). However, due to polymerization interference, this method was not effective for poly(methyl methacrylate) polymer, where coprinting was not possible with rifampicin or vancomycin (Inzana et al., 2015).

Furthermore, 3D-printed hydrogels were prepared with polyglycidol and HA incorporating mesoporous silica nanoparticles. Surface particle charges were one of the reasons for drug release inside the 3D-printed hydrogels (Baumann et al., 2017). Recently, both fibers and particles were included for the spatially controlled delivery of the drugs in the printed scaffolds (Trachtenberg et al., 2013). Compared with nanofibers, microfibers can release the drugs in a more sustainable way (Trachtenberg et al., 2013).

When stimulated by a laser, microcapsules implanted in the matrix of a hydrogel released bioactive cues from a shell of PLGA. Solid hydrophobic surfaces were used to print biomolecules, enzymes and dyes, and PLGA shells containing gold nanorods were printed on the hydrogel matrices and were used to release those biomolecules, dyes and enzymes (Gupta et al., 2015). When the laser was used, selective rupturing of the microcapsules took place because of the functionalization on the capsules. Therefore, there was a release of the bioactive cues in a spatial and temporal manner from the microcapsules (Gupta et al., 2015).

Bioprinting affects the biological activity of the drugs loaded in the scaffold similar to growth factors; the activity reduced by between 18% and 1% for vancomycin and heparin followed by spraying through the ink jet nozzles (Vorndran et al., 2010). When vancomycin was included into a cement, the biological activity reduced by around 11% (Vorndran et al., 2010). To avoid a detrimental influence on the postprinting drug delivery, printing parameters such as printing pressure, temperature and the time between two layers must be tailored for both bioinks and composite inks (Trachtenberg et al., 2013).

Liposomes are highly employed as drug delivery carriers due to their capacity to transport and protect a wide spectrum of compounds over time. They have been used as carriers for the spatially controlled delivery of bioactive cues such as drugs, genetic materials and growth factors into a scaffold, which helps in cell proliferation (Janeczek et al., 2017; Monteiro et al., 2014; Olekson et al., 2015). Furthermore, hydrogels loaded with liposomes (e.g. dextran, gelatin, chitosan) were developed (Grijalvo et al., 2016) to reduce the burst-release in the hydrogels. Their biocompatibility, as well as their rheological and physical features, have enhanced their therapeutic promise in the area of regenerative medicine (Zylberberg & Matosevic, 2017).

Additional research has been conducted on cyclodextrin drug delivery in regenerative medicine as well as in bioprinting. For example, g-cyclodextrins were immobilized onto a hydrogel that released osteogenic agents (such as dexamethasone) to human-adipose-derived stem cells and also enhanced bone growth (Lima et al., 2014). Furthermore, fibrous scaffolds containing gelatin and PLLA were designed. The osteogenic agent adamantylamine-loaded b-cyclodextrin was used to coat hydroxyapatite particles and simvastatin-loaded b-cyclodextrin onto this scaffold. This system enabled the sustained release of simvastatin by two to four times, increasing in vitro and in vivo bone regeneration (Lee et al., 2016). Cyclodextrins were tested for printability in other applications (Loebel et al., 2017).

In conclusion, prevalent pharmacological forms like microparticles and nanoparticles are known for the delivery of bioactive cues. When fibers are loaded with bioactive cues, it allows the combined delivery of bioactive cues with the suitable nanotopography for optimal cell adherence. Table 8.2 summarizes the applications of bioprinting to deliver bioactive cues in a spatially controlled manner for bone tissue engineering.

TABLE 8.2
Scaffolds for the Spatially Controlled Delivery of Bioactive Cues by 3D Bioprinting

Bioink Material	Animal Model	Bioactive Cues	Bioprinting Technique	Reference
Core-shell PLGA nanospheres	-	Growth factor TGF-β1	SLA & electrospraying	Trachtenberg et al. (2013)
Synthetic nanosilicate clays (Laponite) blended with an alginate and methylcellulose bioink	-	BSA and VEGF	Extrusion printing	Ahlfeld et al. (2017)
Collagen microfibers	-	Growth factor BMP-2	Extrusion printing	Du et al. (2015)
Gelatin microspheres	Mice	Growth factor BMP-2	Extrusion printing	Poldervaart et al. (2013)
Mesoporous bioactive glass and mesoporous silica nanoparticles	Rabbit	Isoniazid and rifampicin drug	Extrusion printing	Li et al. (2015c)
Mesoporous silica nanoparticles incorporated in a polyglycidol and HA hydrogel	-	Drug	Extrusion printing	Baumann et al. (2017)

Bioprinting is a popular technique in bone tissue engineering and bone regeneration. Various bioprinting technologies are available such as particle fusion, inkjet printing, extrusion and light-assisted methods. Bioink design needs to be optimized according to the printing method chosen (Guvendiren et al., 2016). These different technologies are discussed in the supplementary material.

8.6.3 Layer by Layer

Thin film coating layers are created layer by layer (LbL), a manufacturing method that functionalizes surfaces (Qian et al., 2018; Song et al., 2020). LbL assembly is a quick and efficient method for surface modification (Ma et al., 2021). The process, which primarily relies on electrostatic binding, entails the adsorption of electrolytes with opposing charges to a substrate to produce single layers one by one that can be progressively deposited to create multilayer films (Boudou et al., 2010). Apart from electrostatic attraction, van der Waals forces, covalent bonding, hydrophobic interaction, biological recognition or combinations of these forces can also form multilayer films (Tang et al., 2006).

LbL surface functionalization made it possible to create efficient systems for drug delivery with better outcomes. Films made by LbL can provide spatially controlled delivery of the bioactive cues to the tissue (Alkekhia et al., 2020; Boudou et al., 2010; Park et al., 2018). The amount of the growth factors administered to the healing areas is optimized for effectiveness with minimal undesirable adverse effects such as cancer and osteolysis (connected to BMP dosages that are slightly higher than the normal physiological condition) (Guillot et al., 2013; Shah et al., 2011). Growth factors can be incorporated into crosslinked films following LbL assembly that act as protein reservoirs, or inside a multilayer film, they can be included in the multiple layers that are created via electrostatic LbL (Cheng et al., 2019; Collins et al., 2021).

In one study, LbL was used to assemble two polyelectrolytes, Poly-β-aminoester 2, PAA and chondroitin sulfate (CS) that were used as vehicles for the growth factor delivery in a controlled manner (Shah et al., 2011). The authors incorporated two growth factors, namely, osteogenic BMP-2 and angiogenic VEGF. They prepared two tetralayer films by LbL assembly, incorporating one growth factor each to make poly-β-aminoester 2-PAA/BMP-2/PAA and poly-β-aminoester 2-CS/VEGF/CS. Then, the LBL-assembled tetralayer films were deposited onto 3D scaffolds which were osteoconductive, made of macroporous PCL/β-TCP to form $[\text{Poly2/PAA/rhBMP-2/PAA}]_x$ $[\text{Poly2/CS/rhVEGF/CS}]_y$.

By increasing the pH from 5.0 to 7.4, the two growth factors were delivered because of lack of stability and imbalance of charge in the coating. Within two weeks, BMP-2 was released from the coating, but within the first eight days, VEGF was released. Inside the intramuscular region of a rat femur, both growth factors produced ectopic bone development and both the growth factors maintained their potency (Shah et al., 2011). The deposition of LbL-assembled films containing BMP onto a substrate permits for a spatially controlled delivery (Guillot et al., 2013) and can effectively overcome the primary drawback of the present therapeutic delivery strategy for BMP-2 using collagen sponge: fast release without spatial control (Collins et al., 2021; Crouzier et al., 2011).

The LbL approach is very advantageous for deposition of antibiotic coatings onto orthopaedic implants. It can lower the rate of infections caused by implants and can accelerate osteogenesis (Chae et al., 2020; Goodman et al., 2013). Authors applied LbL to coat titanium implants to prevent implant-related infectious disease and also the interactions between bone and cells are increased at the surface of the implant.

In a different study, HA–dopamine/CH multilayered systems were deposited onto titanium alloy (Ti, Nb, Zr) implant surfaces, and the anti-infection properties improved. Differentiation and adhesion of the osteoblast cells were also accelerated compared with titanium implants without any LbL-assembled coating (Zhang et al., 2013). In short, LbL can be useful in maintaining anti-infection, antioxidant and osteogenic potency (Choi et al., 2021).

Researchers have used LbL to assemble multilayered films comprising poly-β-amino ester, PEI and gentamicin sulfate; the films were deposited as a coating on titanium implants to treat an infection in a rabbit bone model (Moskowitz et al., 2010). Within the first three days, 70% of the gentamicin was released from the coating in vitro in an aqueous environment. The release of gentamicin was carried forward through a diffusion mechanism. The drug release was continued for the next four weeks, but the degradation products are nontoxic towards preosteoblast cells MC3T3-E1. For in vivo, when the coated 3D titanium implants were compared with the uncoated titanium implant, it was observed that viable bacteria count was significantly decreased in coated titanium implants. These titanium implants were used to treat staphylococcus aureus infection in a rabbit bone model (Moskowitz et al., 2010).

Growth factors and cell adhesion peptides were also delivered via the LbL method (Wang et al., 2016). Positively charged chitosan (CH) was deposited with negatively charged oxidized alginate (OAlg), and BMP-2 was incorporated into BSA-based nanoparticles to form positively charged BSA–BMP-2 nanoparticles. Those nanoparticles were assembled by LbL together with peptide layers, which were negatively charged.

Further, the cell proliferation and adhesion behaviour of glycine-arginine-glycine-aspartate-serine (GRGDS) peptide grafted on OAlg/CH films were studied (Wang et al., 2016). Deposition of BMP-2 and GRGD onto porous titanium scaffolds helped in bone tissue growth. Sustained release of BMP-2 was observed from the coatings for 28 days. This long release span was caused because BSA obstructed the diffusion of BMPs. These two bioactive cues, GRGDS and BMP, improved MSC adhesion, differentiation and proliferation, and helped in bone tissue generation (Wang et al., 2016).

In another study, a nanoscale barrier was formed by the deposition of exponentially growing polycationic poly L-lysine (PLL)/HA and linearly growing poly(diallyldimethylammonium chloride)/poly(styrene sulfonate). These barriers were basically nano-valves that were mechanically active; the nanopores present in the film opened up by a mechanical stimulus, and PLL diffusion took place through the barrier. This phenomenon of closing and opening of the pores depends on the magnitude of the mechanical deformation (Mertz et al., 2007).

Salt concentration and pH can also affect the drug release behaviour. For example, methylene blue dye was incorporated into the poly(acrylic acid)/poly(allylamine hydrochloride) (PAA/PAH) bilayer assembly at pH of 2.5. At low pH 2.5, there were disruptions between the dye and PAA interactions enabling the release of the dye (Chung & Rubner, 2002).

Additionally, a system for the delivery of two growth factors was fabricated using electrospinning and LbL assembly together. A nanofibrous film of silk fibroin (SF), PCL and polyvinyl alcohol (PVA) core shell was prepared. The nanofibers were loaded with BMP-2, and connective tissue growth factor (CTGF) was incorporated into the LbL-assembled film surface. This resulted in effective delivery of CTGF and BMP-2. Angiogenesis and osteogenesis was also enhanced, which is confirmed by both in vitro and in vivo studies (Cheng et al., 2019). Additionally, researchers demonstrated that LbL-assembled film made from glycosaminoglycan HA and PLL showed similar interactions to those found between the ECM and the cells. This significantly improved the cell's affinity from various lineages (Domínguez-Arca et al., 2021). In short, integrating osteogenic

TABLE 8.3
Scaffolds for Spatially Controlled Delivery of Bioactive Cues by LbL

LBL Assembly Material	Animal Model	Bioactive Cues	Reference
poly(β-amino ester)/polyanion/ growth factor/polyanion	Rat	Growth factors rhBMP and rhVEGF	Shah et al. (2011)
Poly-β-amino ester/PEI/ gentamicin sulfate	Rabbit	Drug gentamycin	Moskowitz et al. (2010)
CH/OAlg/BSA-BMP-2/OAlg HA/dopamine/CH	-	Growth factor BMP-2	Zhang et al. (2013)
SF/PCL/PVA nanofibrous film	Mice	BMP-2/CTGF	Cheng et al. (2019)
PAA/PAH bilayer		Methylene blue dye	Chung & Rubner (2002)

growth factors and functional exosomes into LBL-assembled films, is a viable strategy to imitate the structure of the host, enhance biological capabilities and improve the distribution of growth factors (Zha et al., 2021). Table 8.3 summarized the applications of LbL assembly to deliver bioactive cues in a spatially controlled manner for bone tissue engineering.

SUMMARY AND FUTURE DIRECTIONS

The spatially controlled delivery of bioactive cues plays a vital role in bone tissue engineering. Biomaterials are combined to control the release profiles of the bioactive cues over spatiotemporal delivery. This field needs a more progressive understanding of the signalling process of native bioactive molecules during bone regeneration and healing. Spatially controlled delivery requires the determining bioactive cue concentrations and their temporal and spatial distributions, taking into consideration the local interaction with target cells and microvascular and interstitial flow.

To provide the spatiotemporally controlled release of the bioactive cues and accelerate bone regeneration, different types of delivery systems along with various delivery techniques have been developed from nano to macro scale. Integrating delivery systems with biomaterials is leading to advanced bone tissue engineering applications. The clinical necessity of developing delivery systems with spatially controlled distribution of growth factors is due to adverse effects associated with direct applications of growth factors. Encapsulation of bioactive cues in scaffolds can be useful for controlling their release kinetics.

The spatial presentation of bioactive cues has been extensively investigated to understand the in vitro cell responses, but it will be a challenge to maintain these presentations in the complex biological environments of real bone fractures. Protein adsorption and local cell responses influence the spatially controlled release of bioactive cues from scaffolds. As the effects of spatial presentation differ significantly between in vitro and in vivo studies, it is very important to investigate in vivo effects of spatial presentation of bioactive cues.

As technologies proceed towards clinical translation, a balance needs to be established between the spatially controlled delivery of bioactive cues and fabrication complexity. Complex fabrication processes with multicomponent systems can increase the costs of therapy. Animal studies and finally clinical trials will be a crucial step that will demonstrate therapeutic value for repairing bone defects. Technology for spatially controlled bioactive cues has progressed rapidly, and further advancements in this field are anticipated to have substantial impacts on the clinical success of bone tissue engineering applications in the future.

ACKNOWLEDGMENTS

The authors are thankful to the Indian Institute of Technology Roorkee for providing its infrastructure and facilities. We would like to express gratitude to support for all the personnel from Department of Metallurgical and Materials Engineering and Centre for Nanotechnology.

LIST OF ABBREVIATIONS

BMPs	Bone morphogenetic proteins
BSA	Bovine serum albumin
CaP	Calcium phosphate
CTGF	Connective tissue growth factor
ECM	Extracellular matrix
FGF	Fibroblast growth factor
GRGDS	Glycine-arginine-glycine-aspartate-serine
IFN-γ	Interferon gamma
IL-4	Interleukin 4

LBL	Layer-by-layer
MSCs	Mesenchymal stem cells
OAlg	Oxidized alginate
PA	Peptide amphiphiles
PAA	Polyacrylic acid
PCL	Polycaprolactone
PDGF	Platelet-derived growth factor
PEG	Poly (ethylene glycol)
PEI	Polyethyleneimine
PGA	Polyglycolic acid
PLA	Poly (L-lactic acid)
PLGA	Poly (lactic-co-glycolic acid)
PLL	Poly-L-lysine
PVA	Polyvinyl alcohol
SF	Silk fibroin
SLA	Stereolithography
TCP	Tricalcium phosphate
TGF-β	Transforming growth factor beta
VEGF	Vascular endothelial growth factor

REFERENCES

Adams, C. S., Antoci Jr, V., Harrison, G., Patal, P., Freeman, T. A., Shapiro, I. M., Parvizi, J., Hickok, N. J., Radin, S., & Ducheyne, P. (2009). Controlled release of vancomycin from thin sol-gel films on implant surfaces successfully controls osteomyelitis. *J. Orthop. Res.* 27: 701–709.

Ahlfeld, T., Cidonio, G., Kilian, D., Duin, S., Akkineni, A. R., Dawson, J. I., Yang, S., Lode, A., Oreffo, R. O. C., & Gelinsky, M. (2017). Development of a clay based bioink for 3D cell printing for skeletal application. *Biofabrication.* 9: 34103.

Alkekhia, D., Hammond, P. T., & Shukla, A. (2020). Layer-by-layer biomaterials for drug delivery. *Annu. Rev. Biomed. Eng.* 22: 1–24.

Amjadian, S., Seyedjafari, E., Zeynali, B., & Shabani, I. (2016). The synergistic effect of nano-hydroxyapatite and dexamethasone in the fibrous delivery system of gelatin and poly (l-lactide) on the osteogenesis of mesenchymal stem cells. *Int. J. Pharm.* 507: 1–11.

Baumann, B., Jungst, T., Stichler, S., Feineis, S., Wiltschka, O., Kuhlmann, M., Lindén, M., & Groll, J. (2017). Control of nanoparticle release kinetics from 3D printed hydrogel scaffolds. *Angew. Chem. Int. Ed. Engl.* 56: 4623–4628.

Becker, S. T., Bolte, H., Schünemann, K., Seitz, H., Bara, J. J., Beck-Broichsitter, B. E., Russo, P. A. J., Wiltfang, J., & Warnke, P. H. (2012). Endocultivation: The influence of delayed vs. simultaneous application of BMP-2 onto individually formed hydroxyapatite matrices for heterotopic bone induction. *Int. J. Oral Maxillofac Surg.* 41: 1153–1160.

Bittner, S. M., Guo, J. L., & Mikos, A. G. (2018). Spatiotemporal control of growth factors in three-dimensional printed scaffolds. *Bioprinting.* 12: e00032.

Boudou, T., Crouzier, T., Ren, K., Blin, G., & Picart, C. (2010). Multiple functionalities of polyelectrolyte multilayer films: New biomedical applications. *Adv. Mater.* 22: 441–467.

Cai, Y., Yu, J., Kundu, S. C., & Yao, J. (2016). Multifunctional nano-hydroxyapatite and alginate/gelatin based sticky gel composites for potential bone regeneration. *Mater. Chem. Phys.* 181: 227–233.

Castro, N. J., O'Brien, C. M., & Zhang, L. G. (2014). Biomimetic biphasic 3-D nanocomposite scaffold for osteochondral regeneration. *AIChE J.* 60: 432–442.

Chae, K., Jang, W. Y., Park, K., Lee, J., Kim, H., Lee, K., Lee, C. K., Lee, Y., Lee, S. H., & Seo, J. (2020). Antibacterial infection and immune-evasive coating for orthopedic implants. *Sci. Adv.* 6: eabb0025.

Chang, P. C., Seol, Y. J., Cirelli, J. A., Pellegrini, G., Jin, Q., Franco, L. M., Goldstein, S. A., Chandler, L. A., Sosnowski, B., & Giannobile, W. V. (2010). PDGF-B gene therapy accelerates bone engineering and oral implant osseointegration. *Gene Ther.* 17: 95–104.

Chen, X., Tan, B., Bao, Z., Wang, S., Tang, R., Wang, Z., Chen, G., Chen, S., Lu, W. W., Yang, D., & Peng, S. (2021). Enhanced bone regeneration via spatiotemporal and controlled delivery of a genetically engineered BMP-2 in a composite Hydrogel. *Biomaterials*. 277: 121117.

Chen, X., Wang, W., Cheng, S., Dong, B., & Li, C. Y. (2013). Mimicking bone nanostructure by combining block copolymer self-assembly and 1D crystal nucleation. *ACS Nano*. 7: 8251–8257.

Cheng, G., Yin, C., Tu, H., Jiang, S., Wang, Q., Zhou, X., Xing, X., Xie, C., Shi, X., & Du, Y. (2019). Controlled co-delivery of growth factors through layer-by-layer assembly of core—Shell nanofibers for improving bone regeneration. *ACS Nano*. 13: 6372–6382.

Choi, S., Jo, H. S., Song, H., Kim, H. J., Oh, J. K., Cho, J. W., Park, K., & Kim, S. E. (2021). Multifunctional tannic acid-alendronate nanocomplexes with antioxidant, anti-inflammatory, and osteogenic potency. *Nanomaterials*. 11: 1812.

Chung, A. J., & Rubner, M. F. (2002). Methods of loading and releasing low molecular weight cationic molecules in weak polyelectrolyte multilayer films. *Langmuir*. 18: 1176–1183.

Chung, B. G., Kang, L., & Khademhosseini, A. (2007). Micro-and nanoscale technologies for tissue engineering and drug discovery applications. *Expert Opin. Drug Discov*. 2: 1653–1668.

Collins, M. N., Ren, G., Young, K., Pina, S., Reis, R. L., & Oliveira, J. M. (2021). Scaffold fabrication technologies and structure/function properties in bone tissue engineering. *Adv. Funct. Mater*. 31: 2010609.

Cornelsen, M., Petersen, S., Dietsch, K., Rudolph, A., Schmitz, K., Sternberg, K., & Seitz, H. (2013). Infiltration of 3D printed tricalciumphosphate scaffolds with biodegradable polymers and biomolecules for local drug delivery. *BME—BMT*. 58: 000010151520134090.

Corradetti, B., Taraballi, F., Powell, S., Sung, D., Minardi, S., Ferrari, M., Weiner, B. K., & Tasciotti, E. (2015). Osteoprogenitor cells from bone marrow and cortical bone: Understanding how the environment affects their fate. *Stem Cells Dev*. 24: 1112–1123.

Cross, M., & Dexter, T. M. (1991). Growth factors in development, transformation, and tumorigenesis. *Cell*. 64: 271–280.

Crouzier, T., Sailhan, F., Becquart, P., Guillot, R., Logeart-Avramoglou, D., & Picart, C. (2011). The performance of BMP-2 loaded TCP/HAP porous ceramics with a polyelectrolyte multilayer film coating. *Biomaterials*. 32: 7543–7554.

Dahabreh, Z., Calori, G. M., Kanakaris, N. K., Nikolaou, V. S., & Giannoudis, P. V. (2009). A cost analysis of treatment of tibial fracture nonunion by bone grafting or bone morphogenetic protein-7. *Int. Orthop*. 33: 1407–1414.

Dalton, P. D., Derby, B., Forgacs, G., & Li, Q. (2016). Biofabrication: Reappraising the definition of an evolving field. *Biofabrication*. 8: 013001.

D'Andrea, L. D., Iaccarino, G., Fattorusso, R., Sorriento, D., Carannante, C., Capasso, D., Trimarco, B., & Pedone, C. (2005). Targeting angiogenesis: Structural characterization and biological properties of a de novo engineered VEGF mimicking peptide. *Proc. Natl. Acad. Sci*. 102: 14215–14220.

Dang, M., Saunders, L., Niu, X., Fan, Y., & Ma, P. X. (2018). Biomimetic delivery of signals for bone tissue engineering. *Bone Res*. 6: 1–12.

David Roodman, G. (2003). Role of stromal-derived cytokines and growth factors in bone metastasis. *Cancer*. 97: 733–738.

De la Riva, B., Sánchez, E., Hernández, A., Reyes, R., Tamimi, F., López-Cabarcos, E., Delgado, A., & Évora, C. (2010). Local controlled release of VEGF and PDGF from a combined brushite—Chitosan system enhances bone regeneration. *J. Control. Release*. 14: 45–52.

De Witte, T. M., Fratila-Apachitei, L. E., Zadpoor, A. A., & Peppas, N. A. (2018). Bone tissue engineering via growth factor delivery: From scaffolds to complex matrices. *Regen. Biomater*. 5: 197–211.

Dimitriou, R., Tsiridis, E., & Giannoudis, P. V. (2005). Current concepts of molecular aspects of bone healing. *Injury*. 36: 1392–1404.

Ding, Z., Fan, Z., Huang, X., Lu, Q., Xu, W., & Kaplan, D. L. (2016). Silk—Hydroxyapatite nanoscale scaffolds with programmable growth factor delivery for bone repair. *ACS Appl. Mater. Interfaces*. 8: 24463–24470.

Domínguez-Arca, V., Costa, R. R., Carvalho, A. M., Taboada, P., Reis, R. L., Prieto, G., & Pashkuleva, I. (2021). Liposomes embedded in layer by layer constructs as simplistic extracellular vesicles transfer model. *Mater. Sci. Eng. C*. 121: 111813.

Du, M., Chen, B., Meng, Q., Liu, S., Zheng, X., Zhang, C., Wang, H., Li, H., Wang, N., & Dai, J. (2015). 3D bioprinting of BMSC-laden methacrylamide gelatin scaffolds with CBD-BMP2-collagen microfibers. *Biofabrication*. 7: 44104.

Eivazzadeh-Keihan, R., Chenab, K. K., Taheri-Ledari, R., Mosafer, J., Hashemi, S. M., Mokhtarzadeh, A., Maleki, A., & Hamblin, M. R. (2020). Recent advances in the application of mesoporous silica-based nanomaterials for bone tissue engineering. *Mater. Sci. Eng. C*. 107: 110267.

El Bialy, I., Jiskoot, W., & Reza Nejadnik, M. (2017). Formulation, delivery and stability of bone morphogenetic proteins for effective bone regeneration. *Pharm. Res.* 34: 1152–1170.

Evans, C. H., Ghivizzani, S. C., & Robbins, P. D. (2012). Orthopedic gene therapy—Lost in translation? *J. Cell. Physiol.* 227: 416–420.

Farokhi, M., Mottaghitalab, F., Samani, S., Shokrgozar, M. A., Kundu, S. C., Reis, R. L., Fatahi, Y., & Kaplan, D. L. (2018). Silk fibroin/hydroxyapatite composites for bone tissue engineering. *Biotechnol. Adv.* 36: 68–91.

Farokhi, M., Mottaghitalab, F., Shokrgozar, M. A., Ai, J., Hadjati, J., & Azami, M. (2014). Bio-hybrid silk fibroin/calcium phosphate/PLGA nanocomposite scaffold to control the delivery of vascular endothelial growth factor. *Mater. Sci. Eng. C*. 35: 401–410.

Feng, K., Sun, H., Bradley, M. A., Dupler, E. J., Giannobile, W. V., & Ma, P. X. (2010). Novel antibacterial nanofibrous PLLA scaffolds. *J. Control. Release*. 146: 363–369.

Franceschi, R. T. (2005). Biological approaches to bone regeneration by gene therapy. *J. Dent. Res.* 84: 1093–1103.

Freeman, F. E., Pitacco, P., van Dommelen, L. H. A., Nulty, J., Browe, D. C., Shin, J. Y., Alsberg, E., & Kelly, D. J. (2020). 3D bioprinting spatiotemporally defined patterns of growth factors to tightly control tissue regeneration. *Sci. Adv.* 6: eabb5093.

Friedlaender, G. E., Perry, C. R., Cole, J. D., Cook, S. D., Cierny, G., Muschler, G. F., Zych, G. A., Calhoun, J. H., LaForte, A. J., & Yin, S. (2001). Osteogenic protein-1 (bone morphogenetic protein-7) in the treatment of tibial nonunions: A prospective, randomized clinical trial comparing rhOP-1 with fresh bone autograft. *J Bone Joint Surg. Am.* 83: S151.

Gan, Q., Zhu, J., Yuan, Y., Liu, H., Qian, J., Li, Y., & Liu, C. (2015). A dual-delivery system of pH-responsive chitosan-functionalized mesoporous silica nanoparticles bearing BMP-2 and dexamethasone for enhanced bone regeneration. *J Mater. Chem. B*. 3: 2056–2066.

Gbureck, U., Vorndran, E., Müller, F. A., & Barralet, J. E. (2007). Low temperature direct 3D printed bioceramics and biocomposites as drug release matrices. *J. Control. Release*. 122: 173–180.

Geuze, R. E., Theyse, L. F. H., Kempen, D. H. R., Hazewinkel, H. A. W., Kraak, H. Y. A., Öner, F. C., Dhert, W. J. A., & Alblas, J. (2012). A differential effect of bone morphogenetic protein-2 and vascular endothelial growth factor release timing on osteogenesis at ectopic and orthotopic sites in a large-animal model. *Tissue Eng. Part A*. 18: 2052–2062.

Ghadakzadeh, S., Mekhail, M., Aoude, A., Hamdy, R., & Tabrizian, M. (2016). Small players ruling the hard game: SiRNA in bone regeneration. *J. Bone Miner. Res.* 31: 475–487.

Gibbs, D. M. R., Black, C. R. M., Dawson, J. I., & Oreffo, R. O. C. (2016). A review of hydrogel use in fracture healing and bone regeneration. *J. Tissue Eng. Regen. Med.* 10: 187–198.

Glass, G. E., Chan, J. K., Freidin, A., Feldmann, M., Horwood, N. J., & Nanchahal, J. (2011). TNF-α promotes fracture repair by augmenting the recruitment and differentiation of muscle-derived stromal cells. *Proc. Natl. Acad. Sci.* 108: 1585–1590.

Gonzalez-Fernandez, T., Rathan, S., Hobbs, C., Pitacco, P., Freeman, F. E., Cunniffe, G. M., Dunne, N. J., McCarthy, H. O., Nicolosi, V., & O'Brien, F. J. (2019). Pore-forming bioinks to enable spatio-temporally defined gene delivery in bioprinted tissues. *J. Control. Release*. 301: 13–27.

Gonzalez-Fernandez, T., Tierney, E. G., Cunniffe, G. M., O'Brien, F. J., & Kelly, D. J. (2016). Gene delivery of TGF-β3 and BMP2 in an MSC-laden alginate hydrogel for articular cartilage and endochondral bone tissue engineering. *Tissue Eng. Part A*. 22: 776–787.

Goodman, S. B., Yao, Z., Keeney, M., & Yang, F. (2013). The future of biologic coatings for orthopaedic implants. *Biomaterials*. 34: 3174–3183.

Grijalvo, S., Mayr, J., Eritja, R., & Díaz, D. D. (2016). Biodegradable liposome-encapsulated hydrogels for biomedical applications: A marriage of convenience. *Biomater. Sci.* 4: 555–574.

Guihard, P., Boutet, M. A., Brounais-Le Royer, B., Gamblin, A. L., Amiaud, J., Renaud, A., Berreur, M., Rédini, F., Heymann, D., & Layrolle, P. (2015). Oncostatin m, an inflammatory cytokine produced by macrophages, supports intramembranous bone healing in a mouse model of tibia injury. *Am. J. Pathol.* 185: 765–775.

Guillot, R., Gilde, F., Becquart, P., Sailhan, F., Lapeyrere, A., Logeart-Avramoglou, D., & Picart, C. (2013). The stability of BMP loaded polyelectrolyte multilayer coatings on titanium. *Biomaterials*. 34: 5737–5746.

Guler, H. P., Zapf, J., & Froesch, E. R. (1987). Short-term metabolic effects of recombinant human insulin-like growth factor I in healthy adults. *N. Engl. J. Med.* 317: 137–140.

Guo, P., Coban, O., Snead, N. M., Trebley, J., Hoeprich, S., Guo, S., & Shu, Y. (2010). Engineering RNA for targeted siRNA delivery and medical application. *Adv. Drug Deliv. Rev.* 62: 650–666.

Gupta, M. K., Meng, F., Johnson, B. N., Kong, Y. L., Tian, L., Yeh, Y. W., Masters, N., Singamaneni, S., & McAlpine, M. C. (2015). 3D printed programmable release capsules. *Nano Lett.* 15: 5321–5329.

Guvendiren, M., Molde, J., Soares, R. M. D., & Kohn, J. (2016). Designing biomaterials for 3D printing. *ACS Biomater. Sci. Eng.* 2: 1679–1693.

Habraken, W., Wolke, J. G. C., & Jansen, J. A. (2007). Ceramic composites as matrices and scaffolds for drug delivery in tissue engineering. *Adv. Drug Deliv. Rev.* 59: 234–248.

He, C., Xiao, G., Jin, X., Sun, C., & Ma, P. X. (2010). Electrodeposition on nanofibrous polymer scaffolds: Rapid mineralization, tunable calcium phosphate composition and topography. *Adv. Funct. Mater.* 20: 3568–3576.

He, S., Fang, J., Zhong, C., Wang, M., & Ren, F. (2022). Spatiotemporal delivery of pBMP2 and pVEGF by a core—Sheath structured fiber-hydrogel gene-activated matrix loaded with peptide-modified nanoparticles for critical-sized bone defect repair. *Adv. Healthc. Mater.* 11: 2201096.

He, W., Reaume, M., Hennenfent, M., Lee, B. P., & Rajachar, R. (2020). Biomimetic hydrogels with spatial-and temporal-controlled chemical cues for tissue engineering. *Biomater. Sci.* 8: 3248–3269.

Hettiaratchi, M. H., Krishnan, L., Rouse, T., Chou, C., McDevitt, T. C., & Guldberg, R. E. (2020). Heparin-mediated delivery of bone morphogenetic protein-2 improves spatial localization of bone regeneration. *Sci. Adv.* 6: eaay1240.

Hoare, T. R., & Kohane, D. S. (2008). Hydrogels in drug delivery: Progress and challenges. *Polymer.* 49: 1993–2007.

Hoffman, A. S. (2012). Hydrogels for biomedical applications. *Adv. Drug Deliv. Rev.* 64: 18–23.

Hu, Y., Cai, K., Luo, Z., Xu, D., Xie, D., Huang, Y., Yang, W., & Liu, P. (2012). TiO2 nanotubes as drug nanoreservoirs for the regulation of mobility and differentiation of mesenchymal stem cells. *Acta Biomater.* 8: 439–448.

Inzana, J. A., Olvera, D., Fuller, S. M., Kelly, J. P., Graeve, O. A., Schwarz, E. M., Kates, S. L., & Awad, H. A. (2014). 3D printing of composite calcium phosphate and collagen scaffolds for bone regeneration. *Biomaterials.* 35: 4026–4034.

Inzana, J. A., Trombetta, R. P., Schwarz, E. M., Kates, S. L., & Awad, H. A. (2015). 3D printed bioceramics for dual antibiotic delivery to treat implant-associated bone infection. *Eur. Cells Mater.* 30: 232.

Jacob, J., Haponiuk, J. T., Thomas, S., & Gopi, S. (2018). Biopolymer based nanomaterials in drug delivery systems: A review. *Mater. Today Chem.* 9: 43–55.

Janeczek, A. A., Scarpa, E., Horrocks, M. H., Tare, R. S., Rowland, C. A., Jenner, D., Newman, T. A., Oreffo, R. O. C., Lee, S. F., & Evans, N. D. (2017). PEGylated liposomes associate with Wnt3A protein and expand putative stem cells in human bone marrow populations. *Nanomedicine.* 12: 845–863.

Jantz, L. M. (1999). The Cambridge encyclopedia of human growth and development. *Am. J. Phys. Anthropol.* 110: 473–474.

Jeon, O., Song, S. J., Yang, H. S., Bhang, S. H., Kang, S. W., Sung, M. A., Lee, J. H., & Kim, B. S. (2008). Long-term delivery enhances in vivo osteogenic efficacy of bone morphogenetic protein-2 compared to short-term delivery. *Biochem. Biophys. Res. Commun.* 369: 774–780.

Kanakaris, N. K., Lasanianos, N., Calori, G. M., Verdonk, R., Blokhuis, T. J., Cherubino, P., De Biase, P., & Giannoudis, P. V. (2009). Application of bone morphogenetic proteins to femoral non-unions: A 4-year multicentre experience. *Injury.* 40: S54–S61.

Kang, M. S., Kim, J. H., Singh, R. K., Jang, J. H., & Kim, H. W. (2015). Therapeutic-designed electrospun bone scaffolds: Mesoporous bioactive nanocarriers in hollow fiber composites to sequentially deliver dual growth factors. *Acta Biomatr.* 16: 103–116.

Kempen, D. H. R., Lu, L., Heijink, A., Hefferan, T. E., Creemers, L. B., Maran, A., Yaszemski, M. J., & Dhert, W. J. A. (2009). Effect of local sequential VEGF and BMP-2 delivery on ectopic and orthotopic bone regeneration. *Biomaterials.* 30: 2816–2825.

Ker, E. D. F., Chu, B., Phillippi, J. A., Gharaibeh, B., Huard, J., Weiss, L. E., & Campbell, P. G. (2011). Engineering spatial control of multiple differentiation fates within a stem cell population. *Biomaterials.* 32: 3413–3422.

Kim, B. S., Yang, S. S., & Kim, C. S. (2018). Incorporation of BMP-2 nanoparticles on the surface of a 3D-printed hydroxyapatite scaffold using an ε-polycaprolactone polymer emulsion coating method for bone tissue engineering. *Colloids Surf. B.* 170: 421–429.

Kim, H. D., Amirthalingam, S., Kim, S. L., Lee, S. S., Rangasamy, J., & Hwang, N. S. (2017). Biomimetic materials and fabrication approaches for bone tissue engineering. *Adv. Healthc. Mater.* 6: 1700612.

Krebs, M. D., & Alsberg, E. (2011). Localized, targeted, and sustained siRNA delivery. *Chem. Eur. J.* 17: 3054–3062.

Kwon, D. H., Lee, S. J., Wikesjö, U. M. E., Johansson, P. H., Johansson, C. B., & Sul, Y. (2017). Bone tissue response following local drug delivery of bisphosphonate through titanium oxide nanotube implants in a rabbit model. *J. Clin. Periodontol.* 44: 941–949.

Lee, E. A., Yim, H., Heo, J., Kim, H., Jung, G., & Hwang, N. S. (2014). Application of magnetic nanoparticle for controlled tissue assembly and tissue engineering. *Arch. Pharm. Res.* 37: 120–128.

Lee, J. B., Kim, J. E., Balikov, D. A., Bae, M. S., Heo, D. N., Lee, D., Rim, H. J., Lee, D., Sung, H., & Kwon, I. K. (2016). Poly (l-lactic acid)/gelatin fibrous scaffold loaded with simvastatin/beta-cyclodextrin-modified hydroxyapatite inclusion complex for bone tissue regeneration. *Macromol. Biosci.* 16: 1027–1038.

Lee, J. S., Lee, J. S., & Murphy, W. L. (2010). Modular peptides promote human mesenchymal stem cell differentiation on biomaterial surfaces. *Acta Biomatr.* 6: 21–28.

Lee, S. S., Fyrner, T., Chen, F., Álvarez, Z., Sleep, E., Chun, D. S., Weiner, J. A., Cook, R. W., Freshman, R. D., & Schallmo, M. S. (2017). Sulfated glycopeptide nanostructures for multipotent protein activation. *Nat. Nanotechnol.* 12: 821–829.

Lee, S. S., Hsu, E. L., Mendoza, M., Ghodasra, J., Nickoli, M. S., Ashtekar, A., Polavarapu, M., Babu, J., Riaz, R. M., & Nicolas, J. D. (2015). Gel scaffolds of BMP-2-binding peptide amphiphile nanofibers for spinal arthrodesis. *Adv. Healthc. Mater.* 4: 131–141.

Lee, S. S., Huang, B. J., Kaltz, S. R., Sur, S., Newcomb, C. J., Stock, S. R., Shah, R. N., & Stupp, S. I. (2013). Bone regeneration with low dose BMP-2 amplified by biomimetic supramolecular nanofibers within collagen scaffolds. *Biomaterials.* 34: 452–459.

Li, C., Armstrong, J. P., Pence, I. J., Kit-Anan, W., Puetzer, J. L., Carreira, S. C., Moore, A. C., & Stevens, M. M. (2018). Glycosylated superparamagnetic nanoparticle gradients for osteochondral tissue engineering. *Biomaterials.* 176: 24–33.

Li, C., Ouyang, L., Armstrong, J. P., & Stevens, M. M. (2021b). Advances in the fabrication of biomaterials for gradient tissue engineering. *Trends Biotechnol.* 39: 150–164.

Li, K., Zhu, M., Xu, P., Xi, Y., Cheng, Z., Zhu, Y., & Ye, X. (2015c). Three-dimensionally plotted MBG/PHBHHx composite scaffold for antitubercular drug delivery and tissue regeneration. *J. Mater. Sci. Mater. Med.* 26: 1–8.

Li, L., Zuo, Y., Zou, Q., Yang, B., Lin, L., Li, J., & Li, Y. (2015b). Hierarchical structure and mechanical improvement of an n-HA/GCO—PU composite scaffold for bone regeneration. *ACS Appl. Mater. Interfaces.* 7: 22618–22629.

Li, L., Zhou, G., Wang, Y., Yang, G., Ding, S., & Zhou, S. (2015a). Controlled dual delivery of BMP-2 and dexamethasone by nanoparticle-embedded electrospun nanofibers for the efficient repair of critical-sized rat calvarial defect. *Biomaterials.* 37: 218–229.

Li, Y., Liu, Y., Li, R., Bai, H., Zhu, Z., Zhu, L., Zhu, C., Che, Z., Liu, H., Wang, J., & Huang, L. (2021a). Collagen-based biomaterials for bone tissue engineering. *Mater. Des.* 210: 110049.

Liang, P., Zheng, J., Zhang, Z., Hou, Y., Wang, J., Zhang, C., & Quan, C. (2019). Bioactive 3D scaffolds self-assembled from phosphorylated mimicking peptide amphiphiles to enhance osteogenesis. *J. Biomater. Sci. Polym. Ed.* 30: 34–48.

Liang, Y., & Kiick, K. L. (2014). Heparin-functionalized polymeric biomaterials in tissue engineering and drug delivery applications. *Acta Biomatr.* 10: 1588–1600.

Lima, A. C., Puga, A. M., Mano, J. F., Concheiro, A., & Alvarez-Lorenzo, C. (2014). Free and copolymerized γ-cyclodextrins regulate the performance of dexamethasone-loaded dextran microspheres for bone regeneration. *J. Mater. Chem. B.* 2: 4943–4956.

Lin, X., Elliot, J. J., Carnes, D. L., Fox, W. C., Pena, L. A., Campion, S. L., Takahashi, K., Atkinson, B. L., & Zamora, P. O. (2007). Augmentation of osseous phenotypes in vivo with a synthetic peptide. *J. Orthop. Res.* 25: 531–539.

Lin, X., Takahashi, K., Campion, S. L., Liu, Y., Gustavsen, G. G., Pena, L. A., & Zamora, P. O. (2006). Synthetic peptide F2A4-K-NS mimics fibroblast growth factor-2 in vitro and is angiogenic in vivo. *Int. J. Mol. Med.* 17: 833–839.

Lin, Y. H., Chiu, Y. C., Shen, Y. F., Wu, Y. H. A., & Shie, M. Y. (2018). Bioactive calcium silicate/poly-ε-caprolactone composite scaffolds 3D printed under mild conditions for bone tissue engineering. *J. Mater. Sci.: Mater. Med.* 29: 1–13.

Liu, J. M. H., Zhang, X., Joe, S., Luo, X., & Shea, L. D. (2018). Evaluation of biomaterial scaffold delivery of IL-33 as a localized immunomodulatory agent to support cell transplantation in adipose tissue. *J. Immunol. Regener. Med.* 1: 1–12.

Liu, L., Bhatia, R., & Webster, T. J. (2017). Atomic layer deposition of nano-TiO2 thin films with enhanced biocompatibility and antimicrobial activity for orthopedic implants. *Int. J. Nanomed.* 12: 8711.

Liu, X., Smith, L. A., Hu, J., & Ma, P. X. (2009). Biomimetic nanofibrous gelatin/apatite composite scaffolds for bone tissue engineering. *Biomaterials.* 30: 2252–2258.

Liu, Y., Li, X., & Liang, A. (2022). Current research progress of local drug delivery systems based on biodegradable polymers in treating chronic osteomyelitis. *Front. Bioeng. Biotech.* 10: 2215.

Liu, Y., Luo, D., & Wang, T. (2016). Hierarchical structures of bone and bioinspired bone tissue engineering. *Small.* 12: 4611–4632.

Loebel, C., Rodell, C. B., Chen, M. H., & Burdick, J. A. (2017). Shear-thinning and self-healing hydrogels as injectable therapeutics and for 3D-printing. *Nat. Protoc.* 12: 1521–1541.

Lynn, D. M., & Langer, R. (2000). Degradable poly (β-amino esters): Synthesis, characterization, and self-assembly with plasmid DNA. *J. Am. Chem. Soc.* 122: 10761–10768.

Ma, C., Jing, Y., Sun, H., & Liu, X. (2015). Hierarchical nanofibrous microspheres with controlled growth factor delivery for bone regeneration. *Adv. Healthc. Mater.* 4: 2699–2708.

Ma, X., Wu, G., Dai, F., Li, D., Li, H., Zhang, L., & Deng, H. (2021). Chitosan/polydopamine layer by layer self-assembled silk fibroin nanofibers for biomedical applications. *Carbohydr. Polym.* 251: 117058.

Madl, C. M., Mehta, M., Duda, G. N., Heilshorn, S. C., & Mooney, D. J. (2014). Presentation of BMP-2 mimicking peptides in 3D hydrogels directs cell fate commitment in osteoblasts and mesenchymal stem cells. *Biomacromolecules.* 15: 445–455.

Madrigal, J. L., Sharma, S. N., Campbell, K. T., Stilhano, R. S., Gijsbers, R., & Silva, E. A. (2018). Microgels produced using microfluidic on-chip polymer blending for controlled released of VEGF encoding lentivectors. *Acta Biomatr.* 69: 265–276.

Magrez, A., Horváth, L., Smajda, R., Salicio, V., Pasquier, N., Forro, L., & Schwaller, B. (2009). Cellular toxicity of TiO2-based nanofilaments. *Acs Nano.* 3: 2274–2280.

Makadia, H. K., & Siegel, S. J. (2011). Poly Lactic-Co-Glycolic Acid (PLGA) as biodegradable controlled drug delivery carrier. *Polymers.* 3: 1377–1397.

McClellan, J. W., Mulconrey, D. S., Forbes, R. J., & Fullmer, N. (2006). Vertebral bone resorption after transforaminal lumbar interbody fusion with bone morphogenetic protein (rhBMP-2). *Clin. Spine Surg.* 19: 483–486.

McKay, B., & Sandhu, H. S. (2002). Use of recombinant human bone morphogenetic protein-2 in spinal fusion applications. *Spine.* 27: S66–S85.

McKay, W. F., Peckham, S. M., & Badura, J. M. (2007). A comprehensive clinical review of recombinant human bone morphogenetic protein-2 (INFUSE® Bone Graft). *Int. Orthop.* 31: 729–734.

McMillan, A., Nguyen, M. K., Gonzalez-Fernandez, T., Ge, P., Yu, X., Murphy, W. L., Kelly, D. J., & Alsberg, E. (2018). Dual non-viral gene delivery from microparticles within 3D high-density stem cell constructs for enhanced bone tissue engineering. *Biomaterials.* 161: 240–255.

Mehta, M., Schmidt-Bleek, K., Duda, G. N., & Mooney, D. J. (2012). Biomaterial delivery of morphogens to mimic the natural healing cascade in bone. *Adv. Drug Deliv. Rev.* 64: 1257–1276.

Mertz, D., Hemmerlé, J., Mutterer, J., Ollivier, S., Voegel, J. C., Schaaf, P., & Lavalle, P. (2007). Mechanically responding nanovalves based on polyelectrolyte multilayers. *Nano Lett.* 7: 657–662.

Minardi, S., Corradetti, B., Taraballi, F., Byun, J. H., Cabrera, F., Liu, X., Ferrari, M., Weiner, B. K., & Tasciotti, E. (2016b). IL-4 release from a biomimetic scaffold for the temporally controlled modulation of macrophage response. *Ann. Biomed. Eng.* 44: 2008–2019.

Minardi, S., Fernandez-Moure, J. S., Fan, D., Murphy, M. B., Yazdi, I. K., Liu, X., Weiner, B. K., & Tasciotti, E. (2020). Biocompatible PLGA-mesoporous silicon microspheres for the controlled release of BMP-2 for bone augmentation. *Pharmaceutics.* 12: 118.

Minardi, S., Pandolfi, L., Taraballi, F., De Rosa, E., Yazdi, I. K., Liu, X., Ferrari, M., & Tasciotti, E. (2015). PLGA-mesoporous silicon microspheres for the in vivo controlled temporospatial delivery of proteins. *ACS Appl. Mater. Interfaces.* 7: 16364–16373.

Minardi, S., Taraballi, F., Pandolfi, L., & Tasciotti, E. (2016a). Patterning biomaterials for the spatiotemporal delivery of bioactive molecules. *Front. Bioeng. Biotech.* 4: 45.

Mohammadi, M., Alibolandi, M., Abnous, K., Salmasi, Z., Jaafari, M. R., & Ramezani, M. (2018). Fabrication of hybrid scaffold based on hydroxyapatite-biodegradable nanofibers incorporated with liposomal formulation of BMP-2 peptide for bone tissue engineering. *Nanomed. Nanotechnol. Biol. Med.* 14: 1987–1997.

Monteiro, N., Martins, A., Reis, R. L., & Neves, N. M. (2014). Liposomes in tissue engineering and regenerative medicine. *J. R. Soc. Interface*. 11: 20140459.

Moroni, L., Boland, T., Burdick, J. A., De Maria, C., Derby, B., Forgacs, G., Groll, J., Li, Q., Malda, J., & Mironov, V. A. (2018). Biofabrication: A guide to technology and terminology. *Trends Biotechnol*. 36: 384–402.

Moskowitz, J. S., Blaisse, M. R., Samuel, R. E., Hsu, H. P., Harris, M. B., Martin, S. D., Lee, J. C., Spector, M., & Hammond, P. T. (2010). The effectiveness of the controlled release of gentamicin from polyelectrolyte multilayers in the treatment of staphylococcus aureus infection in a rabbit bone model. *Biomaterials*. 31: 6019–6030.

Mouriño, V., & Boccaccini, A. R. (2010). Bone tissue engineering therapeutics: Controlled drug delivery in three-dimensional scaffolds. *J. R. Soc. Interface*. 7: 209–227.

Nie, T., Baldwin, A., Yamaguchi, N., & Kiick, K. L. (2007). Production of heparin-functionalized hydrogels for the development of responsive and controlled growth factor delivery systems. *J. Control. Release*. 122: 287–296.

Nitta, S. K., & Numata, K. (2013). Biopolymer-based nanoparticles for drug/gene delivery and tissue engineering. *Int. J. Mol. Sci*. 14: 1629–1654.

Novais, A., Chatzopoulou, E., Chaussain, C., & Gorin, C. (2021). The potential of FGF-2 in craniofacial bone tissue engineering: A review. *Cells*. 10: 932.

Nurkesh, A., Jaguparov, A., Jimi, S., & Saparov, A. (2020). Recent advances in the controlled release of growth factors and cytokines for improving cutaneous wound healing. *Front. Cell Dev. Biol*. 8: 638.

O'Brien, F. J., Harley, B. A., Yannas, I. V., & Gibson, L. (2004). Influence of freezing rate on pore structure in freeze-dried collagen-GAG scaffolds. *Biomaterials*. 25: 1077–1086.

Olekson, M. A. P., Faulknor, R., Bandekar, A., Sempkowski, M., Hsia, H. C., & Berthiaume, F. (2015). SDF-1 liposomes promote sustained cell proliferation in mouse diabetic wounds. *Wound Repair Regen*. 23: 711–723.

Oliveira, É. R., Nie, L., Podstawczyk, D., Allahbakhsh, A., Ratnayake, J., Brasil, D. L., & Shavandi, A. (2021). Advances in growth factor delivery for bone tissue engineering. *Int. J. Mol. Sci*. 22: 903.

Oliveira, P. N., Montembault, A., Sudre, G., Alcouffe, P., Marcon, L., Gehan, H., Lux, F., Albespy, K., Centis, V., & Campos, D. (2019). Self-crosslinked fibrous collagen/chitosan blends: Processing, properties evaluation and monitoring of degradation by bi-fluorescence imaging. *Int. J. Biol. Macromol*. 131: 353–367.

Park, J. Y., Shim, J. H., Choi, S. A., Jang, J., Kim, M., Lee, S. H., & Cho, D. W. (2015). 3D printing technology to control BMP-2 and VEGF delivery spatially and temporally to promote large-volume bone regeneration. *J. Mater. Chem. B*. 3: 5415–5425.

Park, S. H., Han, U., Choi, D., & Hong, J. (2018). Layer-by-layer assembled polymeric thin films as prospective drug delivery carriers: Design and applications. *Biomater. Res*. 22: 1–13.

Park, S. H., Yun, B. G., Won, J. Y., Yun, W. S., Shim, J. H., Lim, M. H., Kim, D. H., Baek, S. A., Alahmari, Y. D., & Jeun, J. H. (2017). New application of three-dimensional printing biomaterial in nasal reconstruction. *The Laryngoscope*. 127: 1036–1043.

Penheiter, S. G., Mitchell, H., Garamszegi, N., Edens, M., Doré Jr, J. J. E., & Leof, E. B. (2002). Internalization-dependent and-independent requirements for transforming growth factor β receptor signaling via the Smad pathway. *Mol. Cell. Biol*. 22: 4750–4759.

Poldervaart, M. T., Gremmels, H., van Deventer, K., Fledderus, J. O., Öner, F. C., Verhaar, M. C., Dhert, W. J. A., & Alblas, J. (2014). Prolonged presence of VEGF promotes vascularization in 3D bioprinted scaffolds with defined architecture. *J. Control. Release*. 184: 58–66.

Poldervaart, M. T., Wang, H., van der Stok, J., Weinans, H., Leeuwenburgh, S. C. G., Öner, F. C., Dhert, W. J. A., & Alblas, J. (2013). Sustained release of BMP-2 in bioprinted alginate for osteogenicity in mice and rats. *PloS One*. 8: e72610.

Qian, Y., Li, L., Song, Y., Dong, L., Chen, P., Li, X., Cai, K., Germershaus, O., Yang, L., & Fan, Y. (2018). Surface modification of nanofibrous matrices via layer-by-layer functionalized silk assembly for mitigating the foreign body reaction. *Biomaterials*. 164: 22–37.

Quinlan, E., López-Noriega, A., Thompson, E., Kelly, H. M., Cryan, S. A., & O'Brien, F. J. (2015a). Development of collagen—Hydroxyapatite scaffolds incorporating PLGA and alginate microparticles for the controlled delivery of rhBMP-2 for bone tissue engineering. *J. Control. Release*. 198: 71–79.

Quinlan, E., Partap, S., Azevedo, M. M., Jell, G., Stevens, M. M., & O'Brien, F. J. (2015b). Hypoxia-mimicking bioactive glass/collagen glycosaminoglycan composite scaffolds to enhance angiogenesis and bone repair. *Biomaterials*. 52: 358–366.

Raiche, A. T., & Puleo, D. A. (2004). In vitro effects of combined and sequential delivery of two bone growth factors. *Biomaterials*. 25: 677–685.

Rittipakorn, P., Thuaksuban, N., Mai-Ngam, K., Charoenla, S., & Noppakunmongkolchai, W. (2021). Bioactivity of a novel polycaprolactone-hydroxyapatite scaffold used as a carrier of low dose bmp-2: An in vitro study. *Polymers*. 13: 466.

Rodell, C. B., Rai, R., Faubel, S., Burdick, J. A., & Soranno, D. E. (2015). Local immunotherapy via delivery of interleukin-10 and transforming growth factor β antagonist for treatment of chronic kidney disease. *J. Control. Release*. 206: 131–139.

Romagnoli, C., D'Asta, F., & Brandi, M. L. (2013). Drug delivery using composite scaffolds in the context of bone tissue engineering. *Clin. Cases. Miner. Bone Metab*. 10: 155.

Schlessinger, J., & Ullrich, A. (1992). Growth factor signaling by receptor tyrosine kinases. *Neuron*. 9: 383–391.

Shadjou, N., & Hasanzadeh, M. (2015). Bone tissue engineering using silica-based mesoporous nanobiomaterials: Recent progress. *Mater. Sci. Eng. C*. 55: 401–409.

Shah, N. J., Macdonald, M. L., Beben, Y. M., Padera, R. F., Samuel, R. E., & Hammond, P. T. (2011). Tunable dual growth factor delivery from polyelectrolyte multilayer films. *Biomaterials*. 32: 6183–6193.

Shen, X., Zhang, Y., Gu, Y., Xu, Y., Liu, Y., Li, B., & Chen, L. (2016). Sequential and sustained release of SDF-1 and BMP-2 from silk fibroin-nanohydroxyapatite scaffold for the enhancement of bone regeneration. *Biomaterials*. 106: 205–216.

Singh, R. K., Jin, G. Z., Mahapatra, C., Patel, K. D., Chrzanowski, W., & Kim, H. W. (2015). Mesoporous silica-layered biopolymer hybrid nanofibrous scaffold: A novel nanobiomatrix platform for therapeutics delivery and bone regeneration. *ACS Appl. Mater. Interfaces*. 7: 8088–8098.

Sithole, M. N., Kumar, P., Du Toit, L. C., Erlwanger, K. H., Ubanako, P. N., & Choonara, Y. E. (2023). A 3D-printed biomaterial scaffold reinforced with inorganic fillers for bone tissue engineering: In vitro assessment and in vivo animal studies. *Int. J. Mol. Sci*. 24: 7611.

Peltola, S. M., Melchels, F. P., Grijpma, D. W., & Kellomäki, M. (2008). A review of rapid prototyping techniques for tissue engineering purposes. *Ann. Med*. 40: 268–280.

Smucker, J. D., Rhee, J. M., Singh, K., Yoon, S. T., & Heller, J. G. (2006). Increased swelling complications associated with off-label usage of rhBMP-2 in the anterior cervical spine. *Spine*. 31: 2813–2819.

Snoddy, B., & Jayasuriya, A. C. (2016). The use of nanomaterials to treat bone infections. *Mater. Sci. Eng. C*. 67: 822–833.

Song, J., Winkeljann, B., & Lieleg, O. (2020). Biopolymer-based coatings: Promising strategies to improve the biocompatibility and functionality of materials used in biomedical engineering. *Adv. Mater. Interfaces*. 7: 2000850.

Spiller, K. L., Nassiri, S., Witherel, C. E., Anfang, R. R., Ng, J., Nakazawa, K. R., Yu, T., & Vunjak-Novakovic, G. (2015). Sequential delivery of immunomodulatory cytokines to facilitate the M1-to-M2 transition of macrophages and enhance vascularization of bone scaffolds. *Biomaterials*. 37: 194–207.

Stevens, M. M., & George, J. H. (2005). Exploring and engineering the cell surface interface. *Science*. 310: 1135–1138.

Subbiah, R., Ruehle, M. A., Klosterhoff, B. S., Lin, A. S. P., Hettiaratchi, M. H., Willett, N. J., Bertassoni, L. E., García, A. J., & Guldberg, R. E. (2021). Triple growth factor delivery promotes functional bone regeneration following composite musculoskeletal trauma. *Acta Biomatr*. 127: 180–192.

Sun, T., Zhou, K., Liu, M., Guo, X., Qu, Y., Cui, W., Shao, Z., Zhang, X., & Xu, S. (2018). Loading of BMP-2-related peptide onto three-dimensional nano-hydroxyapatite scaffolds accelerates mineralization in critical-sized cranial bone defects. *J. Tissue Eng. Regener. Med*. 12: 864–877.

Tang, Z., He, C., Tian, H., Ding, J., Hsiao, B. S., Chu, B., & Chen, X. (2016). Polymeric nanostructured materials for biomedical applications. *Prog. Polym. Sci*. 60: 86–128.

Tang, Z., Wang, Y., Podsiadlo, P., & Kotov, N. A. (2006). Biomedical applications of layer-by-layer assembly: From biomimetics to tissue engineering. *Adv. Mater*. 18: 3203–3224.

Tarafder, S., Koch, A., Jun, Y., Chou, C., Awadallah, M. R., & Lee, C. H. (2016). Micro-precise spatiotemporal delivery system embedded in 3D printing for complex tissue regeneration. *Biofabrication*. 8: 25003.

Tibbitt, M. W., & Anseth, K. S. (2009). Hydrogels as extracellular matrix mimics for 3D cell culture. *Biotechnol. Bioeng*. 103: 655–663.

Trachtenberg, J. E., Mountziaris, P. M., Kasper, F. K., & Mikos, A. G. (2013). Fiber-based composite tissue engineering scaffolds for drug delivery. *Isr. J. Chem*. 53: 646–654.

Udomluck, N., Lee, H., Hong, S., Lee, S. H., & Park, H. (2020). Surface functionalization of dual growth factor on hydroxyapatite-coated nanofibers for bone tissue engineering. *Appl. Surf. Sci*. 520: 146311.

Vo, T. N., Kasper, F. K., & Mikos, A. G. (2012). Strategies for controlled delivery of growth factors and cells for bone regeneration. *Adv. Drug Deliv. Rev*. 64: 1292–1309.

Von Einem, S., Schwarz, E., & Rudolph, R. (2010). A novel TWO-STEP renaturation procedure for efficient production of recombinant BMP-2. *Protein Expr. Purif.* 73: 65–69.

Vorndran, E., Klammert, U., Ewald, A., Barralet, J. E., & Gbureck, U. (2010). Simultaneous immobilization of bioactives during 3D powder printing of bioceramic drug-release matrices. *Adv. Funct. Mater*. 20: 1585–1591.

Wang, B., Guo, Y., Chen, X., Zeng, C., Hu, Q., Yin, W., Li, W., Xie, H., Zhang, B., & Huang, X. (2018). Nanoparticle-modified chitosan-agarose-gelatin scaffold for sustained release of SDF-1 and BMP-2. *Int. J. Nanomed*. 13: 7395.

Wang, J., Xie, B., Zhu, Z., Xie, G., & Luo, B. (2021). 3D-printed construct from hybrid suspension as spatially and temporally controlled protein delivery system. *J. Biomater. Appl*. 36: 264–275.

Wang, Z., Dong, L., Han, L., Wang, K., Lu, X., Fang, L., Qu, S., & Chan, C. W. (2016). Self-assembled biodegradable nanoparticles and polysaccharides as biomimetic ECM nanostructures for the synergistic effect of RGD and BMP-2 on bone formation. *Sci. Rep*. 6(1): 25090.

Wei, G., & Ma, P. X. (2006). Macroporous and nanofibrous polymer scaffolds and polymer/bone-like apatite composite scaffolds generated by sugar spheres. *J. Biomed. Mater. Res. A*. 78: 306–315.

Wei, S., Jian, C., Xu, F., Bao, T., Lan, S., Wu, G., Qi, B., Bai, Z., & Yu, A. (2018). Vancomycin—impregnated electrospun polycaprolactone (PCL) membrane for the treatment of infected bone defects: An animal study. *J. Biomater. Appl*. 32: 1187–1196.

Whitesides, G. M., Mathias, J. P., & Seto, C. T. (1991). Molecular self-assembly and nanochemistry: A chemical strategy for the synthesis of nanostructures. *Science*. 254: 1312–1319.

Wohl, B. M., & Engbersen, J. F. J. (2012). Responsive layer-by-layer materials for drug delivery. *J. Control. Release*. 158: 2–14.

Wubneh, A., Tsekoura, E. K., Ayranci, C., & Uludağ, H. (2018). Current state of fabrication technologies and materials for bone tissue engineering. *Acta Biomatr*. 80: 1–30.

Xie, G., Sun, J., Zhong, G., Liu, C., & Wei, J. (2010). Hydroxyapatite nanoparticles as a controlled-release carrier of BMP-2: Absorption and release kinetics in vitro. *J. Mater. Sci. Mater. Med*. 21: 1875–1880.

Xue, J., Xie, J., Liu, W., & Xia, Y. (2017). Electrospun nanofibers: New concepts, materials, and applications. *Acc. Chem. Res*. 50: 1976–1987.

Yang, F., Wolke, J. G. C., & Jansen, J. A. (2008). Biomimetic calcium phosphate coating on electrospun poly (ε-caprolactone) scaffolds for bone tissue engineering. *Chem. Eng. J*. 137: 154–161.

Yao, Q., Liu, Y., Selvaratnam, B., Koodali, R. T., & Sun, H. (2018). Mesoporous silicate nanoparticles/3D nanofibrous scaffold-mediated dual-drug delivery for bone tissue engineering. *J. Control. Release*. 279: 69–78.

Yi, H., Ur Rehman, F., Zhao, C., Liu, B., & He, N. (2016). Recent advances in nano scaffolds for bone repair. *Bone Res*. 4: 1–11.

Yun, Y. P., Kim, S. E., Kang, E. Y., Kim, H. J., Park, K., & Song, H. R. (2013). The effect of Bone Morphogenic Protein-2 (BMP-2)-immobilizing heparinized-chitosan scaffolds for enhanced osteoblast activity. *Tissue Eng. Regen. Med*. 10: 122–130.

Zha, Y., Li, Y., Lin, T., Chen, J., Zhang, S., & Wang, J. (2021). Progenitor cell-derived exosomes endowed with VEGF plasmids enhance osteogenic induction and vascular remodeling in large segmental bone defects. *Theranostics*. 11: 397.

Zhang, K., Wang, S., Zhou, C., Cheng, L., Gao, X., Xie, X., Sun, J., Wang, H., Weir, M. D., & Reynolds, M. A. (2018). Advanced smart biomaterials and constructs for hard tissue engineering and regeneration. *Bone Res*. 6: 31.

Zhang, X., Li, Y., Chen, Y. E., Chen, J., & Ma, P. X. (2016). Cell-free 3D scaffold with two-stage delivery of miRNA-26a to regenerate critical-sized bone defects. *Nat. Commun*. 7: 10376.

Zhang, X., Li, Z., Yuan, X., Cui, Z., & Yang, X. (2013). Fabrication of dopamine-modified hyaluronic acid/chitosan multilayers on titanium alloy by layer-by-layer self-assembly for promoting osteoblast growth. *Appl. Surf. Sci*. 284: 732–737.

Zhou, K., Yu, P., Shi, X., Ling, T., Zeng, W., Chen, A., Yang, W., & Zhou, Z. (2019). Hierarchically porous hydroxyapatite hybrid scaffold incorporated with reduced graphene oxide for rapid bone ingrowth and repair. *ACS Nano*. 13: 9595–9606.

Zhou, P., Wu, J., Xia, Y., Yuan, Y., Zhang, H., Xu, S., & Lin, K. (2018). Loading BMP-2 on nanostructured hydroxyapatite microspheres for rapid bone regeneration. *Int. J. Nanomed.* 13: 4083–4092.

Zhou, X., Feng, W., Qiu, K., Chen, L., Wang, W., Nie, W., Mo, X., & He, C. (2015). BMP-2 derived peptide and dexamethasone incorporated mesoporous silica nanoparticles for enhanced osteogenic differentiation of bone mesenchymal stem cells. *ACS Appl. Mater. Interfaces*. 7: 15777–15789.

Zhu, H., Zheng, K., & Boccaccini, A. R. (2021). Multi-functional silica-based mesoporous materials for simultaneous delivery of biologically active ions and therapeutic biomolecules. *Acta Biomater*. 129: 1–17.

Zhu, L., Liu, Y., Wang, A., Zhu, Z., Li, Y., Zhu, C., Che, Z., Liu, T., Liu, H., & Huang, L. (2022). Application of BMP in bone tissue engineering. *Front. Bioeng. Biotech.* 10: 810880.

Zhu, M., Li, K., Zhu, Y., Zhang, J., & Ye, X. (2015). 3D-printed hierarchical scaffold for localized isoniazid/rifampin drug delivery and osteoarticular tuberculosis therapy. *Acta Biomater*. 16: 145–155.

Zhu, W., Cui, H., Boualam, B., Masood, F., Flynn, E., Rao, R. D., Zhang, Z. Y., & Zhang, L. G. (2018). 3D bioprinting mesenchymal stem cell-laden construct with core—Shell nanospheres for cartilage tissue engineering. *Nanotechnology*. 29: 185101.

Zylberberg, C., & Matosevic, S. (2017). Bioengineered liposome—Scaffold composites as therapeutic delivery systems. *Ther. Deliv*. 8: 425–445.

9 Nanotechnology Advancements for Improved Bone Metabolism, Regeneration and Treatment of Bone Diseases

Vianni Chopra, Diana Arredondo Bernal, Gaurav Chauhan, Sergio Omar Martinez Chapa, and Deepa Ghosh

9.1 INTRODUCTION

Bone is the second-most transplanted organ after blood, and the cost of surgeries and post-surgery-related treatment is very high (Qiao et al., 2022). The amount of money spent on all bone-related products, including pins, grafts, prosthetics, etc., comes to around USD 5.5 billion annually. According to the Global Burden of Diseases, Injuries, and Risk Factors Study in 2019, there were a total of 178 million bone fractures (102 million in men and 76.4 million in women) (Wu et al., 2021).

Langer and Vacanti coined the term "tissue engineering" as an interdisciplinary field that applies the principles of engineering and life sciences toward the development of biological substitutes that restore, maintain, or improve tissue function or a whole organ (Chu et al., 2014). The development of new advanced materials has accelerated the translation of tissue engineering technologies from bench to bedside (Gadekar et al., 2021). In recent decades, the emergence of technologies based on nanoscience has led to significant improvements in the areas of engineering, industry, and healthcare (Yu et al., 2017b). The era of nanotechnology has shown that material advancements can lead to the development of structures that can closely mimic the size and morphological requirements of naturally occurring bone tissues (Hajiali et al., 2021). Figure S9.1 shows the hierarchical structure of bone depicting its macro, micro and nano architectures.

In the past decade, there has been an extensive exploration of various nanostructured materials as shown in Figure 9.1 such as micelles (Yan et al., 2018), nanoparticles (Das et al., 2015; Hasan et al., 2018; Liu et al., 2017), nanofibers (Maharjan et al., 2021; Shams et al., 2020), and thin films (La et al., 2013; Ren et al., 2017) in both biological and medical fields. Through surface chemical modifications, these materials can be tailored to exhibit specific properties. For instance, nanostructured materials have recently found positive applications in bone-related diseases; nanoparticles and micelle-based drug carriers with functional ligands have been developed to achieve bone-targeting due to their high specific surface area, enabling them to pass through the smallest capillary vessels. Due to their small size, nanoparticles can quickly respond to external stimuli from the environment, such as ultrasound, magnetic field, pH, and even X-ray exposure (Li et al., 2019; J Hill et al., 2019).

DOI: 10.1201/9781003307310-11

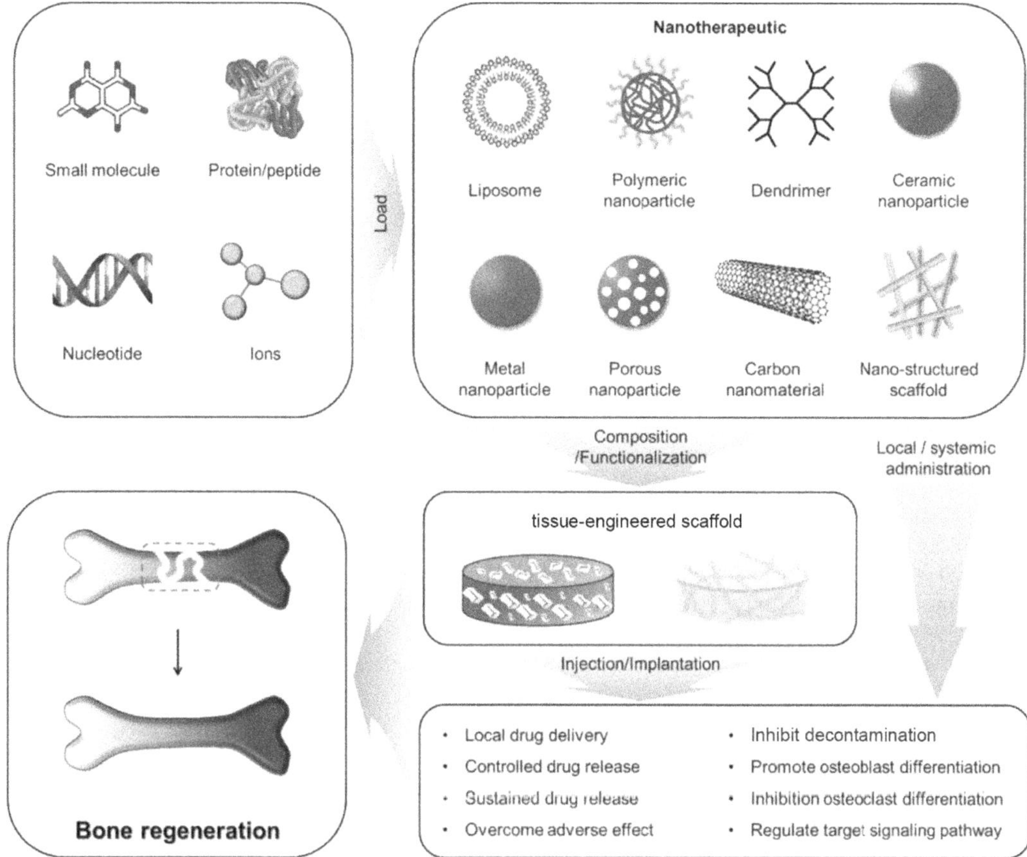

FIGURE 9.1 A concise summary of the approaches for using materials-based nanotherapeutics to treat diseased and injured bone tissue is as follows: therapeutic molecules, including small molecular drugs, protein molecules, genetic molecules, and ions, can influence the signaling processes of bone-associated cells. These molecules are integrated into various materials-based nano-structures to create nanotherapeutics that can be administered locally or systemically to affected bone tissue. Additionally, nanotherapeutics can be combined with 3D tissue engineering scaffolds to replicate the host microenvironment (reproduced with permission from Lee, C. S., Singh, R. K., Hwang, H. S., Lee, N. H., Kurian, A. G., Lee, J. H., Kim, H. S., Lee, M. & Kim, H. W.: Materials-based nanotherapeutics for injured and diseased bone. Prog. Mater. Sci. 2023. 135. 101087. Copyright 2023 Elsevier).

9.2 NANOMATERIALS USED IN BONE REGENERATION

Nanomaterials have gained significant attention in the field of bone regeneration due to their unique properties, such as the high surface-area-to-volume ratio, tunable size and shape, and biocompatibility. These properties allow them to mimic the natural extracellular matrix (ECM) of bone and provide a suitable environment for cell adhesion, proliferation, and differentiation. Nanomaterials such as nanoparticles, nanofibers, and nanocomposites have been explored for their potential applications in bone tissue engineering (BTE). They can be used to deliver therapeutic agents such as growth factors and drugs to promote bone regeneration.

Additionally, they can be incorporated into scaffolds to enhance their mechanical properties and improve the structural integrity of the newly formed bone tissue. Figure 9.2 details the effect of various dimensionalities of nanomaterials on bone regeneration. These have broadly been classified as nanoparticles, nanofibers and nanocomposites.

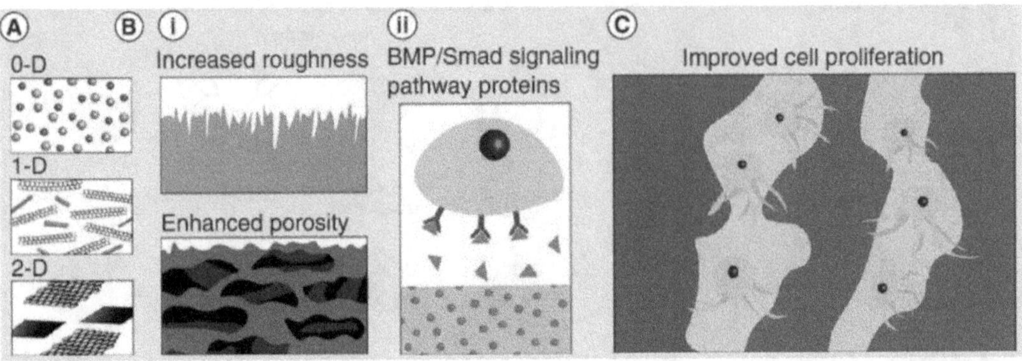

FIGURE 9.2 (A) Bone tissue engineering scaffolds incorporate various nanomaterial structures, including zero-dimensional (0D) materials like AuNP and magnetic nanoparticles (NPs); one-dimensional (1D) NPs such as carbon nanotubes and gold nanorods; and two-dimensional (2D) structures such as graphene. (B) The incorporation of nanomaterials in scaffold design allows for the introduction of surface roughness, nanoporosity, and higher stiffness, which mimics native bone tissue. NPs can also modify the protein corona formed around the scaffold and activate the BMP signaling pathway for stem cells. (C) By incorporating NPs into scaffolds, enhanced cell proliferation is achieved through both mechanical and biological mechanisms induced by the NPs (reproduced with permission from Hill, M. J., Qi, B., Bayaniahangar, R., Araban, V., Bakhtiary, Z., Doschak, M. R., Goh, B. C., Shokouhimehr, M., Vali, H., Presley, J. F. & Zadpoor, A. A.: Nanomaterials for bone tissue regeneration: updates and future perspectives. Nanomedicine. 2019. 14. 2987–3006. Copyright 2019 Future Science Group).

9.2.1 Nanoparticles

Nanoparticles have emerged as a promising approach for bone regeneration due to their ability to target and deliver therapeutic agents to the site of injury or defect and their potential to enhance the regenerative capacity of bone cells. Therapeutic molecules used for bone repair and regeneration include small molecular drugs; protein molecules such as growth factors and peptides; genetic molecules including DNAs, RNAs, and oligonucleotides; and metal ions such as silicate, cobalt, and copper. To deliver these therapeutic molecules, a range of nanomaterials including liposomes, polymeric nanoparticles, metallic nanoparticles, and carbon nanomaterials are utilized through various processing techniques.

9.2.1.1 Polymeric Nanoparticles

PLGA nanoparticles: PLGA nanoparticles have been shown to promote osteogenic differentiation of mesenchymal stem cells (MSCs) and to enhance bone regeneration in vivo (Ghavimi et al., 2020; Jin et al., 2021; Ilhan et al., 2022).

Chitosan nanoparticles: Chitosan nanoparticles have been shown to promote bone regeneration by enhancing the proliferation and differentiation of osteoblasts and MSCs (Sruthi et al., 2020; Raftery et al., 2017; Li et al., 2017)

Gelatin nanoparticles: Gelatin nanoparticles have been shown to promote osteogenic differentiation of MSCs and to enhance bone regeneration in vivo (Mu et al., 2020; Farbod et al., 2016).

9.2.1.2 Inorganic Nanoparticles

Inorganic nanoparticles are also being investigated for their potential use in bone regeneration due to their unique physical and chemical properties. For example, silica nanoparticles have been shown to promote osteogenic differentiation of MSCs and enhance bone regeneration in vivo. Silica nanoparticles also have antibacterial properties, which can prevent infection during bone healing process (Hosseinpour et al., 2021; Lei et al., 2019; Castro et al., 2018).

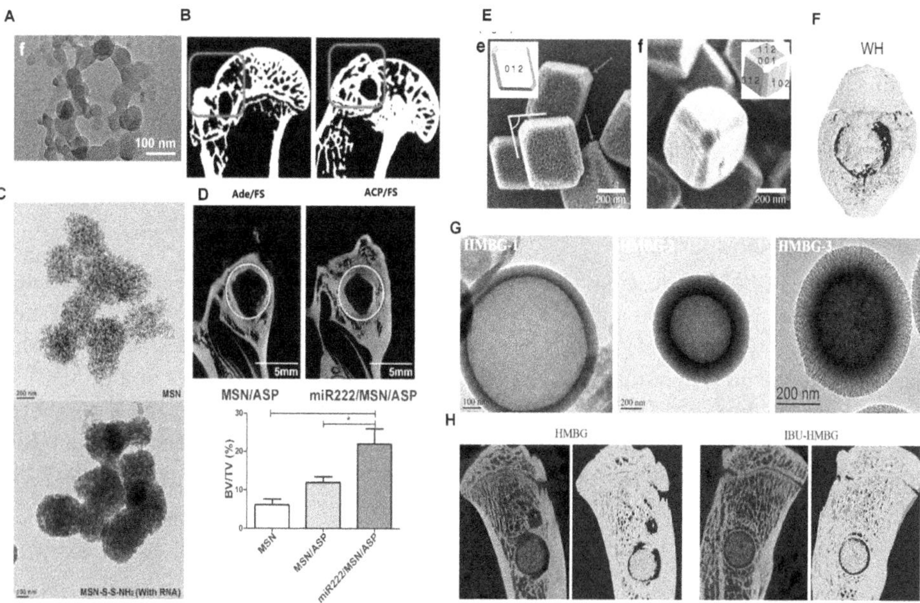

FIGURE 9.3 (A) Amorphous calcium phosphate nanoparticles prepared using $CaCl_2$ as precursor; panel shows TEM; (B) micro-CT images of femur after eight weeks (reproduced under the terms of CC-BY 4.0 (https://creativecommons.org/licenses/by/4.0/) International License from Liao, H., Yu, H. P., Song, W., Zhang, G., Lu, B., Zhu, Y. J., Yu, W. & He, Y.: Amorphous calcium phosphate nanoparticles using adenosine triphosphate as an organic phosphorus source for promoting tendon—bone healing. J. Nanobiotechnol. 2021. 19. 1–17. Copyright 2021 Liao et al., published by Springer Nature). (C) TEM images of morphology of MSN(a) and miR222/MSNs (lower panel); (D) micro-CT scan of bone in the mandibular defect areas of rats in the MSN, MSN/ASP, and miR222/MSN/ASP microsphere hydrogel groups (upper panel) and bone volume (BV)/tissue volume (TV) % showing significant more new bone formation (lower panel) (reproduced with permission from Lei, L., Liu, Z., Yuan, P., Jin, R., Wang, X., Jiang, T., & Chen, X.: Injectable colloidal hydrogel with mesoporous silica nanoparticles for sustained corelease of microRNA-222 and aspirin to achieve innervated bone regeneration in rat mandibular defects. J. Mater. Chem. B. 2019. 7. 2722–2735. Copyright 2019 Royal Society of Chemistry). (E) Rhombohedral habit of whitlockite (WH: $Ca_{18}Mg_2(HPO_4)_2(PO_4)_{12}$) crystal and field emission scanning electron microscope image of WH nanoparticles; (F) in vivo cranial bone regeneration shown by micro-CT (reproduced with permission from Kim, H. D., Jang, H. L., Ahn, H. Y., Lee, H. K., Park, J., Lee, E. S., Lee, E. A., Jeong, Y. H., Kim, D. G., Nam, K. T. & Hwang, N. S.: Biomimetic whitlockite inorganic nanoparticles-mediated in situ remodeling and rapid bone regeneration. Biomaterials. 2017. 112. 31–43. Copyright 2017 Elsevier). (G) The TEM images of HMBG nanoparticles; (H) micro-CT evaluation of bone regeneration in the rat tibia defects with implantation of HMBG and IBU-HMBG samples after 4 weeks; (reproduced under the terms of CC-BY 4.0 (https://creativecommons.org/licenses/by/4.0/) International License from Wang, Y., Pan, H., & Chen, X.: The preparation of hollow mesoporous bioglass nanoparticles with excellent drug delivery capacity for bone tissue regeneration. Front. Chem. 2019. 7. 283. Copyright 2019 Wang et al., published by Frontiers).

9.2.1.3 Ceramic Nanoparticles

Ceramic-based nanoparticles have been extensively investigated for their potential use in bone regeneration due to their biocompatibility, mechanical strength, and ability to stimulate bone growth. Some types of ceramic nanoparticles that have been studied for bone regeneration are shown in Figure 9.3.

Hydroxyapatite (Hap) nanoparticles: Hap is a natural mineral component of bone and has been extensively studied for its ability to promote bone regeneration in vitro and in vivo (Huang et al., 2022; Kim et al., 2017).

Calcium phosphate (CaP) nanoparticles: CaP is another natural mineral component of bone, and it has been shown to enhance the proliferation and differentiation of osteoblasts and to promote bone regeneration in vitro and in vivo (Liao et al., 2021; Levingstone et al., 2019).

Bioglass nanoparticles: Bioglass is a bioactive glass that has been shown to promote bone regeneration by enhancing the activity of osteoblasts and stimulating angiogenesis in vitro and in vivo (Wu et al., 2022; Wang et al., 2019).

Zirconia (ZrO_2) nanoparticles: Zirconia is a ceramic material with high mechanical strength and biocompatibility. ZrO_2 nanoparticles have been shown to aid bone regeneration in vitro and in vivo (Mabrouk et al., 2022; Wang et al., 2016a).

9.2.1.4 Carbon Nanoparticles

Carbon nanotubes (CNTs) are cylindrical carbon molecules with high mechanical strength and unique electrical and thermal properties. CNTs have been shown to help in bone regeneration both in vitro and in vivo (Zhang et al., 2019a). Graphene oxide (GO) nanoparticles have been shown to enhance the osteogenic differentiation of MSCs in vitro and in vivo. Chopra et al. (2020) synthesized zinc-doped hydroxyapatite (HapZ) nanorods on the surface of rGO using a one-pot hydrothermal method. There was an in situ reduction of GO to rGO, accompanied by the nucleation and formation of HapZ on the rGO surface. The final composite, G_3HapZ, showed enhanced protein adsorption and continuous zinc release as shown in Figure 9.4.

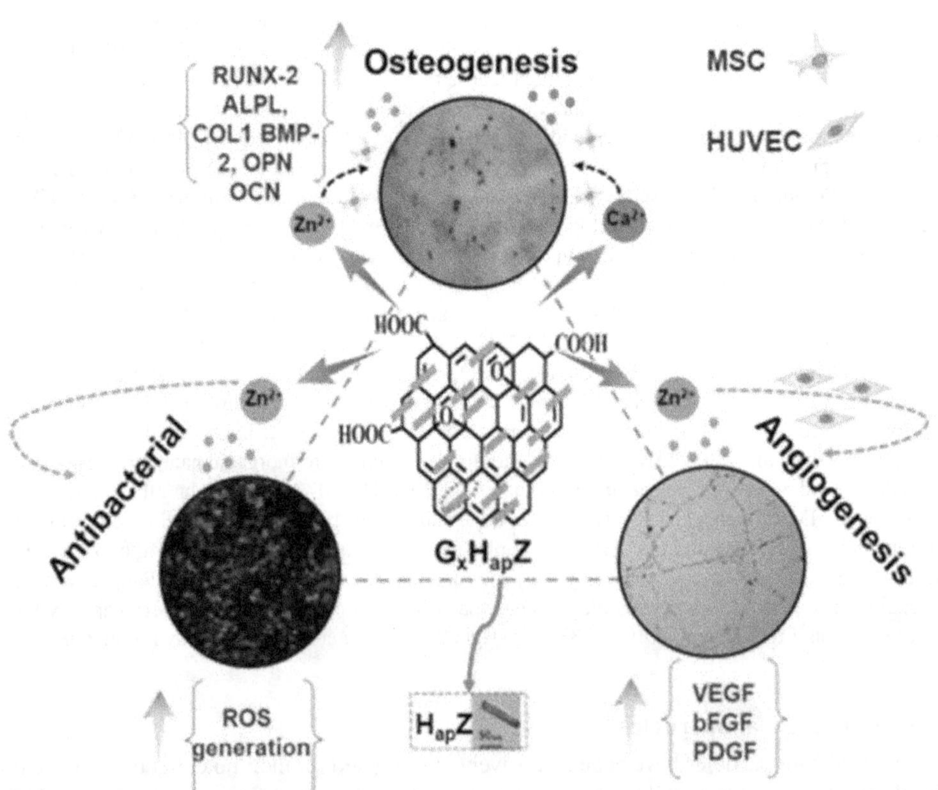

FIGURE 9.4 Zinc-doped hydroxyapatite nanorods on rGO surface show osteogenic, angiogenic, and antimicrobial properties (reproduced with permission from Chopra, V., Thomas, J., Sharma, A., Panwar, V., Kaushik, S., Sharma, S., Porwal, K., Kulkarni, C., Rajput, S., Singh, H. & Jagavelu, K.: Synthesis and evaluation of a zinc eluting rGO/hydroxyapatite nanocomposite optimized for bone augmentation. ACS Biomater. Sci. Eng. 2020. 6. 6710–6725. Copyright 2020 American Chemical Society).

This biocompatible composite displayed its osteoconductive potential in biomineralization studies. The osteoinductive property was confirmed by its ability to upregulate RUNX-2, alkaline phosphatase, COL-1, osteocalcin, and osteopontin in human umbilical mesenchymal stem cells (MSCs). Whereas the vascularization potential was displayed by its ability to induce endothelial cell migration, attachment, and proliferation, the antimicrobial activity was confirmed by its ability to inhibit bacterial attachment and biofilm formation. Further, the accelerated bone regeneration and neovascularization observed in a rat animal model could be attributed to the release of zinc ions.

9.2.2 Nanofibers

Nanofibers have been studied extensively for their potential applications in bone regeneration. As discussed in previous sections, these are ultrafine fibers with diameters in the range of tens to hundreds of nanometers that mimic the structure and mechanical properties of the natural ECM in bone tissue. Nanofibers can be used as scaffolds to support the growth and differentiation of bone cells such as osteoblasts and osteocytes. The high surface-area-to-volume ratio and porosity of the nanofibers allow for enhanced cell adhesion, proliferation, and differentiation. The nanofiber scaffolds can also provide mechanical support for the new bone tissue and promote its integration with the surrounding tissues.

Hong-Pei et al. (2015) incorporated HA/GO in gelatin/chitosan composite nanofiber scaffold by electrospinning that showed uniform and smooth morphology and a good antibacterial effect against *Staphylococcus aureus* and *Escherichia coli*. Ma et al. (2012) developed Hap/GO-based porous polylactic acid (PLA) scaffold using electrospinning. Wu et al. (2015) prepared 3D-printed GO-modified β-tricalcium phosphate scaffolds that had more significant bone formation in a critical-sized calvarial defect in New Zealand white male rabbits.

Shuai et al. (2022) prepared GO/Hap 3D-printed poly-L-lactide scaffolds having improved cohesive strength and mechanical properties and were cytocompatible. Peng et al. (2017) incorporated GO in Hap/polyetheretherketone composites and showed improved mechanical properties and enhanced healing in an in vivo rabbit radius bone injury model. Wang et al. (2020) made a tricomponent scaffold with silk fibroin (SF), nano-hydroxyapatite (nHap), and GO, which showed promising in vitro osteogenic potential in bone marrow-derived mesenchymal stem cells (BMSCs).

Chopra et al. (2022) employed gelatin nanofibers to incorporate zinc-doped nano-hydroxyapatite (ZnHp) decorated with rGO platelets (ZnHp@rGO) and pristine ZnHp as shown in Figure 9.5(A). The mechanical properties were improved, and degradation rates were delayed due to the incorporation of rGO in the nanofibers. On in vitro evaluation, the respective gelatin nanofibers appeared to aid the accelerated differentiation of MSCs toward the osteogenic lineage without the need for any exogenous osteogenic supplement in the milieu. The biomimetic cues provided by ZnHp and ZnHp@rGO also favored angiogenesis, as reflected by the enhanced CD-31 expression and iNOS levels. The ability of these nanofibers to induce vascularization was confirmed using an in vivo model and an in ovo model. Apart from their osteoinductive and angiogenic properties, the nanofibers exhibited favorable anti-biofilm activity by preventing the growth of *S. aureus*.

9.2.3 Nanocomposites

Nanocomposites are materials that combine nanoparticles with other materials such as polymers, ceramics, or metals to create hybrid structures with enhanced properties. In the context of bone healing, nanocomposites can be used to improve the mechanical strength, biocompatibility, and regenerative capacity of bone substitutes and implants. In this section, we present some examples of how nanocomposites can be used for bone healing.

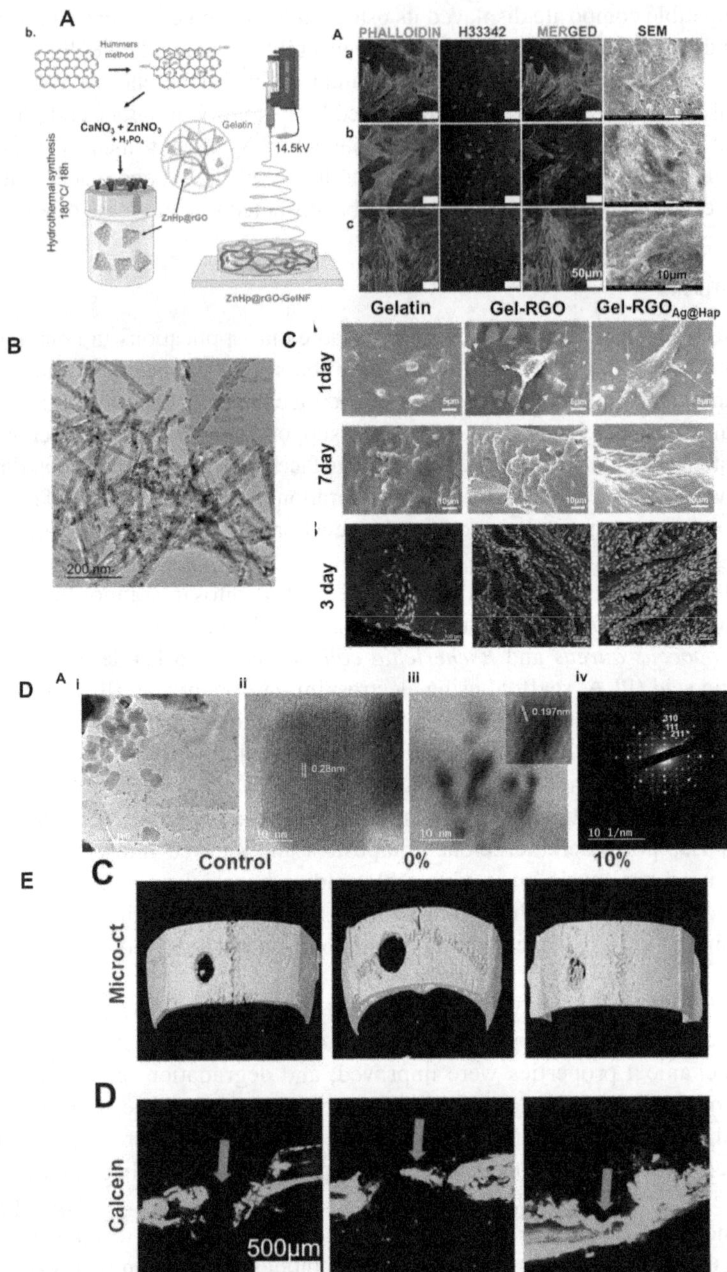

FIGURE 9.5 (A) Synthesis scheme of ZnHp on rGO incorporated in gelatin nanofibers (shown as b) and cellular attachment of MSCs on these nanofibers using Actin/H-33342 and SEM (shown as A). Here, a represents gelatin nanofibers, b represents ZnHp in gelatin nanofibers, and c denotes ZnHp on rGO incorporated in gelatin nanofibers (reproduced with permission from Chopra, V., Thomas, J., Chauhan, G., Kaushik, S., Rajput, S., Guha, R., Chattopadhyay, N., Martinez-Chapa, S. O. & Ghosh, D.: Gelatin Nanofibers Loaded with Zinc-Doped Hydroxyapatite for Osteogenic Differentiation of Mesenchymal Stem Cells. ACS Appl. Nano Mater. 2022. 5. 2414–2428. Copyright 2022 American Chemical Society). (B) TEM and (C) cellular attachment using SEM on gelatin, gelatin-GO, and silver-Hap gel-GO cryogels and live dead assay of MG-63 cells cultured over a period of 14 days on these cryogels (reproduced with permission from Chopra, V., Thomas, J., Sharma, A., Panwar, V., Kaushik, S., & Ghosh, D.: A bioinspired, ice-templated multifunctional 3D cryogel composite crosslinked through in situ reduction of GO displayed improved mechanical, osteogenic and antimicrobial properties. Mater.

Sci. Eng. C. 2021. 119. 111584. Copyright 2021 Elsevier). (D) TEM (i), high-resolution transmission electron microscopy (ii and iii), and selected area (electron) diffraction spectra (iv) of gold nanodots and Iohydroxyapatite nanorods on rGO surface and (E) in vivo bone regeneration potential of gold nanodots and nanohydroxyapatite nanorods on rGO surface incorporated in injectable calcium sulfate bone cements. Here, C shows the micro-CT images and BV/TV ratio of newly formed callus of control, 0% and 10% bone cements; D shows confocal images of calcein stained and labelled calvarial sections (reproduced with permission from Chopra, V., Thomas, J., Kaushik, S., Rajput, S., Guha, R., Mondal, B., Naskar, S., Mandal, D., Chauhan, G., Chattopadhyay, N. & Ghosh, D.: Injectable Bone Cement Reinforced with Gold Nanodots Decorated rGO-Hydroxyapatite Nanocomposites, Augment Bone Regeneration. Small. 2023. 19. e2204637. Copyright 2023 Wiley-VCH GmbH).

9.2.3.1 Polymeric Nanocomposites

Polymeric nanocomposites are materials that combine nanoparticles with polymers, such as PLA, polyethylene glycol (PEG), and chitosan. These materials can be used as scaffolds for BTE or as coatings for bone implants. The addition of nanoparticles, such as Hap or GO, can improve the mechanical properties and bioactivity of the polymeric matrix, as well as promote cell adhesion, proliferation, and differentiation.

The in situ synthesis of Hap on GO (Zhao et al., 2013), chitosan-GO (Li et al., 2013), and rGO (Neelgund et al., 2013) surfaces has been carried out by mixing the chemical precursors in a pH-dependent environment and letting them age for the complete transformation of apatite into hydroxy-apatite. During the synthesis, the oxygen functionalities act as nucleating sites for calcium ions via electrostatic interactions; these Ca^{2+} sites then interact with the phosphate ions and crystallize into apatite nanoparticles. The GO/rGO surfaces have been functionalized with various bioactive materials for enhanced mineralization, like gelatin (Liu et al., 2014a), polydopamine (Liu et al., 2012), fibrinogen (Wang et al., 2014), or other molecules.

Hydrothermal synthesis uses the formation of apatite crystals on GO/rGO surfaces at high temperatures and pressures. This technique improves the crystallinity of Hap and the stoichiometric composition that imparted the necessary biophysical and biochemical cues for cellular attachment and improved biological activity on MC3T3-E1 cells (Fan et al., 2014). Liu et al. (2012) showed the biocompatibility and increased mitochondrial activities of L929 cells on rGO/HA using MTT assay. Bone grafts of rGO/Ha prepared using hydrothermal synthesis by Lee et al. (2015) showed greater bone density in bone defects (6 mm in diameter and 2.5 mm in depth) in the parietal bone of rabbits in comparison with control/Hap groups. Nie et al. (2017) showed that the self-assembly of GO and Hap at high temperatures led to the in situ reduction of GO to rGO and formed a scaffolding structure. This structure showed in vitro osteogenic potential and bone-healing capacity in an in vivo rabbit calvarial defect.

Chopra et al. (2021) explored the role of silver-ion-doped Hap as an osteoinductive and antimicrobial agent in a scaffold system. Biopolymeric 3D scaffolds often lack biochemical cues and mechanical strength to encourage bone tissue regeneration, as shown in Figure 9.5(B–E). Chemical crosslinkers have been extensively used to impart strength but have been found to be toxic at the site of implantation and lack physical strength.

This was addressed by engineering a self-crosslinked polymer through the in situ reduction of GO in a gelatin cryogel using ice as a template to create pores. The cryogels had superior mechanical properties (2.4 MPa) over their reported counterparts (mostly in the kPa range) and were also comparable with the properties of cancellous bone (2–20 MPa). The optimized biocompatible cryogel favored bone cells' adhesion and proliferation over a period of 14 days.

The osteoconductive and osteoinductive potential of the cryogel was confirmed through biomineralization and osteogenic differentiation of MG-63 cells. Furthermore, these cryogels showed prolonged antimicrobial activity against *S. aureus*. The superior crosslinking achieved between gelatin and GO, in addition to its ability to support bone formation and prevent infection make this an attractive approach for BTE application.

TABLE 9.1
The Antibacterial, Osteogenic, Angiogenic, and Osteointegrative Properties of Various Metals Used for BTE

	Properties							Reference
Cation	Nontoxic	Antibacterial	Drug Delivery Capacity	Osteoinductive	Angiogenesis	Mechanical/ Electrical Property	Osteointegration	
Silver	Y	Y	Y	Y	N	Y	N	Stanić et al. (2011) Devi & Vijayalakshmi (2020) Chambard et al. (2020) Saini et al. (2019) Anjaneyulu et al. (2017) Xu et al. (2016) Erdem et al. (2022)
Zinc	Y	Y	Y	Y	Y	Y	N	Jin et al. (2014) Xiong et al. (2017) Yang et al. (2018) Pan et al. (2020) Fernandes et al. (2020) Yang et al. (2017) Komarova et al. (2020) Xie et al. (2019) Xiao et al. (2018)
Gold	Y	Y	Y	Y	N	Y	N	Yi et al. (2010) Li et al. (2016) Banerjee et al. (2018)
Strontium	Y	N (with antibiotics)	Y	Y	Y (growth factors)	Y	N	Huang et al. (2013) Zhou et al. (2015) Yu et al. (2017a) Curran et al. (2011) Zhang et al. (2019c)
Cobalt	Y	N	Y	N	Y	Y	N	Kargozar et al. (2017) Mani (2016) Kulanthaivel et al. (2021) Kulanthaivel et al. (2016) Kahaie Khosrowshahi et al. (2021) Lin et al. (2019)
Magnesium	Y	N (with antibiotics)	Y	Y	N	Y	N	Predoi et al. (2019) Singh et al. (2015) Bose et al. (2018) Swetha et al. (2021) Yedekçi et al. (2022)

Y = yes and N = no

9.2.3.2 Metallic Nanocomposites

Metallic nanocomposites are materials that combine nanoparticles with metals, such as titanium (Ti) or magnesium (Mg). These materials can be used as implants or coatings for bone healing. Table 9.1 shows the various properties of different metal ions for bone regeneration. GO/Hap has been deposited over Ti substrates using electrophoretic, electrochemical, and thermal spray techniques (Zhao et al., 2011; Fu et al., 2015; Chavez-Valdez et al., 2013). By controlling the thickness, morphology, and crystallinity of apatite, there was increased adhesive and cohesive strength, fracture toughness, and biological activity.

Zanin et al. (2013) prepared globular nano-Hap onto rGO by electrodeposition that was found biocompatible with MSC. Oyefusi et al. (2014) established more cellular proliferation and a greater osteogenic response of human fetal osteoblastic cell line on GO/Hap coatings than did bare Ti substrate. Functional bioactive coatings over the metallic implant impart various properties to them. Metallic, polymeric, ceramic, and carbon based have shown significant improvement in the osteogenic potential of bare implants. The addition or substitution of various cations and anions impart certain functionalities and biological modalities to make the otherwise osteoconductive Hap into osteoinductive. Liu et al. (2014b) cultured osteoblast cells on the composite coatings showing a higher proliferation rate and better stretching behavior on the Hap-based coatings than on bare Ti. Adding nanoparticles, such as silver (Ag) or zinc (Zn), can improve the antimicrobial properties and biocompatibility of the metallic matrix as well as enhance the bone-forming ability and angiogenic potential.

9.2.3.3 Ceramic Nanocomposites

Ceramic nanocomposites are materials that combine nanoparticles with ceramics, such as HA, calcium sulphates, CaP, or TCP. These materials can be used as bone substitutes or coatings for bone implants. Adding nanoparticles can improve the mechanical strength, bioactivity, and osteoinductivity of the ceramic matrix, as well as enhance the bone-bonding ability and antibacterial properties.

To enhance the physical, osteogenic, and angiogenic properties of calcium-sulfate-based bone cement, Chopra et al. (2023) synthesized gold nanodots and nanohydroxyapatite-decorated rGO sheets (AuHp@rGO) and incorporated them in the chitosan (CS) system (Figure 9.5). These sheets were further functionalized with vancomycin (used as a model drug) to provide antibacterial activity. The modified CS displayed favorable timing for setting and injectability, along with superior mechanical properties and slower degradation rates than existing cement formulations. MSCs and human umbilical vein endothelial cells (HUVECs) showed good bioactivity, antimicrobial property, and biocompatibility.

Additionally, due to the local release of calcium and gold ions, there was a paracrine signaling mediated crosstalk between MSCs and HUVECs seeded on these cements. This resulted in the upregulation of various markers like BMP-2 and RUNX-2. These bone cements also showed improvement in bone volume/total volume ratio and bone remodeling in the rat cranial defect model and enhanced CD31/endomucin staining for vascularized bone formation. The cement also exhibited enhanced endothelial cell recruitment in an in vivo wound model. Overall, the results showed the synergistic and strengthening effects of AuHp@rGO nanosheets and calcium sulfate hemihydrate-based injectable bone cement for bone defect repair. In brief, nanocomposites offer a promising approach for bone healing due to their ability to combine the advantages of different materials and achieve synergistic effects. However, the design and optimization of nanocomposites for bone healing require careful consideration of their composition, structure, and processing parameters, as well as their biocompatibility and safety.

9.3 BONE DISEASES

Bone-related diseases pose a significant threat to the health of people worldwide; the most prevalent bone-related illnesses are osteoporosis, osteoarthritis, bone metastasis, osteomyelitis, myeloma, and bone defects, with each disease requiring a distinct treatment approach. For osteoporosis and osteoarthritis, medications such as estrogen substitutes, calcitonin, chondroitin sulfate, or glucosamine are commonly used. On the other hand, bisphosphonates, denosumab, and cytotoxic agents are commonly used to treat bone metastasis and myeloma, along with radiotherapy (Lee et al., 2023). When treating bone damage, substitute materials such as titanium alloys are used to fill or replace the damaged area (Pan et al., 2020). While these treatments have been effective, they come with inherent problems such as short drug retention time, low drug protection, low accumulation at the lesion site, and implant-related infection or nondegradable issues.

9.3.1 Osteosarcoma

Osteosarcoma is a type of bone cancer that arises from bone-forming cells called osteoblasts. It typically occurs in children, teenagers, and young adults and is the most common type of primary bone cancer (Luetke et al., 2014). Osteosarcoma can develop in any bone but most commonly occurs in the long bones of the arms or legs, particularly near the knee.

The exact cause of osteosarcoma is not known, but certain risk factors have been identified including a history of radiation therapy, certain inherited genetic conditions, and certain bone diseases such as Paget's disease. Symptoms of osteosarcoma include pain and swelling in the affected area as well as difficulty moving the affected limb. Treatment for osteosarcoma typically involves a combination of surgery, chemotherapy, and sometimes radiation therapy. The specific treatment plan will depend on the location and extent of the tumor, as well as the age and overall health of the patient. The prognosis for osteosarcoma varies depending on the stage and location of the tumor, but overall, the outlook has improved in recent years with advances in treatment (Gill & Gorlick, 2021). Table S9.2 classifies the various types of nanomaterials and the active moieties used for osteosarcoma therapy. Some examples are illustrated in Figure 9.6.

9.3.2 Osteoporosis

Primary osteoporosis (OSP) is characterized by hormonal changes and aging, while in secondary OSP, bone loss is caused by underlying medical conditions or medication use (Clayton & Hochberg, 2013). This musculoskeletal disease affects many individuals, leading to fragile and brittle bones, increased risk of fractures, and reduced quality of life (Wei et al., 2016). Dysregulation of normal bone homeostasis is a hallmark of OSP, where increased osteoclast activity leads to accelerated bone turnover and decreased bone mineral density. Additionally, pro-inflammatory proteins and cytokines contribute to bone resorption and slow bone formation. Depending on the underlying cause, OSP can be classified as primary or secondary. Table S9.3 shows the various nanotechniques used and Figure 9.7 illustrates some examples.

9.3.3 Osteoarthritis

Osteoarthritis (OA) is a common joint disease that affects millions of people worldwide. It is a chronic condition that occurs when the cartilage that cushions the joints wears down over time, leading to pain, stiffness, and a limited range of motion in the affected joint. OA can affect any joint in the body, but it is most commonly found in the knees, hips, and hands. It is often associated with aging, but it can also occur due to injury, repetitive use, or a genetic predisposition (Bottini et al., 2016).

OA causes degeneration of the joints; it occurs when chondrocytes, which are the cells responsible for generating and maintaining cartilage, shift from their normal, cartilage-generating state to a cartilage-breaking down, or catabolic, state. In this catabolic state, the chondrocytes engage in autophagy, which is a natural protective mechanism that allows the cells to break down damaged proteins and organelles. OA is also typically associated with hypertrophy, which refers to an increase in cell volume (Holyoak et al., 2016). The different nanoparticles and nanocomposites used are described in Figure 9.8.

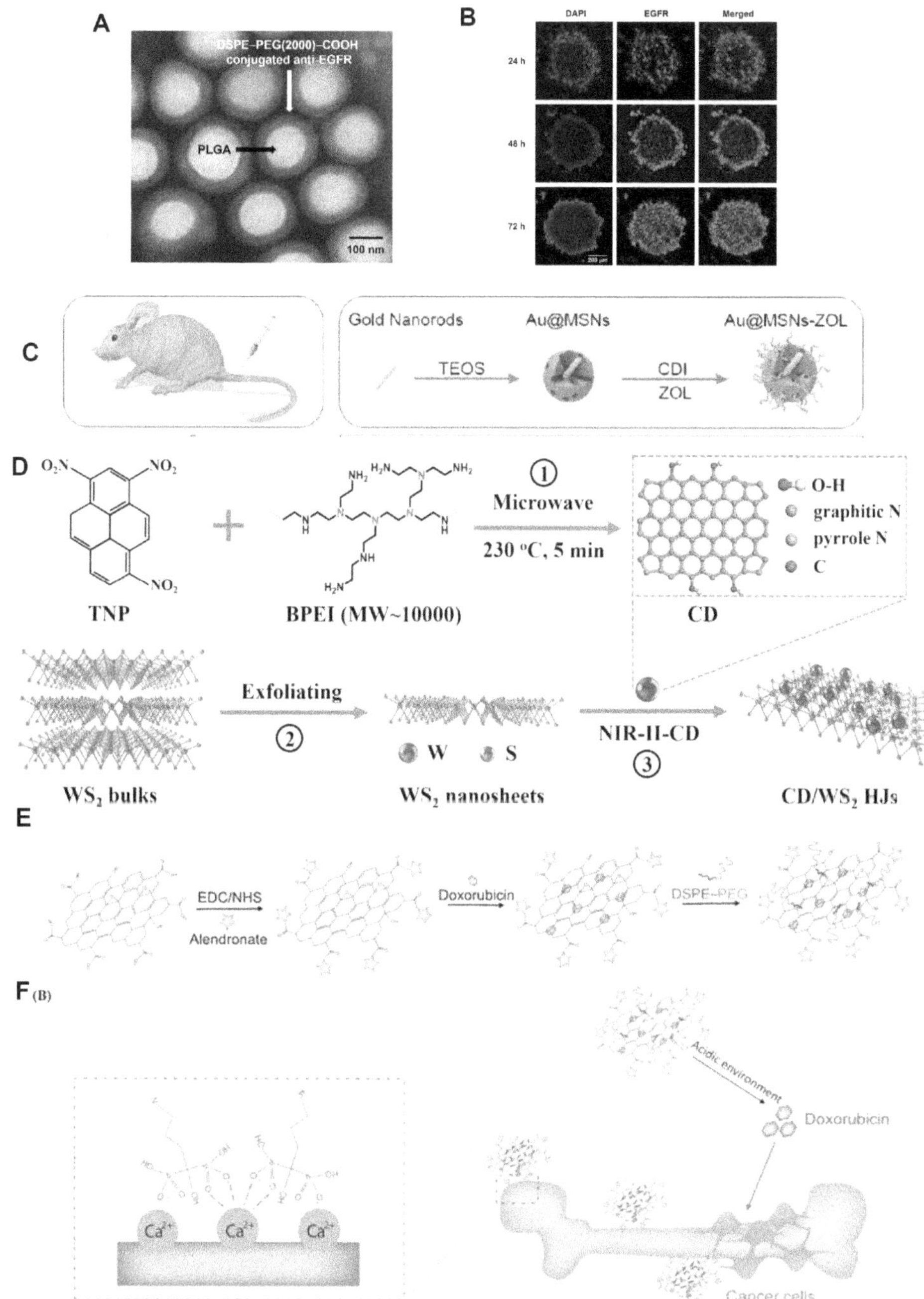

FIGURE 9.6 (A) TEM image that shows the core-shell structure of doxorubicin, sodium 131- iodide, and anti-EGFR-loaded in PLGA nanoparticles (DIE-NPs), with a scale bar of 100 nm. (B) The penetration of the DIE-NPs in a 3D human MG-63 tumor spheroid; the spheroids are treated at different incubation times (24, 48, and 72 h) with Alexa Fluor 647 antihuman EGFR antibody conjugated to the surface of the DIE-NPs, which appears as red fluorescence in the images. The scale bar is 200 μm (reproduced under the terms of CC-BY 4.0 (https://creativecommons.org/licenses/by/4.0/) International License from Marshall, S. K., Saelim, B., Taweesap, M., Pachana, V., Panrak, Y., Makchuchit, N., & Jaroenpakdee, P.: Anti-EGFR Targeted Multifunctional I-131 Radio-Nanotherapeutic for Treating Osteosarcoma: In Vitro 3D Tumor Spheroid Model. Nanomaterials. 2022. 12. 3517. Copyright 2022 Marshall et al., published by MDPI). (C) Gold nanorods enclosed inside mesoporous

silica nanoparticles (Au@MSNs) conjugated to zoledronate for breast cancer photothermal therapy (reproduced with permission from Sun, W., Ge, K., Jin, Y., Han, Y., Zhang, H., Zhou, G., Yang, X., Liu, D., Liu, H., Liang, X.J. & Zhang, J.: Bone-targeted nanoplatform combining zoledronate and photothermal therapy to treat breast cancer bone metastasis. ACS Nano. 2019. 13. 7556–7567. Copyright 2019 American Chemical Society). (D) Synthesis of carbon dot/WS2 heterojunctions for NIR-II enhanced photothermal therapy of osteosarcoma (reproduced with permission from Geng, B., Qin, H., Shen, W., Li, P., Fang, F., Li, X., Pan, D. & Shen, L.: Carbon dot/WS2 heterojunctions for NIR-II enhanced photothermal therapy of osteosarcoma and bone regeneration. Chem. EngI. 2020. 383. 123102. Copyright 2020 Elsevier). (E) Scheme of synthesis of DOX@PEG-NGO-AL complexes and (F) targeted delivery of doxorubicin to bone tumor microenvironment by strong chelation of alendronate functionalized NGOs with hydroxyapatite (reproduced with permission from Pham, T. T., Nguyen, H. T., Dai Phung, C., Pathak, S., Regmi, S., Ha, D. H., Kim, J. O., Yong, C. S., Kim, S. K., Choi, J. E. & Yook, S.: Targeted delivery of doxorubicin for the treatment of bone metastasis from breast cancer using alendronate-functionalized graphene oxide nanosheets. J. Ind. Eng. Chem. 2019. 76. 310–317. Copyright 2019 Elsevier).

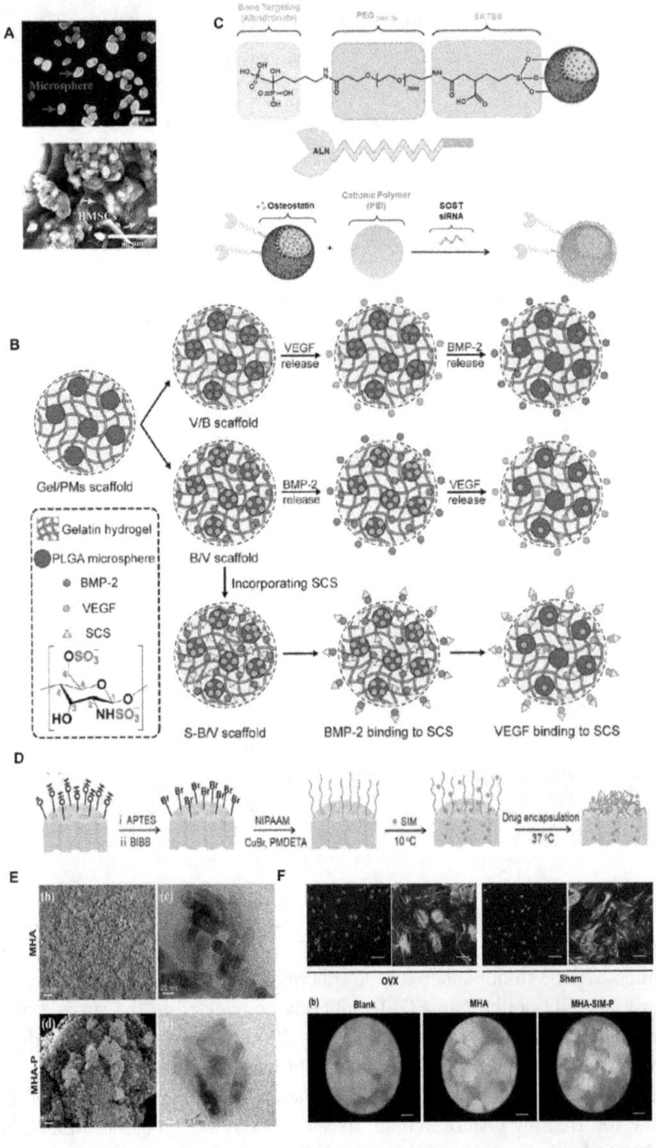

FIGURE 9.7 (A) Composite microspheres of n-HA/resveratrol/chitosan with synergistic anti-inflammatory and osteogenic properties for regenerating osteoporotic bone (reproduced under the terms of CC-BY 4.0

(https://creativecommons.org/licenses/by/4.0/) International License from Li, L., Yu, M., Li, Y., Li, Q., Yang, H., Zheng, M., Han, Y., Lu, D., Lu, S. & Gui, L.: Synergistic anti-inflammatory and osteogenic n-HA/resveratrol/chitosan composite microspheres for osteoporotic bone regeneration. Bioact. Mater. 2021. 6. 1255–1266. Copyright 2021 Li et al., published by Elsevier). (B) Sequential release of BMP-2 and VEGF was achieved through the preparation of VEGF in hydrogel and BMP in PLGA microsphere (V/B) and BMP in hydrogel and VEGF in PLGA microsphere (B/V) scaffolds. The SCS and BMP in hydrogel and VEGF in PLGA microsphere B/V scaffolds (S-B/V) scaffold demonstrated superior binding efficiency and sustained release dynamics, attributed to the interaction between SCS and BMP-2-VEGF (reproduced with permission from Zhang, S., Chen, J., Yu, Y., Dai, K., Wang, J., & Liu, C.: Accelerated bone regenerative efficiency by regulating sequential release of BMP-2 and VEGF and synergism with sulfated chitosan. ACS Biomater. Sci. Eng. 2019b. 5. 1944–1955. Copyright 2019 American Chemical Society). (C) Alendronate-modified PEG was used to functionalize the surface of mesoporous silica nanoparticles. Osteostatin was loaded onto the nanoparticles, which were then coated with a cationic polymer and bound to sclerostin short-interfering RNA to form the final system, which showed osteoporosis remission and new bone formation (reproduced under the terms of CC-BY 4.0 (https://creativecommons.org/licenses/by/4.0/) International License from Mora-Raimundo, P., Lozano, D., Benito, M., Mulero, F., Manzano, M., & Vallet-Regí, M.: Osteoporosis remission and new bone formation with mesoporous silica nanoparticles. Adv. Sci. 2021. 8. e2101107. Copyright 2021 Mora-Raimundo et al., published by Wiley-VCH GmbH). (D) The synthesis of mesoporous hydroxyapatite (MHA), poly(N-isopropylacrylamide and simvastatin conjugated mesoporous hydroxyapatite (MHA-SIM-P). (E) TEM images of MHA and MHA-SIM-P scale bar is 20 nm. and (F) the cellular skeleton of ovariectomized mice model (OVX) and sham BMSCs were imaged using fluorescence microscopy (a; bar = 100 μm). Alizarin Red staining was performed on OVX BMSCs in Blank, MHA, or MHA-SIM-P osteogenic medium for 14 days and imaged (b; bar = 200 μm) (reproduced under the terms of CC-BY 4.0 (https://creativecommons.org/licenses/by/4.0/) International License from Wu, T., Sun, J., Tan, L., Yan, Q., Li, L., Chen, L., Liu, X. & Bin, S.: Enhanced osteogenesis and therapy of osteoporosis using simvastatin loaded hybrid system. Bioact. Mater. 2020. 5. 348–357. Copyright 2020 Wu et al., published by Elsevier).

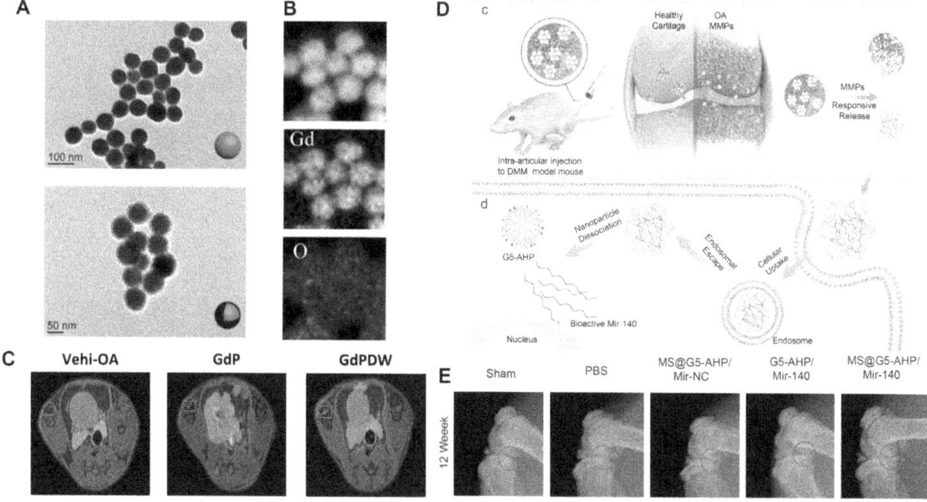

FIGURE 9.8 (A) TEM images that illustrate the typical morphology of two types of nanoparticles (NPs): $Gd_2(CO_3)_3$ and $Gd_2(CO_3)_3$@PDA (GdP). (B) EDX element mapping that illustrates the spatial distribution of Gd and O in GdP. (C) The ability of different NPs to target cartilage in vivo was assessed in anterior cruciate ligament transection-induced osteoarthritis (OA) mice using T1-weighted magnetic resonance imaging (reproduced with permission from Ouyang, Z., Tan, T., Liu, C., Duan, J., Wang, W., Guo, X., Zhang, Q., Li, Z., Huang, Q., Dou, P. & Liu, T.: Targeted delivery of hesperetin to cartilage attenuates osteoarthritis by bimodal imaging with $Gd_2(CO_3)_3$@ PDA nanoparticles via TLR-2/NF-κB/Akt signaling. Biomaterials. 2019. 205. 50–63. Copyright 2019 Elsevier). (D) To alleviate OA progression, c) MS@G5-AHP/miR-140 was introduced into the articular cavity. d) Uptake of G5-AHP/miR-140 polypIIs by endocytosis and subsequent miR-140 release. (E) Mouse knee joints were imaged using

X-ray radiography to display the administration of phosphate-buffered saline, MS@G5-AHP/miR-NC, G5-AHP/miR-140, and MS@G5-AHP/miR-140 within the intra-articular space for treating osteoarthritis induced by destabilization of the medial meniscus. The radiographs were captured at 12 weeks following the surgery (reproduced under the terms of CC-BY 4.0 (https://creativecommons.org/licenses/by/4.0/) International License from Li, B., Wang, F., Hu, F., Ding, T., Huang, P., Xu, X., Liang, J., Li, C., Zhou, Q., Lu, M. & Deng, L.: Injectable "nano-micron" combined gene-hydrogel microspheres for local treatment of osteoarthritis. NPG Asia Mater. 2022. 14. 1. Copyright 2022 Li et al., published by Nature Portfolio).

9.4 CHALLENGES

Nanotechnology has emerged as a promising approach for bone regeneration due to its unique ability to manipulate materials at the nanoscale level. However, there are several challenges faced by nanotechnology in bone regeneration.

Biocompatibility: One of the most significant challenges in using nanomaterials for bone regeneration is ensuring their biocompatibility. Nanomaterials can trigger an immune response in the body, leading to inflammation and tissue damage.

Toxicity: Some nanoparticles have been shown to be toxic to cells and tissues. The toxicity of nanomaterials can depend on their size, shape, surface charge, and composition.

Regulating cell behavior: The interaction between nanomaterials and cells is complex and still needs to be fully understood. It is crucial to design nanomaterials that can regulate cell behavior, such as promoting cell adhesion, proliferation, and differentiation, to achieve optimal bone regeneration.

Achieving optimal mechanical properties: The mechanical properties of nanomaterials play a critical role in their effectiveness in bone regeneration. However, achieving optimal mechanical properties while maintaining biocompatibility and minimizing toxicity is challenging.

Cost-effectiveness: Developing and producing nanomaterials for bone regeneration can be expensive, which can limit their accessibility and widespread use.

Clinical translation: The lack of appropriate and standard procedures before clinical trials, physiological differences in animal models and lack of in vitro–in vivo correlation has led to difficulties in clinical translation.

CONCLUSION

Nanotechnology has shown great promise in the field of bone tissue engineering, as seen above, which involves the use of biomaterials and cells to regenerate or repair damaged bone tissue. Nanoparticles can be engineered to carry drugs or growth factors that stimulate bone growth and repair. These NPs can be designed to release their cargo at a specific time or location, providing a controlled and sustained release of the therapeutic agent.

Nanofibers and nanocomposites made from materials such as collagen, hydroxyapatite, and polymers have been developed to mimic the structure of natural bone. These materials can be used as scaffolds to support the growth and differentiation of stem cells into bone tissue. NPs can be used to improve the imaging of bone tissue. For example, magnetic NPs can be used in magnetic resonance imaging to provide a clearer picture of bone structure and regeneration.

Nanomechanical testing can be used to analyze the mechanical properties of bone at the nanoscale level, providing insights into the bone's strength and potential for regeneration. Nanotechnology can be used to modify the surface properties of materials used in BTE, such as increasing their hydrophilicity, which can improve cell adhesion and proliferation. Overall, nanotechnology has the potential to revolutionize BTE by improving the efficiency and effectiveness of therapeutic agents and enhancing the mechanical properties of scaffolds, leading to better outcomes for patients with bone injuries and diseases.

ACKNOWLEDGEMENTS

The authors (V.C and D.G) thank the Science and Engineering Research Board, India, for funding (CRG/2018/000213, SPF/2021/000151. The authors thank the Institute of Nanoscience and Technology, Mohali, India, for providing support for the doctoral program and infrastructure. V.C and S.O.M.C acknowledge funding from the Federico Bauer Foundation (ILST002–21ID14002).

LIST OF ABBREVIATIONS

BMPs	Bone morphogenetic proteins
CaP	Calcium phosphate
DOX	Doxorubicin
ECM	Extracellular matrix
EGFR	Epidermal growth factor receptor
GO	Graphene oxide
HA	Hydroxyapatite
iNOS	Inducible nitric oxide synthase
M2	Alternatively activated macrophages
MBG	Mesoporous bioactive glass
MHA	Mesoporous hydroxyapatite
micro-CT	Computerized microtomography
MRI	Magnetic resonance imaging
MSCs	Mesenchymal stem cells
NC	Nanocement
NIR	Near-infrared imaging
OA	Osteoarthritis
OSP	Osteoporosis
PEG	Polyethylene glycol
rGO	Reduced graphene oxide
RUNX2	Runt-related transcription factor 2
SA	Sodium alginate
SEM	Scanning electron microscope
SIM	Simvastatin
TCP	Tricalcium phosphate
TEM	Transmission electron microscopy
TGF	Transforming growth factor
VEGF	Vascular endothelial growth factor

REFERENCES

Ai, F., Chen, L., Yan, J., Yang, K., Li, S., Duan, H., Cao, C., Li, W., & Zhou, K. (2020). Hydroxyapatite scaffolds containing copper for bone tissue engineering. *J. Sol-Gel Sci. Technol.* 95: 168–179.

Anjaneyulu, U., Priyadarshini, B., Nirmala Grace, A., & Vijayalakshmi, U. (2017). Fabrication and characterization of Ag doped hydroxyapatite-polyvinyl alcohol composite nanofibers and its in vitro biological evaluations for bone tissue engineering applications. *J. Sol-Gel Sci. Technol.* 81: 750–761.

Azeena, S., Subhapradha, N., Selvamurugan, N., Narayan, S., Srinivasan, N., Murugesan, R., Chung, T. W., & Moorthi, A. (2017). Antibacterial activity of agricultural waste derived wollastonite doped with copper for bone tissue engineering. *Mater. Sci. Eng. C.* 71: 1156–1165.

Banerjee, S., Bagchi, B., Bhandary, S., Kool, A., Hoque, N. A., Thakur, P., & Das, S. (2018). A facile vacuum assisted synthesis of nanoparticle impregnated hydroxyapatite composites having excellent antimicrobial properties and biocompatibility. *Ceram. Int.* 44: 1066–1077.

Bose, S., Vu, A. A., Emshadi, K., & Bandyopadhyay, A. (2018). Effects of polycaprolactone on alendronate drug release from Mg-doped hydroxyapatite coating on titanium. *Mater. Sci. Eng. C.* 88: 166–171.

Bottini, M., Bhattacharya, K., Fadeel, B., Magrini, A., Bottini, N., & Rosato, N. (2016). Nanodrugs to target articular cartilage: An emerging platform for osteoarthritis therapy. *Nanomedicine: NBM*. 12: 255–268.

Castro, A. G., Diba, M., Kersten, M., Jansen, J. A., van den Beucken, J. J., & Yang, F. (2018). Development of a PCL-silica nanoparticles composite membrane for guided bone regeneration. *Mater. Sci. Eng. C*. 85: 154–161.

Chambard, M., Remache, D., Balcaen, Y., Dalverny, O., Alexis, J., Siadous, R., Bareille, R., Catros, S., Fort, P., Grossin, D., & Gitzhofer, F. (2020). Effect of silver and strontium incorporation route on hydroxyapatite coatings elaborated by rf-SPS. *Materialia*. 12: 100809.

Chavez-Valdez, A. R. B. A., Shaffer, M. S., & Boccaccini, A. R. (2013). Applications of graphene electrophoretic deposition: A review. *J. Phys. Chem. B*. 117: 1502–1515.

Chopra, V., Thomas, J., Chauhan, G., Kaushik, S., Rajput, S., Guha, R., Chattopadhyay, N., Martinez-Chapa, S. O., & Ghosh, D. (2022). Gelatin nanofibers loaded with zinc-doped hydroxyapatite for osteogenic differentiation of mesenchymal stem cells. *ACS Appl. Nano Mater*. 5: 2414–2428.

Chopra, V., Thomas, J., Kaushik, S., Rajput, S., Guha, R., Mondal, B., Naskar, S., Mandal, D., Chauhan, G., Chattopadhyay, N., & Ghosh, D. (2023). Injectable bone cement reinforced with gold nanodots decorated rGO-hydroxyapatite nanocomposites, augment bone regeneration. *Small*. 19: e2204637.

Chopra, V., Thomas, J., Sharma, A., Panwar, V., Kaushik, S., & Ghosh, D. (2021). A bioinspired, ice-templated multifunctional 3D cryogel composite crosslinked through in situ reduction of GO displayed improved mechanical, osteogenic and antimicrobial properties. *Mater. Sci. Eng. C*. 119: 111584.

Chopra, V., Thomas, J., Sharma, A., Panwar, V., Kaushik, S., Sharma, S., Porwal, K., Kulkarni, C., Rajput, S., Singh, H., & Jagavelu, K. (2020). Synthesis and evaluation of a zinc eluting rGO/hydroxyapatite nanocomposite optimized for bone augmentation. *ACS Biomater. Sci. Eng*. 6: 6710–6725.

Chu, T. M. G., Liu, S. S. Y., & Babler, W. J. (2014). Craniofacial biology, orthodontics, and implants. In *Basic and Applied Bone Biology*. D. B. Burr, and M. R. Allen, Eds. Massachusetts: Elsevier, pp. 225–242.

Clayton, E. S., & Hochberg, M. C. (2013). Osteoporosis and osteoarthritis, rheumatoid arthritis and spondyloarthropathies. *Curr. Osteoporos. Rep*. 11: 257–262.

Curran, D. J., Fleming, T. J., Towler, M. R., & Hampshire, S. (2011). Mechanical parameters of strontium doped hydroxyapatite sintered using microwave and conventional methods. *J. Mech. Behav. Biomed. Mater*. 4: 2063–2073.

Das, A., Kumar, A., Patil, N. B., Viswanathan, C., & Ghosh, D. (2015). Preparation and characterization of silver nanoparticle loaded amorphous hydrogel of carboxymethylcellulose for infected wounds. *Carbohydr. Polym*. 130: 254–261.

Devi, P. S., & Vijayalakshmi, K. A. (2020). Analysis of antibacterial activity and cytotoxicity of silver oxide doped hydroxyapatite exposed to DC glow discharge plasma. *Mater. Today: Proc*. 26: 3604–3608.

Erdem, R., Yavuz, E., Akarsu, E., Akarsu, M., Yılmaz, Ö. E., & Coşgun, A. (2022). Electrospinning of antibacterial scaffolds composed of poly (L-lactide-co-ε-caprolactone)/collagen type I/silver doped hydroxyapatite particles: Potential material for bone tissue engineering. *J. Text. Inst*. 114: 1–14.

Fan, Z., Wang, J., Wang, Z., Ran, H., Li, Y., Niu, L., Gong, P., Liu, B., & Yang, S. (2014). One-pot synthesis of graphene/hydroxyapatite nanorod composite for tissue engineering. *Carbon*. 66: 407–416.

Farbod, K., Diba, M., Zinkevich, T., Schmidt, S., Harrington, M. J., Kentgens, A. P., & Leeuwenburgh, S. C. (2016). Gelatin nanoparticles with enhanced affinity for calcium phosphate. *Macromol. Biosci*. 16: 717–729.

Fernandes, M. H., Alves, M. M., Cebotarenco, M., Ribeiro, I. A., Grenho, L., Gomes, P. S., Carmezim, M. J., & Santos, C. F. (2020). Citrate zinc hydroxyapatite nanorods with enhanced cytocompatibility and osteogenesis for bone regeneration. *Mater. Sci. Eng. C*. 115: 111147.

Fu, C., Song, B., Wan, C., Savino, K., Wang, Y., Zhang, X., & Yates, M. Z. (2015). Electrochemical growth of composite hydroxyapatite coatings for controlled release. *Surf. Coat. Technol*. 276: 618–625.

Gadekar, V., Borade, Y., Kannaujia, S., Rajpoot, K., Anup, N., Tambe, V., Kalia, K., & Tekade, R. K. (2021). Nanomedicines accessible in the market for clinical interventions. *J. Control. Release*. 330: 372–397.

Geng, B., Qin, H., Shen, W., Li, P., Fang, F., Li, X., Pan, D., & Shen, L. (2020). Carbon dot/WS2 heterojunctions for NIR-II enhanced photothermal therapy of osteosarcoma and bone regeneration. *Chem. Eng. J*. 383: 123102.

Ghavimi, M. A., Bani Shahabadi, A., Jarolmasjed, S., Memar, M. Y., Maleki Dizaj, S., & Sharifi, S. (2020). Nanofibrous asymmetric collagen/curcumin membrane containing aspirin-loaded PLGA nanoparticles for guided bone regeneration. *Sci. Rep*. 10: 1–15.

Gill, J., & Gorlick, R. (2021). Advancing therapy for osteosarcoma. *Nat. Rev. Clin. Oncol*. 18: 609–624.

Hajiali, H., Ouyang, L., Llopis-Hernandez, V., Dobre, O., & Rose, F. R. (2021). Review of emerging nanotechnology in bone regeneration: Progress, challenges, and perspectives. *Nanoscale*. 13: 10266–10280.

Hasan, A., Waibhaw, G., Saxena, V., & Pandey, L. M. (2018). Nano-biocomposite scaffolds of chitosan, carboxymethyl cellulose and silver nanoparticle modified cellulose nanowhiskers for bone tissue engineering applications. *Int. J. Biol. Macromol.* 111: 923–934.

Heidari, F., Bahrololoom, M. E., Vashaee, D., & Tayebi, L. (2015). In situ preparation of iron oxide nanoparticles in natural hydroxyapatite/chitosan matrix for bone tissue engineering application. *Ceram. Int.* 41: 3094–3100.

Holyoak, D. T., Tian, Y. F., van der Meulen, M. C., & Singh, A. (2016). Osteoarthritis: Pathology, mouse models, and nanoparticle injectable systems for targeted treatment. *Ann. Biomed. Eng.* 44: 2062–2075.

Hong-Pei, L., Yingbo, W., Zhi, S., Xiong, L., & Wang, S. (2015). Electrospinning gelatin/chitosan/hydroxyapatite/graphene oxide composite nanofibers with antibacterial properties. *J. Inorg. Mater.* 30: 516–522.

Hosseinpour, S., Walsh, L. J., & Xu, C. (2021). Modulating osteoimmune responses by mesoporous silica nanoparticles. *ACS Biomater. Sci. Eng.* 8: 4110–4122.

Huang, B., Chen, M., Tian, J., Zhang, Y., Dai, Z., Li, J., & Zhang, W. (2022). Oxygen-carrying and antibacterial fluorinated nano-hydroxyapatite incorporated hydrogels for enhanced bone regeneration. *Adv. Healthc. Mater.* 11: 2102540.

Huang, Y., Yan, Y., Pang, X., Ding, Q., & Han, S. (2013). Bioactivity and corrosion properties of gelatin-containing and strontium-doped calcium phosphate composite coating. *Appl. Surf. Sci.* 282: 583–589.

Ilhan, M., Kilicarslan, M., & Orhan, K. (2022). Effect of process variables on in vitro characteristics of clindamycin phosphate loaded PLGA nanoparticles in dental bone regeneration and 3D characterization studies using nano-CT. *J. Drug Deliv. Sci. Technol.* 76: 103710.

J Hill, M., Qi, B., Bayaniahangar, R., Araban, V., Bakhtiary, Z., Doschak, M. R., Goh, B. C., Shokouhimehr, M., Vali, H., Presley, J. F., & Zadpoor, A. A. (2019). Nanomaterials for bone tissue regeneration: Updates and future perspectives. *Nanomedicine*. 14: 2987–3006.

Jin, G., Qin, H., Cao, H., Qian, S., Zhao, Y., Peng, X., Zhang, X., Liu, X., & Chu, P. K. (2014). Synergistic effects of dual Zn/Ag ion implantation in osteogenic activity and antibacterial ability of titanium. *Biomaterials*. 35: 7699–7713.

Jin, S., Xia, X., Huang, J., Yuan, C., Zuo, Y., Li, Y., & Li, J. (2021). Recent advances in PLGA-based biomaterials for bone tissue regeneration. *Acta Biomater.* 127: 56–79.

Kargozar, S., Lotfibakhshaiesh, N., Ai, J., Mozafari, M., Milan, P. B., Hamzehlou, S., Barati, M., Baino, F., Hill, R. G., & Joghataei, M. T. (2017). Strontium-and cobalt-substituted bioactive glasses seeded with human umbilical cord perivascular cells to promote bone regeneration via enhanced osteogenic and angiogenic activities. *Acta Biomater.* 58: 502–514.

Khosrowshahi, A. K., Khoshfetrat, A. B., Khosrowshahi, Y. B., & Maleki-Ghaleh, H. (2021). Cobalt content modulates characteristics and osteogenic properties of cobalt-containing hydroxyapatite in in-vitro milieu. *Mater. Today Commun.* 27: 102392.

Kim, H. D., Jang, H. L., Ahn, H. Y., Lee, H. K., Park, J., Lee, E. S., Lee, E. A., Jeong, Y. H., Kim, D. G., Nam, K. T., & Hwang, N. S. (2017). Biomimetic whitlockite inorganic nanoparticles-mediated in situ remodeling and rapid bone regeneration. *Biomaterials*. 112: 31–43.

Komarova, E. G., Sharkeev, Y. P., Sedelnikova, M. B., Prymak, O., Epple, M., Litvinova, L. S., Shupletsova, V. V., Malashchenko, V. V., Yurova, K. A., Dzyuman, A. N., & Kulagina, I. V. (2020). Zn-or Cu-containing CaP-based coatings formed by micro-arc oxidation on titanium and Ti-40Nb alloy: Part II—Wettability and biological performance. *Materials*. 13: 4366.

Kulanthaivel, S., Agarwal, T., Rathnam, V. S., Pal, K., & Banerjee, I. (2021). Cobalt doped nano-hydroxyapatite incorporated gum tragacanth-alginate beads as angiogenic-osteogenic cell encapsulation system for mesenchymal stem cell based bone tissue engineering. *Int. J. Biol. Macromol.* 179: 101–115.

Kulanthaivel, S., Roy, B., Agarwal, T., Giri, S., Pramanik, K., Pal, K., Ray, S. S., Maiti, T. K., & Banerjee, I. (2016). Cobalt doped proangiogenic hydroxyapatite for bone tissue engineering application. *Mater. Sci. Eng. C*. 58: 648–658.

La, W. G., Park, S., Yoon, H. H., Jeong, G. J., Lee, T. J., Bhang, S. H., Han, J. Y., Char, K., & Kim, B. S. (2013). Delivery of a therapeutic protein for bone regeneration from a substrate coated with graphene oxide. *Small*. 9: 4051–4060.

Lee, C. S., Singh, R. K., Hwang, H. S., Lee, N. H., Kurian, A. G., Lee, J. H., Kim, H. S., Lee, M., & Kim, H. W. (2023). Materials-based nanotherapeutics for injured and diseased bone. *Prog. Mater. Sci.* 135: 101087.

Lee, J. H., Shin, Y. C., Lee, S. M., Jin, O. S., Kang, S. H., Hong, S. W., Jeong, C. M., Huh, J. B., & Han, D. W. (2015). Enhanced osteogenesis by reduced graphene oxide/hydroxyapatite nanocomposites. *Sci. Rep.* 5: 18833.

Lei, L., Liu, Z., Yuan, P., Jin, R., Wang, X., Jiang, T., & Chen, X. (2019). Injectable colloidal hydrogel with mesoporous silica nanoparticles for sustained co-release of microRNA-222 and aspirin to achieve innervated bone regeneration in rat mandibular defects. *J. Mater. Chem. B.* 7: 2722–2735.

Levingstone, T. J., Herbaj, S., & Dunne, N. J. (2019). Calcium phosphate nanoparticles for therapeutic applications in bone regeneration. *Nanomaterials.* 9: 1570.

Li, A., Xie, J., & Li, J. (2019). Recent advances in functional nanostructured materials for bone-related diseases. *J. Mater. Chem. B.* 7: 509–527.

Li, B., Wang, F., Hu, F., Ding, T., Huang, P., Xu, X., Liang, J., Li, C., Zhou, Q., Lu, M., & Deng, L. (2022). Injectable "nano-micron" combined gene-hydrogel microspheres for local treatment of osteoarthritis. *NPG Asia Mater.* 14: 1.

Li, H., Ji, Q., Chen, X., Sun, Y., Xu, Q., Deng, P., Hu, F., & Yang, J. (2017). Accelerated bony defect healing based on chitosan thermosensitive hydrogel scaffolds embedded with chitosan nanoparticles for the delivery of BMP2 plasmid DNA. *J. Biomed. Mater. Res. A.* 105: 265–273.

Li, J., Zhang, J., Wang, X., Kawazoe, N., & Chen, G. (2016). Gold nanoparticle size and shape influence on osteogenesis of mesenchymal stem cells. *Nanoscale.* 8: 7992–8007.

Li, L., Yu, M., Li, Y., Li, Q., Yang, H., Zheng, M., Han, Y., Lu, D., Lu, S., & Gui, L. (2021). Synergistic anti-inflammatory and osteogenic n-HA/resveratrol/chitosan composite microspheres for osteoporotic bone regeneration. *Bioact. Mater.* 6: 1255–1266.

Li, M., Wang, Y., Liu, Q., Li, Q., Cheng, Y., Zheng, Y., Xi, T., & Wei, S. (2013). In situ synthesis and biocompatibility of nano hydroxyapatite on pristine and chitosan functionalized graphene oxide. *J. Mater. Chem. B.* 1: 475–484.

Liao, H., Yu, H. P., Song, W., Zhang, G., Lu, B., Zhu, Y. J., Yu, W., & He, Y. (2021). Amorphous calcium phosphate nanoparticles using adenosine triphosphate as an organic phosphorus source for promoting tendon—Bone healing. *J. Nanobiotechnol.* 19: 1–17.

Lin, W. C., Yao, C., Huang, T. Y., Cheng, S. J., & Tang, C. M. (2019). Long-term in vitro degradation behavior and biocompatibility of polycaprolactone/cobalt-substituted hydroxyapatite composite for bone tissue engineering. *Dent. Mater.* 35: 751–762.

Liu, C., Shen, J., Yeung, K. W. K., & Tjong, S. C. (2017). Development and antibacterial performance of novel polylactic acid-graphene oxide-silver nanoparticle hybrid nanocomposite mats prepared by electrospinning. *ACS Biomater. Sci. Eng.* 3: 471–486.

Liu, H., Cheng, J., Chen, F., Bai, D., Shao, C., Wang, J., Xi, P., & Zeng, Z. (2014a). Gelatin functionalized graphene oxide for mineralization of hydroxyapatite: Biomimetic and in vitro evaluation. *Nanoscale.* 6: 5315–5322.

Liu, H., Xi, P., Xie, G., Shi, Y., Hou, F., Huang, L., Chen, F., Zeng, Z., Shao, C., & Wang, J. (2012). Simultaneous reduction and surface functionalization of graphene oxide for hydroxyapatite mineralization. *J. Phys. Chem. C.* 116: 3334–3341.

Liu, Y., Dang, Z., Wang, Y., Huang, J., & Li, H. (2014b). Hydroxyapatite/graphene-nanosheet composite coatings deposited by vacuum cold spraying for biomedical applications: Inherited nanostructures and enhanced properties. *Carbon.* 67: 250–259.

Luetke, A., Meyers, P. A., Lewis, I., & Juergens, H. (2014). Osteosarcoma treatment—Where do we stand? A state of the art review. *Cancer Treat. Rev.* 40: 523–532.

Ma, H., Su, W., Tai, Z., Sun, D., Yan, X., Liu, B., & Xue, Q. (2012). Preparation and cytocompatibility of polylactic acid/hydroxyapatite/graphene oxide nanocomposite fibrous membrane. *Chin. Sci. Bull.* 57: 3051–3058.

Ma, Y., Li, Y., Hao, J., Ma, B., Di, T., & Dong, H. (2019). Evaluation of the degradation, biocompatibility and osteogenesis behavior of lithium-doped calcium polyphosphate for bone tissue engineering. *Bio-Med. Mater. Eng.* 30: 23–36.

Mabrouk, M., Moaness, M., & Beherei, H. H. (2022). Fabrication of mesoporous zirconia and titania nanomaterials for bone regeneration and drug delivery applications. *J. Drug Deliv. Sci. Technol.* 78: 103957.

Maharjan, B., Park, J., Kaliannagounder, V. K., Awasthi, G. P., Joshi, M. K., Park, C. H., & Kim, C. S. (2021). Regenerated cellulose nanofiber reinforced chitosan hydrogel scaffolds for bone tissue engineering. *Carbohydr. Polym.* 251: 117023.

Mani, G. (2016). Metallic biomaterials: Cobalt-chromium alloys. In *Handbook of Biomaterial Properties*. W. Murphy, J. Black, and G. Hastings, Eds. New York: Springer, pp. 159–166.

Marshall, S. K., Saelim, B., Taweesap, M., Pachana, V., Panrak, Y., Makchuchit, N., & Jaroenpakdee, P. (2022). Anti-EGFR targeted multifunctional I-131 radio-nanotherapeutic for treating osteosarcoma: In vitro 3D tumor spheroid model. *Nanomaterials*. 12: 3517.

Mayer, I., Cuisinier, F. J., Popov, I., Schleich, Y., Gdalya, S., Burghaus, O., & Reinen, D. (2006). Phase relations between β-tricalcium phosphate and hydroxyapatite with manganese(II): Structural and spectroscopic properties. *Eur. J. Inorg. Chem.* 2006: 1460–1465.

Mora-Raimundo, P., Lozano, D., Benito, M., Mulero, F., Manzano, M., & Vallet-Regí, M. (2021). Osteoporosis remission and new bone formation with mesoporous silica nanoparticles. *Adv. Sci.* 8: e2101107.

Mu, Z., Chen, K., Yuan, S., Li, Y., Huang, Y., Wang, C., Zhang, Y., Liu, W., Luo, W., Liang, P., & Li, X. (2020). Gelatin nanoparticle-injectable platelet-rich fibrin double network hydrogels with local adaptability and bioactivity for enhanced osteogenesis. *Adv. Healthc. Mater.* 9: 1901469.

Neelgund, G. M., Oki, A., & Luo, Z. (2013). In situ deposition of hydroxyapatite on graphene nanosheets. *Mater. Res. Bull.* 48: 175–179.

Nie, W., Peng, C., Zhou, X., Chen, L., Wang, W., Zhang, Y., Ma, P. X., & He, C. (2017). Three-dimensional porous scaffold by self-assembly of reduced graphene oxide and nano-hydroxyapatite composites for bone tissue engineering. *Carbon*. 116: 325–337.

Ouyang, Z., Tan, T., Liu, C., Duan, J., Wang, W., Guo, X., Zhang, Q., Li, Z., Huang, Q., Dou, P., & Liu, T. (2019). Targeted delivery of hesperetin to cartilage attenuates osteoarthritis by bimodal imaging with Gd2(CO3)3@PDA nanoparticles via TLR-2/NF-κB/Akt signaling. *Biomaterials*. 205: 50–63.

Oyefusi, A., Olanipekun, O., Neelgund, G. M., Peterson, D., Stone, J. M., Williams, E., Carson, L., Regisford, G., & Oki, A. (2014). Hydroxyapatite grafted carbon nanotubes and graphene nanosheets: Promising bone implant materials. *Spectrochim. Acta A*. 132: 410–416.

Pan, C., Hu, Y., Gong, Z., Yang, Y., Liu, S., Quan, L., Yang, Z., Wei, Y., & Ye, W. (2020). Improved blood compatibility and endothelialization of titanium oxide nanotube arrays on titanium surface by zinc doping. *ACS Biomater. Sci. Eng.* 6: 2072–2083.

Peng, S., Feng, P., Wu, P., Huang, W., Yang, Y., Guo, W., Gao, C., & Shuai, C. (2017). Graphene oxide as an interface phase between polyetheretherketone and hydroxyapatite for tissue engineering scaffolds. *Sci. Rep.* 7: 46604.

Pham, T. T., Nguyen, H. T., Dai Phung, C., Pathak, S., Regmi, S., Ha, D. H., Kim, J. O., Yong, C. S., Kim, S. K., Choi, J. E., & Yook, S. (2019). Targeted delivery of doxorubicin for the treatment of bone metastasis from breast cancer using alendronate-functionalized graphene oxide nanosheets. *J. Ind. Eng. Chem.* 76: 310–317.

Predoi, D., Iconaru, S. L., Predoi, M. V., Stan, G. E., & Buton, N. (2019). Synthesis, characterization, and antimicrobial activity of magnesium-doped hydroxyapatite suspensions. *Nanomaterials*. 9: 1295.

Priya, B. A., Senthilguru, K., Agarwal, T., Narayana, S. G. H., Giri, S., Pramanik, K., Pal, K., & Banerjee, I. (2015). Nickel doped nanohydroxyapatite: Vascular endothelial growth factor inducing biomaterial for bone tissue engineering. *RSC Adv.* 5: 72515–72528.

Qiao, K., Xu, L., Tang, J., Wang, Q., Lim, K. S., Hooper, G., Woodfield, T. B., Liu, G., Tian, K., Zhang, W., & Cui, X. (2022). The advances in nanomedicine for bone and cartilage repair. *J. Nanobiotechnol.* 20: 141.

Raftery, R. M., Castaño, I. M., Chen, G., Cavanagh, B., Quinn, B., Curtin, C. M., Cryan, S. A., & O'Brien, F. J. (2017). Translating the role of osteogenic-angiogenic coupling in bone formation: Highly efficient chitosan-pDNA activated scaffolds can accelerate bone regeneration in critical-sized bone defects. *Biomaterials*. 149: 116–127.

Ren, N., Li, J., Qiu, J., Yan, M., Liu, H., Ji, D., Huang, J., Yu, J., & Liu, H. (2017). Growth and accelerated differentiation of mesenchymal stem cells on graphene-oxide-coated titanate with dexamethasone on surface of titanium implants. *Dent. Mater.* 33: 525–535.

Saini, R. K., Bagri, L. P., & Bajpai, A. K. (2019). Nano-silver hydroxyapatite based antibacterial 3D scaffolds of gelatin/alginate/poly (vinyl alcohol) for bone tissue engineering applications. *Colloids Surf. B*. 177: 211–218.

Saxena, V., & Pandey, L. M. (2021). Design and characterization of biphasic ferric hydroxyapatite-zincite nanoassembly for bone tissue engineering. *Ceram. Int.* 47: 28274–28287.

Shams, M., Nezafati, N., Poormoghadam, D., Zavareh, S., Zamanian, A., & Salimi, A. (2020). Synthesis and characterization of electrospun bioactive glass nanofibers-reinforced calcium sulfate bone cement and its cell biological response. *Ceram. Int.* 46: 10029–10039.

Shuai, C., Peng, B., Feng, P., Yu, L., Lai, R., & Min, A. (2022). In situ synthesis of hydroxyapatite nanorods on graphene oxide nanosheets and their reinforcement in biopolymer scaffold. *J. Adv. Res.* 35: 13–24.

Singh, G., Singh, R. P., & Jolly, S. S. (2020). Customized hydroxyapatites for bone-tissue engineering and drug delivery applications: A review. *J. Sol-Gel Sci. Technol.* 94: 505–530.

Singh, J., Singh, H., & Batra, U. (2015). Magnesium doped hydroxyapatite: Synthesis, characterization and bioactivity evaluation. In *Biomaterials Science: Processing, Properties, and Applications V: Ceramic Transactions*. R. Narayan, S. Bose, and A. Bandyopadhyay, Eds. Pennsylvania: The American Ceramic Society, pp. 161–174.

Sruthi, R., Balagangadharan, K., & Selvamurugan, N. (2020). Polycaprolactone/polyvinylpyrrolidone coaxial electrospun fibers containing veratric acid-loaded chitosan nanoparticles for bone regeneration. *Colloids Surf. B.* 193: 111110.

Stanić, V., Janaćković, D., Dimitrijević, S., Tanasković, S. B., Mitrić, M., Pavlović, M. S., Krstić, A., Jovanović, D., & Raičević, S. (2011). Synthesis of antimicrobial monophase silver-doped hydroxyapatite nanopowders for bone tissue engineering. *Appl. Surf. Sci.* 257: 4510–4518.

Sun, W., Ge, K., Jin, Y., Han, Y., Zhang, H., Zhou, G., Yang, X., Liu, D., Liu, H., Liang, X. J., & Zhang, J. (2019). Bone-targeted nanoplatform combining zoledronate and photothermal therapy to treat breast cancer bone metastasis. *ACS Nano.* 13: 7556–7567.

Swetha, S., Balagangadharan, K., Lavanya, K., & Selvamurugan, N. (2021). Three-dimensional-poly(lactic acid) scaffolds coated with gelatin/magnesium-doped nano-hydroxyapatite for bone tissue engineering. *Biotechnol. J.* 16: 2100282.

Tripathi, A., Saravanan, S., Pattnaik, S., Moorthi, A., Partridge, N. C., & Selvamurugan, N. (2012). Bio-composite scaffolds containing chitosan/nano-hydroxyapatite/nano-copper—Zinc for bone tissue engineering. *Int. J. Biol. Macromol.* 50: 294–299.

Ullah, I., Zhang, W., Yang, L., Ullah, M. W., Atta, O. M., Khan, S., Wu, B., Wu, T., & Zhang, X. (2020). Impact of structural features of Sr/Fe co-doped HAp on the osteoblast proliferation and osteogenic differentiation for its application as a bone substitute. *Mater. Sci. Eng. C.* 110: 110633.

Wang, J., Wang, H., Wang, Y., Li, J., Su, Z., & Wei, G. (2014). Alternate layer-by-layer assembly of graphene oxide nanosheets and fibrinogen nanofibers on a silicon substrate for a biomimetic three-dimensional hydroxyapatite scaffold. *J. Mater. Chem. B.* 2: 7360–7368.

Wang, J., Yin, W., He, X., Wang, Q., Guo, M., & Chen, S. (2016a). Good biocompatibility and sintering properties of zirconia nanoparticles synthesized via vapor-phase hydrolysis. *Sci. Rep.* 6: 1–9.

Wang, L., Fang, M., Xia, Y., Hou, J., Nan, X., Zhao, B., & Wang, X. (2020). Preparation and biological properties of silk fibroin/nano-hydroxyapatite/graphene oxide scaffolds with an oriented channel-like structure. *RSC Adv.* 10: 10118–10128.

Wang, Y., Pan, H., & Chen, X. (2019). The Preparation of hollow mesoporous bioglass nanoparticles with excellent drug delivery capacity for bone tissue regeneration. *Front. Chem.* 7: 283.

Wang, Y., Yang, X., Gu, Z., Qin, H., Li, L., Liu, J., & Yu, X. (2016b). In vitro study on the degradation of lithium-doped hydroxyapatite for bone tissue engineering scaffold. *Mater. Sci. Eng. C.* 66: 185–192.

Wei, D., Jung, J., Yang, H., Stout, D. A., & Yang, L. (2016). Nanotechnology treatment options for osteoporosis and its corresponding consequences. *Curr. Osteoporos. Rep.* 14: 239–247.

Wu, A. M., Bisignano, C., James, S. L., Abady, G. G., Abedi, A., Abu-Gharbieh, E., Alhassan, R. K., Alipour, V., Arabloo, J., Asaad, M., & Asmare, W. N. (2021). Global, regional, and national burden of bone fractures in 204 countries and territories, 1990–2019: A systematic analysis from the global burden of disease study 2019. *Lancet Healthy Longev.* 2: e580–e592.

Wu, C., Xia, L., Han, P., Xu, M., Fang, B., Wang, J., Chang, J., & Xiao, Y. (2015). Graphene-oxide-modified β-tricalcium phosphate bioceramics stimulate in vitro and in vivo osteogenesis. *Carbon.* 93: 116–129.

Wu, T., Sun, J., Tan, L., Yan, Q., Li, L., Chen, L., Liu, X., & Bin, S. (2020). Enhanced osteogenesis and therapy of osteoporosis using simvastatin loaded hybrid system. *Bioact. Mater.* 5: 348–357.

Wu, Z., Bai, J., Ge, G., Wang, T., Feng, S., Ma, Q., Liang, X., Li, W., Zhang, W., Xu, Y., & Guo, K. (2022). Regulating macrophage polarization in high glucose microenvironment using lithium-modified bioglass-hydrogel for diabetic bone regeneration. *Adv. Healthc. Mater.* 11: 2200298.

Xiao, D., Yang, F., Zhao, Q., Chen, S., Shi, F., Xiang, X., Deng, L., Sun, X., Weng, J., & Feng, G. (2018). Fabrication of a Cu/Zn co-incorporated calcium phosphate scaffold-derived GDF-5 sustained release system with enhanced angiogenesis and osteogenesis properties. *RSC Adv.* 8: 29526–29534.

Xie, L., Yang, Y., Fu, Z., Li, Y., Shi, J., Ma, D., Liu, S., & Luo, D. (2019). Fe/Zn-modified Tricalcium Phosphate (TCP) biomaterials: Preparation and biological properties. *RSC Adv.* 9: 781–789.

Xiong, K., Wu, T., Fan, Q., Chen, L., & Yan, M. (2017). Novel reduced graphene oxide/zinc silicate/calcium silicate electroconductive biocomposite for stimulating osteoporotic bone regeneration. *ACS Appl. Mater. Interfaces*. 9: 44356–44368.

Xu, Z. L., Lei, Y., Yin, W. J., Chen, Y. X., Ke, Q. F., Guo, Y. P., & Zhang, C. Q. (2016). Enhanced antibacterial activity and osteoinductivity of Ag-loaded strontium hydroxyapatite/chitosan porous scaffolds for bone tissue engineering. *J. Mater. Chem. B*. 4: 7919–7928.

Yan, S., Ren, J., Jian, Y., Wang, W., Yun, W., & Yin, J. (2018). Injectable maltodextrin-based micelle/hydrogel composites for simvastatin-controlled release. *Biomacromolecules*. 19: 4554–4564.

Yang, H., Qu, X., Lin, W., Wang, C., Zhu, D., Dai, K., & Zheng, Y. (2018). In vitro and in vivo studies on zinc-hydroxyapatite composites as novel biodegradable metal matrix composite for orthopedic applications. *Acta Biomater*. 71: 200–214.

Yang, Y. C., Chen, C. C., Wang, J. B., Wang, Y. C., & Lin, F. H. (2017). Flame sprayed zinc doped hydroxyapatite coating with antibacterial and biocompatible properties. *Ceram. Int*. 43: S829–S835.

Yedekçi, B., Tezcaner, A., Yılmaz, B., Demir, T., & Evis, Z. (2022). 3D porous PCL-PEG-PCL/strontium, magnesium and boron multi-doped hydroxyapatite composite scaffolds for bone tissue engineering. *J. Mech. Behav. Biomed. Mater*. 125: 104941.

Yi, C., Liu, D., Fong, C. C., Zhang, J., & Yang, M. (2010). Gold nanoparticles promote osteogenic differentiation of mesenchymal stem cells through p38 MAPK pathway. *ACS Nano*. 4: 6439–6448.

Yu, L., Rowe, D. W., Perera, I. P., Zhang, J., Suib, S. L., Xin, X., & Wei, M. (2020). Intrafibrillar mineralized collagen—Hydroxyapatite-based scaffolds for bone regeneration. *ACS Appl. Mater. Interfaces*. 12: 18235–18249.

Yu, N., Cai, S., Wang, F., Zhang, F., Ling, R., Li, Y., Jiang, Y., & Xu, G. (2017a). Microwave assisted deposition of strontium doped hydroxyapatite coating on AZ31 magnesium alloy with enhanced mineralization ability and corrosion resistance. *Ceram. Int*. 43: 2495–2503.

Yu, X., Tang, Z., Sun, D., Ouyang, L., & Zhu, M. (2017b). Recent advances and remaining challenges of nanostructured materials for hydrogen storage applications. *Prog. Mater. Sci*. 88: 1–48.

Zanin, H., Saito, E., Marciano, F. R., Ceragioli, H. J., Granato, A. E. C., Porcionatto, M., & Lobo, A. O. (2013). Fast preparation of nano-hydroxyapatite/superhydrophilic reduced graphene oxide composites for bioactive applications. *J. Mater. Chem. B*. 1: 4947–4955.

Zhang, S., Chen, J., Yu, Y., Dai, K., Wang, J., & Liu, C. (2019b). Accelerated bone regenerative efficiency by regulating sequential release of BMP-2 and VEGF and synergism with sulfated chitosan. *ACS Biomater. Sci. Eng*. 5: 1944–1955.

Zhang, X. Y., Chen, Y. P., Han, J., Mo, J., Dong, P. F., Zhuo, Y. H., & Feng, Y. (2019c). Biocompatiable silk fibroin/carboxymethyl chitosan/strontium substituted hydroxyapatite/cellulose nanocrystal composite scaffolds for bone tissue engineering. *Int. J. Biol. Macromol*. 136: 1247–1257.

Zhang, X. Y., Yin, X., Luo, J., Zheng, X., Wang, H., Wang, J., Xi, Z., Liao, X., Machuki, J. O. A., Guo, K., & Gao, F. (2019a). Novel hierarchical nitrogen-doped multiwalled carbon nanotubes/cellulose/nano-hydroxyapatite nanocomposite as an osteoinductive scaffold for enhancing bone regeneration. *ACS Biomater. Sci. Eng*. 5: 294–307.

Zhao, H., Dong, W., Zheng, Y., Liu, A., Yao, J., Li, C., Tang, W., Chen, B., Wang, G., & Shi, Z. (2011). The structural and biological properties of hydroxyapatite-modified titanate nanowire scaffolds. *Biomaterials*. 32: 5837–5846.

Zhao, Y., Sun, K. N., Wang, W. L., Wang, Y. X., Sun, X. L., Liang, Y. J., Sun, X. N., & Chui, P. F. (2013). Microstructure and anisotropic mechanical properties of graphene nanoplatelet toughened biphasic calcium phosphate composite. *Ceram. Int*. 39: 7627–7634.

Zhou, H., Kong, S., Pan, Y., Zhang, Z., & Deng, L. (2015). Microwave-assisted fabrication of strontium doped apatite coating on Ti6Al4V. *Mater. Sci. Eng. C*. 56: 174–180.

10 Osteoblast and Osteoclast Crosstalk during Osteo-Homeostasis and Biotherapeutic Interventions

Harishkumar Madhyastha, Radha Madhyastha, Kaushita Banerjee, Yuichi Nakajima, Masugi Maruyama and Nozomi Watanabe

10.1 INTRODUCTION

Skeleton mass is a vital organ in the maintenance of the human body. The adult skeleton has bones in multiple categories, for instance 126 appendicular bones, 74 axial bones and 6 auditory ossicles, and it is a dynamic connective tissue that has multiple physiological and biomechanical functions in all vertebrates. They are generally classified as long, short, flat or irregular bones according to location and general functions in the body (Buckwalter & Cooper, 1987).

Clavicles, humeri, radii, ulnae, metacarpals, femurs, tibiae, fibulae, metatarsals and phalanges are long bones. Tarsal and carpal bones are recognized as short bones, and small portions of membranous bones are flat bones; each type of bone serves a specialized function. In total, the skeleton supports the body shape, helps in movement and locomotion, protect the internal organs, maintain the mineral hemostasis, and maintain the hematopoiesis (Clarke, 2008).

The human skeleton consists of 80% and 20% cortical and trabecular bone, respectively. Dense and solid cortical bone surrounds the marrow space, which comprises honeycomb-like networks of trabecular and cortical structure with osteons called the Haversian canals (Cooper et al., 2004). Cortical bone consists of outer periosteal and inner endosteal surfaces. The periosteal surface helps in appositional growth and fracture repair of bone by the continuous formation of osteoblasts.

However, bone resorption by osteoclasts takes place mainly in the endosteal surface with the progress of age of organisms. Cortical and trabecular bones are oriented in lamellar patterns with collagen fibril arrangements similar to the plywood structure, whereas in woven bone, this orientation is absent; it forms in a disorganized manner and is thereby weaker than laminar bone, and it is often seen in diseases that involve high bone turnover such as osteitis fibrosa cystica and Paget's disease (Paget, 1877). In periosteum regions of bone except in joints, the fibrous connective tissues sheath surrounds the cortical surface with blood vessels, nerve fibers and serval bone cells. Thick collagen fibers called Sharpey's fibers connect the periosteum with the outer cortical surface, and disorders at these junctions (Benjamin et al., 2002) are called enthesopathies; two common sports-related ones are skeletal hyperostosis and seronegative spondyloarthropathies, known, respectively, as tennis elbow and jumper's knee.

Over the course of life, bone undergoes continuous remodeling, including longitudinal, especially during childhood and adolescence. Longitudinal expansion occurs at growth plates with cartilage proliferation in the epiphyseal and metaphyseal regions of long bone and subsequent mineralization to form neo-primary bone. The influence of age and physiologic functions continuously changes the shape of the bone during the modeling and remodeling stage.

DOI: 10.1201/9781003307310-12

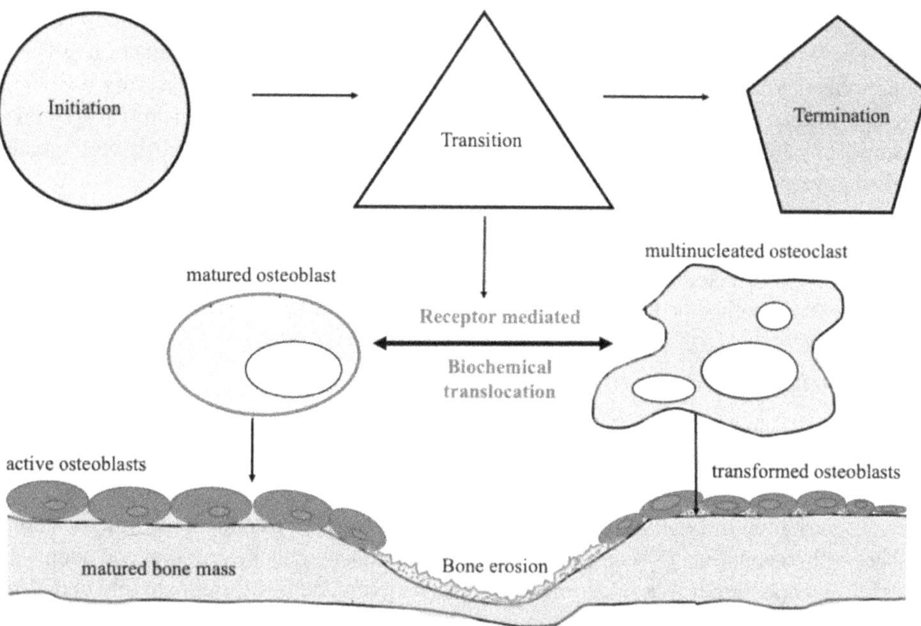

FIGURE 10.1 Chronology of osteoporosis due to intra-communication signaling during bone etiology.

Due to biomechanical skeletal forces, the bone may change its shape by widening the growth axis. During the modeling phase, the physiological tensile stresses of loading highly regulate the actions of bone cell response according to Wolff's law to change the organization of bone trabeculae (Greer, 1993). Bone remodeling is the process by which bone is renewed according to mineral homeostasis to maintain bone strength and generally progresses with age over four sequential phases: development, activation, resorption and reversal. Complete bone formation happens within four to six months, and old bone degenerates constantly due to age and osteopathically related complications in three intermittent phases: initiation, transition and termination. Matured osteoblast continuously helps in new bone formation. However, negative osteoclast feedback ignites bone resorption due to an imbalance in biochemical pathways (Figure 10.1).

These two processes are mainly governed by master bone cells, osteoblasts and osteoclasts. Collagenous matrix synthesis and its mineralization regulation is governed by the releasing of small, membrane-bound vesicles to concentrate calcium and phosphate in matrix and is negatively percussed by mineralization inhibitors such as pyrophosphate and proteoglycans (Anderson, 2003). Bone mechanical strength is, therefore, mainly preserved by calcium and phosphate hemostasis and this increased demand is negatively met by osteoclasts, bone resorption cells.

Bone extracellular matrix mainly comprises collagenous proteins like type III, type V and fibril-associated collagens with interrupted triple helices. Osteoblasts mainly synthesize and secrete these collagenous proteins in a molar basis as proteoglycans, glycosylated proteins, and ©-carboxylated (gla) proteins. The specific role of each collagen protein is not well documented, but the proteins are known to have direct relevance in many metabolic bone-related syndromes like osteogenesis imperfecta, Ehlers-Danlos syndrome and hypophosphatasia (El Demellawy et al., 2018).

Along with matrix proteins, bone minerals play an essential role in bone health. Typical healthy bone has 5 to 70% mineral, 20 to 40% organic matrix, up to 10% water and less than 3% lipids. The critical marker minerals of bone are hydroxyapatite, carbonates (CO_3), magnesium (Mg) and acid phosphate. The expression of alkaline phosphatase and many noncollagenous proteins like osteocalcin, osteopontin and sialoprotein directly regulates hydroxyapatite crystal formation with coordinated activity with osteocytes. Terminally differentiated osteoblasts, namely osteocytes, function as networking cells that are active during the osteolysis process and function as lysosome-dependent phagocytic cells. Regarding osteocyte and osteoblast interactions during bone development, recent studies indicate that bone mechanochemical signaling communications are dependent on dynamic physiological interactions between these two cells with a multilateral metabolism mechanism governed by the central nervous system (Meunier et al., 1973).

Several nano-aided therapeutic interventions are currently in use, but the gap between knowledge and applications remains significant (Pham, 2011). Unlike a traditional chemical-based drug, nanomedicine is designed as a site-directed drug to avoid potential unwanted effects. In the chapter, we comprehensively evaluate the nanotherapeutic aspects of controlling the pathogenesis of bone cell-related disorders.

10.1.1 Osteoblasts and Osteoclast Crosstalk

Cartilage and bone are formed by chondrocytes and osteoblasts, respectively. Figure 10.2 explains the basic communication scenario between two master cells of bone biogenesis and bone consumption molecular regulation. Intramembranous and endochondral ossification during embryonic development help in bone formation through the differentiation of bone-forming osteoblasts within the connective tissue sheet with the continuous secretion of osteoids, which later become mineralized compact bone.

However, in endochondral ossification, some mesenchymal cells differentiate into chondrocytes, which later become cartilages. Since chondrocytes and osteoblasts share a single progenitor, it is interesting to explore the pathway-directed differentiation between the two. Transcription factors like Sox9, Sox5 and ®-catenin are essential for chondrogenic ignition (Akiyama et al., 2004), and cbfa1, runt-related transcription factor-2 (RUNX2), osterix (Osx) and activating transcription factor 4 are necessary for osteoblast formation (Kobayashi & Kronenberg, 2005). Other factors like the WNT signaling pathway, which is activated by WNT10B protein, promote osteoblast differentiation (Bennett et al., 2005). Osteoblasts with overexpressed WNT10B increase bone mineral density and the volume and number of trabecular bones in particular, but WNT10B-deficient mice showed loweredn trabecular bone mass with a decrease in osteocalcin content in serum (Bennett et al., 2007), suggesting the coupling factors of WNT10B.

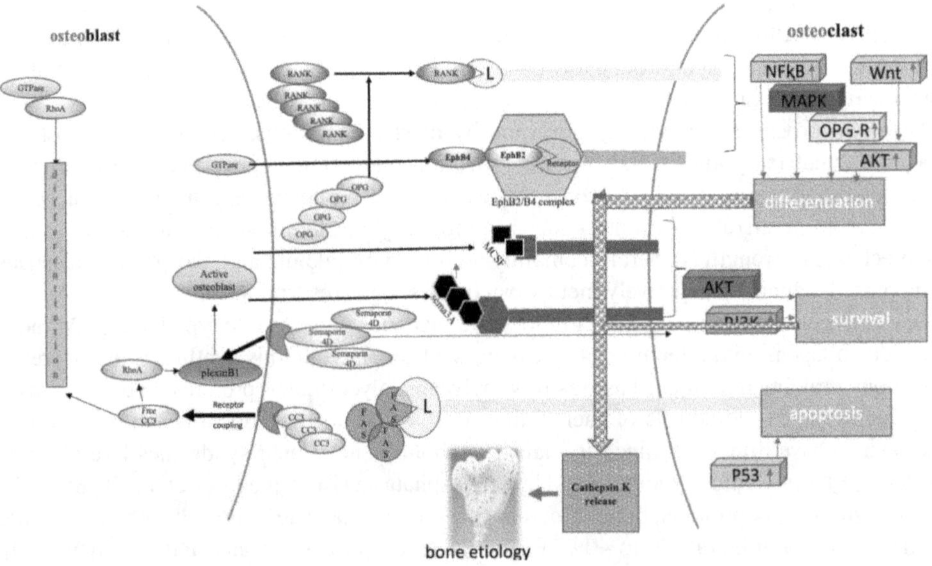

FIGURE 10.2 Molecular-mediated osteoblast and osteoclast communication in bone etiology.

Another essential protein that regulates bone modeling is TGF-β1 commonly found in bone matrix osteoblast cells. TGF-β1 binds to latency-associated protein mistakenly to keep TGF-β1 in latency state and temporarily inactivates the TGF-β1 which triggers the osteoclastic bone resorption cells. Another growth factor, namely IGF-1 accumulates in bone matrix binds to insulin growth factor binding protein mainly during the physiological disturbances during the acidic pH range (Kim et al., 2020).

In aging human women, menopause is a critical phase with rapid turnover of bone mass and significant changes in bone macrostructure and micro-architecture; it features various immune and metabolic changes and can be associated with complications. Bone remodeling and mass balance is a dynamic process wherein old or damaged bone is continuously removed by bone-consuming cells called osteoclasts. Bone-resorbing cells originate from homeopathic stem cells, and bone erosion takes place by continuous secretion of acidic and proteolytic enzymes (namely cathepsin-K) by degrading or dissolving the collagen or other matrix protein.

Therefore, balanced osteoblast–osteoclast communications is key for fine tuning bone formation and bone resorption. The interaction between these two cells is governed by the ephrin signaling pathway. Ephrin B1, B2 and B3 bind to the tyrosine kinase receptor EPBH (B1, B2, B3, B4, B5 or B6) through bidirectional signaling transduction initiated by EPHB4-mediated C-FOS/NFATC1 cascade. Mismatch between micro communication between two cells results in abnormal bone etiology like secondary osteoporosis in postmenopausal women and diabetes-associated and glucocorticoid-dependent osteoporosis (Tonna et al., 2016).

Another molecule that plays an important role in osteoblast-to-osteoclast communication is macrophage colony-stimulating Factor 1 (M-CSF), a hematopoietic growth factor that allows the ssurvival, proliferation, differentiation and mobility of osteoclasts. M-CSF deficiency mouse with thymidine inserted in the Csf1 gene showed few osteoclasts when the mice were young, but this phenomenon disappeared as the mice aged, indicating the importance of M-CSF in osteoclast formation. Osteoclast differentiation factor, namely nuclear factor B ligand (RANKL), is TNF ligand superfamily member II.

RANKL is highly expressed in osteoblasts, osteocytes and activated lymphocytes and binds to its respective cognate receptor activator of NF-κB (RANK) on surface, leading to osteoclast formation, fusion and activation (Yasuda, 2021). Osteoclastogenesis inhibition factors like osteoprotegerin (OPG) and TNF alpha superfamily 11B members (TNFRSF11B) play an important role in regulating osteoclast formation. Postnatal bone loss was noticed in TNFRSF11B-deficient mice hence considered as essential regulator marker protein in osteoclast genesis biology.

Sphingosine kinase helps in the phosphorylation of sphingosine to generate sphingosine 1 phosphate (SIP), which is overexpressed in osteoclast precursor cells. Subsequently, SIP-activated osteoblast overexpress RANKL, which finally augments osteoclastogenesis during the stress (Hodun et al., 2021). Soluble protein, collagen triple helix repeat containing 1 (CTHRC1) in mature osteoclast induces osteoblast differentiation. Upregulation of CTHRC1 was noticed in osteoblasts when osteoclasts communicated with hydroxyapatite and calcium content.

In short, it is quite evident that cell-to-cell communication governs through several factors like direct contact mechanism, cytokines and extracellular matrix interaction with the overexpression of several well-coordinated signaling pathways like OPG/RANKL/RANK, RANKL/LGR4/RANK, ephrin/EPHB4, FAS/FASL, MAPK, P13K, AKT and NF-κB. In addition, osteoclasts also indirectly influence osteoblast-mediated bone formation by d_2 isoforms of vacuolar (H^+) Atpase 9v-ATPase) V0 domain (Atp6v0d_2), semaporin 4D and some microRNAs like miRNA377, miRNA335 and miRNA 503 (Mediero et al., 2018). As we have described with these cell communication systems, one of the most fundamental and enduring challenges in developing increasingly influential skeletal therapeutics is overcoming the osteoblast/osteoclast interaction. Effective drugs that often blunt the activity of both antiresorptive and anabolic drugs could be developed, but osteoporotic drug therapeutics studies are limited due to healthcare resources.

10.2 OSTEOBLAST- AND OSTEOCLAST-DEPENDENT BONE PATHOLOGY

Osteoporosis is a skeletal fragility syndrome of increased bone turnover with decreased bone mass, and one in two women and one in five men will experience this syndrome in their lifetime. Bone cell turnover rate determines the healthiness of bone. Within bone mass, 90% of bone cells consist of primary osteocytes, which send signals to either osteoblasts or osteoclasts to remodel or maintain the net mass. Some of the common bone-related diseases are listed in Table 10.1.

A mismatch between osteoblast and osteoclast micro communication leads to osteoporosis and many other critical bone pathologies in human beings. When abnormal metabolic balances ignite the initial osteoporosis and osteopetrosis, there is direct contact between osteoblasts and osteoclasts that is governed by micro-gap junctions (Everts et al., 2002). After osteoporosis, Paget's disease is the second most common bone focal disorder in the world (Appelman-Dijkstra & Papapoulos, 2018); it arises due to the increased recruitment of osteoclasts in the bone-forming region. Patients with Paget's disease show high levels of matrix metalloproteinase, IL-6 and RANKL and calcitriol in pelvis, spine, femora and skull bones. Missense mutations of the ZNF687 gene also lead to the giant bone cell tumors in Paget's disease (Divisato et al., 2016).

Treatment with pharmacologically active bisphosphonate significantly reduces the severity of Paget's disease. However, joint pain like hip arthroplasty and back pain in lumbar vertebrae is frequent with other parts of the body due to decreases in calcium metabolism, especially with elderly people. Another side effect of continuous bisphosphonate treatment is the impaired mineralization of newly formed bone, called osteomalacia. Therefore, the benefit and risk balance of bisphosphonate treatment should be carefully monitored.

TABLE 10.1
Different Marker Molecules of Bone Pathology with Specific Morphological Syndromes

Disease Name	Syndrome	Marker Molecule	Reference
Paget's disease	Losing the mechanical strength of bone	BMP fluctuations	Appelman-Dijkstra & Papapoulos (2018)
Van Bunchem disease	Autoimmune disorder (AID)	Increased ALP, PINP, OC and SOST mutations	Uitterlinden et al. (2004)
Rheumatoid arthritis	AID with inflammatory index	Increased levels of CTX-1, TRAP5b and PYD	Smolen et al. (2016)
Tumor-induced osteomalacia	Rare disorder	Increased levels of FGF23, ALP and OC	Minisola et al. (2022)
Primary osteoporosis	Joint pain and fracture	Higher ®CTX-1, PYD, DPYR, TRAP5b, BALP and OC	Glaser & Kaplan (1997)
Vanishing bone disease	Maxillofacial disorder	VEGF1 mutation	Gorham & Stout (1955)
Adamantinoma of jaw	Rare malignant maxillofacial region tumor	MAPK kinase mutation	Fisher (1913)
Spondylitis (vertebral osteomyelitis)	Neck bone pain	IL-3	Jaramillo-de la Torre et al. (2006)
Ankylosing spondylitis	Axial joint pain Uveal tract pain	HLA-B27	Braun & Sieper (2007)
Traction apophysitis	Micro trauma	Unknown	Micheli (1987)
Proteus bone disorder	Abnormal bone	AKT1 mutation	Buser et al. (2020)
Ossifying fibroma	Dysplasia of tibia and fibula	unknown	Manes et al. (2013)
Osteogenesis imperfecta	Brittle bone formation	Mutation in Col1A1 and Col1A2.	Adam et al. (1993)

Van Buchem disease (VBD) is the rarest autosomal recessive disease, with cranial nerve paralysis, neuralgic pain, sensorineural hearing loss and visual impairment (Uitterlinden et al., 2004). Enlargement of the forehead and overgrowth of the mandible are general symptoms of VBD etiology. Mutation in the SOST gene and defective synthesis of sclerostin are main reasons for VBD progression. The current treatment option is surgery, with very little or nil progress with pharmacologic sclerostin inhibitor intervention.

The chronic inflammatory joint disease rheumatoid arthritis causes cartilage and bone damage with permanent disability (Smolen et al., 2016). It is a heterogeneous disorder with presence of seropositive autoantibodies and is caused by infections of *E. coli* and other pathogenic bacteria. The complex cytokines and chemokines in activated fibroblasts, activated T and B cells and macrophages trigger osteoclast turnover due to infections that lead to aggravations of TNF, IL-6, GM-CSF and IL-1. Disease-modifying antirheumatic drugs and nonsteroidal anti-inflammatory drugs (NSAIDS) can only reduce pain and improve physical function for a while; they will not interfere with inflammatory hot spots. The possible future therapy angle for rheumatoid arthritis is still not precise and currently under investigation.

Another type of bone pathology is ultra-rare paraneoplastic syndrome, also known as tumor-induced osteomalacia (TIO), caused by the overproduction of FGF23. TIO morbidity is high, but it progresses slowly; however, it is difficult to diagnose (Minisola et al., 2022). The primary diagnosis involves checking blood phosphate levels, which will be chronically low due to the loss of phosphate in the kidney. The X-linked FGF23 mutation is a major prevalent cause of hypophosphatemia (YIO). Genotypically, TIO is initiated by the fusion of FN1 (fibronectin-encoding gene) FGFR1 (fibroblast growth factor receptor-encoding gene). Collectively, mis-fusion of FN1 and FGFR1 increases tubular phosphate secretion, which leads to osteomalacia, loss of muscle function and, ultimately, proximal myopathy. Total body MRI has been advocated for TIO location in the body, and surgery is the best practice for fine management of TIO. In YIO, the FGF23-blocking IgG monoclonal antibody KRN23, in a clinically directed randomized human trial, showed meaningful increases in serum phosphate and 1,25(OH)2D levels (Carpenter et al., 2014).

Primary osteoporosis is a silent disease phase that occurs prior to bone fracture and is commonly found in postmenopausal women and 50 years or older aged men (Klibanski et al., 2001). Decreased mass/volume density of mineralized bone is the primary cause of osteoporosis, with acute back pain with compressed vertebral fracture. Juvenile diabetics and suboptimal lifestyle-related food disorders are the main reasons for primary osteoporosis in younger adults (Glaser & Kaplan, 1997; Rozenberg et al., 2020).

Osteoporosis is diagnosed clinically with X-ray absorptiometry following the international standard of δ 2.5 BMD. Currently, the bisphosphonates denosumab, teriparatide and abaloparatide are the available standard drugs (Lorentzon, 2019), but the gold standard to treat primary osteoporosis is still under investigation. One rare lymphatic vessel-related maxillofacial bone disease is known as vanishing bone disease (VBD), also known as massive osteolysis, Gorhams's disease, phantom bone disease, progressive osteolysis, hemangiomatosis and lymphangiomatosis (Gorham & Stout, 1955). The rapid proliferation of vascular tissue with high circulating PDGF BB and hypoxic and/or acidosis-mediated enzyme hydrolysis is the main cause of VBD. It is diagnosed with plain radiographs, radio-isotope bone scans, computed tomography and MRI scans. Simple osteogenic nutrients like calcium, phosphorous and vitamin D are the standard prevention method.

Other tibia disorders are adamantinoma or ameloblastoma, commonly termed jaw tumor (Fisher, 1913). This is a local, invasive, slow-growing tumor of odontogenic epithelium which arises from enamel tissue The common symptoms of this disease are swelling, redness and sensitivity loss in the mandibular region where the tumor is growing. Histologically, ameloblastoma comprises two types of cells: peripherally located columnar basal cells called ameloblasts and slowly growing, deeply situated epithelial cells that look like stellate reticulum. Mutations of BRAFV600E in MAPK and smoothened mutation in sonic Hedgehog signaling pathways leads to etiology of adamantinoma (Ghai, 2022).

Many inherited bone deformities in the neck and head are complicated by secondary infections, mainly from inflammation-igniting organisms like *S. aureus* and *M. tuberculosis*. Vertebral osteomyelitis (VO) is one such etiology that progresses in regions of osseous space, neural arch gaps, epidural space and paraspinal soft tissue areas. The incidence of VO began increasing in recent decades (Jaramillo-de la Torre et al., 2006), and at present, NSAIDs along with bisphosphonate are the keystone of its management.

Ankylosing spondylitis (AS) is an inflammatory rheumatic disease of the axial skeleton (Braun & Sieper, 2007); currently, physiotherapy-aided NSAIDS treatment remains the most-recommended long-term AS management. Joint overuse injuries in children is known as traction apophysitis (Micheli, 1987), and a rare inherited connective tissue disorder known as osteogenesis imperfecta is a common dental and other bone disorder caused by slicing mutations of collagens A1, A2 and A7 (Adam et al., 1993). Autosomal disorder is caused by a mismatch of alpha1(1) and alpha2(1) of type 1 collagen, found abundantly in bone, skin and tendon extracellular matrix (Marini et al., 2017).

Meanwhile, ossifying fibroma (OF) is a rare, nonneoplastic abnormal gingival outgrowth in the area of interdental papillae. There are several types of OF—namely, central, peripheral, mandibular and psammomatoid—depending on the degree and etiology of mandibular inflammation (Manes et al., 2013). A mosaic appearance associated with bone cancer known as proteus disorder and caused by a somatic variant in AKT1 c.49G that is overexpressed compared with its counterpart, phosphorylated p (Glu17Lys) (Buser et al., 2020). Some less-common bone diseases that include Iselin's disease, so-called Little League elbow, Osgood-Schlatter disease, Sever's disease and Sinding-Larsen-Johansson disease are yet to be explored and pose a high degree of challenge to clinicians and biologists (Grabowski, 2009).

10.3 BIOENGINEERING INTERVENTIONS IN OSTEOPATHOLOGY

Bone bioengineering incorporates cells like MC3T3-E1, MG-63 and SaOs-2 along with human, bovine, rat and mouse osteoblasts and osteoclasts. Several intrinsic biological factors like choice of cell, cellular metabolic engineering, overactivated stem cell influences and supporting media are important in osteo-cell-mediated bone repair (Czekanska et al., 2012). Figure 10.3 depicts some reconstructions of damaged bone with various biotechnological and molecular-mediated routes.

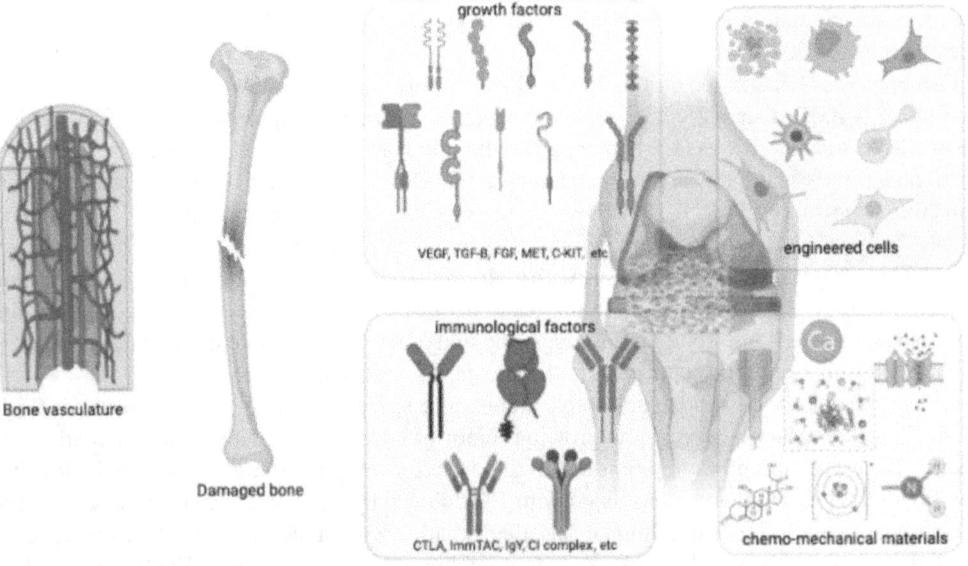

FIGURE 10.3 Damaged bone reconstruction incorporating various growth factors, immunological factors and cell engineering with chemo-mechanical materials.

It was earlier believed that osteoblasts and osteoclasts were the major bone cells involved in osteo-hemostasis, but now, more emphasis is being placed on other cells, like mesenchymal stem cell (MSC) osteoblast lineage cells and monocyte-macrophage osteoclast primary cells; the process of bone healing is biologically intertwined with continuous cross-communications between all these master cells at the site of injury. Tightly coordinated interplay between various cells and the injury site is the signature event in the process of fracture healing. Otherwise, hematomas and plasma coagulation with acute inflammation lead to secondary bone infections. Organic bone matrix-induced bone mineralization by osteoblasts helps in primary bone formation by secreting differentiation factors like RUNX2 and Osx; however, in the final phase, osteoclasts with high-expression RANKL activator starts the process of bone reabsorption. Another avenue of bone regeneration targets the senescence-associated secretory phenotypes (SASP) with the help of senotherapeutics models, such as using senomorphic and senolytic agents to inhibit SASP.

10.3.1 Artificial Scaffolds

Autologous bone grafts are the gold standard of bone replacement therapy in humans due to its advantages, such as osteoinductivity, osteoconductivity, surface topography matching and less irritability. Nevertheless, autologous implants have caveats like host durability and immunoreaction, infection and poor mechanical strength. Scaffolds are artificial substrates prepared either by chemical synthesis or by natural source that are highly biocompatible and nontoxic to cells and that have superior mechanical, flexible, biodegradable properties.

Various preclinical implantable models are being developed in animals to study the process of bone formation and repair during healing. For example, researchers have studied drug-loaded hydrogels and other injectables in a hind limb regeneration model to investigate tendon bone pathology (Luca et al., 2010; Sharma et al., 2022). Electrospinning is also being studied as an alternate scaffold-aided technique for bone fracture repair, and microfibers and nanofibers synthesized by chemical or biological means have high mechanical properties; their large surface area is being used as nests to hold cells in place during implantation at the site of injury.

Three-dimensional (3D) and 4D engineered bone tissues have a variety of functions in terms of cell adhesion, growth and differentiation in bone transplantation (Kumari et al., 2022a, 2022b). Recent years have seen tremendous achievements in musculoskeletal defect regeneration using natural silk biopolymers from lepidopteran insects like *Bombyx mori*, *Antheraea pernyi* and *Nephila clavipes* with high biocompatibility (Bhattacharjee et al., 2017). Other naturally derived biomaterials like collagen, hyaluronic acid, polyhydroxyalkanoate and chitosan are being studied and utilized in bone tissue scaffold engineering using cryogelation with start materials like agarose, polyvinyl alcohol, polyethylene glycol, laminin and cellulose. Cryogel can respond to various stimuli like electricity and oxygen-releasing antioxidants, as described by many investigators (Shiekh et al., 2018; Tyshkunova et al., 2022).

10.3.2 Engineered Hydrogels

Hydrogels of alginates, pluronic acid, chitosan, and fibrin glues form semisolid and viscous scaffolds that have been extensively researched in tissue engineering. They are crosslinked polymeric compounds with the capacity to absorb high aqueous volumes. During chemical synthesis, synthetic or natural polymers will be modified with reactive functional groups.

In osteochondral tissue engineering, multilayered hydrogels are being used with cell sandwich systems during the repair of articular joints and cranium defects (Moreira Teixeira et al., 2014). Hydrogel degradability after implantation is crucial in tissue engineering. Degradability can be achieved by two routes: hydrolytic or enzymatic. Adding ester linker materials like lactic acid groups during the synthesis increases the rate of hydrolytic degradation, but some proteins have protease cleavage sites; during the extracellular matrix turnover, hydrogels will be degraded through this enzymatic mechanism.

Drug-conjugated hydrogels are being considered as versatile platforms in cartilage engineering. Some commonly studied hydrogels that can be conjugated for cartilage regeneration are insulin-like growth factor 1; transforming growth factor beta 1, 2, and 3 (TGF-β1, β2, β3); basic fibroblast-derived growth factor 1, platelet-derived growth factor BB and bone morphogenetic protein 2 (Moreira Teixeira et al., 2014). Bone-adhesive hydrogels are excellent alternatives for noncompatible pins, screws and plates during the fracture joints. This glue-like adhesive material possesses excellent cohesive mechanical properties in terms of strength, stiffness and toughness issues between two joints. For example, crosslinking between N-hydroxysuccinimide functionalized poly(2-oxazoline) s with amine-functionalized poly(2-oxazoline) with calcium ions in reaction buffer serves the excellent glue materials (Sánchez-Fernández et al., 2021).

Proper nutrient and oxygen supply are crucial for bone healing through the proper vascular systems, but one challenge with bone healing is reduced vasculature during the regeneration. Researchers have developed injectable hydrogels with chitin and butylene succinate loaded with fibrin nanoparticles and magnesium-doped bioglass and observed good resurgence of irregular bone defects (Priya et al., 2016). A great deal of research has addressed cell-encapsulated hydrogel spheroids in bone tissue engineering. For instance, 3D cell spheroids are considered excellent in vitro models for studying bone regeneration due to their bio-mimics and near tissue-like morphology. Scientists developed revascularized bone tissue composite with MSCs with umbilical vein endothelial cell hydrogel spheroids and studied the osteogenic potentiation and nature of vasculature in collagen-laden spheroids (Anthon & Valente, 2022; Benavides et al., 2015).

10.3.3 3D Bioprinting

Layer-by-layer material deposition by artificial guided robotic arm printing describes the process of 3D bioprinting using bioinks. Intralayer bonding and adhesion can be increased with heat transfer, UV light and also crosslinking materials and have great advantages in ortho-engineering techniques. At present, three types of bioprinters are currently available: laser assisted, injection and micro-extrusion. Laser-guided printers have high resolution—from picometer to micrometer scale—offering highly precise bioprinting with cell loading up to 200 cells/mL. In contrast, inkjet and extrusion printing involve secreting droplets onto a solid surface by thermal actuation principle. Although these printing techniques have the advantages of low cost and mass production, the shear stress on living cells is an issue.

In all three cases, the nature of bioinks in terms of homogeneity, rheological properties, viscosity, crosslinking ability and surface tension plays a major role in the printed final products. Bioinks are made of either natural or synthetic polymers like chitosan, fibrin, gellan gum, agarose, collagen, PCL/extracellular matrix, polyethylene glycol, methacrylated hyaluronic acid, hyaluronic acid/poly(glucidol)/PCL, polylactic acid, (PLA) and polyglycolic acid with cell-culture-compatible medium and growth factors. The first task of 2D bioprinting is designing the desired construct with the aid of computer-aided design software that integrates G-code programming language to deliver a 3D construction. This technique has been successfully demonstrated in chondrocyte-mediated chondrogenesis in vitro, but its effective translation to clinical application remains daunting due to complexity in chondrogenesis biochemical pathways and in vivo antigenicity issues.

10.3.4 Nanotechnologies in Orthopedics

Nanotechnologies in orthopedics are mainly focused on the therapeutic delivery of nano drugs and nano detection methods. Iontophoresis, the application of low-ampere direct monophasic electric current for transdermal drug delivery, is being studied for delivering anti-inflammatory drugs such as dexamethasone in bone joints. Tendinopathy healing is being effectively promoted with the successful application of gold nanoparticles through iontophoresis in rodent models (Dohnert et al., 2012).

A nanocrystal polymer particle, kratogenin, showed more promising results in a murine osteoarthritis model than did the kratogenin solution or its ionic form (Maudens et al., 2018). Nanosphere conjugate forms of kratogenin combined with chitosan oligosaccharide-pluronic F127 carboxyl diclofenac were studied in osteoarthritis therapy because of the excellent thermo responsive properties of this nanosphere (Kang et al., 2016). Immediate release of diclofenac at the site of injury and sustained secondary release of kratogenin in response to local tissue temperature suggest the dual function of the nanosphere.

In comparison with free drug treatment, nanomedicine has played an important role in the treatment of many osteopathologies. For example, in osteosarcoma, a common primary malignant bone neoplasm, chemotherapy is limited, and patients have severe drug-resistant syndrome, but a cisplatin–doxorubicin-crosslinked nanogel was reported to cure osteosarcoma. A pH-responsive calcium zolendronate nanogel with folic acid targeted delivery was studied to combat bone cancer cell metastasis, and the zoledronate uptake increased to 80% to 85% (Reid et al., 2020). Nanotechnology-based antibiotic drug delivery through surface and morphology modifications have often shown proven efficacy (Kumar & Madhyastha, 2017; Sahoo et al., 2020).

Bioglass prepared by quenching or solution-in-gel process contains mainly calcium oxide, silicates, borate and phosphorus. Osteointegration greatly increases osteoblast activation to form new bones. Conductive nanomaterials like piezoelectric and magnetic materials have great applications in bone regeneration. Some of the well-studied piezoelectric materials for bone regeneration are barium titanate, boron nitride and zinc oxide, which show high osteoinduction activity since bone itself is a natural piezoelectric material.

Some of the piezoelectric polymers have also received increased attention in recent years. Among these, polyvinylidene fluoride, PCL (poly(Σ-caprolactone), PLA and poly-3-hydroxybutarate-3-hydroxy valerate have excellent biocompatibility, but resistance to biodegradation limits the clinical use of these polymers. Researchers have debated the use of electrical stimulation and subsequent nanomedicine to heal fractures and spinal arthrodesis. However, persistent lacunae are optimized by adding graphene or metallic nanoparticles (Munir et al., 2019).

Functional group modification with carbon atoms in nanoparticles prepared by graphene oxide has excellent osteogenic, chondrogenic, adipogenic and neurogenic differentiation of stem cells. Being a carbon-based material, graphene stereochemically changes into fullerene if warped, becomes a carbon nanotube if rolled and changes into graphite if stacked in layers (Geim, 2009). Graphene materials are being used in patient-specific nanoconstructs by additive manufacturing to produce custom-sized bone replacement models for defects (Meneses et al., 2022).

Implantable alloys tend to erode and corrode over time, but metallic ortho-implants are being used as a stable and most promising strategy to overcome the degenerative and fracture resilience issues. For instance, surface-modified titanium is an alternate mode for fractured bone replacement. Rutile, brookite and anatase are oxide forms of titanium and are being used as orthopedic implants in total hip arthroplasty in the acetabular and femoral regions (Naziri et al., 2013), total knee arthroplasty (Agarwal et al., 2013) and fracture fixation in the humerus (Bandalović et al., 2014).

Human bone is an anisotropic biomaterial with viscoelastic behavior. The elastic properties depend on the direction of bone, which stretches and bends according to the body's movements. The properties are measured by Young's modulus along with the longitudinal axis of bone (Bonfield & Grynpas, 1977).

Knowledge of the mechanical properties of bone is key for drug designers and medical prosthetic manufacturers, and mismatched Young's moduli between bone and artificial implants are a major issue in orthopedic biology that leads to stress shielding. After implantation surgery, bone tries to balance the load between the original organ with artificial implants to minimize the stress-shielding phenomenon (Kaur & Singh, 2019; Tian et al., 2019). Naturally, bone tries to adjust the stress shielding by distributing the loads.

Poor-quality, poorly designed implants have adverse effects on natural bone: Bone with high load induces osteoblasts to increase bone mass, and bone with less load decreases in mass, in turn rejecting implants. Therefore, the processing parameters of titanium or any other alloys (e.g., vanadium, aluminum, magnesium), proper design and proper surface modifications are important in implant biology. Other implant issues include continuous corrosion and allergic reactions in the highly reactive body environment, but stable, anticorrosive coating of oxide film on metallic alloy may prevent corrosion.

CONCLUSION

The prevalence of metabolic illnesses like osteo-related issues are a global burden related to metabolism and the bioenergetics patterns of osteo cells. Bone-related pathologies cause significant morbidity, mortality and human psychological discomfort, although the burden of osteoporosis varies from country to country; gaps in knowledge need to be filled by proper awareness, social counseling, advanced research and scientific inputs.

Osteoporosis and other bone-related diseases are highly researched; understanding the fine-tuned metabolic functions in the skeletal system has inspired new lines of research through nanoengineering modules. Targeting the senescence-associated secretory phenotypes by ROS harvesting nanomaterial is an increasing option to treat osteoporosis in recent years. Along with nano-mediated treatment options, injectable biocomposites seem to be a novel therapeutic option for bone aging prevention. Control of bone regeneration with bone-mimicking substances will offer a cost-effective, low-morbidity option for skeletal repair.

LIST OF ABBREVIATIONS

BMP2	Bone morphogenetic protein 2
$BRAF^{V600E}$	B-Rapidly accelerated Fibrosarcoma V 600 E
C-FOS	Fos Proto-Oncogene Transcription Factor Subunit
Csf	Colony-stimulating factor
FAS	Fatty Acid Synthase
FASL	Fatty Acid Synthase Ligand
FGF23	Fibroblast growth factor 23
IL-6	Interleukin 6
MAPK	Mitogen Activated Protein Kinase
MRI	Magnetic Resonance Imaging
MSC	Mesenchymal stem cell
NF-κB	Nuclear factor kappa B
NFATC1	Nuclear Factor of Activated T cells 1
P13K	Phosphoinositide 3 -Kinase
PCL	poly-Σ-caprolactone
PVA	Poly Vinyl Alcohol
RANKL	Receptor Activator of Nuclear factor k B Ligand
RUNX2	Runt-related transcription factor-2
SOST	Sclerostin protein
Sox5	SRY-box transcription factor 5
Sox9	SRY-box transcription factor 9
TGF-β1	Transforming Growth Factor beta-1
TIO	Tumor induced osteomalacia
VO	Vertebral Osteomyelitis
WNT	Wingless/integrated

REFERENCES

Adam, M. P., Ardinger, H. H., Pagon, R. A., Wallace, S. E., Bean, L. J., Gripp, K. W., & Amemiya, A. (1993). *GeneReviews®*. Seattle, WA: University of Washington.

Agarwal, S., Azam, A., & Morgan-Jones, R. (2013). Metal metaphyseal sleeves in revision total knee replacement. *Bone Joint J.* 95-B: 1640–1644.

Akiyama, H., Lyons, J. P., Mori-Akiyama, Y., Yang, X., Zhang, R., Zhang, Z., Deng, J. M., Taketo, M. M., Nakamura, T., Behringer, R. R., & de Crombrugghe, B. (2004). Interactions between Sox9 and beta-catenin control chondrocyte differentiation. *Genes Dev.* 18: 1072–1087.

Anderson, H. C. (2003). Matrix vesicles and calcification. *Curr. Rheumatol. Rep.* 5: 222–226.

Anthon, S. G., & Valente, K. P. (2022). Vascularization strategies in 3D cell culture models: From scaffold-free models to 3D bioprinting. *Int. J. Mol. Sci.* 23: 14582.

Appelman-Dijkstra, N. M., & Papapoulos, S. E. (2018). Paget's disease of bone. *Best Pract. Res. Clin. Endocrinol. Metab.* 32: 657–668.

Bandalović, A., Cukelj, F., Knežević, J., Ostojić, M., Pavić, A., Parać, Z., & Rošin, M. (2014). The results of internal fixation of proximal humeral osteoporotic fractures with PHILOS locking plate. *Psychiatr. Danubina.* 2: 376–381.

Benavides, O. M., Quinn, J. P., Pok, S., Petsche Connell, J., Ruano, R., & Jacot, J. G. (2015). Capillary-like network formation by human amniotic fluid-derived stem cells within fibrin/poly(ethylene glycol) hydrogels. *Tissue Eng. Part A.* 21: 1185–1194.

Benjamin, M., Kumai, T., Milz, S., Boszczyk, B. M., Boszczyk, A. A., & Ralphs, J. R. (2002). The skeletal attachment of tendons—Tendon "entheses". *Comp. Biochem. Physiol. Part A Mol. Integr. Physiol.* 133: 931–945.

Bennett, C. N., Longo, K. A., Wright, W. S., Suva, L. J., Lane, T. F., Hankenson, K. D., & MacDougald, O. A. (2005). Regulation of osteoblastogenesis and bone mass by Wnt10b. *Proc. Natl. Acad. Sci. U. S. A.* 102: 3324–3329.

Bennett, C. N., Ouyang, H., Ma, Y. L., Zeng, Q., Gerin, I., Sousa, K. M., Lane, T. F., Krishnan, V., Hankenson, K. D., & MacDougald, O. A. (2007). Wnt10b increases postnatal bone formation by enhancing osteoblast differentiation. *J. Bone Miner. Res.* 22: 1924–1932.

Bhattacharjee, P., Kundu, B., Naskar, D., Kim, H. W., Maiti, T. K., Bhattacharya, D., & Kundu, S. C. (2017). Silk scaffolds in bone tissue engineering: An overview. *Acta Biomater.* 63: 1–17.

Bonfield, W., & Grynpas, M. D. (1977). Anisotropy of the young's modulus of bone. *Nature.* 270: 453–454.

Braun, J., & Sieper, J. (2007). Ankylosing spondylitis. *Lancet.* 369: 1379–1390.

Buckwalter, J. A., & Cooper, R. R. (1987). Bone structure and function. *Instr. Course Lect.* 36: 27–48.

Buser, A., Lindhurst, M. J., Kondolf, H. C., Yourick, M. R., Keppler-Noreuil, K. M., Sapp, J. C., & Biesecker, L. G. (2020). Allelic heterogeneity of proteus syndrome. *Cold Spring Harb. Mol. Case Stud.* 6: a005181.

Carpenter, T. O., Imel, E. A., Ruppe, M. D., Weber, T. J., Klausner, M. A., Wooddell, M. M., Kawakami, T., Ito, T., Zhang, X., Humphrey, J., & Peacock, M. (2014). Randomized trial of the anti-FGF23 antibody KRN23 in X-linked hypophosphatemia. *J. Clin. Invest.* 124: 1587–1597.

Clarke, B. (2008). Normal bone anatomy and physiology. *Clin. J. Am. Soc. Nephrol.* 3: S131–S139.

Cooper, D. M., Matyas, J. R., Katzenberg, M. A., & Hallgrimsson, B. (2004). Comparison of microcomputed tomographic and microradiographic measurements of cortical bone porosity. *Calcif. Tissue Int.* 74: 437–447.

Czekanska, E. M., Stoddart, M. J., Richards, R. G., & Hayes, J. S. (2012). In search of an osteoblast cell model for in vitro research. *Eur. Cells Mater.* 24: 1–17.

Divisato, G., Formicola, D., Esposito, T., Merlotti, D., Pazzaglia, L., Del Fattore, A., Siris, E., Orcel, P., Brown, J. P., Nuti, R., & Gianfrancesco, F. (2016). ZNF687 mutations in severe paget disease of bone associated with giant cell tumor. *Am. J. Hum. Genet.* 98: 275–286.

Dohnert, M. B., Venâncio, M., Possato, J. C., Zeferino, R. C., Dohnert, L. H., Zugno, A. I., De Souza, C. T., Paula, M. M., & Luciano, T. F. (2012). Gold nanoparticles and diclofenac diethylammonium administered by iontophoresis reduce inflammatory cytokines expression in Achilles tendinitis. *Int. J. Nanomed.* 7: 1651–1657.

El Demellawy, D., Davila, J., Shaw, A., & Nasr, Y. (2018). Brief review on metabolic bone disease. *Acad. Forensic Pathol.* 8: 611–640.

Everts, V., Delaissé, J. M., Korper, W., Jansen, D. C., Tigchelaar-Gutter, W., Saftig, P., & Beertsen, W. (2002). The bone lining cell: Its role in cleaning Howship's lacunae and initiating bone formation. *J. Bone Miner. Res*. 17: 77–90.

Fisher, B. (1913). Primary adamantinoma of the tibia. *Z. Pathol*. 12: 422–441.

Geim, A. K. (2009). Graphene: Status and prospects. *Science*. 324: 1530–1534.

Ghai, S. (2022). Ameloblastoma: An updated narrative review of an enigmatic tumor. *Cureus*. 14: e27734.

Glaser, D. L., & Kaplan, F. S. (1997). Osteoporosis: Definition and clinical presentation. *Spine*. 22: 12S–16S.

Gorham, L. W., & Stout, A. P. (1955). Massive osteolysis (acute spontaneous absorption of bone, phantom bone, disappearing bone); its relation to hemangiomatosis. *JBJS*. 37: 985–1004.

Grabowski, P. (2009). Physiology of bone. In *Calcium and Bone Disorders in Children and Adolescents*. J. Allgrove, and N. Shaw, Eds. Basel: Karger, pp. 32–48.

Greer, R. B. (1993). Wolff's law. *Orthop. Rev*. 22: 1087–1088.

Hodun, K., Chabowski, A., & Baranowski, M. (2021). Sphingosine-1-phosphate in acute exercise and training. *Scand. J. Med. Sci. Sports*. 31: 945–955.

Jaramillo-de la Torre, J. J., Bohinski, R. J., & Kuntz, C. (2006). Vertebral osteomyelitis. *Neurosurg. Clin*. 17: 339–351.

Kang, M. L., Kim, J. E., & Im, G. I. (2016). Thermoresponsive nanospheres with independent dual drug release profiles for the treatment of osteoarthritis. *Acta Biomater*. 39: 65–78.

Kaur, M., & Singh, K. (2019). Review on titanium and titanium based alloys as biomaterials for orthopaedic applications. *Mater. Sci. Eng. C*. 102: 844–862.

Kim, J. M., Lin, C., Stavre, Z., Greenblatt, M. B., & Shim, J. H. (2020). Osteoblast-osteoclast communication and bone homeostasis. *Cells*. 9: 2073.

Kobayashi, T., & Kronenberg, H. (2005). Minireview: Transcriptional regulation in development of bone. *Endocrinology*. 146: 1012–1017.

Kumar, S. A., & Madhyastha, H. (2017). Polymeric nanoparticles for vaccine delivery. In *Integrating Biologically-Inspired Nanotechnology Into Medical Practice*. B. K. Nayak, A. Nanda, and M. A. Bhat, Eds. Hershey, PA: IGI-Global, pp. 32–49.

Kumari, G., Abhishek, K., Singh, S., Hussain, A., Altamimi, M. A., Madhyastha, H., Webster, T. J., & Dev, A. (2022a). A voyage from 3D to 4D printing in nanomedicine and healthcare: Part I. *Nanomedicine*. 17: 237–253.

Kumari, G., Abhishek, K., Singh, S., Hussain, A., Altamimi, M. A., Madhyastha, H., Webster, T. J., & Dev, A. (2022b). A voyage from 3D to 4D printing in nanomedicine and healthcare: Part II. *Nanomedicine*. 17: 255–270.

Lorentzon, M. (2019). Treating osteoporosis to prevent fractures: Current concepts and future developments. *J. Intern. Med*. 285: 381–394.

Luca, L., Rougemont, A. L., Walpoth, B. H., Gurny, R., & Jordan, O. (2010). The effects of carrier nature and pH on rhBMP-2-induced ectopic bone formation. *J. Control. Release*. 147: 38–44.

Manes, R. P., Ryan, M. W., Batra, P. S., Mendelsohn, D., Fang, Y. V., & Marple, B. F. (2013). Ossifying fibroma of the nose and paranasal sinuses. *Int. Forum. Allergy Rhinol*. 3: 161–168.

Marini, J. C., Forlino, A., Bächinger, H. P., Bishop, N. J., Byers, P. H., Paepe, A., Fassier, F., Fratzl-Zelman, N., Kozloff, K. M., Krakow, D., Montpetit, K., & Semler, O. (2017). Osteogenesis imperfecta. *Nat. Rev. Dis. Primers*. 3: 17052.

Maudens, P., Seemayer, C. A., Thauvin, C., Gabay, C., Jordan, O., & Allémann, E. (2018). Nanocrystal-polymer particles: Extended delivery carriers for osteoarthritis treatment. *Small*. 14: 1703108.

Mediero, A., Wilder, T., Shah, L., & Cronstein, B. N. (2018). Adenosine A. *FASEB J*. 32: 3487–3501.

Meneses, J., van de Kemp, T., Costa-Almeida, R., Pereira, R., Magalhães, F. D., Castilho, M., & Pinto, A. M. (2022). Fabrication of polymer/graphene biocomposites for tissue engineering. *Polymers*. 14: 1038.

Meunier, P., Courpron, P., Edouard, C., Bernard, J., Bringuier, J., & Vignon, G. (1973). Physiological senile involution and pathological rarefaction of bone: Quantitative and comparative histological data. *Clin. Endocrinol. Metab*. 2: 239–256.

Micheli, L. J. (1987). The traction apophysitises. *Clin. Sports Med*. 6: 389–404.

Minisola, S., Fukumoto, S., Xia, W., Corsi, A., Colangelo, L., Scillitani, A., Pepe, J., Cipriani, C., & Thakker, R. V. (2022). Tumor-induced osteomalacia: A comprehensive review. *Endocr. Rev*. 4: 323–353.

Moreira Teixeira, L. S., Patterson, J., & Luyten, F. P. (2014). Skeletal tissue regeneration: Where can hydrogels play a role? *Int. Orthop*. 38: 1861–1876.

Munir, K. S., Wen, C., & Li, Y. (2019). Carbon nanotubes and graphene as nanoreinforcements in metallic biomaterials: A review. *Adv. Biosyst.* 3: e1800212.

Naziri, Q., Issa, K., Pivec, R., Harwin, S. F., Delanois, R. E., & Mont, M. A. (2013). Excellent results of primary THA using a highly porous titanium cup. *Orthopedics.* 36: e390–e394.

Klibanski, A., Adams-Campbell, L., Bassford, T., Blair, S. N., Boden, S. D., Dickersin, K., & Russell, W. E. (2001). Osteoporosis prevention, diagnosis, and therapy. *J. Am. Med. Assoc.* 285: 785–795.

Paget, J. (1877). On a form of chronic inflammation of bones (osteitis deformans). *Med. Chir. Trans.* 60: 37–64.9.

Pham, C. T. (2011). Nanotherapeutic approaches for the treatment of rheumatoid arthritis. *Wiley Interdiscip. Rev. Nanomed. Nanobiotechnol.* 3: 607–619.

Priya, M. V., Sivshanmugam, A., Boccaccini, A. R., Goudouri, O. M., Sun, W., Hwang, N., Deepthi, S., Nair, S. V., & Jayakumar, R. (2016). Injectable osteogenic and angiogenic nanocomposite hydrogels for irregular bone defects. *Biomed. Mater.* 11: 035017.

Reid, I. R., Green, J. R., Lyles, K. W., Reid, D. M., Trechsel, U., Hosking, D. J., Black, D. M., Cummings, S. R., Russell, R. G. G., & Eriksen, E. F. (2020). Zoledronate. *Bone.* 137: 115390.

Rozenberg, S., Bruyère, O., Bergmann, P., Cavalier, E., Gielen, E., Goemaere, S., Kaufman, J. M., Lapauw, B., Laurent, M. R., De Schepper, J., & Body, J. J. (2020). How to manage osteoporosis before the age of 50. *Maturitas.* 138: 14–25.

Sahoo, P. R., Madhyastha, H., Madhyastha, R., Maruyama, M., & Nakajima, Y. (2020). Recent progress in nanotheranostic medicine. In *Nanopharmaceuticals: Principles and Applications* (Vol. 3). V. K. Yata, S. Ranjan, N. Dasgupta, and E. Lichtfouse, Eds. Cham, Switzerland: Springer, pp. 317–334.

Sánchez-Fernández, M. J., Rutjes, J., Félix Lanao, R. P., Bender, J. C. M. E., van Hest, J. C. M., & Leeuwenburgh, S. C. G. (2021). Bone-adhesive hydrogels based on dual crosslinked poly(2-oxazoline)s. *Macromol. Biosci.* 21: e2100257.

Sharma, S., Madhyastha, H., Kirwale, S. S., Sakai, K., Katakia, Y. T., Majumder, S., & Roy, A. (2022). Dual antibacterial and anti-inflammatory efficacy of a chitosan-chondroitin sulfate-based in-situ forming wound dressing. *Carbohydr. Polym.* 298: 120126.

Shickh, P. A., Singh, A., & Kumar, A. (2018). Oxygen-releasing antioxidant cryogel scaffolds with sustained oxygen delivery for tissue engineering applications. *ACS Appl. Mater. Interfaces.* 10: 18458–18469.

Smolen, J. S., Aletaha, D., & McInnes, I. B. (2016). Rheumatoid arthritis. *Lancet.* 388: 1984.

Tian, L., Tang, N., Ngai, T., Wu, C., Ruan, Y., Huang, L., & Qin, L. (2019). Hybrid fracture fixation systems developed for orthopaedic applications: A general review. *J. Orthop. Translat.* 16: 1–13.

Tonna, S., Poulton, I. J., Taykar, F., Ho, P. W., Tonkin, B., Crimeen-Irwin, B., Tatarczuch, L., McGregor, N. E., Mackie, E. J., Martin, T. J., & Sims, N. A. (2016). Chondrocytic ephrin B2 promotes cartilage destruction by osteoclasts in endochondral ossification. *Development.* 143: 648–657.

Tyshkunova, I. V., Poshina, D. N., & Skorik, Y. A. (2022). Cellulose cryogels as promising materials for biomedical applications. *Int. J. Mol. Sci.* 23: 2037.

Uitterlinden, A. G., Arp, P. P., Paeper, B. W., Charmley, P., Proll, S., Rivadeneira, F., Fang, Y., van Meurs, J. B., Britschgi, T. B., Latham, J. A., & Brunkow, M. E. (2004). Polymorphisms in the sclerosteosis/van Buchem disease gene (SOST) region are associated with bone-mineral density in elderly whites. *Am. J. Hum. Genet.* 75: 1032–1045.

Yasuda, H. (2021). Discovery of the RANKL/RANK/OPG system. *J. Bone Miner. Metab.* 39: 2–11.

11 Modulatory Effects of Phytobioactives in Bone Metabolism and Regeneration

Archita Gupta, Rahul Deka, Sanjay Kumar Mehta, Kanishka Kunal, and Sneha Singh

11.1 INTRODUCTION

The human body is an interconnected network of various systems, among which the most important is the musculoskeletal system, which consists mainly of bones and connective tissue. The primary function of the musculoskeletal system is to provide a definite internal shape and structure. Bones are organs constructed from dense connective tissues, primarily collagen, a durable protein. In addition, the bone stores essential nutrients, minerals, and lipids and produces blood cells that play a critical role in protecting the body from extraneous materials (Hadjidakis & Androulakis, 2006; Olszta et al., 2007).

Bones are stiff and rigid due to the deposition of calcium and other mineral salts in the tissues. The cellular framework comprising osteoblasts, osteoclasts, osteocytes, and osteoprogenitor cells is essential for maintaining bone homeostasis (Berendsen & Olsen, 2015). Disorders affect the bones in many ways, from traumatic fractures to progressive cancerous tissue formation. Bone abnormalities may contribute to chronic pain and disability without proper therapy.

Common bone diseases in adults and children include osteoporosis involving low bone density, osteogenesis imperfecta turning bones brittle, Paget's disease making the bones weaker, bone infections, bone tuberculosis, and bone cancer (Rodan & Martin, 2000). Apart from bone diseases, critical fractures arising from sports activities, heavy lifting, and accidents can become a grave concern for the normal functioning of the body (Fazzalari, 2011). The treatment options for bone fractures include ultrasound therapy, which stimulates bone growth through higher neuroreceptors at the site of the fracture; bone morphogenic proteins (BMPs), which stimulate bone extracellular matrix (ECM) regeneration; growth hormones to increase osteoblastic activity; and tissue-engineered scaffolds at fracture sites that contain osteoconductive and biocompatible materials for bones such as hydroxyapatite, calcium sulfate, type I collagen, and β- tricalcium phosphate (β-TCP).

Although autografts remain the benchmark for bone fracture healing, their widespread availability remains a matter of concern (Roberts & Rosenbaum, 2012). This leads us to alternatives such as orthobiologics. Orthobiologics refers to integrating bioactive substances and regenerative stem cells with bone substitutes for efficient healing of the bone. Bone regeneration is a rigorous, well-ordered operation that encompasses a myriad of cellular components and other bioactive materials (Singh et al., 2020), and orthobiologics encompass bioactive substances such as BMPs, bisphosphonates, and other osteoinductive molecules.

However, despite their exhaustive utilization for regulating osteoblastic and osteoclastic activity, they often display side effects that need to be kept in check. Some of the well-documented adverse effects of such synthetic formulations are chronic hypocalcemia, wherein low calcium reduces bone mineral density; chronic inflammation followed by extreme pain and swelling in the bones; disruptive cancer formation; ectopic bone formation in nonosseous tissues such as muscles; enhanced

DOI: 10.1201/9781003307310-13

osteoclast-mediated bone remodeling; and cervical lymph node swelling that makes diagnosis and treatment difficult (Allen, 2008; James et al., 2016). This required utilization of alternative treatment medicines for efficient bone regeneration with no side effects.

From the annals of history to modern-day usage, herbal medicines have always had a strong foothold in the treatment regimes of humans. Plants are known for their bioactive phytoconstituents, forming the basis of treatment for many diseases (Das et al., 2021). Recent research applying phytobioactives has shown them to be cost-effective and easily accessible and show few complexities; they have shown promising potential and gathered significant attention (Gupta et al., 2021).

Considering the challenges and side effects of conventional methods of bone fracture healing, the use of phytobioactives has great potential. Their wide scale, economic availability, and lesser side effects make phytobioactives better for treating bone-related injuries (Gupta et al., 2023a). This chapter provides a comprehensive review of the key secondary metabolites of plants and their roles in bone regeneration, which could be advantageous for producing functional, efficient bone scaffolds. This chapter also highlights several extraction methods for phytobioactives and underlying modes of distribution. Further, we discussed various biomaterial- and nanomaterial-based delivery systems for phytobioactives as advanced bone regeneration strategies.

11.2 PHYTOBIOACTIVES IN BONE REGENERATION

The twenty-first century consists of many health issues that have made people's lives no less than a battlefield. Reports link the continuous prescription of allopathic drugs to unwanted side effects, raising alarms over their use (Marian et al., 2008). The World Health Organization (WHO), with the vision of creating awareness and broader acceptability of traditional medicine, launched the WHO Traditional Medicine Strategy 2014–2023 in 2013, which advanced traditional medicine from around the globe such as Ayurveda, Traditional Chinese Medicine, and Unani and promoted their rapid development and globalization (Burton et al., 2015).

Phytobioactives is a broad term that encompasses plant extracts, phytoconstituents, and their formulations (Wen et al., 2019). More than half of the world's population relies on some form of phytobioactives in their daily life. Excessive population growth, drug resistance, and expensive treatment modalities have compelled society to incorporate phytobioactive-based medications to treat diseases.

Traditional medicine utilization dates to 7000 BCE and has diverse values and traditions and a wide scope of use across the Indian subcontinent. Although British colonization created hurdles in the spread of traditional medicine-related information, the rural population relied on using traditional medicine for treating diseases (Jaiswal & Williams, 2017). In the Indian medicine market, it is estimated that more than 50% of modern-day drug formulations are derived from compounds with a plant baseline. According to statistics, well over 60% of cancer medications currently on the market or in clinical trials are composed of phytobioactives (Greenwell & Rahman, 2015). Around 80% of cardiovascular, anticancer, immunosuppressive, and antibacterial medications come from plant origin. Numerous clinical trials of such drug formulations composed of plant origin are going on globally, and the widescale acceptability of traditional medicine will bring new treatment regimes (Petrovska, 2012).

The world, encompassing developing and developed countries, has an enormous reservoir of valuable medicinal plants; the WHO estimates that this is more than 20,000. Extraction remains the primary step in evaluating plant extracts for biological activity from natural sources. Different plant parts like leaves, stem, flower, fruits, and roots can be utilized for extracting different phytobioactives (Figure 11.1).

Various extraction methods have been implemented that consider the chemical composition of the bioactive compound to be extracted. This aids in the specific isolation, identification, and further screening of the compounds. For better bioactivity, various solvent solutions of varying polarity are incorporated into crude plant extracts (Shakoor et al., 2023; Singh et al., 2020). In the case

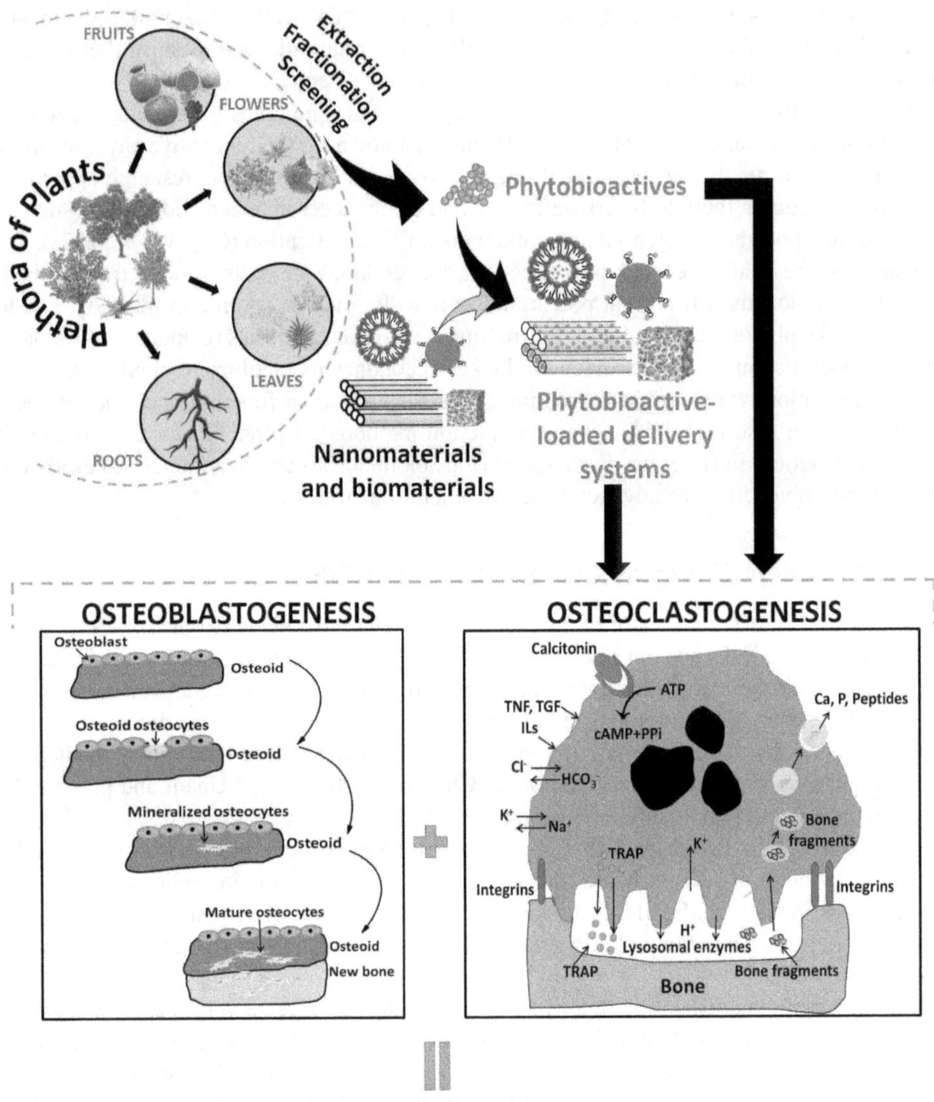

FIGURE 11.1 Bone remodeling potential of phytobioactives and phytobioactive-loaded delivery systems. The phytobioactives obtained by extraction, fractionation, and screening can either be directly used in the bone remodeling process or loaded into nanomaterial- and/or biomaterial-based delivery systems for efficient bone remodeling (reproduced with permission from Gupta, A., Mehta, S. K., Kumar, A., & Singh, S.: Advent of phytobiologics and nano-interventions for bone remodeling: a comprehensive review. Crit. Rev. Biotechnol. 2021. 3. 142–169. Copyright 2021 Taylor & Francis).

of nonpolar compounds, extraction can be performed using hexane and ethyl acetate as solvents (Awotedu et al., 2020); for polar compounds, extraction can be performed using methanol (Abd Aziz et al., 2021); for organic compounds, extraction can be performed using chloroform (Jones & Kinghorn, 2012); for lipophilic compounds, extraction can be performed using dichloromethane or a 1:1 mix of methanol and dichloromethane (Marrelli et al., 2012).

Although conventional techniques such as Soxhlet extraction and maceration are used extensively, technology advances have led to the development of more sophisticated techniques such as supercritical fluid extraction, microwave-assisted extraction, and ultrasound-assisted extraction. They offer less loss of bioactive compounds, better stability, reduced use of organic solvents, preliminary filtration regarding sample cleanup, and preferable extraction kinetics (Xu et al., 2017). However, phytobioactives research lacks interaction-related information, and their complex compositions and extraction processes make it difficult to identify their bioactive constituents. Therefore, the shift towards a more targeted drug research approach is the need of the hour. A systems biology approach is being tried to identify bioactive phytoconstituents from crude extracts. Modern-day techniques like gas chromatography, thin layer chromatography, ultraviolet, and mass spectroscopy have aimed to better classify phytobioactives, opening up new avenues in studying crosstalk between phytoconstituents (Mobasseri et al., 2020).

Phytobioactives exhibit efficient antioxidant (Vaiserman et al., 2020), anticancer (Ganesan et al., 2018), antimicrobial (Kuo et al., 2020), antiosteoporotic (Shen et al., 2018), and cardioprotective (Houacine et al., 2020) effects among others. Some well-known phytobioactives are polyphenols, terpenoids, steroids, vitamins, and alkaloids. Phytobioactives, as a whole, are considered potent, nontoxic, and cost-efficient alternatives to synthetic bioactive molecules. Research is advancing expeditiously on their healing action in bone and bone-related injuries (Gupta et al., 2021).

There are two important cells, osteoblasts and osteoclasts, that are prominently involved in bone remodeling, and phytobioactives significantly influence the activity of these two cells through different mechanisms. Osteoblasts are involved in bone formation, and phytobioactives activate the well-regulated process of osteoblastogenesis; they allow for differentiating osteoblasts and the enhanced expression of osteoblastic genes. Osteoblasts differentiate into osteocytes and facilitate calcium deposition and tissue mineralization, entrapping the osteocytes within the mineralized tissue and resulting in new bone (Figure 11.1).

Phytobioactives extracted using polar solvents are reported to enhance the formation of soft bone callus followed by osteoblastogenesis triggered by the upregulation of alkaline phosphatase (ALP) and Runt-related transcription factor-2 (Runx2) through different signaling pathways (Toor et al., 2019). Phytobioactives also ameliorate fractures and promote the formation of soft bone tissue around the injury site (Khedgikar et al., 2017). They additionally regulate the activity of osteoclasts, which are involved in bone resorption. Phytobioactives inhibit the expression of such osteoclastic genes, thereby maintaining bone density.

Resveratrol, a prominent phytobioactive molecule, has been shown to slow down the activity of the nuclear factor kappa-light-chain enhancer of activated B cells (NF-κB) pathway induced by the receptor activator of nuclear factor kappa-B ligand (RANKL) and the downregulation of inflammatory markers necessary for osteoclastogenesis (He et al., 2010). An important phytobioactive obtained from tea has been shown to enhance the rate of osteoclast apoptosis via the downregulation of the RANKL-JNK pathway (Tominari et al., 2015). Although traditional medicine is widely available for treating bone-related disorders or fractures, its underlying mechanisms are not well explored, posing the need to explore the potential of phytobioactives for treating bone disorders and healing.

The different classes of phytobioactives (e.g., terpenoids, steroids, alkaloids, polyphenols) are studied for their effects on regulating bone metabolic pathways and other factors, and various methods have been utilized to extract potential phytobioactives; specific classes call for specific extraction methods. Traditional medicine lacks clear information regarding its underlying molecular mechanisms. Information regarding molecule-to-molecule interaction, chemical structures, and biosynthetic pathways of phytobioactives can be crucial in developing more advanced and better formulations to stimulate bone regeneration. In the supplementary material provided with this chapter, we discuss in detail different phytobioactives, their biosynthetic pathways, the specific extraction process, and the chemical structures essential in regulating bone regeneration.

11.2.1 Terpenoids and Steroids

Plants are complex like other living organisms, regulated by different physiological processes. Plants are factories of a wide range of primary and secondary metabolites. Secondary metabolites are phytobioactives that are not directly responsible for normal physiological processes in plants (Olivoto et al., 2017). One such class of secondary metabolites is terpenoids. Terpenes constitute a class of simple hydrocarbons, and terpenoids form a modified class of terpenes.

More than 10,000 terpenoids have been documented; many more are yet to be investigated. A significant proportion of terpene concentration is available from plants and fungal origin, and a limited amount derives from bacterial strains. The occurrence of terpenoids can be traced way back in history, having their presence in fossils and age-specific sedimentary particles (de Lima et al., 2019).

The role of terpenoids and steroids has been reported by several researchers in studies on antimicrobial (Gutiérrez-del-Río et al., 2018), anticancer (Chen et al., 2021), antidiabetic (Smitha Grace et al., 2019), and immunomodulatory (Raphael & Kuttan, 2003) activity and most recently in the field of bone modulation (Xu et al., 2021). Scientists have reported the bone modulation properties of terpenoids in terms of their defensive role against the loss of bone cells and maintaining bone homeostasis (Figure 11.2 and Figure 11.3).

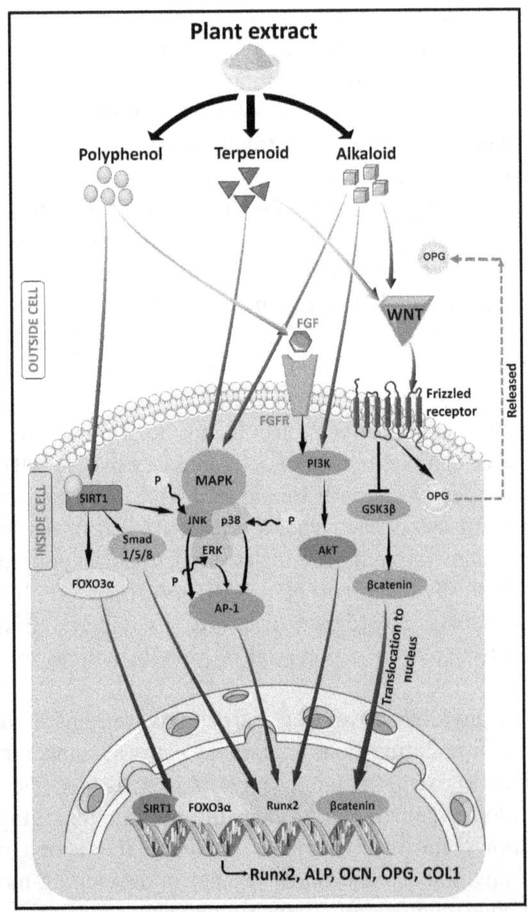

FIGURE 11.2 Mechanistic pathway involved in osteoblastogenesis by terpenoids, alkaloids, and polyphenols. Different classes of phytobioactives obtained from plant extracts can interact with the osteoblast receptor or cellular proteins to enhance the expression of osteoblastic proteins like Runx2, ALP, OCN, OPG, and COL1.

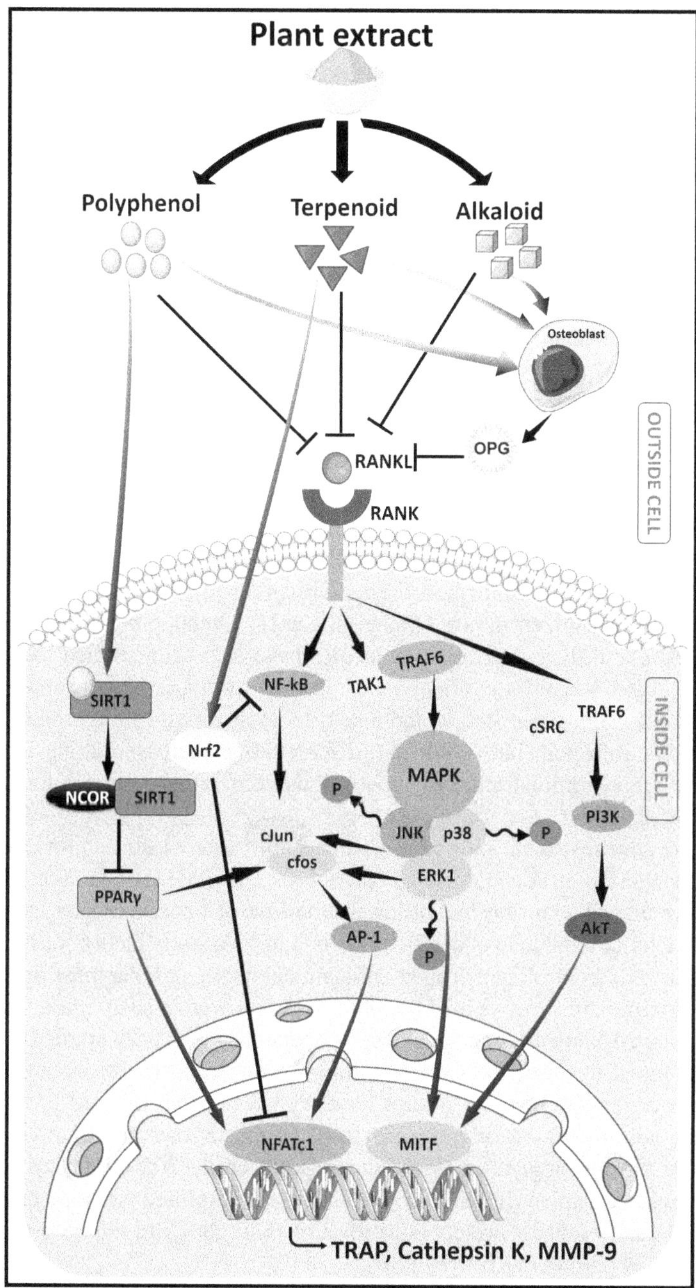

FIGURE 11.3 Mechanistic pathway involved in osteoclastogenesis by terpenoids, alkaloids, and polyphenols. Different classes of phytobioactives obtained from plant extracts interact with RANKL or cellular proteins of osteoclasts to inhibit the expression of osteoclastic proteins like TRAP, Cathepsin K, and MMP-9.

In vitro reports have shown that monoterpenoids can impact the differentiation of both osteoblasts (bone-forming cells) and osteoclasts (bone-resorbing cells) via the same pathways (Dolder et al., 2006; Mühlbauer et al., 2003). The proliferation of bone marrow mesenchymal cells (BMSCs) was shown to increase with the application of iridoid glycosides, namely, monotropein, swertiamarin, and catalpol with the eventual stimulation of the Wnt pathway and obstructing NF-κB (Cheng et al., 2020). Another study showed higher anti-osteoclast activity after applying swertiamarin in osteoblast–osteoclast cocultures. The researchers observed that swertiamarin obtained from methanol extract of *Enicostema axillare* decreased the expression of RANKL and receptor activator of nuclear factor kappa-B (RANK) expression, elevating the levels of osteoprotegerin, thus favoring the anti-osteoclast activity (Hairul-Islam et al., 2017). Additionally, bakuchiol obtained from the extract of *Psoralea corylifolia L.* hinders the phosphorylation of Akt and the nuclear translocation of phosphorylated c-jun, which affects the RANKL-stimulated differentiation of osteoclasts (Chai et al., 2018). An in vivo study incorporating ovariectomized mice showed that catalpol obtained from *Rehmannia glutinosa* extract stimulated the bone regeneration capability of BMSCs (Yang et al., 2021).

Similar to monoterpenoids, the activity of diterpenoids like abietic acids, kir, cafestol, and kahweol has been studied with respect to bone remodeling. Experimental studies reflect that cafestol and kahweol activate Nrf-2, which decreases osteoclast differentiation (Fukuma et al., 2015). The NF-κB and mitogen-activated protein kinase (MAPK) pathways influence a wide range of bone-related deformities (Kramer & Goodyear, 2007). Abietic acid, kahweol, and cafestol inhibit osteoclast differentiation and reduce their bone resorption ability by inducing oxidative stress as a consequence of NF-κB downregulation and inhibition of p38 MAPK phosphorylation (Choi et al., 2019).

In vitro and in vivo studies showed that after the application of kir, the RANKL-induced NF-κB p65 pathway, caveolin-1 expression, and Ca^{2+} oscillation were downregulated, compromising bone osteoclastogenesis; the authors confirmed their findings on microcomputed tomography (micro-CT) scans of the ovariectomized mouse (Zou et al., 2021). Comparably, triterpenoids like lupeol, oleanolic acid, alisol, and their derivative molecules have also been studied for bone remodeling (Kushwaha et al., 2016). Lupeol and alisol were reported to hinder NF-κB and MAPK pathways conferring their use for anti-osteoporotic and anti-osteoclast activity (Şöhretoğlu & Renda, 2020). Experimental studies reflected that osteoblast differentiation increased along with a decrease in osteoclast activity after administration of lupeol, thus conferring their use for anti-osteoporotic activity (Nguyen et al., 2021).

Similarly, lupeol administration showed pronounced anti-osteoclastic activity in 1α,25(OH)2D3-induced osteoclastogenesis in a coculture of osteoblasts and BMSCs (Wang et al., 2016). Mouse model studies have also shown that lupeol lowers the loss of bone, thus confirming their use for anti-osteoporotic activity (Chauhan et al., 2018). In one in vivo study incorporating ovariectomized mice, alisol significantly controlled estrogen-deficient decreases in bone mass density and induced changes in bone microarchitecture; Th-17 lymphocyte levels were also affected (Lee et al., 2010).

One of the most well-known tetraterpenoids, lycopene, has also been studied for bone remodeling activities and found to lower the oxidative stress experienced by osteoblasts, thus conferring a protective effect on bones. In vitro studies have shown that NF-κB and MAPK pathways are inhibited with the administration of lycopene, thus delimiting osteoclast activity; these findings were supported by the histological analysis (Odes-Barth et al., 2020; Palozza et al., 2012). The oxygenated terpenoid derivative limonoid was also recently explored for bone modulation studies. Findings indicated that limonoids protect bone through their ability to inhibit osteoclast activity by modulating the MAPK pathway (Kimira, 2019).

Limonin, a limonoid compound, was administered to analyze its effect on osteoblasts. In vitro studies incorporating MC3T3-E1 cell lines showed that limonin could modulate the extracellular signal-regulated kinase (ERK) and p38-MAPK signaling pathway, thus inducing osteoblast differentiation (Park et al., 2021). Micro-CT analysis for ovariectomized mice models showed elevated bone mass density and enhanced bone microarchitecture after administering limonin (Lee et al., 2016).

Saponins are steroidal compounds consisting of triterpenoid units interlinked to one or more polysaccharide chains. In vitro studies incorporating MC3T3-E1 cell lines showed that H_2O_2-stimulated oxidative stress was lowered by using a saponin called ophiopogonin D obtained from roots of *Dioscorea batatas*, thus regaining their osteoblast differentiation activity (Sautour et al., 2007). This correlated to the fact that ophiopogonin D is a better antioxidant that directly affects the FOXO3α-β-catenin signaling pathways (Huang et al., 2015). Similarly, another saponin called diosgenin, mainly found in *Dioscorea villosa* wild yam tubers, has been reported for anti-osteoporotic activity (An et al., 2016). A mouse model showed that diosgenin administration enhanced osteoblast differentiation and bone microarchitecture, conferring its potential use for osteoporosis treatment (Ge et al., 2021).

Cardiac glycosides (digoxin, digitoxin) and phytosterol (β-sitosterol, β-ecdysone) come under the class of steroids. Reports suggest their beneficial use for postmenopausal women due to their estrogen-mimicking properties and bone protection properties (Dean et al., 2017). β-ecdysone, a well-known phytosteroid obtained from alcoholic extract of *Tinospora cordifolia* has been reported for enhancing osteoblasts differentiation (Singh et al., 2020). An in vitro study incorporating the MG-63 cell line showed that β-ecdysone administration increased bone cell formation (Abiramasundari et al., 2018).

11.2.2 Alkaloids and Other Nitrogen-Containing Compounds

The class of natural compounds called alkaloids are also considered an important class of secondary metabolites produced by plants. The term *alkaloids* was coined by W. Meissner and is derives from the Greek 'alkal' referring to 'alkali' and 'oides', meaning 'like', which translates to 'alkali-like compounds' considering their favorable nitrogen content. Stereochemical conformations of the phytoconstituents significantly impact the biological properties governed by the molecules.

The role of alkaloids and other nitrogen-containing compounds has been reported by several researchers regarding antifungal (Qihua et al., 2001), antitumor (Zhang & Kanakkanthara, 2020), anticholinergic (Cornelissen et al., 2020), and antimalarial (Liu et al., 2020) effect, and most recently, alkaloids have been incorporated into bone remodeling studies (Umashankar, 2020). The canonical Wnt/β-catenin signaling pathway is an essential pathway for the direct functioning of BMSCs and the indirect functioning of osteoblasts. Experimental studies have shown that berberine, an isoquinoline alkaloid extracted from plants such as *Berberis pruinosa* was able to upregulate the Wnt/β-catenin signaling pathway (Figure 11.2) (Tao et al., 2016).

Transcription factors play a significant role in the differentiation of osteoblasts. Runx2 is a principal osteogenic transcription factor that was shown to be upregulated through the p38-MAPK pathway after the administration of berberine. The PI3K/Akt pathway is responsible for migrating BMSCs to sites of skeletal damage, and this process was also elevated after adding berberine to the experimental model (Wong et al., 2020a). Reports have shown that berberine can inhibit the interaction of RANKL/RANK, which in turn controls the level of osteoclast differentiation (Figure 11.3) (Zhou et al., 2015a). The effect of berberine was also studied with respect to the osteoclast–miRNA relationship. Investigators reported that miRNA-23a regulated the RANKL-associated glycogen synthase kinase-3 beta (GSK3β) pathway. Specifically, berberine inhibited RANKL, which indirectly modulates the GSK3β pathway, thus controlling the differentiation of osteoclasts (Sujitha & Rasool, 2019).

In an experimental study of osteoporotic menopausal women, carboline alkaloids extracted from the seed of *Peganum harmala* were reported to enhance the bone mineral density of the study population (Hafshejani et al., 2021). Similarly, harmine, yet another carboline alkaloid extracted from *Peganum harmala*, showed potential in upregulating the Runx2, Ost, and BMP signaling pathways, ultimately enhancing osteoblast differentiation (Yonezawa et al., 2011). In vitro studies revealed that piperine, an alkaloid of medical importance obtained from *Piper nigrum*, could upregulate the expression of the Runx2 transcription factor, subsequently enhancing osteoblastic differentiation of MC3T3-E1 and C3H10T1/2 cell lines (Kim et al., 2018). Another in vitro study reported enhanced osteogenesis with increased ALP expression post-administration of piperine (Li et al., 2019). Benzophenanthridine alkaloid extracted from *Sanguinaria canadensis* was also evaluated for its anti-osteoporotic activity. A series of in vitro studies incorporating MC3T3-E1 cell lines showed inhibition of NF-κB and ERK signaling pathways, leading to the attenuation of bone osteoclast functioning (Zhang et al., 2018).

11.2.3 Polyphenols

Everyone is highly advised to eat at least five servings of fruits and vegetables daily for a healthy life. Drinking green tea and red wine and eating chocolates occasionally also increase well-being and life expectancy. The answer to these recommendations lies within the biggest class of phyto-bioactives: polyphenols.

Curcuma longa is a rhizome most commonly found in the Indian subcontinent, also known as turmeric (Bose et al., 2018). Four types of curcuminoids are present in *Curcuma longa*, curcumin I, II, III, and cyclocurcumin, of which curcumin I constitutes the highest percentage in the rhizome (Ahangari et al., 2019). Numerous medicinal properties have been reported for curcumin, such as antioxidant, antitumor, antimicrobial, anti-arthritic, and anti-inflammatory (Bose et al., 2018; Ahangari et al., 2019) effects.

Curcumin is also known to regulate different signaling pathways and molecular targets such as NF-κB, tumor necrosis factor-α (TNF-α), cytokines, and vascular endothelial growth factor (VEGF). These signaling pathways and molecular targets assist in bone turnover in some way or the other, in which NF-κB plays a vital role in regulating osteoclast cells and maintaining bone density (Bose et al., 2018). Therefore, curcumin has been extensively used recently to treat diseases related to bones and tendons.

Curcumin was tested on Sprague–Dawley rats to check its efficacy in healing patellar tendon window defects created in two groups of rats. It was observed that the group of rats administered 100 mg/kg body weight of curcumin orally showed better recovery and healing of tendons than the control group (Jiang et al., 2016). In a recent study, bone formation due to the use of curcumin in type-2 diabetic mice was also reported. The group of diabetic mice administered 10 μmol/L of curcumin showed decreased bone destruction and enhanced bone density. Hence curcumin could be used to treat osteoporosis arising from diabetes (He et al., 2020).

Naringin, another polyphenol, is a flavanone and is most commonly derived from the pericarp of citrus fruits. Naringin has several pharmaceutical properties, such as antitumor, anti-inflammatory, antioxidant, antidiabetic, and immunomodulatory (Kiran et al., 2017) effects. Researchers also used naringin to increase bone mass among rats suffering from retinoic acid-induced osteoporosis (Wong et al., 2007) and found that it enhances the protein content, alkaline phosphatase activity, and proliferation of UMR106 cells (osteoblast-like cells) among rats (Leena et al., 2017). Silibinin is a flavonoid extracted from the seeds and fruits of *Silybum marianum* and is well-known for its anticancer, antihepatotoxic, and anti-inflammatory properties (Kvasnička et al., 2003; Jia et al., 2010; Salamone et al., 2012).

Researchers have recently discovered that silibinin induces the osteogenic differentiation of stem cells, osteoblast differentiation, and osteoclast inhibition. Although silibinin has good pharmaceutical properties, its use is limited due to its hydrophobic nature and low bioavailability. Resveratrol is a stilbene obtained from *Polygonum cuspidatum* belonging to the class of flavonols and has very high antioxidant properties (Gupta et al., 2020a). It is known to activate Sirtuin 1 (Sirt1), a nicotine adenine dinucleotide-dependent deacetylase that plays a major role in increasing enzymatic activity in bone cells (Figure 11.2).

Resveratrol meditates the differentiation of mesenchymal stem cells (MSCs) for osteoblast formation through direct or indirect participation. In the indirect mechanism, Sirt1 activated by resveratrol interacts with nuclear receptor corepressor, which inhibits peroxisome proliferator-activated receptor gamma (PPARγ) and subsequently osteoclastogenesis (Shakibaei et al., 2011). The inhibition of PPARγ affects the kinetics of the nuclear factor of activated T-cells (NFATc1) directly and indirectly by preventing the expression of activator protein-1 (AP-1) through deactivating the transcription of cJun and cfos transcription factor. The downregulation of NFATc1 through Sirt1 leads to the inhibition of osteoclastogenesis.

Likewise, resveratrol interacts with Sirt1 and regulates the process of osteoblastogenesis by interacting with various downstream molecules. Sirt1 activates the transcription of Runx2, which leads to the formation of the Sirt1-Runx2 complex. The activation of Sirt1 by resveratrol also contributes to the increased phosphorylation of various downstream kinases like suppressor of mothers against decapentaplegic (SMAD1/5/8), MAPKs, PKB/Akt, and AMPK, which contributes to the osteoblastic differentiation (Lee et al., 2011; Shakibaei et al., 2011).

Sirt1 also regulates Runx2 through the phosphorylation of SMAD1/5/8 and expression of AP-1 by activating the JNK pathway. Expression of Runx2 is also known to be stimulated by the activation of the PI3K/Akt pathway when polyphenol interacts with fibroblast growth factor ligands (Fernández-Arroyo et al., 2015). The upregulation of Runx2 by polyphenol induces osteoblast differentiation and proliferation. Sirt1 also interacts with the FOXO3α gene, resulting in the expression of the Sirt1/FOXO3α complex in DNA, which induces osteoblastogenesis.

In another such process, polyphenols inhibit the binding of RANKL to the RANK receptor, which results in downstream deactivation of NF-κB and MAPKs (Figure 11.3). The inhibition of NF-κB and MAPKs prevents the expression of JNK, p38, ERK1, and AP-1, thereby downregulating the expression of NFATc1 and inhibiting osteoclastogenesis. Polyphenols are also known to enhance the expression of osteoprotegerin (OPG) marker protein within osteoblasts. OPG inhibits the activity of RANKL, resulting in the downregulation of osteoclastogenesis (Shakibaei et al., 2011).

Quercetin is a common phytobioactive that is mostly found in fruits and vegetables. It is known to enhance bone cell activity without affecting the proliferation property and, therefore, is one of the most suitable phytobioactives that can be used for bone formation and repairing bone defects. Researchers studied quercetin in animal models and determined that it could heal bone defects in 14 days (Wong et al., 2008). Catechin is primarily obtained by consuming tea, and epigallocatechin-3-gallate (EGCG), a catechin majorly found in green tea, shows the strongest antioxidant and antitumor effect (Bors & Saran, 1987; Yang et al., 2002). Very few studies have been carried out to know the effect of EGCG on bone health and metabolism, but it is reported that catechins activate osteogenic differentiation among MSCs and improve the alkaline phosphatase activity of osteoblasts; the researchers also reported that EGCG inhibits osteoclast differentiation by inhibiting the expression of RANKL (Vali et al., 2007).

RANKL is an important factor for osteoclast differentiation and bone resorption; EGCG inhibits bone resorption by suppressing RANKL activity (Tominari et al., 2015). In one study, EGCG suppressed the differentiation of RAW2647 macrophage into osteoclast cells (Lin et al., 2009). Rutin is also known as vitamin P and is a type of bioflavonoid that is known for its antioxidant, anti-inflammatory, and anticancer activity (Lee et al., 2020). Rutin can be found in abundance in different fruits and vegetables, but grapes and buckwheat remain the major sources of rutin (Frutos et al., 2019; Kreft et al., 2006). Sugar moiety attached to the phenolic group of rutin makes the bioflavonoid hydrophilic, and its various properties have led to its use for different treatments such as cardiovascular, tumor, cerebrovascular diseases, and inflammation (Frutos et al., 2019; Zhao et al., 2019).

Rutin is a dietary glycoside that gets converted into quercetin by the bacteria present in the large intestine (Hyun et al., 2014; Tamura et al., 1980). The high antioxidant activity of the molecule has attracted researchers' interest in its use in the inhibition of osteoclast differentiation and the promotion of osteoblast differentiation. The reactive oxygen species (ROS) level is linked with bone metabolism. Studies have shown that a high ROS level can increase osteoclast differentiation, which can decrease bone mass (Kyung et al., 2008).

In one study, rutin was used to control the level of ROS and TNF-α to inhibit osteoclast differentiation. The researchers concluded that rutin inhibits the formation of RANKL-induced TNF-α and the activation of NF-κB and controls the release of ROS, which helped inhibit osteoclast formation (Kyung et al., 2008). The double planar benzene ring present in rutin is similar to naturally occurring estrogen, allowing rutin to act like estrogen by binding to estrogen receptors (Zhao et al., 2020).

Researchers also reported that rutin enhances bone mass in osteopenia rats by inducing osteoblast differentiation and inhibiting osteoclast formation. Wistar rats were used for the experiment, in which 20 rats were ovariectomized (OVX) and 10 were sham-operated controls. The authors reported that a dose of 0.25% rutin in the diet of OVX rats inhibited femoral trabecular bone loss by enhancing osteoblast differentiation and decreasing bone resorption rate among rats

(Horcajada-Molteni et al., 2000). Researchers have also studied the effects of rutin derived from watercress (*N. officinale*) on human MG-63 osteoblasts. The rutin enhanced cell proliferation and alkaline phosphatase activity, as well as stimulating collagen formation in MG-63 cells (Hyun et al., 2014).

11.3 CHALLENGES FACED DURING PHYTOBIOACTIVE USAGE

Plants are considered factories of numerous medicinally active phytobioactives. Phytobioactives of primary and secondary origin exhibit immense potential in tackling or preventing diseases. Such compounds can range from phenol-containing polyphenols to nitrogen-containing alkaloids as well as diversely modified lipids like terpenoids and much more. Phytobioactives have been used for ages, but several issues have restricted them from being clinically used as approved drugs. The primary issues that persist with using phytobioactives is pharmacokinetic issues like bioavailability, multiple drug interactions, and metabolic instability (Dominguez et al., 2017). Phytobioactives also encounter low aqueous solubility (Cao et al., 2020) and inaccessibility to the site of action (McClements & Öztürk, 2021).

Phytobioactives have challenging pharmacokinetic profiles regulating absorption, distribution, metabolism, excretion, and toxicity (ADMET). ADMET issues are generally identified by the low solubility of the compounds, poor gastrointestinal absorption, and excessive hepatic metabolism (Amawi et al., 2017). Phytobioactive absorption sites vary in different areas of the gastrointestinal tract (Figure 11.4). The phytobioactives are generally absorbed from the small intestine after being hydrolyzed by intestinal enzymes and colonic microflora.

Phytobioactives, when ingested with other materials, can result in the complexation of the phytoconstituents, thereby limiting their absorption. Phytobioactives in the body can also undergo glucuronidation, methylation, and sulfation, making the highly polar complexes extremely susceptible to excretion or elimination from the body (Spencer, 2003). As a result, the metabolites that reach the different organs through systemic circulation are structurally different from the initial phytobioactive, making it difficult to determine their pharmacological effects (Pandey & Rizvi, 2009).

Phytobioactive metabolites usually circulate in the body bound to albumin, resulting in their nonspecific delivery and in much lower concentrations of phytobioactives reaching the site of action (Parhi et al., 2020). Moreover, after reaching the colon, the unabsorbed phytobioactives experience significant degradation via hydrolysis and ring fission through microflora (Murota et al., 2018; Marín et al., 2015). Reports have indicated that flavanols degrade completely within hours when incubated with intestinal secretions (Thilakarathna & Rupasinghe, 2013).

The use of curcumin, a polyphenol, is limited due to its hydrophobic nature, very low bioavailability of about 11 ng/mL, and rapid metabolism (Gupta et al., 2020c). Similarly, quercetin, a flavanol, degrades rapidly within 6 h under normal physiological pH, resulting in only 20–30% bioavailability of its oral dose (Kandemir et al., 2022). The limited bioavailability of the phytobioactives significantly reduces their pharmacological effects.

Low solubility is another issue faced by phytobioactives due to their hydrophobic nature (Pereira et al., 2015). An appropriate dosage of the phytoformulation needs to be administered for an effective therapeutic potential. Low concentrations below the optimum dosage will result in inefficacy. Such limitations faced by phytobioactives pose a significant barrier in clinical development that cannot be overcome by increasing their doses. Moreover, high doses can cause countereffects by increasing inflammatory reactions (Akindele et al., 2014).

Therefore, it is necessary to enhance the research to meet the challenges faced by the systemic delivery of phytobioactives. A comprehensive and systematic approach for precise and prolonged delivery is highly required. Different delivery systems for the phytobioactives are advancements in bone regeneration, enhancing the overall solubility, bioavailability, delivery, and optimal dosage (Verma et al., 2019b).

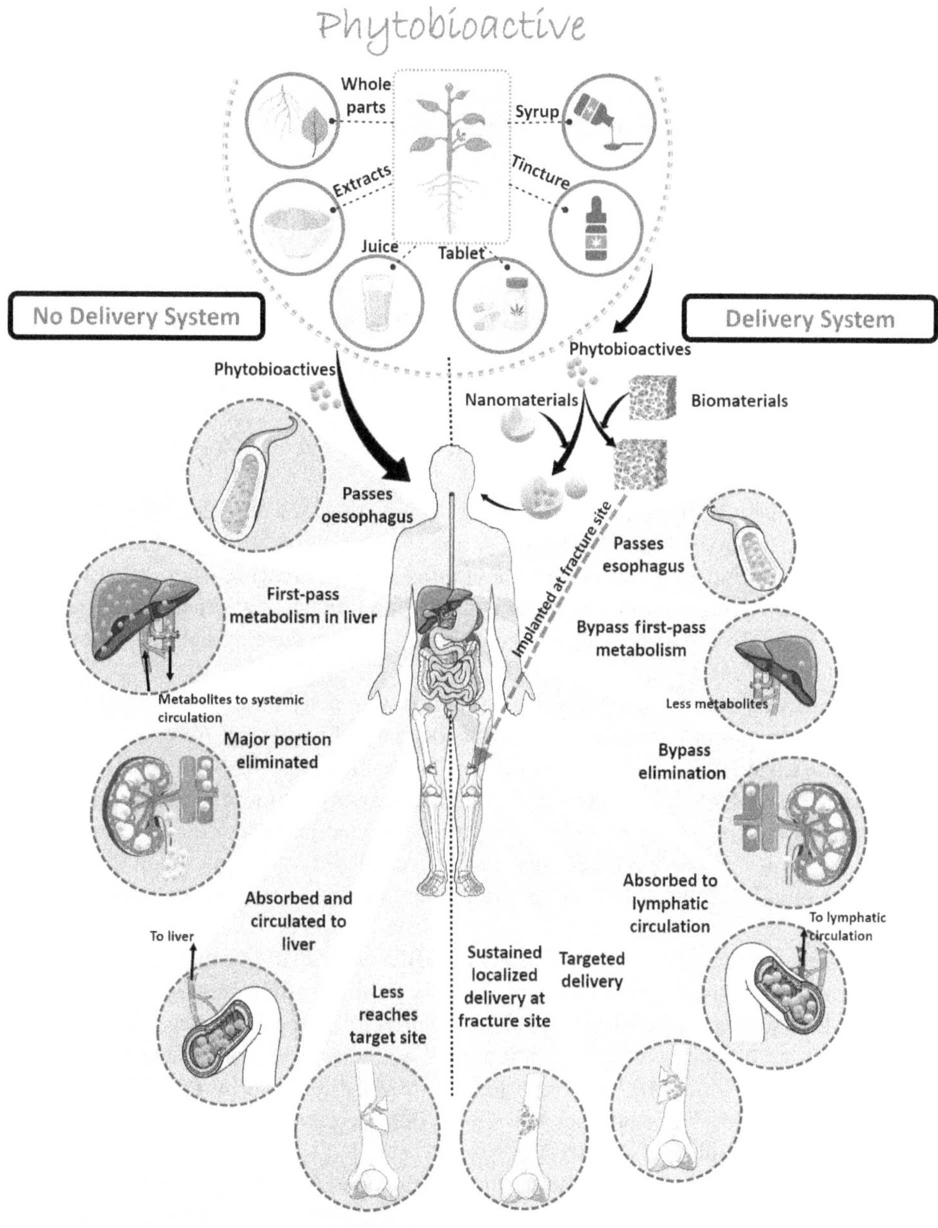

FIGURE 11.4 Fate of phytobioactives in the human body with no delivery system and with nano-material- and biomaterial-based delivery systems used for fracture healing.

11.4 DELIVERY SYSTEMS FOR PHYTOBIOACTIVES

11.4.1 Nanomaterial-Based Delivery Systems

Nanomaterial-based delivery systems (NDS), in the 1–100 nm size range, act as carriers of phytobioactives to sites of action. NDS comes in different shapes and compositions, bringing unique modes of action (Gu et al., 2013; Gupta & Singh, 2022). They can comprise polymeric nanoparticles, inorganic nanoparticles, nanoemulsions, nano-scaled spheres, and lipidemic nanoparticles among others (Wilczewska et al., 2012).

The phytobioactives can be loaded via different techniques ranging from hydrophobic loading into the polymeric matrix of organic nanoparticles to hydrophilic functionalization onto the surface of inorganic nanoparticles (Gupta et al., 2021). NDS for phytobioactives are necessary to overcome their low bioavailability, instability, and low solubility. Once loaded into the NDS, phytobioactives can easily overcome the barriers to their direct administration, facilitating their site-directed delivery (Figure 11.4).

The NDS facilitates the sustained and prolonged release of phytobioactives to the body tissues. After the uptake of phytobioactive-loaded NDS, the phytobioactive passes through the gastrointestinal tract, eluding the acidic environment, and reaches the colon. The NDS also prevents the degradation of phytobioactives by the colonic microbiota, thereby leading to maximum absorption (Patra et al., 2018). The site-directed delivery through an NDS allows the phytobioactives to evade the first-pass metabolism, and slower excretion out of the system leads to better efficacy at lower concentrations (Suri et al., 2007).

Different NDS have been synthesized and are under research to enhance the bioavailability, stability, and efficacy of phytobioactives in bone tissue engineering. Berberine, an alkaloid derivative of isoquinoline, is a well-known phytobioactive for treating osteoarthritis. However, its poor bioavailability, low solubility in an aqueous medium, and short half-life have limited its clinical use and delivery to the targeted site, leading to the development of different carrier vehicles.

Liposomes are well-established NDS due to their low toxicity and biodegradable nature, and they are one of the most-considered carriers for the delivery of berberine. A comparison study was conducted to investigate the efficiency of PEGylated liposomes carrying berberine with PEGylated liposomes carrying miRNA-23a (Sujitha et al., 2020). An arthritis mouse model study showed that berberine-loaded liposomes were more efficient in the targeted entry into the disease site than the miRNA-23a liposomes. The effects were the result of reduced RANKL secretion in the talocrural joint, which eventually limits osteoclast differentiation and excessive loss of calcium (Sujitha & Rasool, 2019).

Berberine-coated mannosylated liposomes (ML-BBR) were also formulated, and their efficacy against bone marrow-derived monocytes/macrophages (BMMs) stimulated by RANKL was studied. When BMMs were treated with ML-BBR as opposed to free berberine, p-GSK3, NFATc1, and calcineurin were downregulated, which inhibited osteoclastogenesis (Sujitha & Rasool, 2019). Further high expression of MMP9 was reported in BMMs stimulated by RANKL and led to the degradation of the ECM. The study showed diminishing expression of MMP9 among the cells treated with ML-BBR (Sujitha et al., 2018).

Chitosan nanoparticles loaded with berberine (BBR-loaded CNs) have also been used for their efficient delivery and anti-apoptosis of chondrocytes in an osteoarthritis rat model. The delivery of berberine by BBR-loaded CNs increased the level of berberine and its retention time in rat plasma compared with the rat model administered with free berberine. The treatment with BBR-loaded CNs also decreased the expression of caspase-3 and Bax and increased the expression of Bcl-2, resulting in anti-apoptosis of chondrocytes in the articular cartilage region of the rats (Zhou et al., 2015b).

Curcumin, an essential phytobioactive extracted from the rhizomes of *Curcuma longa L.*, is known to regulate NF-κβ at the cellular level (Aggarwal et al., 2009; Bose et al., 2018). NF-κβ plays an important role in bone remodeling, and various studies have shown that curcumin downregulates osteoclastogenesis by inactivating NF-κβ and stopping its entry into the nucleus. However, curcumin's rapid metabolism, low absorption, and low bioavailability have limited its use for bone remodeling. To overcome the mentioned issues, studies have been carried out for local and targeted delivery of curcumin (Bose et al., 2018).

The local delivery of curcumin helps to eliminate the issues with oral delivery, such as the need for a high dosage of curcumin due to its poor bioavailability. In one such study, kappa-carrageenan (κ-Carr) nanoparticles were synthesized to deliver curcumin efficiently. The κ-Carr nanoparticles loaded with curcumin (CUR@Carr) showed better viability and differentiation of osteoblast than the free curcumin when studied in MC3T3-E1. The CUR@Carr enhanced osteogenesis, tissue-nonspecific alkaline phosphatase activity, and ECM formation, whereas free curcumin at the same concentration was more toxic and showed negligible osteogenesis and mineralization (Nogueira et al., 2022).

A group of researchers also explored the local delivery of curcumin using an alendronate/curcumin (ALN/CUR) nanoparticle formulation coated with hyaluronic acid (HA-ALN/CUR) and its efficacy against MC3T3-E1 osteoblasts. HA-ALN/CUR nanoparticles promoted the efficient proliferation and differentiation of MC3T3-E1 cells and high mineralization. The researchers also reported upregulation of Runx2, BMP, and osteocalcin (OCN) in the group of cell lines treated with HA-ALN/CUR (Dong et al., 2018).

Bioceramics are known to mimic bone architecture, so carbonated apatite (CA) was derived from egg shells and is used as a nanocarrier for the delivery of curcumin. This curcumin-loaded CA was tested against MG-63 human osteosarcoma cells. It was observed that the nanocarrier could treat the osteosarcoma cell, prevent post-cancer inflammation, and aid in bone healing and regeneration (Verma et al., 2019a). Curcumin bioavailability was increased by encapsulating it in a liposome, which was further incorporated into a three-dimensional (3D)-printed calcium phosphate scaffold. When encapsulated curcumin was tested on human fetal osteoblasts, the results showed increased cell viability and proliferation (Sarkar & Bose, 2019).

To improve the bioavailability of EGCG, CNs loaded with EGCG were synthesized in another study. The efficiency of the nanoparticles was tested by culturing MSCs derived from the human umbilical cord to promote osteogenic differentiation. The study showed that the sustained release of EGCG for 16 days enhanced osteoblast differentiation by activating the Wnt/β-catenin signaling pathway (Wang et al., 2021).

Quercetin (Que), one of the most abundant phytobioactives in many plants, is known for its potent antioxidant, anti-inflammatory, and osteogenic properties (Lesjak et al., 2018; Wong et al., 2020b; Han et al., 2022). Que is extensively studied because of its ability to inhibit different cytokines like nitric oxide, TNF-α, and interleukin-1β released from RAW 264.7 (Jantan et al., 2015; Han et al., 2022). Que downregulates the polarization of M1 macrophage by inhibiting the NF-κB pathway, whereas it upregulates the polarization of M2 macrophage through the activation of Akt and AMPK pathways. Que is also known to inhibit osteoclastogenesis by inactivating the RANKL pathway.

The anti-inflammatory ability of Que and its interaction with various pathways makes it a promising polyphenol for bone remodeling and regeneration (Napimoga et al., 2013). Its traits make it eco-friendly and economical for treating various bone-related issues, but its hydrophobic nature and poor stability limit its clinical application. Various efforts have been made to address Que's low solubility and stability so that it can be used to its full potential.

Solid lipid nanoparticles (SLNs) are highly biocompatible and efficient in targeted drug delivery. An SLN loaded with Que was encapsulated in a hyaluronic acid–poly (ε-caprolactone-co-lactide)-b-poly (ethylene glycol)-b-poly (ε-caprolactone-co-lactide) hydrogel (HA-PCLA), and its in vivo and in vitro efficacy was studied to evaluate its bone repairing ability (Zhou et al., 2023). The Que-SLN@HA-PCLA hydrogel showed better new bone formation in eight weeks and vascularization than did the free quercetin (Que-@HA-PCLA) and the hydrogel with no Que (HA-PCLA). Through immunofluorescence staining of the cranial section, it was reported that Que-SLN@HA-PCLA showed lower expression of M1 macrophage and higher expression of M2 macrophage, which might be the reason behind the more efficient bone-repairing ability of the Que-@HA-PCLA hydrogel (Zhou et al., 2023).

Oral administration of Que-loaded solid lipid nanoparticles (QSLNs) has also been conducted to check its efficacy among OVX rats. The QSLNs were compared with free Que to evaluate the efficiency of Que in restoring the bone mass density of the femur, tibia, and lumbar spine in different groups of OVX rats. The study reported a 3.5-fold increase in serum Que levels in the OVX rats when administered orally with QSLNs. Overall, the group treated with QSLNs showed better bone mass recovery than those treated with free Que. However, free Que and QSLNs downregulated osteoclastogenesis by inhibiting NF-κB ligands and had no hyperplasic effect among the OVX rats (Ahmad et al., 2016).

Different carrying agents have been used to efficiently deliver rutin to the targeted site for minimum drug loss. One of the most common drug delivery vehicles for rutin is nanoparticles. CNs, one of the most common nanoparticles, have been used to encapsulate rutin. One study shows that rutin-loaded CNs enhanced rutin's anticarcinogenic and antimicrobial properties, which can be applied in treating dental disorders (Patil & Jobanputra, 2015).

The therapeutic application of silibinin is limited by its poor aqueous solubility and low bioavailability when administered orally (Cho et al., 2012). To overcome this issue, Leena et al. (2017) used an alternative method to deliver silibinin. They loaded silibinin on chitosan nanoparticles (SCNs) and encapsulated it in an alginate/gelatin scaffold and studied the efficacy of this scaffold for its ability to differentiate mouse MSCs into osteoblasts; specifically, they studied the expression of different markers that indicate osteoblast differentiation. MSCs, when treated with the Alg/Gel–50 μM SCN scaffold, increased the expression of Runx2, Col-1, ALP, and OCN compared with the scaffold in which silibinin was absent (Leena et al., 2017).

Bioactive glass (BG)-based biomaterials do not inhibit inflammatory responses or delay bone healing. Recently, Mo et al. (2022) synthesized naringin-loaded mesoporous BG nanoparticles to control the inflammatory response and promote osteogenesis. In vitro studies revealed that the naringin-loaded nanoparticles more effectively inhibited the inflammatory response than did the nonloaded nanoparticles, thereby synergistically facilitating osteogenesis and inhibiting osteoclastogenesis. In vivo, studies on rat femoral defect models suggested the upregulation of osteogenic genes in the presence of naringin-loaded nanoparticles. The findings show that combining BG and naringin offers a novel idea for good bone immunomodulatory properties.

11.4.2 Biomaterial-Based Delivery Systems

The current biomedical approaches to address bone-related deformities are either healthy bone transplantation (Shegarfi & Reikeras, 2009) or derivative bone transplantation (Grigolo et al., 2001). Major complications following such approaches are a heterologous immune response, possible dissemination of bone diseases, an inadequate pool of donor tissues, and post-surgical pain at the translocation site (Schmidt, 2021). Targeting injury sites with phytobioactive agents is crucial for enhanced healing, but phytobioactives face the issue of nonspecific binding and pharmacokinetics profile leading to lower concentrations of the drug reaching the target site.

To overcome such issues, different biomaterials have been widely investigated for their bone regeneration capabilities (Gupta et al., 2020b). Biomaterials like fibrous and nonfibrous mats, hydrogels, ceramic materials, metallic implants, multilayered scaffolds, 3D-printed scaffolds, and composite scaffolds are recently under study for bone tissue engineering. Biomaterial-based delivery systems (BDS) for phytobioactives could be a better alternative and provide better bone regeneration capabilities than traditional methods.

BDS help in localizing treatment to any injury site, with less involvement in normal pharmacokinetics and sustained release of phytobioactives overcoming burst release onto the site of injury (Figure 11.4) (Yang et al., 2020). For the successful regeneration of bone, biomaterials should combine appropriate mechanical, chemical, and biological properties. The prominent characteristics include biomaterial compatibility and release patterns, as well as their physicochemical and interfacial aspects (Cezar & Mooney, 2015).

BDS comprise two broad categories: affinity-based systems in which interactions between the loaded phytobioactives and the delivery system determine the release kinetics and reservoir-based systems such as hydrogels, composite materials, microspheres, and nanofibrous scaffold in which the biomaterial determines the kinetics of the phytobioactives' release to the site of action (Mohtaram et al., 2013).

An in vitro study showed that porous scaffolds significantly improve osteoporotic bone regeneration. Scaffolds were synthesized using the electrospinning technique, incorporating hydroxyapatite and berberine alkaloids into cellulose acetate nanofibers. The prepared heterogeneous scaffold showed better osteoblast proliferation capacity and enhanced cell surface mineralization. Upregulation of various osteoblast differentiation pathways was also reported, namely Wnt/β-cat, Runx2, and p38-MAPK (Shaban et al., 2021).

Likewise, a scaffold prepared from hydroxyapatite/polyamide 66 with a coating of berberine gave promising bone-regenerative properties (Huang et al., 2011). Both cartilage and subchondral bone are necessary for keeping the bones intact. Scaffolds prepared using a combination of sodium hyaluronate, sodium alginate, and berberine showed potential in regenerating damaged cartilage and subchondral tissues by activating the Wnt signaling pathway (Sujitha & Rasool, 2019). Open bone fracture is a critical problem that can lead to nonspecific infections. An injectable BDS was prepared using a nano-hydroxyapatite (nHap)/chitosan functionalized with berberine to counter this. The scaffold eradicated microbial infection and simultaneously affected bone regeneration (Sujitha & Rasool, 2019).

Bone regeneration is greatly influenced by angiogenesis, or the formation of new blood vessels to support its growth process. BDS can enhance angiogenesis for better bone regeneration properties. Cucurbitacin B, a tetraterpenoid extracted from plants belonging to the Cucurbitaceae family, has shown the potential to promote the formation of new blood vessels in vitro (Ma et al., 2021b).

A mouse model study incorporating cucurbitacin B into a biomaterial scaffold composed of poly(lactic-co-glycolic acid) (PLGA) and β-TCP showed potential in enhancing angiogenesis and, eventually, osteogenesis for countering bone defects in the skull region of the mouse. Further, cytotoxicity testing, tube formation assay, and immunoblotting highlighted the safe dose for cucurbitacin B and its agonistic effect on vascular endothelial growth factor receptor 2 (VEGFR2) for a prospective therapeutic agent for bone-related deformities (Cheng et al., 2021).

A sodium alginate composite hydrogel was prepared using cannabidiol, a terpenoid extracted from *Cannabis sativa*, and the cannabidiol-based hydrogel enhanced thermal stability and mechanobiological properties. Further analysis showed that there was an upregulation of osteogenic genes such as OCN, Runx2, and angiogenic VEGFR genes (Qi et al., 2022). Bone tissue engineering is a fascinating field with an immense scope for phytobioactives to be better therapeutic agents than other compounds.

Vancomycin is used as a first-line treatment for treating complicated bone-related infections. Scaffolds are extensively used as a delivery system for the sustained and targeted release of drugs, but premature degradation limits their potential. To counter that, scaffolds prepared using cross-linked glutaraldehyde and piperine exhibited better environmental stability for releasing vancomycin for promoting bone-related deformities (Ranganathan et al., 2019).

Berberine-loaded polycaprolactone/polyvinylpyrrolidone electrospun nanofibers were synthesized and coated on a bilayer membrane of collagen and chitosan. In vitro studies indicate that the electrospun nanofibers help in the adhesion and proliferation of osteoblasts and improve the cell–cell communication and migration required for bone regeneration. Additionally, in vivo tests showed that bone healing was stimulated when berberine was loaded in the nanofibers and implanted into a femoral defect in adult rats for four and eight weeks (Zhang et al., 2021).

Similarly, in another study, a berberine/polycaprolactone/collagen (BBR/PCL/COL) scaffold was synthesized using electrospinning by varying the concentration of BBR (Ma et al., 2021a). The BBR/PCL/COL scaffold had suitable biocompatibility and considerably enhanced the proliferation and differentiation of dental stem cells. Further, the synthesized scaffold was implanted into a bone lesion in rats to investigate its bone healing potential. The histological study of the BBR/PCL/COL scaffold showed angiogenesis, neo-bone formation, deeper H&E staining, and more readily discernible newly formed collagen (Ma et al., 2021a).

Que is a plant flavanol with a broad range of biological effects, such as stimulating bone regeneration and acting as an antioxidant and anti-inflammatory (Lesjak et al., 2018; Wong et al., 2020b). Composite microspheres were synthesized comprising quercetin, nHap, and PCL, and the developed composite stimulated osteogenic differentiation, as evidenced by the elevated ALP, OCN, and Runx2 bone-forming markers. Additionally, the quercetin-loaded microspheres showed good bone regeneration potential in vivo. It was observed that osteogenesis and immunoregulation work together to promote bone healing over time (Han et al., 2022).

Gelatin, tragacanth, and nHap were used to develop a highly porous scaffold loaded with quercetin. The MTT assay showed 84% cell viability in the scaffold loaded with quercetin. The researchers also observed that the sustained release of quercetin from the scaffold upregulated osteogenic genes, Col-1, Runx2, BGLAP, basic fibroblast derived growth factor 1, SP7, and SPP1 (Madani et al., 2022).

Another group developed a biocompatible and functionalized periosteum membrane of PLGA/MgO/Que. Its efficacy was checked on BMSCs and observed to stimulate osteogenic cell proliferation, migration, and differentiation (He et al., 2022b). Recently, a biodegradable ceramic composite with a polyurethane membrane loaded with polyphenolic phytobioactives of *Cissus quadrangularis* was synthesized for managing periosteum and enhancing bone formation in a tumor resection model of osteosarcoma (Gupta et al., 2023b). The membrane helped develop the periosteum and mineralize the osseous tissues to prevent further fracture due to osteosarcoma.

The delivery of resveratrol at defect sites can be achieved by loading it in a scaffold for bone growth and development. Researchers developed a composite hydrogel consisting of resveratrol-loaded gelatin methacrylate (Res-SLNs/GelMA) for bone regeneration. In vitro and in vivo studies showed that Res-loaded hydrogel can promote efficient bone regeneration through osteogenic differentiation of BMSCs. The synthesized functionalized hydrogel has the potential to be used in bone tissue engineering due to the sustained release of Res exhibiting good osteoconduction, osteoinduction, and biocompatibility (Wei et al., 2021).

The nHap has been widely used in bone tissue engineering and has achieved great success in reconstructing bone defects. Chitosan- and nHap-based composite microspheres were loaded with resveratrol, and up-regulation of bone markers like ALP, Runx2, Col-1, and OCN was observed in the presence of functionalized microspheres evidencing their potential to promote osteo-differentiation (Li et al., 2021). A scaffold prepared using nHap/silk fibroin was functionalized with naringin-loaded gelatin microspheres. The scaffold accelerated the healing of critical-size vertebral bone defects in osteoporotic rats. The new bone formation was observed through H&E staining, fast green staining, micro-CT, X-rays, and bone protein marker levels of BMP-2, Runx2, and OCN (Yu et al., 2021). The sustained release of naringin from a nHap/collagen scaffold at the defect site stimulated osteogenesis, tissue reconstruction, and early repair of skull defects in rats (Zuo et al., 2022).

The potential biological activities of zinc–silibinin complexes on osteoblasts were also investigated. Increased calcium deposition and osteoblast markers such as ALP and Runx2 confirmed osteoblast differentiation. Furthermore, the zinc–silibinin complexes had high antibacterial activity, which is useful in bone tissue engineering (Vimalraj et al., 2018).

Researchers found that biocompatible zinc–curcumin (Zn-CUR) composite nanofibers have better cellular adhesion and proliferation than drug-free nanofibers due to their osteogenic ability and cytocompatibility. Furthermore, adding Zn-CUR-loaded composite to scaffold increases ALP activity and mineralization. The composite nanofiber also has antibacterial activity, which can help to reduce postoperative infection (Sedghi et al., 2018).

EGCG was loaded in polylactic/gelatin electrospun nanofiber, and the bone regeneration property of the nanofibrous membrane was studied for eight weeks against control. The composite electrospun nanofiber showed biocompatibility, antibacterial property, osteoinductivity, and sustained release of EGCG over one week. The EGCG-loaded nanofiber induced 70% bone regeneration at the defect area and showed better bone regeneration capability when compared to the control group (Song et al., 2022).

EGCG/duck's feet collagen/hydroxyapatite (EGCG/DC/Hap) sponge was synthesized by a group of researchers to test its capability to enhance bone tissue regeneration. The EGCG/DC/Hap sponge was tested by culturing BMSCs on the sponge isolated from rabbits, and the in vivo tests were carried out by implantation of the sponge in nude mice. The histological staining confirmed that the EGCG/DC/Hap sponge enhanced cell proliferation, cell attachment, and expression of ALP, and the study indicated high biocompatibility of the synthesized sponge (Kook et al., 2018).

In a different study, hesperidin's role in developing organic bone matrix was reported for the first time. The researchers synthesized a collagenous scaffold loaded with hesperidin BMP2, in which the dosage of BMP2 was suboptimal. The in vivo experiment with the scaffold showed more nonectopic and controlled bone formation than ectopic bone formation due to the large dosage of BMP2 for repairing critical-size defects. The picrosirius red staining of the bone regeneration showed that hesperidin induced bone mineral formation and bone matrix organization and was also responsible for maintaining matrix-to-mineral ratio in addition to osteoblast differentiation. This study showed that hesperidin could significantly influence controlled bone regeneration (Miguez et al., 2021).

Polyethylene glycol (PEG)-coated nHap was used to develop a catalpol-loaded delivery system (PEG-nHap/CTP). In vitro studies indicate that PEG-nHap/CTP can promote the proliferation of MC3T3-E1 and increase ALP secretion and nodule formation (He et al., 2022a). To examine the local inflammation and ectopic bone formation, CTP was loaded onto an electrospun polylactide/gelatin composite fibrous mesh and subcutaneously implanted. The findings revealed that CTP modulates cellular behavior via cell paracrine to strengthen intercellular communication. It modulates the signaling between BMSCs and macrophages, which polarizes M1/M2 and inhibits osteoclast differentiation, inducing osteogenic differentiation and angiogenesis. Thus, CTP-loaded composite material could be a promising bioactive stimulator for bone tissue engineering (Zhang et al., 2022).

Nanofibers synthesized using electrospinning also serve as a good delivery vehicle for curcumin. CUR-loaded collagen nanofiber was fabricated. In vitro and in vivo nanofiber studies revealed that the fabricated nanofiber shows good antimicrobial activity and early defect healing within 28 days (Ghavimi et al., 2020). Poly (ε-caprolactone) nanofibers were fabricated and loaded with curcumin using a similar technique. The study showed increased cell proliferation of MC3T3-E1 as the concentration of curcumin was increased in the nanofiber (Jain et al., 2016). Graphene oxide and Zn-CUR nanofiber also showed similar traits as they helped enhance the osteogenic process and showed good antibacterial activity (Sedghi et al., 2018).

CONCLUSION

Remedies are essential for severe structural anomalies in complex bone fractures brought on by a variety of illnesses and traumas. Although autografts continue to be the benchmark in orthopedics because of their potency and high biological stability, they are not always readily available. Thus, it is imperative to create substitutes for bone tissue regeneration that are secure, economical, and demonstrates quicker restoration.

Throughout prehistory, Ayurvedic therapeutic practices employed multiple phytobioactives. Numerous plant species have been shown to be beneficial in treating bone-related issues, and combinatorial formulations are used to strengthen bones and speed the process of recuperating from damage. Despite being used extensively in herbal remedies, phytobioactives' potential value and effective mechanism are yet undefined; many phytobioactives with bone regeneration attributes are acknowledged as being present, and there are still many more that need to be investigated.

Although there aren't any known side effects from using traditional medications, it is nevertheless essential to understand how they participate with the body's organs and tissues through preclinical and clinical experiments. Aside from this, detailed ADMET pharmacokinetic profiling is the main area that requires research and analysis in phytobiology. Many studies have been conducted, some of which claim that complete raw extract has better effects on bone regeneration than purified components, whereas others claim the opposite. Further analysis and inferences are required to establish which phytobioactive crude extract or individual phytoconstituent has higher potency in terms of promoting bone regeneration.

Although phytobioactives have a well-documented list of benefits, they suffer from targeted delivery or limited bioavailability. The field of nanotechnology has numerous benefits in terms of delivering bioactive compounds; nanomaterial- and biomaterial-based delivery can be of great benefit in treating bone-related issues. The era of phyto-delivery systems is booming, and its wide-scale application in bone regeneration is advancing. There is still room down the line for further investigations into the effects of phytobioactives on the bone metabolic pathways or integrating phytobioactives with scaffolds to produce biofunctionalized tissues for bone regeneration or utilizing nano-based delivery for better healing effects.

ACKNOWLEDGEMENTS

S.S. would like to acknowledge the Department of Science and Technology (DST), Ministry of Science and Technology, Government of India (Project# DST/NM/NT-2018/48) and Science & Engineering Research Board (SERB) (Project# CRG/2021/002179) for funding the work. A.G. and R.D. would like to acknowledge SERB (Project# CRG/2021/002179), and S.K.M. would like to acknowledge DST (Project# DST/NM/NT-2018/48) for its financial assistance. K.K. would like to acknowledge BIT Mesra for providing the fellowship.

LIST OF ABBREVIATIONS

ALP	Alkaline phosphatase
AP-1	Activator protein 1
BDS	Biomaterial-based delivery systems
BMMs	Bone marrow-derived monocytes/macrophages
BMP	Bone morphogenetic protein
BMSC	Bone marrow mesenchymal cell
CA	Carbonated apatite
CTP	Catalpol
EGCG	epigallocatechin-3-gallate
ERK	Extracellular signal-regulated kinase
JNK	c-Jun N-terminal kinase
MAPK	Mitogen-activated protein kinases
micro-CT	Microcomputed tomography
MSC	Mesenchymal stem cell
NDS	Nanomaterial-based delivery system
NFATc1	Nuclear factor of activated T-cell
NF-κB	Nuclear factor kappa-light-chain enhancer of activated B cells
nHap	Nano-hydroxyapatite
OCN	Osteocalcin
OPG	Osteoprotegerin
OVX	Ovariectomized
QSLN	Quercetin loaded solid lipid nanoparticle
Que	Quercetin
RANK	Receptor activator of nuclear factor kappa-B
RANKL	Receptor activator of nuclear factor kappa-B ligand
ROS	Reactive oxygen species
Runx2	Runt-related transcription factor-2
SCN	Silibinin loaded chitosan nanoparticle
Sirt1	Sirtuin 1

SLN Solid lipid nanoparticle
TNF-α Tumor necrosis factor- α
VEGF Vascular endothelial growth factor

REFERENCES

Abd Aziz, N. A., Hasham, R., Sarmidi, M. R., Suhaimi, S. H., & Idris, M. K. H. (2021). A review on extraction techniques and therapeutic value of polar bioactives from Asian medicinal herbs: Case study on Orthosiphon aristatus, Eurycoma longifolia and Andrographis paniculata. *Saudi Pharm. J.* 29: 143–165.

Abiramasundari, G., Mohan Gowda, C. M., & Sreepriya, M. (2018). Selective estrogen receptor modulator and prostimulatory effects of phytoestrogen β-ecdysone in Tinospora cordifolia on osteoblast cells. *J. Ayurveda Integr. Med.* 9: 161–168.

Aggarwal, B. B., & Sung, B. (2009). Pharmacological basis for the role of curcumin in chronic diseases: An age-old spice with modern targets. *Trends Pharmacol. Sci.* 30: 85–94.

Ahangari, N., Kargozar, S., Ghayour-Mobarhan, M., Baino, F., Pasdar, A., Sahebkar, A., Ferns, G. A. A., Kim, H., & Mozafari, M. (2019). Curcumin in tissue engineering: A traditional remedy for modern medicine. *BioFactors.* 45: 135–151.

Ahmad, N., Banala, V. T., Kushwaha, P., Karvande, A., Sharma, S., Tripathi, A. K., Verma, A., Trivedi, R., & Mishra, P. R. (2016). Quercetin-loaded solid lipid nanoparticles improve osteoprotective activity in an ovariectomized rat model: A preventive strategy for post-menopausal osteoporosis. *RSC Adv.* 6: 97613–97628.

Akindele, A. J., Adeneye, A. A., Salau, O. S., Sofidiya, M. O., & Benebo, A. S. (2014). Dose and time-dependent sub-chronic toxicity study of hydroethanolic leaf extract of Flabellaria paniculata Cav: (Malpighiaceae) in rodents. *Front. Pharmacol.* 5: 78.

Allen, M. R. (2008). Bisphosphonates and osteonecrosis of the jaw: Moving from the bedside to the bench. *Cells Tissues Organs.* 189: 289–294.

Amawi, H., Ashby, C. R., & Tiwari, A. K. (2017). Cancer chemoprevention through dietary flavonoids: What's limiting? *Chin. J. Cancer.* 36: 1–13.

An, J., Yang, H., Zhang, Q., Liu, C., Zhao, J., Zhang, L., & Chen, B. (2016). Natural products for treatment of osteoporosis: The effects and mechanisms on promoting osteoblast-mediated bone formation. *Life Sci.* 147: 46–58.

Awotedu, O. L., Okeke, U. E., Ogunbamowo, P. O., Ariwoola, O. S., & Omolola, T. O. (2020). Extraction of phytochemical compounds of Leea guineensis (G. Don) leaves using non-polar and polar solvents. *Eur. J. Med. Plants.* 31: 24–31.

Berendsen, A. D., & Olsen, B. R. (2015). Bone development. *Bone.* 80: 14–18.

Bors, W., & Saran, M. (1987). Radical scavenging by flavonoid antioxidants. *Free Radic. Res. Commun.* 2: 289–294.

Bose, S., Sarkar, N., & Banerjee, D. (2018). Effects of PCL, PEG and PLGA polymers on curcumin release from calcium phosphate matrix for in vitro and in vivo bone regeneration. *Mater. Today Chem.* 8: 110–120.

Burton, A., Smith, M., & Falkenberg, T. (2015). Building WHO's global strategy for traditional medicine. *Eur. J. Integr. Med.* 7: 13–15.

Cao, J., Cao, J., Wang, H., Chen, L., Cao, F., & Su, E. (2020). Solubility improvement of phytochemicals using (natural) deep eutectic solvents and their bioactivity evaluation. *J. Mol. Liq.* 318: 113997.

Cezar, C. A., & Mooney, D. J. (2015). Biomaterial-based delivery for skeletal muscle repair. *Adv. Drug Deliv. Rev.* 84: 188–197.

Chai, L., Zhou, K., Wang, S., Zhang, H., Fan, N., Li, J., Tan, X., Hu, L., & Fan, X. (2018). Psoralen and bakuchiol ameliorate M-CSF plus RANKL-induced osteoclast differentiation and bone resorption cia inhibition of AKT and AP-1 pathways in vitro. *Cell. Physiol. Biochem.* 48: 2123–2133.

Chauhan, S., Sharma, A., Upadhyay, N. K., Singh, G., Lal, U. R., & Goyal, R. (2018). In-vitro osteoblast proliferation and in-vivo anti-osteoporotic activity of Bombax ceiba with quantification of Lupeol, gallic acid and β-sitosterol by HPTLC and HPLC. *BMC Complement. Altern. Med.* 18: 1–12.

Chen, Y., Zhu, Z., Chen, J., Zheng, Y., Limsila, B., Lu, M., Gao, T., Yang, Q., Fu, C., & Liao, W. (2021). Terpenoids from curcumae rhizoma: Their anticancer effects and clinical uses on combination and versus drug therapies. *Biomed. Pharmacother.* 138: 111350.

Cheng, J., Xu, H. Y., Liu, M. M., Cai, J. P., Wang, L., Hua, Z., Wu, X. D., Huo, W. L., & Lv, N. N. (2020). Catalpol promotes the proliferation and differentiation of osteoblasts induced by high glucose by inhibiting KDM7A. *Diabetes Metab. Syndr. Obes.: Targets Ther.* 13: 705–712.

Cheng, W. X., Liu, Y. Z., Meng, X. B., Zheng, Z. T., Li, L. L., Ke, L. Q., Li, L., Huang, C. S., Zhu, G. Y., Pan, H. D., Qin, L., Wang, X. L., & Zhang, P. (2021). PLGA/β-TCP composite scaffold incorporating cucurbitacin B promotes bone regeneration by inducing angiogenesis. *J. Orthop. Translat.* 31: 41–51.

Cho, J. K., Park, J. W., & Song, S. C. (2012). Injectable and biodegradable poly (organophosphazene) gel containing silibinin: Its physicochemical properties and anticancer activity. *J. Pharm. Sci.* 101: 2382–2391.

Choi, J. H., Hwang, Y. P., Jin, S. W., Lee, G. H., Kim, H. G., Han, E. H., Kim, S. K., Kang, K. W., Chung, Y. C., & Jeong, H. G. (2019). Suppression of PMA-induced human fibrosarcoma HT-1080 invasion and metastasis by kahweol via inhibiting Akt/JNK1/2/p38 MAPK signal pathway and NF-κB dependent transcriptional activities. *Food Chem. Toxicol.* 125: 1–9.

Cornelissen, A. S., Klaassen, S. D., van Groningen, T., Bohnert, S., & Joosen, M. J. A. (2020). Comparative physiology and efficacy of atropine and scopolamine in sarin nerve agent poisoning. *Toxicol. Appl. Pharmacol.* 396: 114994.

Das, A., Pandita, D., Jain, G. K., Agarwal, P., Grewal, A. S., Khar, R. K., & Lather, V. (2021). Role of phytoconstituents in the management of COVID-19. *Chem.-Biol. Interact.* 341: 109449.

Dean, M., Murphy, B. T., & Burdette, J. E. (2017). Phytosteroids beyond estrogens: Regulators of reproductive and endocrine function in natural products. *Mol. Cell. Endocrinol.* 442: 98–105.

de Lima, M. C. F., Silva, L. S., da Wiedemann, L. S. M., & da Veiga, V. F. (2019). A brief history of terpenoids. In *Terpenoids against Human Diseases*. N. D. Roy, Ed. Boca Raton: CRC Press, pp. 1–15.

Dolder, S., Hofstetter, W., Wetterwald, A., Mühlbauer, R. C., & Felix, R. (2006). Effect of monoterpenes on the formation and activation of osteoclasts in vitro. *J. Bone Miner. Res.* 21: 647–655.

Dominguez More, G. P., Cardenas, P. A., Costa, G. M., Simoes, C. M., & Aragon, D. M. (2017). Pharmacokinetics of botanical drugs and plant extracts. *Mini-Rev. Med. Chem.* 17: 1646–1664.

Dong, J., Tao, L., Abourehab, M. A., & Hussain, Z. (2018). Design and development of novel hyaluronate-modified nanoparticles for combo-delivery of curcumin and alendronate: Fabrication, characterization, and cellular and molecular evidences of enhanced bone regeneration. *Int. J. Biol. Macromol.* 116: 1268–1281.

Fazzalari, N. L. (2011). Bone fracture and bone fracture repair. *Osteoporos. Int.* 22: 2003–2006.

Fernández-Arroyo, S., Huete-Toral, F., de Lara, M. J. P., de la Luz Cádiz-Gurrea, M., Legeai-Mallet, L., Micol, V., & Pintor, J. (2015). The impact of polyphenols on chondrocyte growth and survival: A preliminary report. *Food Nutr. Res.* 59: 29311.

Frutos, M. J., Rincón-Frutos, L., & Valero-Cases, E. (2019). Rutin. In *Nonvitamin and Nonmineral Nutritional Supplements*. S. M. Nabavi, and A. S. Silva, Eds. Massachusetts: Elsevier, pp. 111–117.

Fukuma, Y., Sakai, E., Nishishita, K., Okamoto, K., & Tsukuba, T. (2015). Cafestol has a weaker inhibitory effect on osteoclastogenesis than kahweol and promotes osteoblast differentiation. *BioFactors.* 41: 222–231.

Ganesan, P., Ramalingam, P., Karthivashan, G., Ko, Y. T., & Choi, D. K. (2018). Recent developments in solid lipid nanoparticle and surface-modified solid lipid nanoparticle delivery systems for oral delivery of phyto-bioactive compounds in various chronic diseases. *Int. J. Nanomed.* 13: 1569–1583.

Ge, Y., Ding, S., Feng, J., Du, J., & Gu, Z. (2021). Diosgenin inhibits Wnt/β-catenin pathway to regulate the proliferation and differentiation of MG-63 cells. *Cytotechnology.* 73: 169–178.

Ghavimi, M. A., Bani Shahabadi, A., Jarolmasjed, S., Memar, M. Y., Maleki Dizaj, S., & Sharifi, S. (2020). Nanofibrous asymmetric collagen/curcumin membrane containing aspirin-loaded PLGA nanoparticles for guided bone regeneration. *Sci. Rep.* 10: 1–15.

Greenwell, M., & Rahman, P. K. S. M. (2015). Medicinal plants: Their use in anticancer treatment. *Int. J. Pharm. Sci. Res.* 6: 4103–4112.

Grigolo, B., Roseti, L., Fiorini, M., Fini, M., Giavaresi, G., Nicoli Aldini, N., Giardino, R., & Facchini, A. (2001). Transplantation of chondrocytes seeded on a hyaluronan derivative (Hyaff®-11) into cartilage defects in rabbits. *Biomat.* 22: 2417–2424.

Gu, W., Wu, C., Chen, J., & Xiao, Y. (2013). Nanotechnology in the targeted drug delivery for bone diseases and bone regeneration. *Int. J. Nanomed.* 8: 2305–2317.

Gupta, A., Mehta, S. K., Kumar, A., & Singh, S. (2021). Advent of phytobiologics and nano-interventions for bone remodeling: A comprehensive review. *Crit. Rev. Biotechnol.* 3: 142–169.

Gupta, A., Mehta, S. K., Qayoom, I., Gupta, S., Singh, S., & Kumar, A. (2023a). Biofunctionalization with Cissus quadrangularis phytobioactives accentuates nano-hydroxyapatite based ceramic nano-cement for neo-bone formation in critical sized bone defect. *Int. J. Pharm.* 642: 123110.

Gupta, A., Padmanabhan, P., & Singh, S. (2020a). Resveratrol isomeric switching during bioreduction of gold nanoparticles: A gateway for cis-resveratrol. *Nanotechnol.* 31: 465603.

Gupta, A., Padmanabhan, P., & Singh, S. (2020b). Bionanocomposites: Green materials for orthopedic applications. In *Green Polymeric Nanocomposites*. S. E. Jujjavarapu, and K. M. Poluri, Eds. Boca Raton: CRC Press, pp. 209–249.

Gupta, A., & Singh, S. (2022). Multimodal potentials of gold nanoparticles for bone tissue engineering and regenerative medicine: Avenues and prospects. *Small.* 18: 2201462.

Gupta, S., Qayoom, I., Gupta, P., Gupta, A., Singh, P., Singh, S., & Kumar, A. (2023b). Exosome-functionalized, drug-laden bone substitute along with an antioxidant herbal membrane for bone and periosteum regeneration in bone sarcoma. *ACS Appl. Mater. Interfaces.* 15: 8824–8839.

Gupta, T., Singh, J., Kaur, S., Sandhu, S., Singh, G., & Kaur, I. P. (2020c). Enhancing bioavailability and stability of curcumin using solid lipid nanoparticles (CLEN): A covenant for its effectiveness. *Front. Bioeng. Biotech.* 8: 879.

Gutiérrez-del-Río, I., Fernández, J., & Lombó, F. (2018). Plant nutraceuticals as antimicrobial agents in food preservation: Terpenoids, polyphenols and thiols. *Int. J. Antimicrob. Agents.* 52: 309–315.

Hadjidakis, D. J., & Androulakis, I. I. (2006). Bone remodeling. *Ann. N. Y. Acad. Sci.* 1092: 385–396.

Hafshejani, Z. K., Lorigooini, Z., Deris, F., Akbari, N., Farahbod, F., Fazelian, S., Moradi, F., & Dehghan, M. (2021). Effect of oral capsule of Peganum harmala seeds on bone density in menopausal women prone to osteoporosis. *J. Shahrekord Univ. Med. Sci.* 23: 139–145.

Hairul-Islam, M. I., Saravanan, S., Thirugnanasambantham, K., Chellappandian, M., Raj, C. S. D., Karikalan, K., Paulraj, M. G., & Ignacimuthu, S. (2017). Swertiamarin, a natural steroid, prevent bone erosion by modulating RANKL/RANK/OPG signaling. *Int. Immunopharmacol.* 53: 114–124.

Han, C., Guo, M., Bai, J., Zhao, L., Wang, L., Song, W., & Zhang, P. (2022). Quercetin-loaded nanocomposite microspheres for chronologically promoting bone repair via synergistic immunoregulation and osteogenesis. *Mater. Des.* 222: 111045.

He, J., Yang, X., Liu, F., Li, D., Zheng, B., Abdullah, A. O., & Liu, Y. (2020). The impact of curcumin on bone osteogenic promotion of MC3T3 cells under high glucose conditions and enhanced bone formation in diabetic mice. *Coat.* 10: 258.

He, M., Pan, Y. W., Chen, S. Q., Meng, Y. Y., & Ni, X. Y. (2022a). Preparation of hydroxyapatite-based composite system and study of its pro-osteogenic effect. *MRS Commun.* 12: 773–779.

He, X., Andersson, G., Lindgren, U., & Li, Y. (2010). Resveratrol prevents RANKL-induced osteoclast differentiation of murine osteoclast progenitor RAW 264.7 cells through inhibition of ROS production. *Biochem. Biophys. Res. Commun.* 401: 356–362.

He, X., Liu, W., Liu, Y., Zhang, K., Sun, Y., Lei, P., & Hu, Y. (2022b). Nano artificial periosteum PLGA/MgO/Quercetin accelerates repair of bone defects through promoting osteogenic– Angiogenic coupling effect via Wnt/β-catenin pathway. *Mater. Today Bio.* 16: 100348.

Horcajada-Molteni, M. N., Crespy, V., Coxam, V., Davicco, M. J., Rémésy, C., & Barlet, J. P. (2000). Rutin inhibits ovariectomy-induced osteopenia in rats. *J. Bone Miner. Res.* 15: 2251–2258.

Houacine, C., Khan, I., & Yousaf, S. S. (2020). Potential cardio-protective agents: A resveratrol review (2000–2019). *Curr. Pharm. Des.* 27: 2943–2955.

Huang, D., Zuo, Y., Zou, Q., Zhang, L., Li, J., Cheng, L., & Li, Y. (2011). Antibacterial chitosan coating on nano-hydroxyapatite/polyamide66 porous bone scaffold for drug delivery. *J. Biomater. Sci. Polym. Ed.* 22: 931–944.

Huang, Q., Gao, B., Wang, L., Zhang, H. Y., Li, X. J., Shi, J., Wang, Z., Zhang, J. K., Yang, L., Luo, Z. J., & Liu, J. (2015). Ophiopogonin D: A new herbal agent against osteoporosis. *Bone.* 74: 18–28.

Hyun, H., Park, H., Jeong, J., Kim, J., Kim, H., Oh, H. I., & Kim, H. H. (2014). Effects of watercress containing rutin and rutin alone on the proliferation and osteogenic differentiation of human osteoblast-like MG-63 cells. *Korean J. Physiol. Pharmacol.* 18: 347.

Jain, S., Meka, S. R. K., & Chatterjee, K. (2016). Curcumin eluting nanofibers augment osteogenesis toward phytochemical based bone tissue engineering. *Biomed. Mater.* 11: 055007.

Jaiswal, Y. S., & Williams, L. L. (2017). A glimpse of ayurveda—The forgotten history and principles of Indian traditional medicine. *J. Tradit. Complement. Med.* 7: 50–53.

James, A. W., LaChaud, G., Shen, J., Asatrian, G., Nguyen, V., Zhang, X., Ting, K., & Soo, C. (2016). A review of the clinical side effects of bone morphogenetic protein-2. *Tissue Eng. Part B Rev.* 22: 284–297.

Jantan, I., Ahmad, W., & Bukhari, S. N. A. (2015). Plant-derived immunomodulators: An insight on their preclinical evaluation and clinical trials. *Front. Recent Dev. Plant Sci.* 6: 655.

Jia, L., Zhang, D., Li, Z., Duan, C., Wang, Y., Feng, F., & Zhang, Q. (2010). Nanostructured lipid carriers for parenteral delivery of silybin: Biodistribution and pharmacokinetic studies. *Colloids Surf. B.* 80: 213–218.

Jiang, D., Gao, P., Lin, H., & Geng, H. (2016). Curcumin improves tendon healing in rats: A histological, biochemical, and functional evaluation. *Connect. Tissue Res.* 57: 20–27.

Jones, W. P., & Kinghorn, A. D. (2012). Extraction of plant secondary metabolites. *Methods Mol. Biol.* 864: 341–366.

Kandemir, K., Tomas, M., McClements, D. J., & Capanoglu, E. (2022). Recent advances on the improvement of quercetin bioavailability. *Trends Food Sci. Technol.* 119: 192–200.

Khedgikar, V., Kushwaha, P., Ahmad, N., Gautam, J., Kumar, P., Maurya, R., & Trivedi, R. (2017). Ethanolic extract of Dalbergia sissoo promotes rapid regeneration of cortical bone in drill-hole defect model of rat. *Biomed. Pharmacother.* 86: 16–22.

Kim, D. Y., Kim, E. J., & Jang, W. G. (2018). Piperine induces osteoblast differentiation through AMPK-dependent Runx2 expression. *Biochem. Biophys. Res. Commun.* 495: 1497–1502.

Kimira, Y. (2019). Elucidation of osteoporosis prevention mechanism by citrus limonoid. *Impact.* 2019: 12–13.

Kiran, S. D. V. S., Rohini, P., & Bhagyasree, P. (2017). Flavonoid: A review on Naringenin. *J. Pharmacogn. Phytochem.* 6: 2778–2783.

Kook, Y. J., Tian, J., Jeon, Y. S., Choi, M. J., Song, J. E., Park, C. H., & Khang, G. (2018). Nature-derived epigallocatechin gallate/duck's feet collagen/hydroxyapatite composite sponges for enhanced bone tissue regeneration. *J. Biomater. Sci. Polym. Ed.* 29: 984–996.

Kramer, H. F., & Goodyear, L. J. (2007). Exercise, MAPK, and NF-κB signaling in skeletal muscle. *J. Appl. Physiol.* 103: 388–395.

Kreft, I., Fabjan, N., & Yasumoto, K. (2006). Rutin content in buckwheat (Fagopyrum esculentum Moench) food materials and products. *Food Chem.* 98: 508–512.

Kuo, Y. T., Liu, C. H., Li, J. W., Lin, C. J., Jassey, A., Wu, H. N., Perng, G. C., Yen, M. H., & Lin, L. T. (2020). Identification of the phytobioactive Polygonum cuspidatum as an antiviral source for restricting dengue virus entry. *Sci. Rep.* 10: 1–15.

Kushwaha, P., Khedgikar, V., Haldar, S., Gautam, J., Mulani, F. A., Thulasiram, H. V., & Trivedi, R. (2016). Azadirachta indica triterpenoids promote osteoblast differentiation and mineralization in vitro and in vivo. *Bioorg. Med. Chem. Lett.* 26: 3719–3724.

Kvasnička, F., Bıba, B., Ševčík, R., Voldřich, M., & Kratka, J. (2003). Analysis of the active components of silymarin. *J. Chromatogr. A.* 990: 239–245.

Kyung, T. W., Lee, J. E., Shin, H. H., & Choi, H. S. (2008). Rutin inhibits osteoclast formation by decreasing reactive oxygen species and TNF-α by inhibiting activation of NF-κB. *Exp. Mol. Med.* 40: 52–58.

Lee, D. H., Jeon, E. J., Ahn, J., Hwang, J. T., Hur, J., Ha, T. Y., Jung, C. H., & Sung, M. J. (2016). Limonin enhances osteoblastogenesis and prevents ovariectomy-induced bone loss. *J. Funct. Foods.* 23: 105–114.

Lee, H. H., Jang, J. W., Lee, J. K., & Park, C. K. (2020). Rutin improves bone histomorphometric values by reduction of osteoclastic activity in osteoporosis mouse model induced by bilateral ovariectomy. *J. Korean Neurosurg. Soc.* 63: 433–443.

Lee, J. W., Kobayashi, Y., Nakamichi, Y., Udagawa, N., Takahashi, N., Im, N. K., Seo, H. J., Jeon, W. B., Yonezawa, T., Cha, B. Y., & Woo, J. T. (2010). Alisol-B, a novel phyto-steroid, suppresses the RANKL-induced osteoclast formation and prevents bone loss in mice. *Biochem. Pharmacol.* 80: 352–361.

Lee, Y. M., Shin, S. I., Shin, K. S., Lee, Y. R., Park, B. H., & Kim, E. C. (2011). The role of sirtuin 1 in osteoblastic differentiation in human periodontal ligament cells. *J. Periodontal Res.* 46: 712–721.

Leena, R. S., Vairamani, M., & Selvamurugan, N. (2017). Alginate/gelatin scaffolds incorporated with Silibinin-loaded Chitosan nanoparticles for bone formation in vitro. *Colloids Surf. B.* 158: 308–318.

Lesjak, M., Beara, I., Simin, N., Pintać, D., Majkić, T., Bekvalac, K., Orčić, D., & Mimica-Dukić, N. (2018). Antioxidant and anti-inflammatory activities of quercetin and its derivatives. *J. Funct. Foods.* 40: 68–75.

Li, C., Li, Y., Zhang, L., Zhang, S., Yao, W., & Zuo, Z. (2019). The protective effect of piperine on ovariectomy induced bone loss in female mice and its enhancement effect of osteogenic differentiation via Wnt/β-catenin signaling pathway. *J. Funct. Foods.* 58: 138–150.

Li, L., Yu, M., Li, Y., Li, Q., Yang, H., Zheng, M., & Gui, L. (2021). Synergistic anti-inflammatory and osteogenic n-HA/resveratrol/chitosan composite microspheres for osteoporotic bone regeneration. *Bioact. Mater*. 6: 1255–1266.

Lin, R. W., Chen, C. H., Wang, Y. H., Ho, M. L., Hung, S. H., Chen, I. S., & Wang, G. J. (2009). (−)-Epigallocatechin gallate inhibition of osteoclastic differentiation via NF-κB. *Biochem. Biophys. Res. Commun*. 379: 1033–1037.

Liu, T. Y., Qu, X. L., & Yan, B. (2020). A sensitive metal—Organic framework nanosensor with cation-introduced chirality for enantioselective recognition and determination of quinine and quinidine in human urine. *J. Mater. Chem. C*. 8: 14579–14586.

Ma, L., Yu, Y., Liu, H., Sun, W., Lin, Z., Liu, C., & Miao, L. (2021a). Berberine-releasing electrospun scaffold induces osteogenic differentiation of DPSCs and accelerates bone repair. *Sci. Rep*. 11: 1–12.

Ma, Y., Yoshida, T., Matoba, K., Kida, K., Shintani, R., Piao, Y., Jin, J., Nishino, T., & Hanayama, R. (2021b). Identification of small compounds regulating the secretion of extracellular vesicles via a TIM4-affinity ELISA. *Sci. Rep*. 11: 1–13.

Madani, P., Hesaraki, S., Saeedifar, M., & Ahmadi Nasab, N. (2022). The controlled release, bioactivity and osteogenic gene expression of Quercetin-loaded gelatin/tragacanth/nano-hydroxyapatite bone tissue engineering scaffold. *J. Biomater. Sci. Polym. Ed*. 34: 217–242.

Marian, F., Joost, K., Saini, K. D., Von Ammon, K., Thurneysen, A., & Busato, A. (2008). Patient satisfaction and side effects in primary care: An observational study comparing homeopathy and conventional medicine. *BMC Complement. Altern. Med*. 8: 1–10.

Marín, L., Miguélez, E. M., Villar, C. J., & Lombó, F. (2015). Bioavailability of dietary polyphenols and gut microbiota metabolism: Antimicrobial properties. *Biomed. Res. Int*. 2015: 905215.

Marrelli, M., Menichini, F., Statti, G. A., Bonesi, M., Duez, P., Menichini, F., & Conforti, F. (2012). Changes in the phenolic and lipophilic composition, in the enzyme inhibition and antiproliferative activity of Ficus carica L. cultivar Dottato fruits during maturation. *Food Chem. Toxicol*. 50: 726–733.

McClements, D. J., & Öztürk, B. (2021). Utilization of nanotechnology to improve the application and bioavailability of phytochemicals derived from waste streams. *J. Agric. Food Chem*. 70: 6884–6900.

Miguez, P. A., Tuin, S. A., Robinson, A. G., Belcher, J., Jongwattanapisan, P., Perley, K., & Barton, E. R. (2021). Hesperidin promotes osteogenesis and modulates collagen matrix organization and mineralization in vitro and in vivo. *Int. J. Mol. Sci*. 22: 3223.

Mo, Y., Zhao, F., Lin, Z., Cao, X., Chen, D., & Chen, X. (2022). Local delivery of naringin in beta-cyclodextrin modified mesoporous bioactive glass promotes bone regeneration: From anti-inflammatory to synergistic osteogenesis and osteoclastogenesis. *Biomater. Sci*. 10: 1697–1712.

Mobasseri, M., Ostadrahimi, A., Tajaddini, A., Asghari, S., Barati, M., Akbarzadeh, M., Nikpayam, O., Houshyar, J., Roshanravan, N., & Alamdari, N. M. (2020). Effects of saffron supplementation on glycemia and inflammation in patients with type 2 diabetes mellitus: A randomized double-blind, placebo-controlled clinical trial study. *Diabetes Metab. Syndr*. 14: 527–534.

Mohtaram, N. K., Montgomery, A., & Willerth, S. M. (2013). Biomaterial-based drug delivery systems for the controlled release of neurotrophic factors. *Biomed. Mater*. 8: 022001.

Mühlbauer, R. C., Lozano, A., Palacio, S., Reinli, A., & Felix, R. (2003). Common herbs, essential oils, and monoterpenes potently modulate bone metabolism. *Bone*. 32: 372–380.

Murota, K., Nakamura, Y., & Uehara, M. (2018). Flavonoid metabolism: The interaction of metabolites and gut microbiota. *Biosci. Biotechnol. Biochem*. 82: 600–610.

Napimoga, M. H., Clemente-Napimoga, J. T., Macedo, C. G., Freitas, F. F., Stipp, R. N., Pinho-Ribeiro, F. A., & Verri Jr, W. A. (2013). Quercetin inhibits inflammatory bone resorption in a mouse periodontitis model. *J. Nat. Prod*. 76: 2316–2321.

Nguyen, M. T. H., Ngo, Q. V., Nguyen, H. T. T., Pham, Q. M., Dinh, T. H., Nguyen, H. T. T., Tinh, N. V., & Nguyen, P. T. M. (2021). Osteogenic activity of lupeol isolated from clinacanthus nutans Lindau: Activity and mode of action. *J. Chem*. 2021: 6704999.

Nogueira, L. F. B., Cruz, M. A. E., Tovani, C. B., Lopes, H. B., Beloti, M. M., Ciancaglini, P., Bottini, M., & Ramos, A. P. (2022). Curcumin-loaded carrageenan nanoparticles: Fabrication, characterization, and assessment of the effects on osteoblasts mineralization. *Colloids Surf. B*. 217: 112622.

Odes-Barth, S., Khanin, M., Linnewiel-Hermoni, K., Miller, Y., Abramov, K., Levy, J., & Sharoni, Y. (2020). Inhibition of osteoclast differentiation by carotenoid derivatives through inhibition of the NF-κB pathway. *Antioxidants*. 9: 1167.

Olivoto, T., Nardino, M., Carvalho, I. R., Follmann, D. N., Szareski, V. J., Ferrari, M., de Pelegrin, A. J., & de Souza, V. Q. (2017). Plant secondary metabolites and its dynamical systems of induction in response to environmental factors: A review. *Afr. J. Agric. Res.* 12: 71–84.

Olszta, M. J., Cheng, X., Jee, S. S., Kumar, R., Kim, Y. Y., Kaufman, M. J., Douglas, E. P., & Gower, L. B. (2007). Bone structure and formation: A new perspective. *Mat. Sci. Eng. R Rep.* 58: 77–116.

Palozza, P., Catalano, A., Simone, R., & Cittadini, A. (2012). Lycopene as a guardian of redox signalling. *Acta Biochim. Pol.* 59: 21–25.

Pandey, K. B., & Rizvi, S. I. (2009). Plant polyphenols as dietary antioxidants in human health and disease. *Oxid. Med. Cell. Longevity.* 2: 270–278.

Parhi, B., Bharatiya, D., & Swain, S. K. (2020). Application of quercetin flavonoid based hybrid nanocomposites: A review. *Saudi Pharm. J.* 28: 1719–1732.

Park, K. R., Kim, S., Cho, M., & Yun, H. M. (2021). Limonoid triterpene, obacunone increases runt-related transcription factor 2 to promote osteoblast differentiation and function. *Int. J. Mol. Sci.* 22: 2483.

Patil, A. G., & Jobanputra, A. H. (2015). Rutin-chitosan nanoparticles: Fabrication, characterization and application in dental disorders. *Polym.-Plast. Technol. Eng.* 54: 202–208.

Patra, J. K., Das, G., Fraceto, L. F., Campos, E. V. R., Rodriguez-Torres, M. D. P., Acosta-Torres, L. S., Diaz-Torres, L. A., Grillo, R., Swamy, M. K., Sharma, S., Habtemariam, S., & Shin, H. S. (2018). Nano based drug delivery systems: Recent developments and future prospects. *J. Nanobiotechnol.* 16: 1–33.

Pereira, M. C., Hill, L. E., Zambiazi, R. C., Mertens-Talcott, S., Talcott, S., & Gomes, C. L. (2015). Nanoencapsulation of hydrophobic phytochemicals using poly (dl-lactide-co-glycolide) (PLGA) for antioxidant and antimicrobial delivery applications: Guabiroba fruit (Campomanesia xanthocarpa O. Berg) study. *LWT-Food Sci. Technol.* 63: 100–107.

Petrovska, B. B. (2012). Historical review of medicinal plants' usage. *Pharmacogn. Rev.* 6: 5.

Qi, J., Zheng, Z., Hu, L., Wang, H., Tang, B., & Lin, L. (2022). Development and characterization of cannabidiol-loaded alginate copper hydrogel for repairing open bone defects in vitro. *Colloids Surf. B.* 212: 112339.

Qihua, W., Boguang, Z., & Daosen, G. (2001). Isolation and identification of a compound from Thermopsis lanceolata to inhibit plant pathogenic fungi. *J. Nanjing For. Univ.* 44: 85–88.

Ranganathan, S., Balagangadharan, K., & Selvamurugan, N. (2019). Chitosan and gelatin-based electrospun fibers for bone tissue engineering. *Int. J. Biol. Macromol.* 133: 354–364.

Raphael, T. J., & Kuttan, G. (2003). Immunomodulatory activity of naturally occurring monoterpenes carvone, limonene, and perillic acid. *Immunopharmacol. Immunotoxicol.* 25: 285–294.

Roberts, T. T., & Rosenbaum, A. J. (2012). Bone grafts, bone substitutes and orthobiologics. *Organogenesis.* 8: 114–124.

Rodan, G. A., & Martin, T. J. (2000). Therapeutic approaches to bone diseases. *Science.* 289: 1508–1514.

Salamone, F., Galvano, F., Cappello, F., Mangiameli, A., Barbagallo, I., & Volti, G. L. (2012). Silibinin modulates lipid homeostasis and inhibits nuclear factor kappa B activation in experimental nonalcoholic steatohepatitis. *Transl. Res.* 159: 477–486.

Sarkar, N., & Bose, S. (2019). Liposome-encapsulated curcumin-loaded 3D printed scaffold for bone tissue engineering. *ACS Appl. Mater. Interfaces.* 11: 17184–17192.

Sautour, M., Mitaine-Offer, A. C., & Lacaille-Dubois, M. A. (2007). The Dioscorea genus: A review of bioactive steroid saponins. *J. Nat. Med.* 61: 91–101.

Schmidt, A. H. (2021). Autologous bone graft: Is it still the gold standard? *Injury.* 52: S18–S22.

Sedghi, R., Sayyari, N., Shaabani, A., Niknejad, H., & Tayebi, T. (2018). Novel biocompatible zinc-curcumin loaded coaxial nanofibers for bone tissue engineering application. *Polymers.* 142: 244–255.

Shaban, N. Z., Kenawy, M. Y., Taha, N. A., Abd El-Latif, M. M., & Ghareeb, D. A. (2021). Cellulose acetate nanofibers: Incorporating Hydroxyapatite (HA), HA/berberine or HA/moghat composites, as scaffolds to enhance in vitro osteoporotic bone regeneration. *Polymers.* 13: 4140.

Shakibaei, M., Buhrmann, C., & Mobasheri, A. (2011). Resveratrol-mediated SIRT-1 interactions with p300 modulate Receptor Activator of NF-κB Ligand (RANKL) activation of NF-κB signaling and inhibit osteoclastogenesis in bone-derived cells. *J. Biol. Chem.* 286: 11492–11505.

Shakoor, R., Hussain, N., Younas, S., & Bilal, M. (2023). Novel strategies for extraction, purification, processing, and stability improvement of bioactive molecules. *J. Basic Microbiol.* 63: 276–291.

Shegarfi, H., & Reikeras, O. (2009). Review article: Bone transplantation and immune response. *J. Ortho. Surg.* 17: 206–211.

Shen, C. L., Kaur, G., Wanders, D., Sharma, S., Tomison, M. D., Ramalingam, L., Chung, E., Moustaid-Moussa, N., Mo, H., & Dufour, J. M. (2018). Annatto-extracted tocotrienols improve glucose homeostasis and bone properties in high-fat diet-induced type 2 diabetic mice by decreasing the inflammatory response. *Sci. Rep.* 8: 1–10.

Singh, P., Gupta, A., Qayoom, I., Singh, S., & Kumar, A. (2020). Orthobiologics with phytobioactive cues: A paradigm in bone regeneration. *Biomed. Pharmacother.* 130: 110754.

Smitha Grace, S. R., Chandran, G., & Chauhan, J. B. (2019). Terpenoids: An activator of "fuel-sensing enzyme AMPK" with special emphasis on antidiabetic activity. *Plant Hum. Health.* 2: 227–244.

Şöhretoğlu, D., & Renda, G. (2020). Medicinal natural products in osteoporosis. *Annu. Rep. Med. Chem.* 55: 327–372.

Song, L., Xie, X., Lv, C., Sun, Y., Li, R., Yao, J., & Yu, Y. (2022). Electrospun biodegradable nanofibers loaded with epigallocatechin gallate for guided bone regeneration. *Compos. B. Eng.* 238: 109920.

Spencer, J. P. (2003). Metabolism of tea flavonoids in the gastrointestinal tract. *J. Nutr.* 133: 3255S–3261S.

Sujitha, S., Dinesh, P., & Rasool, M. (2018). Berberine modulates ASK1 signaling mediated through TLR4/TRAF2 via upregulation of miR-23a. *Toxicol. Appl. Pharmacol.* 359: 34–46.

Sujitha, S., Dinesh, P., & Rasool, M. (2020). Berberine encapsulated PEG-coated liposomes attenuate Wnt1/β-catenin signaling in rheumatoid arthritis via miR-23a activation. *Eur. J. Pharm. Biopharm.* 149: 170–191.

Sujitha, S., & Rasool, M. (2019). Berberine coated mannosylated liposomes curtail RANKL stimulated osteoclastogenesis through the modulation of GSK3β pathway via upregulating miR-23a. *Int. Immunopharmacol.* 74: 105703.

Suri, S. S., Fenniri, H., & Singh, B. (2007). Nanotechnology-based drug delivery systems. *J. Occup. Med. Toxicol.* 2: 1–6.

Tamura, G., Gold, C., Ferro-Luzzi, A., & Ames, B. N. (1980). Fecalase: A model for activation of dietary glycosides to mutagens by intestinal flora. *Proc. Natl. Acad. Sci.* 77: 4961–4965.

Tao, K., Xiao, D., Weng, J., Xiong, A., Kang, B., & Zeng, H. (2016). Berberine promotes bone marrow-derived mesenchymal stem cells osteogenic differentiation via canonical Wnt/β-catenin signaling pathway. *Toxicol. Lett.* 240: 68–80.

Thilakarathna, S. H., & Rupasinghe, H. V. (2013). Flavonoid bioavailability and attempts for bioavailability enhancement. *Nutrients.* 5: 3367–3387.

Tominari, T., Matsumoto, C., Watanabe, K., Hirata, M., Grundler, F. M. W., Miyaura, C., & Inada, M. (2015). Epigallocatechin Gallate (EGCG) suppresses lipopolysaccharide-induced inflammatory bone resorption, and protects against alveolar bone loss in mice. *FEBS Open Bio.* 5: 522–527.

Toor, R. H., Tasadduq, R., Adhikari, A., Chaudhary, M. I., Lian, J. B., Stein, J. L., Stein, G. S., & Shakoori, A. R. (2019). Ethyl acetate and n-butanol fraction of Cissus quadrangularis promotes the mineralization potential of murine pre-osteoblast cell line MC3T3-E1 (sub-clone 4). *J. Cell. Physiol.* 234: 10300–10314.

Umashankar, D. D. (2020). Plant secondary metabolites as potential usage in regenerative medicine. *J. Phytopharmacol.* 9: 270–273.

Vaiserman, A., Koliada, A., Zayachkivska, A., & Lushchak, O. (2020). Nanodelivery of natural antioxidants: An anti-aging perspective. *Front. Bioeng. Biotech.* 7: 447.

Vali, B., Rao, L. G., & El-Sohemy, A. (2007). Epigallocatechin-3-gallate increases the formation of mineralized bone nodules by human osteoblast-like cells. *J. Nutr. Biochem.* 18: 341–347.

Verma, A. H., Gautam, S. P., Bansal, K. K., Prabhakar, N., & Rosenholm, J. M. (2019b). Green nanotechnology: Advancement in phytoformulation research. *Medicines.* 6: 39.

Verma, A. H., Kumar, T. S., Madhumathi, K., Rubaiya, Y., Ramalingan, M., & Doble, M. (2019a). Curcumin releasing eggshell derived carbonated apatite nanocarriers for combined anti-cancer, anti-inflammatory and bone regenerative therapy. *J. Nanosci. Nanotechnol.* 19: 6872–6880.

Vimalraj, S., Rajalakshmi, S., Saravanan, S., Preeth, D. R., Vasanthi, R. L., Shairam, M., & Chatterjee, S. (2018). Synthesis and characterization of zinc-silibinin complexes: A potential bioactive compound with angiogenic, and antibacterial activity for bone tissue engineering. *Colloids Surf. B.* 167: 134–143.

Wang, J., Sun, Q., Wei, Y., Hao, M., Tan, W. S., & Cai, H. (2021). Sustained release of epigallocatechin-3-gallate from chitosan-based scaffolds to promote osteogenesis of mesenchymal stem cell. *Int. J. Biol. Macromol.* 176: 96–105.

Wang, W. H., Chuang, H. Y., Chen, C. H., Chen, W. K., & Hwang, J. J. (2016). Lupeol acetate ameliorates collagen-induced arthritis and osteoclastogenesis of mice through improvement of microenvironment. *Biomed. Pharmacother.* 79: 231–240.

Wei, B., Wang, W., Liu, X., Xu, C., Wang, Y., Wang, Z., & Mao, Y. (2021). Gelatin methacrylate hydrogel scaffold carrying resveratrol-loaded solid lipid nanoparticles for enhancement of osteogenic differentiation of BMSCs and effective bone regeneration. *Regener. Biomater.* 8: rbab044.

Wen, L., Zhang, Z., Sun, D. W., Sivagnanam, S. P., & Tiwari, B. K. (2019). Combination of emerging technologies for the extraction of bioactive compounds. *Crit. Rev. Food Sci. Nutr.* 60: 1826–1841.

Wilczewska, A. Z., Niemirowicz, K., Markiewicz, K. H., & Car, H. (2012). Nanoparticles as drug delivery systems. *Pharmacol. Rep.* 64: 1020–1037.

Wong, R. W. K., & Rabie, A. B. M. (2008). Effect of quercetin on preosteoblasts and bone defects. *Open J. Orthop.* 2: 27.

Wong, R. W. K., Rabie, B., Bendeus, M., & Hägg, U. (2007). The effects of Rhizoma Curculiginis and Rhizoma Drynariae extracts on bones. *Chin. Med.* 2: 1–7.

Wong, S. K., Chin, K. Y., & Ima-Nirwana, S. (2020a). Berberine and musculoskeletal disorders: The therapeutic potential and underlying molecular mechanisms. *Phytomed.* 73: 152892.

Wong, S. K., Chin, K. Y., & Ima-Nirwana, S. (2020b). Quercetin as an agent for protecting the bone: A review of the current evidence. *Int. J. Mol. Sci.* 21: 6448.

Xu, C. C., Wang, B., Pu, Y. Q., Tao, J. S., & Zhang, T. (2017). Advances in extraction and analysis of phenolic compounds from plant materials. *Chin. J. Nat. Med.* 15: 721–731.

Xu, Q., Cao, Z., Xu, J., Dai, M., Zhang, B., Lai, Q., & Liu, X. (2021). Effects and mechanisms of natural plant active compounds for the treatment of osteoclast-mediated bone destructive diseases. *J. Drug Target.* 30: 394–412.

Yang, C. S., Blum, N. T., Lin, J., Qu, J., & Huang, P. (2020). Biomaterial scaffold-based local drug delivery systems for cancer immunotherapy. *Sci. Bull.* 65: 1489–1504.

Yang, C. S., Maliakal, P., & Meng, X. (2002). Inhibition of carcinogenesis by tea. *Annu. Rev. Pharmacol. Toxicol.* 42: 25–54.

Yang, F., Hou, Z. F., Zhu, H. Y., Chen, X. X., Li, W. Y., Cao, R. S., Li, Y. X., Chen, R., & Zhang, W. (2021). Catalpol protects against pulmonary fibrosis through inhibiting TGF-β1/Smad3 and Wnt/β-Catenin signaling pathways. *Front. Pharmacol.* 11: 594139.

Yonezawa, T., Lee, J. W., Hibino, A., Asai, M., Hojo, H., Cha, B. Y., Teruya, T., Nagai, K., Chung, U. Il, Yagasaki, K., & Woo, J. T. (2011). Harmine promotes osteoblast differentiation through bone morphogenetic protein signaling. *Biochem. Biophys. Res. Commun.* 409: 260–265.

Yu, X., Shen, G., Shang, Q., Zhang, Z., Zhao, W., Zhang, P., & Jiang, X. (2021). A Naringin-loaded gelatin-microsphere/nano-hydroxyapatite/silk fibroin composite scaffold promoted healing of critical-size vertebral defects in ovariectomised rat. *Int. J. Biol. Macromol.* 193: 510–518.

Zhang, D., & Kanakkanthara, A. (2020). Beyond the paclitaxel and vinca alkaloids: Next generation of plant-derived microtubule-targeting agents with potential anticancer activity. *Cancers.* 12: 1721.

Zhang, F., Xie, J., Wang, G., Zhang, G., & Yang, H. (2018). Anti-osteoporosis activity of Sanguinarine in preosteoblast MC3T3-E1 cells and an ovariectomized rat model. *J. Cell. Physiol.* 233: 4626–4633.

Zhang, Y., Du, Z., Li, D., Wan, Z., Zheng, T., Zhang, X., & Cai, Q. (2022). Catalpol modulating the crosstalking between mesenchymal stromal cells and macrophages via paracrine to enhance angiogenesis and osteogenesis. *Exp. Cell Res.* 418: 113269.

Zhang, Y., Wang, T., Li, J., Cui, X., Jiang, M., Zhang, M., & Liu, Z. (2021). Bilayer membrane composed of mineralized collagen and chitosan cast film coated with berberine-loaded PCL/PVP electrospun nanofiber promotes bone regeneration. *Front. Bioeng.* 9: 684335.

Zhao, B., Xiong, Y., Zhang, Y., Jia, L., Zhang, W., & Xu, X. (2020). Rutin promotes osteogenic differentiation of periodontal ligament stem cells through the GPR30-mediated PI3K/AKT/mTOR signaling pathway. *Exp. Biol. Med.* 245: 552–561.

Zhao, B., Zhang, Y., Xiong, Y., & Xu, X. (2019). Rutin promotes the formation and osteogenic differentiation of human periodontal ligament stem cell sheets in vitro. *Int. J. Mol. Med.* 44: 2289–2297.

Zhou, L., Song, F., Liu, Q., Yang, M., Zhao, J., Tan, R., Xu, J., Zhang, G., Quinn, J. M. W., Tickner, J., & Xu, J. (2015a). Berberine sulfate attenuates osteoclast differentiation through RANKL induced NF-κB and NFAT pathways. *Int. J. Mol. Sci.* 16: 27087–27096.

Zhou, P., Yan, B., Wei, B., Fu, L., Wang, Y., Wang, W., Zhang, L., & Mao, Y. (2023). Quercetin-solid lipid nanoparticle-embedded hyaluronic acid functionalized hydrogel for immunomodulation to promote bone reconstruction. *Regener. Biomater.* 10: rbad025.

Zhou, Y., Liu, S. Q., Peng, H., Yu, L., He, B., & Zhao, Q. (2015b). In vivo anti-apoptosis activity of novel berberine-loaded chitosan nanoparticles effectively ameliorates osteoarthritis. *Int. Immunopharmacol.* 28: 34–43.

Zou, B., Zheng, J., Deng, W., Tan, Y., Jie, L., Qu, Y., Yang, Q., Ke, M., Ding, Z., Chen, Y., Yu, Q., & Li, X. (2021). Kirenol inhibits RANKL-induced osteoclastogenesis and prevents ovariectomized-induced osteoporosis via suppressing the Ca2+-NFATc1 and Cav-1 signaling pathways. *Phytomed.* 80: 153377.

Zuo, Y., Li, Q., Xiong, Q., Li, J., Tang, C., Zhang, Y., & Wang, D. (2022). Naringin release from a nano-hydroxyapatite/collagen scaffold promotes osteogenesis and bone tissue reconstruction. *Polymers.* 14: 3260.

III

Advancement and Application of Tissue Engineering toward Orthopedic Concerns

12 Unraveling Translational Research on Ultra-High Molecular Weight Polyethylene in Total Hip Joint Arthroplasty

A Lab-to-Industry-Scale Pilot Study

Vidushi Sharma, N. H. Gowtham, Biswanath Kundu, Vamsi Krishna Balla, D. C. Sundaresh, and Bikramjit Basu

12.1 INTRODUCTION

Degenerative arthritis, rheumatoid arthritis, other inflammatory arthritis, and intra-articular trauma damage the articular surfaces, causing extreme pain and inflammation-mediated bone loss (Bellare & Cohen, 1996; Ramani & Parasnis, 1998; Truss et al., 1980; Sharma et al., 2022a; Liphardt et al., 2020; Glyn-Jones et al., 2015). Often, these conditions lead to moderate to severe bone loss and loosening of the joint, and under extreme scenarios, surgical intervention is required (Singh, 2011). These orthopedic surgical interventions are termed arthroplasties and come under the category of total joint arthroplasty (TJA). Generally, TJA procedures are named according to the specific joint application, such as total hip joint arthroplasty (THA)/total hip replacement (THR), total knee arthroplasty (TKA), shoulder arthroplasty (SA), total elbow arthroplasty (TEA), total ankle replacement (TAR), and total disc replacement (TDR). In particular, THR is the most revolutionary intervention to date.

In brief, in THR, an artificial joint replaces a worn, deteriorated, or diseased hip joint (Knight et al., 2011; Callaghan et al., 2000; Pramanik et al., 2005). THR plays a vital role in relieving hip pain that cannot be regulated by medicine or alternative treatment. In addition to relieving pain, an ideal prosthesis is also expected to restore hip joint functions, and its longevity depends on how well it integrates with the implantation site. Yet in real-life scenarios, the functions and longevity of implants, especially the acetabular components, are compromised due to the generation of wear particles, which often results in osteolysis and aseptic loosening (Harris, 1994; Bitar & Parvizi, 2015; Gallo et al., 2013; Vallés & Vilaboa, 2019).

In response, biomaterials including metals and their alloys, polymers, and ceramics have been explored in this field to fabricate joint prostheses, especially acetabular liners (ALs) (Basu & Ghosh, 2017). Among these, ultra-high molecular weight polyethylene (UHMWPE) ALs have been extensively used in the last six decades (Sharma et al., 2022a; Brach del Prever et al., 2009; Pietrzak, 2021). UHMWPE is known for its biocompatibility, high mechanical strength, toughness, impact resistance, and wear resistance (Patil et al., 2020; Hussain et al., 2020; Li & Burstein, 1994; Spiegelberg et al., 2016). Despite having high wear resistance and a low coefficient of friction, existing UHMWPE materials (XL-UHMWPE and vitamin-E reinforced XL-UHMWPE) still generate a considerable amount of wear (post-articulation), which ultimately results in poor implant lifespan (~35 years with 44% success) and failure (Fisher, 1994; Jasty et al., 1997; Nine et al., 2014).

DOI: 10.1201/9781003307310-15

BOX 12.1

According to the American Joint Replacement Registry, the number of joint replacements in the United States is increasing significantly, with a 200% surge in total hip joint replacement procedures anticipated between 2005 and 2030. A similar surge was observed by the Indian Society of Hip and Knee Surgeons (2019), with most of the implants procured from Johnson and Johnson (~48%), followed by Zimmer (21%), Stryker (9.5%), Smith & Nephew (7%), and other companies.

In view of the fact that the existing UHMWPE derivatives possess constraints, mostly associated with implant lifespan and functionality, researchers have been exploring the efficacy of the possible blends and composites in much more detail; the possibility of introducing blends/composites in orthopedics holds huge potential to combat aforementioned issues as new AL materials with clinically relevant performance-limiting tribological, mechanical, and biocompatibility properties (Sharma et al., 2020; Bhusari et al., 2019; Sharma et al., 2022b).

BOX 12.2

Crosslinked UHMWPE (XL-UHMWPE) came into existence as a second-generation UHMWPE derivative. Generally, crosslinking of polyethylene chains is performed by electron beam or gamma irradiation. Irradiated crosslinking of polyethylene chains occurs first in its amorphous region through the recombination of free radicals generated through radiation penetration. These free radicals are formed because of C–C or C–H bond breakdown, and the process depends on the radiation dosage. Although the wear resistance of XL-UHMWPE is better than that of conventional UHMWPE, its oxidation resistance is impaired due to the presence of unreacted free radicals. Consequently, vitamin-E reinforced XL-UHMWPE came into existence as a third-generation derivative.

In addition to the properties of new-generation AL materials, attention should also be paid to the processing routes. The processing routes deployed to manufacture/produce ALs play an important role in determining implant functionality and are less explored. So far, the standard processing routes to manufacture UHMWPE-based implants involve many steps, starting from powder consolidation (compression molding of sheets or extruded bar stocks) to the final near-net-shaped prototype (via machining) (Han et al., 1981).

Notably, UHMWPE undergoes significant changes in its physical, chemical, and mechanical properties during its processing (Zachariades & Kanamoto, 1986; Gul & McGarry, 2004), and only a few studies are available to understand the effect of manufacturability on AL performance. Performance characteristics include surface finish, sphericity, roughness, diameter, thickness, and clearance (Sarkar et al., 2016; Cubillos et al., 2018; Scholes et al., 2000; Gispert et al., 2006). For instance, Ito et al. (2001) observed the effect of AL sphericity on the femoral head (FH), where sphericity departure (out-of-roundness) by more than 30 μm led to higher wear rates. Additionally, a significant effect of liner thickness was also noticed on resulting wear rates (Saikko, 1995; Kurtz et al., 1997); researchers observed that inappropriate liner thickness can influence contact stresses and wear (Lee et al., 1999). Similarly, the surface roughness plays a vital role in AL wear at the counterface, as observed with explants and in *in vitro* experiments (Hall et al., 1997; Wang et al., 1998b; Jedenmalm et al., 2009; Chen et al., 2008).

Another perspective is structure linkage. It was reported that XL-UHMWPE (a widely used AL material) exhibited a wear rate around 5.7 times lower than that of unirradiated UHMWPE (Lestari et al., 2021). In another study, crosslinking increased the wear resistance compared with that of conventional UHMWPE. A further improvement in the wear properties and implant longevity was observed by Oral et al. (2006) with vitamin-E reinforced XL-UHMWPE. In addition, a fourfold improvement in fatigue and wear life compared with UHMWPE was also recorded (Yamamoto et al., 2017; Grupp et al., 2014).

Overall, these studies demonstrated improved tribological performance of conventionally manufactured UHMWPE ALs with major focus either on structure or on quality indices (AL performance), but there have been very few or no efforts dedicated to understanding the correlations among processes and properties (Rumpf, 1990). Lestari et al. (2021) evaluated the performance of a CNC-milled AL in terms of crosslinking dosage (50–100 kGy) and applied varying articulating load (maximum 3000 N). They witnessed that 100 kGy irradiated UHMWPE AL exhibited lower wear depth than did 50 kGy irradiated AL.

BOX 12.3

The performance of AL is linked with several factors, including articulating counterface (ceramic-on-metal, metal-on-polymer, and ceramic-on-polymer), material properties, implant design, testing conditions, and lubrication (Bellare & Cohen, 1996; Ramani & Parasnis, 1998; Truss et al., 1980; Sharma et al., 2022b).

A secondary challenge with conventionally manufactured acetabular liners has been realized with the fact that the preclinical/clinical outcomes of many biomaterials and novel implant technologies do not meet expectations (Milošev et al., 2021). As a result, before translation, preclinical testing should account for all the guiding factors and parameters that the prosthesis will encounter *in vivo* (Izmin et al., 2021). Specific to THR, these factors include radial clearance between AL and FH, distribution of contact stresses on AL depending on thickness, and so on.

Keeping in mind the complexity and constraints linked to experimentation, finite element analysis (FEA) is increasingly becoming a significant tool for end-to-end research (Izmin et al., 2021; Larsen et al., 2021; Hua et al., 2014). The specific benefits of FEA include providing reasonable patient-specific findings to better understand both site- and subject-specific *in vivo* scenarios that are generally time-consuming to obtain experimentally due to both practical and ethical constraints (Stops et al., 2012). Therefore, before manufacturing new-generation implant prototypes, their intermediate performance can be effectively evaluated with FEA to lower both time to market and development time/cost by a factor of two or more (National Science and Technology Council, 2011).

Against this backdrop, this chapter discusses the spectrum of the tests and analyses that need to be considered to translate a new-generation biomaterial from lab scale to industrial scale, especially for THR. This chapter also brings in the relevance and criticality of the essential manufacturing properties, biomechanical response, process parameters, and quality indices (in accordance with ISO standards) for prototype development.

12.2 MANUFACTURING RELEVANT THERMOPHYSICAL PROPERTIES

It is well established that due to its higher molecular weight and hence higher melt viscosity, UHMWPE-based products/prototypes are commercially manufactured using conventional techniques (ram extrusion, compression molding, and hot-isotactic pressing, followed by machining).

These approaches are time-consuming and also result in an implant with compromised clinically relevant performance-limiting properties (Zachariades & Kanamoto, 1986; Gul & McGarry, 2004; Tanner et al., 1995). Although these strategies are well adapted for the consolidation and fusion of highly viscous UHMWPE powder particles, often process optimization is challenging (Han et al., 1981; Barnetson & Hornsby, 1995). Therefore, injection molding to manufacture near-net-shaped new-generation ALs can be a difficult but revolutionizing step in the field of orthopedics.

The advantage of injection molding UHMWPE materials is their shorter production time (~1–2 min per cycle), resulting in better reproducibility and large production capacity. The other benefits for the same include higher surface finish, dimensional tolerance, versatile mold, process design, and near-net shaping (Kashyap & Datta, 2015). Injection molding also helps maintain the physicomechanical properties of the polymeric material. However, a close evaluation of the mechanical, thermal, and flow properties is needed to optimize suitable process parameters and achieve implant with required dimensional tolerance/indices. Such assessment will also help researchers and engineers to understand varying stresses, melt temperatures, cooling rates, heat transfer, and total cycle times for processing and molding specific designs and polymers.

This chapter unravels the injection moldability of a new-generation UHMWPE material (HDPE/UHMWPE blend (HU) and composite (HUmGO)) for THR, along with the correlations with its thermophysical properties. The properties of relevance were melt flow index (MFI), specific heat capacity, thermal conductivity, melt viscosity, thermal degradation temperature, and volumetric shrinkage. The MFI of HUmGO was very low (0.14) at an applied load of 2.16 kg, implying that the flow of HU is slower than that of other thermoplastics (inset Figure 12.1(a)). This is primarily because the high melt viscosity of UHMWPE restricting the flow.

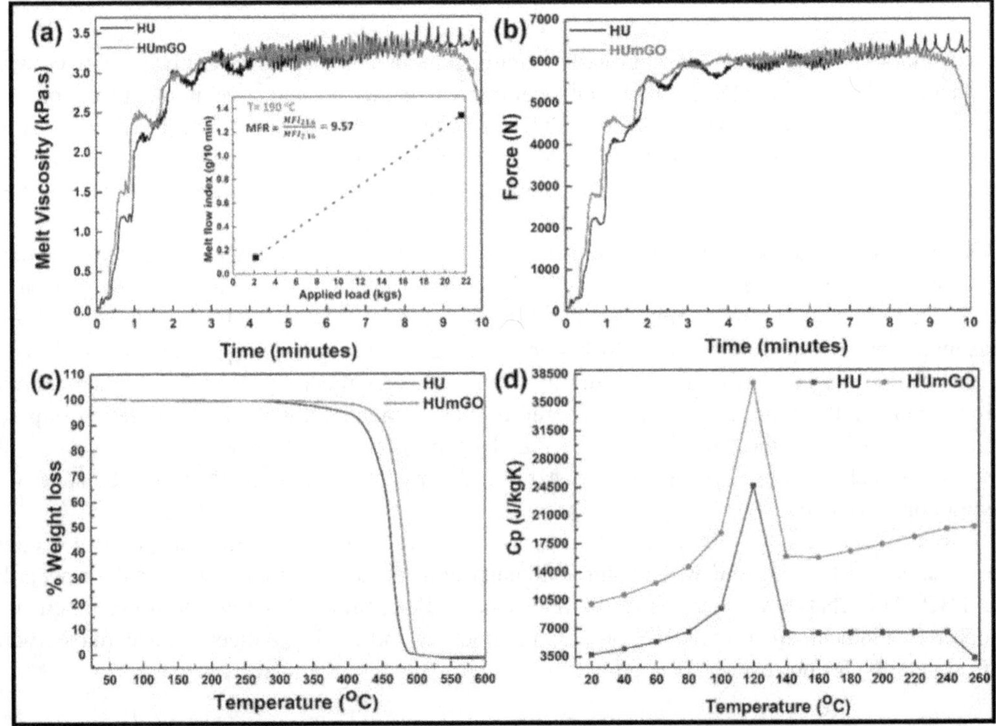

FIGURE 12.1 The flow and thermal properties of new-generation liner materials: (a) melt viscosity as a function of time (s) during extrusion; (b) screw force as a function of time during melt mixing; (c) thermal degradation profile against increasing temperature; and (d) specific heat capacity as a function of temperature. Inset in (a) shows the melt flow rate (MFR) for HUmGO.

Again, considering the simplistic AL prototype design (which we discuss in a later section), we postulate that such low MFI should not significantly affect the HU processing. Similar observations can also be associated with *in situ* melt viscosity and force (Figure 12.1(a,b)): HU and HUmGO exhibited similar flow behavior. The melting temperature (T_m), crystallization temperature (T_c), and % crystallinity (χ_c) of HU and HUmGO are summarized in Table 12.1; we analyzed these outcomes in our previous work (Bhusari et al., 2019). The table clearly shows that adding mGO significantly influenced the thermal properties of the HU matrix. For HUmGO, T_c was 0.9% higher, T_m was 0.6% higher, and χ_c was 32.5% higher w.r.t. HU. An increase (~ 57.6%) in the complex viscosity as a function of angular frequency was also observed (Bhusari et al., 2019). The observable increment in both T_m and % χ_c (Bhusari et al., 2019) with respect to the pristine HDPE and UHMWPE (Table 12.1), can be attributed to the recrystallization of defective polyethylene lamellae into bigger crystals as the blend is heated (Tanem & Stori, 2001). In brief, recrystallization is defined as the partial or complete melting of the initial lamellae prior to melting (at a low-temperature endothermic region) and the development of new, larger lamellae. In addition to recrystallization, the larger crystal lamellae form because of the thickening of lamellae in the solid state before melting (Tanem & Stori, 2000). Herein, the recrystallization or structural reorganization is not expected to be significant enough to alter the overall blend performance as the shift in T_m observed for both HU and HUmGO is less than 3 °C (Table 12.1) (Bhusari et al., 2019). In such a scenario, cocrystallization (a component chain segment diffuses and crystallizes into the lamellae of another component) can also be considered a plausible reason since the T_m values for the two components are almost identical, allowing crystal to form simultaneously (Tanem & Stori, 2000).

The rheological properties of HUmGO show that adding modified GO (mGO) had a significant effect on thermophysical properties. For instance, HUmGO had greater viscosity than HU. Interestingly, the addition of mGO in this newly developed nanocomposite gave two advantages: (a) it acted as a plasticizer, providing a plasticizing effect and better processibility than that of HU and UHMWPE, and (b) its better dispersion resulted in the improved mechanical and thermal properties (Sharma et al., 2020; Bhusari et al., 2019). The melt viscosity of the UHMWPE blend can also be attributed to the entanglement and disentanglement of HDPE and UHMWPE molecular chains under high external forces generated in the barrel during injection molding (Feng et al., 2014). However, a slight alteration in the shear rate due to non-Newtonian behavior can lead to significant changes in their melt viscosity, ultimately affecting process parameters (Kashyap & Datta, 2015).

In addition to rheological properties, thermal properties, namely thermal degradation temperature, melting temperature, thermal conductivity, and specific heat capacity, should also be understood when a highly viscous polymer such as UHMWPE is added to the blend (Huang et al., 2018). These properties must be investigated to optimize heat transfer, processing temperature, and most importantly thermal degradation temperature, since all of these are necessary to estimate the overall process cycle time (Kashyap & Datta, 2015). In the present context, both HU and HUmGO showed weight loss of ~2.5% at 435 °C (Figure 12.1(c)), but weight loss was more significant above that temperature, implying that the HU degrades above 435 °C.

TABLE 12.1
Thermophysical Properties of HU Hybrid and HUmGO Nanocomposite

Composition	Melting Temperature (T_m), °C	Crystallization Temperature (T_c), °C	% Crystallinity (% χ_c)	Complex Viscosity (η), Pa.sec	% Volumetric Shrinkage
HU	131.0	117.4	48.9 ± 5.8	3.3×10^4	2.15
HUmGO	131.9	116.3	55.2 ± 5.9	5.2×10^4	1.17 ± 0.47

In addition to thermal degradation, specific heat capacity provides a better understanding of optimized process cycle times. Figure 12.1(d) shows the variations in specific heat capacity of HU and HUmGO as a function of temperature; the figure shows that HU exhibited a lower C_p of 24706.69 J/kgK, while HUmGO showed a higher C_p of 81756. 2 J/kgK. The Cp was highest near the melting temperatures of both HU and HUmGO (~131 °C). Another thermo-physical property of relevance for injection molding is thermal conductivity, and that of HUmGO (λ_c) is in the range of 0.46 to 0.54 W/mK, indicating the crystalline nature of HUmGO (Hu et al., 2007).

These thermal properties can also help predict the possibilities of molding defects such as sink marks, hot spots, and warpage. Warpage can be a major issue for ALs due to its close relationship with part geometry, especially at higher part thicknesses (>6 mm) (Sánchez et al., 2012). Another critical factor to be considered here is material's volumetric shrinkage, as it directly influences the warpage post-molding (Chang & Faison, 2001). Shrinkage refers to the volume contraction of polymers during the cooling stage of polymer manufacturing.

Most of the shrinkage in plastic molded parts happens during cooling because of the density difference between the polymer's molten state and the cooled state. Moreover, the part may continue to shrink to some extent until the temperature and moisture content stabilize (Chang & Tsaur, 1995). For AL, such considerations become even more substantial as the wall thickness of the AL prototype varies in the range of 8–14 mm, higher than the suggested wall thickness (<6.4 mm) for injection-molded polyethylene. In general, the wall thickness for injection-molded products ranges from 0.8 to 4.8 mm. The % shrinkage can be calculated in accordance with ASTM D955, using the following equation:

$$\%Shrinkage = \frac{V_0 - V_1}{V_0} \tag{12.1}$$

where V_0 is the volume of the injection mold geometry and V_1 is the volume of molded geometry.

For a more reliable interpretation of % shrinkage, triplicates of injection-molded specimens should be considered, and % shrinkage should be reported as mean ± standard deviation. The % shrinkage for HUmGO was found to be 1.17 ± 0.47%, which is less than the range reported for linear shrinkage value for HDPE (2–5%). In contrast, HU showed higher volumetric shrinkage of 2.15%. The shrinkage for both HU and HUmGO can be attributed to the presence of HDPE as well as to the crystalline behavior (Table 12.1). It should be noted that shrinkage is an anisotropic property and will be different in different flow directions (melt flow and radial direction) (Chang & Tsaur, 1995).

12.3 AL DESIGN AND GEOMETRICAL FEATURES

A systematic manufacturing approach should be adopted while developing new-generation AL prototypes. Figure 12.2 shows a typical process flow for developing an AL prototype with clinically relevant performance-limiting properties. Complete prototype development entails developmental activities first in the lab before the final prototyping.

The lab-scale research involves multiple significant steps: 1) optimize the parameters for both processing and sample preparation; 2) assess the physicomechanical and tribological properties; 3) select the most clinically competitive composition; 4) establish biocompatibility both *in vitro* and *in vivo*; 5) fabricate the prototype with the optimized processing parameters, and 6) assess the dimensional aspects and surface properties of the prototype. However, when translating such new-generation biomaterials from bench to bedside, the first step is to design the prototype.In general, a simplistic Ø 44 × 28 mm AL is fabricated by deriving the dimensions (thickness, 8 mm; inner diameter [ID], 28 mm; outer diameter [OD], 44 mm) from suitable clinical models. The derived dimensions are then used as geometrical inputs to design a 3D AL model (generally using Solidworks™ modeling software), as shown in Figure 12.3 (Panel A(a)).

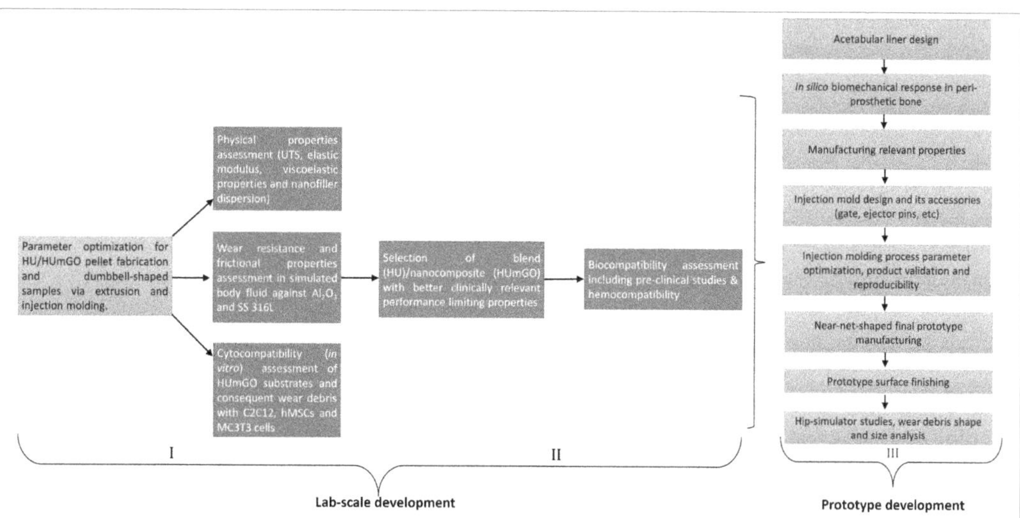

FIGURE 12.2 Process flow for developing new-generation acetabular liner materials (HU and HUmGO); reproduced with permission from Sharma, V., Bose, S., Kundu, B., Bodhak, S., Mitun, D., Balla, V. K. & Basu, B.: Probing the influence of γ-sterilization on the oxidation, crystallization, sliding wear resistance, and cytocompatibility of chemically modified graphene-oxide-reinforced HDPE/UHMWPE nanocomposites and wear debris. ACS Biomater. Sci. Eng. 2020. 6. 1462–1475. Copyright 2020 American Chemical Society; reproduced under the terms of CC-BY 4.0 (https://creativecommons.org/licenses/by/4.0/) International License from Bhusari, S. A., Sharma, V., Bose, S. & Basu, B., HDPE/UHMWPE hybrid nanocomposites with surface functionalized graphene oxide towards improved strength and cytocompatibility. J. R. Soc. Interface. 2019. 16. 20180273. Copyright 2019 Bhusari et al., published by Royal Society).

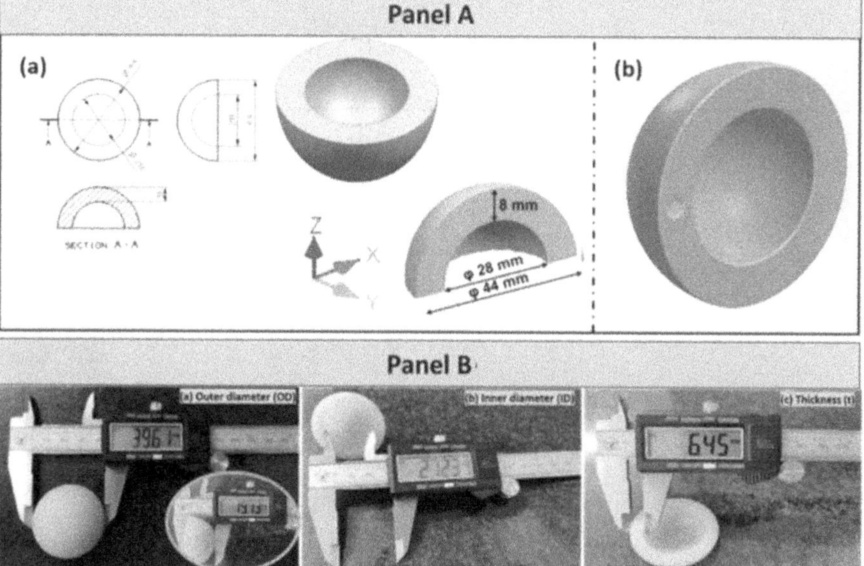

FIGURE 12.3 Panel A–Engineering design aspects and dimensional measurements of the acetabular liner: (a) AL final form and ID, OD, and thickness; (b) additional tolerance at the edges of the ID and OD. Panel B–Dimensional and shape tolerances of processed liners play a key role. Different projected views of surface finished injection-molded acetabular liner: (a) top view with inset showing side view; (b) inner cavity for femoral head accommodation; (c) wall thickness.

In addition to dimensional features, the shrinkage associated with the polymer should also be considered during design. These aspects are linked with additional tolerances (~ 0.5 mm) to be added to both inner and outer edges (refer to yellow highlights on the edges as shown in Figure 12.3 (Panel A(b)). Importantly, from a clinical standpoint and in accordance with ISO 21535:2010, the thickness of the AL should be more than 6 mm. Such thickness is required to accommodate the resultant wear (approximately several microns per year) during its articulation against the FH. Along with thickness, another key geometrical feature is the clearance (~ 0.5 mm) between FH and AL for free rotational motion. After confirming all the geometrical features, a custom-made injection mold should be designed.

12.4 *IN SILICO* BIOMECHANICAL ANALYSIS

In addition to conducting experiments and evaluating their outcomes, FEA is becoming a popular and effective tool for quantifying the preclinical biomechanical responses of the new-generation implants *in silico*. It is also helpful to select materials with relevant performance-limiting properties among different compositions. To perform FEA, a 3D FE model should be created that reconstructs the right side of the hemipelvis along with the articular cartilage and FH. This 3D model is constructed based on the computed tomography (CT) data of the patient. In general, the CT data is in DICOM format (512 × 512 pixels per slice, pixel size: 0.6445, and slice thickness: 1 mm; refer Figure 12.4(a)). The bone components are reconstructed in medical image processing software such as MIMICS®, and all the different elements of the bone are assigned material properties based on X-ray intensity (in Hounsfield units) attenuated in that voxel

In this chapter, we discuss a FE model for different polymeric ALs against a ceramic counterface (ZTA FH; OD Ø 28 mm) with a radial clearance of 40 μm based on several established studies (Mak et al., 2002). The acetabular component is virtually implanted in the reconstructed bony hemipelvis (Figure 12.4(b)), along with the modeling of the natural hemipelvis (for comparison). Virtually, the

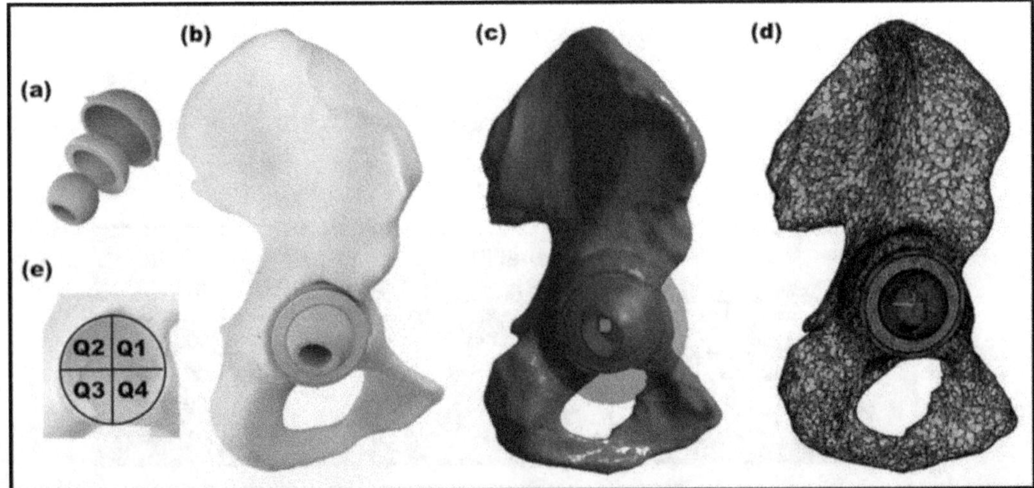

FIGURE 12.4 Finite element models: (a) CAD model of acetabular shell, liner, and femoral head; (b) virtual implantation in 3D-reconstructed hemipelvis; (c) region of interest selection with finer mesh; (d) material property assignment of bone and implant components; and (e) assignment of properties of relevance to virtual hemipelvis and implants.

acetabular region should be reamed to simulate THA during implantation. Throughout FEA simulation, natural bone is considered linearly elastic, isotropic, and homogeneous (Yamako et al., 2014; Jonkers et al., 2008; Chatterjee et al., 2018).

The density varies from 0.95 to 2.11 g/cm^3 for the hemipelvis in consideration. Furthermore, for biomaterials, the properties of relevance are elastic modulus (E) and bone density (ρ). These properties are assigned to each element based on the materials (HU, HUmGO, UHMWPE) in accordance with the following relationships (Ghosh & Gupta, 2014; Anderson & Madigan, 2013; Ghosh et al., 2015; Taddei et al., 2004):

For the hemipelvis,

$$\rho = 1.028 + (0.000769 \times HU) \tag{12.2}$$

$$E = 2349 \times \rho^{2.15} \tag{12.3}$$

For the femoral head,

$$\rho = 0.2389 + (0.0008351 \times HU) \tag{12.4}$$

$$E = 6850\ X\ \rho^{1.49} \tag{12.5}$$

HU in the above equations refers to the Hounsfield units.

In this chapter, we discuss the biomechanical responses of three AL materials: UHMWPE (GUR 1050), HU, and HUmGO. The properties of the various prosthetic materials and articular cartilage are summarized in Table 12.2. The modeled interface between the polymeric (HU, HUmGO, UHMWPE) AL and ceramic FH possesses a frictional contact with a coefficient of friction of 0.08 (Sharma et al., 2020). Herein, the globally adopted 10-noded tetrahedral element size is 1 mm (Figure 12.4(d)).

Additionally, the sacroiliac joint and the pubic symphysis should be fully constrained to replicate physical anatomy (Ghosh et al., 2015; Clarke et al., 2013; Dalstra & Huiskes, 1995; Thompson et al., 2002). The physical activity that is simulated, in general, is normal walking, and the different muscle forces and hip joint forces are divided into eight phases with established magnitudes and locations (Dalstra & Huiskes, 1995; Thompson et al., 2002; Dostal & Andrews, 1981). In the case of the natural model, the hip joint force is applied on a few nodes at the geometric center of the FH; in contrast, for the implanted model, the forces act over an area on the inner surface of the FH. Further, to represent the anatomical geometry, the acetabular anteversion angle and abduction angle for all the other components are taken as 20° and 45°, respectively (Saikko, 2016). For the patient-specific

TABLE 12.2
Material Properties of Various Components of THR and Natural Articular Cartilage. (Poisson's Ratio (υ) for Natural Bone: 0.3)

Components of THR Assembly	Prosthetic Material	Elastic Modulus (GPa)	Poisson's Ratio (υ)	Density (g/cm^3)
Metallic shell	Ti-6Al-4V	116	0.25	4.54
Acetabular liner	UHMWPE	0.676	0.46	0.93
	HU	0.646	0.4	0.96
	HUmGO	0.908	0.4	0.93
Femoral head	ZTA	360	0.23	4.05
Cartilage	–	0.37	0.25	–

components, the different components can be scaled by 0.875 with respect to body centroids to customize the geometry.

The minimum and maximum principal strain at the periprosthetic bone interface are noted and compared for both natural and implanted cases. The difference between the von Mises stress and strain in the natural and implanted models is recorded after each run in a quadrant-wise manner (Q1, Q2, Q3, and Q4) (Figure 12.4(e)).

BOX 12.4

To evaluate the biomechanical response and for analysis ease, the acetabular region is divided into four quadrants: Ql: anteromedial iliac quadrant; Q2: postero-lateral iliac quadrant; Q3: ischial quadrant; and Q4: pubic quadrant.

Of the four quadrants, we used the average von Mises stress in Q2 as the main criterion for comparing the three AL materials, as the stress in Q2 was usually higher due to the direction of hip joint force during the walking gait cycle.

As seen in Figure 12.5(a, b), the differences in the maximum principal strains induced in the periprosthetic bone during the second and sixth phases of the gait cycle—that is, during loading response (LR) and initial swing (ISw)—for UHMWPE and its blend (HU) were comparable, whereas for its composite (HUmGO), the maximum and minimum principal microstrain differences during LR were 210 and 881 and during ISw were 569 and 2474, respectively. For the UHMWPE-implanted model, the microstrain differences ($\times 10^{-6}$) in the LR were 206 and 887, and during the ISw, the differences were 556 and 2457, also both respectively. For the HU-implanted model, the microstrain differences ($\times 10^{-6}$) during the LR were 205 and 877 and were 551 and 2447 during the ISw, respectively. These observations can be visualized using the strain contour maps as well (Figure 12.5(c)). The figure shows that induced strain is more concentrated on Q2 in the acetabulum due to the backward and upward directions of hip joint force exerted by FH on AL.

Interestingly, the strain contour maps show the distribution of the strains during the two important phases of the gait cycle and appear qualitatively similar for UHMWPE, HU, and HUmGO. It is evident that the biomechanical performance of new-generation biomaterials (HU and HUmGO) is comparable with the performance of the clinically used UHMWPE in terms of principal microstrains (both minimum and maximum). Simultaneously, Figure 12.6 shows the von Mises stress in different liner materials in Q2 during various phases of the walking gait cycle.

The average von Mises stress developed in Q2 during LR for UHMWPE AL was 9.0 MPa, whereas for HU and HUmGO ALs, the stresses were 9.7 MPa and 9.6 MPa, respectively. During ISw, the stresses in the UHMWPE and HU ALs were 2.54 MPa and 2.46 MPa, respectively. The maximum recorded von Mises stresses for the UHMWPE and HU ALs were 51.9 MPa and 55.9 MPa, correspondingly, during LR. Notably, the von Mises stresses are higher for Ql and Q2. In particular, the peak stress in Q2 is due to the upward and backward directional forces.

Again, this analysis shows that HU and HUmGO ALs exhibit similar biomechanical performance to that of the clinically used UHMWPE. The principal strains (maximum and minimum) and von Mises stresses developed in the periprosthetic bone were also similar (Figure 12.5). The difference between the average von Mises stresses in the liner Q2 was less than 1 MPa (Figure 12.6). Interestingly, the differences between the implanted and natural models at different gait cycles in different regions of the acetabulum were similar in terms of magnitude (within 100 microstrain). Therefore, the effective load transfer between the FH and acetabulum is not affected by the small differences in the properties of all the liner materials.

Furthermore, the contact stresses in HU are very similar to those of UHMWPE, as evident from von Mises stress (~ <10% difference) developed in the different regions in the liners, possibly because

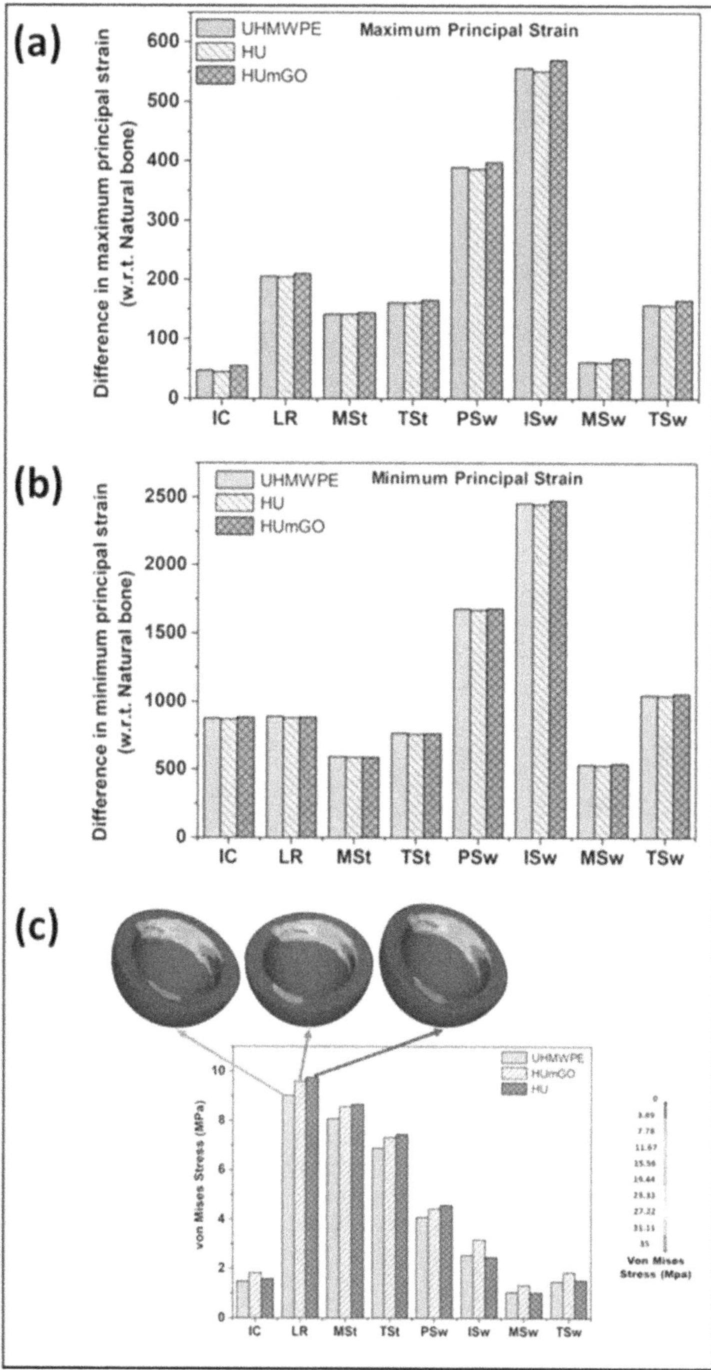

FIGURE 12.5 Strain differences between healthy (natural) and implanted models in terms of (a) maximum and (b) minimum principal strain for the three liner materials (UHMWPE, HU, HUmGO) over the eight phases of walking gait cycle (IC: initial contact, LR: loading response, MSt: mid stance, TSt: terminal stance, PSw: pre-swing, ISw: initial swing, MSw: mid swing, TSw: terminal swing); (c) von Mises stresses developed in virtually implanted liners in Q2 during various phases of the gait cycle. The contour maps show the stress distribution in the liners in the second phase of the cycle. The scale for the contour map is shown on the right.

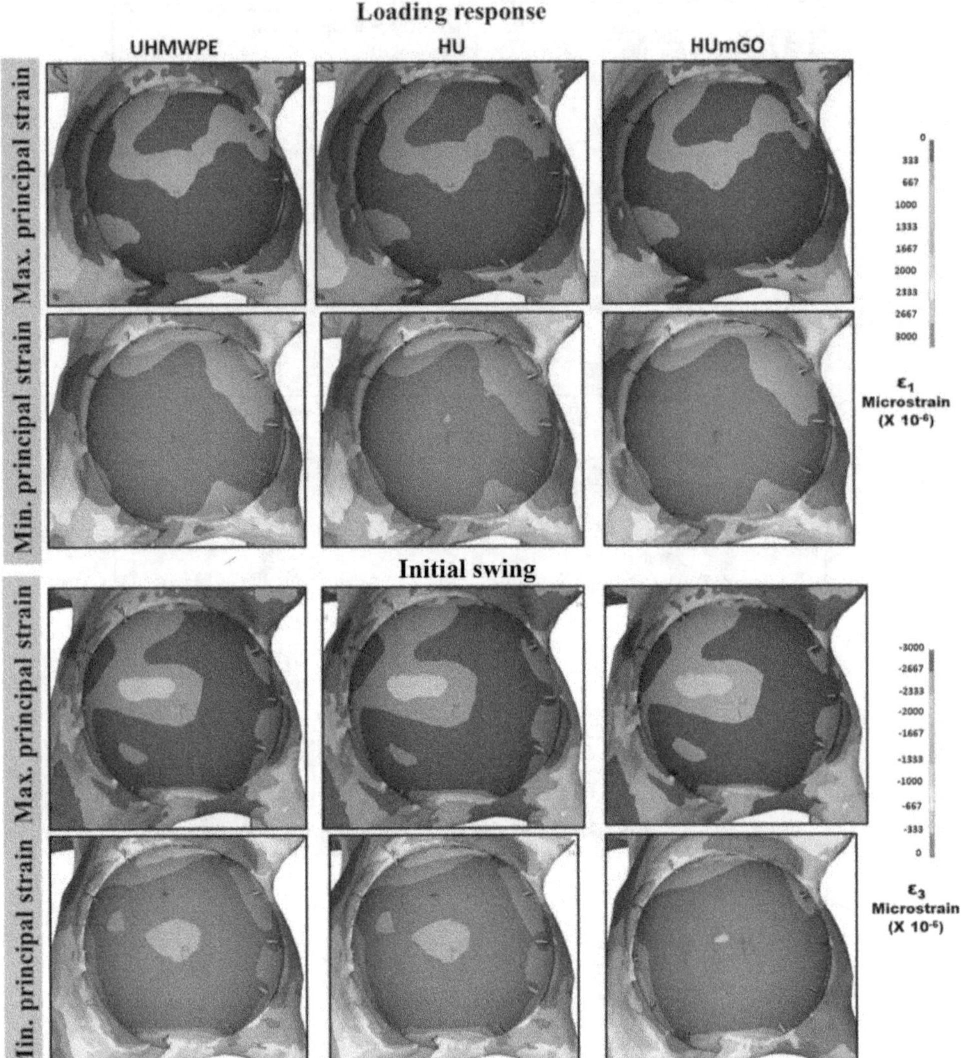

FIGURE 12.6 Contour maps of principal strain reflecting strain distribution in the hemipelvis for the UHMWPE, HU, and HUmGO liners. The upper maps show maximum principal strain (ε_1) distribution in periprosthetic bone, while the lower maps show the minimum principal strain (ε_3) distribution in the periprosthetic bone at two phases of the gait cycle (top panel: LR, bottom panel: ISw).

the elastic modulus and density of different liner materials are quite close. However, approximation in FEA models could lead to ideal results, which are simplistic and do not reflect the real behavior of the material. It is also necessary to estimate the contact mechanics of AL and FH.

Moreover, these simplistic material models do not take into account the possible heterogeneity and anisotropy of the system, which will significantly affect the outcomes. For instance, more material-related information (other than the elastic modulus, density, and Poisson's ratio) should be considered for new biomaterials (HU and HUmGO) to record holistic stress/strain response in periprosthetic bone. In short, the material models need to be improved to reflect structure linkages for both blends and composites. In particular, appropriate material models need to be developed as well to encompass the mechanistic behavior of the fillers, especially in terms of load transfer and wear resistance.

12.5 INJECTION MOLD DESIGN AND AL MOLDING

After critically assessing and evaluating the biomechanical response and thermophysical properties of the new-generation UHMWPE derivatives HU and HUmGO, we selected HU, the basic matrix, first for manufacturing AL prototypes via injection molding; optimizing the processing conditions for HU provided a holistic understanding for both blend and composite. Based on several inputs and investigations, we manufactured a two-cavity integrated mold using machinable metal alloy (such as E7 stainless steel) for AL injection molding.

In brief, an injection mold assembly consists of a separable cavity and a core that in the assembled state holds molten polymer (HU in the present context). Notably, the mold should be designed after carefully accommodating all the geometrical features (possible tolerances and volumetric shrinkage post-processing). Once the mold is ready and loaded, the melt-mixed HU pellets can be injection molded at an injection pressure of 80 MPa and a molding temperature of 240 °C. Simultaneously, the mold temperature can be optimized to provide an appropriate temperature for the gradual cooling of the molten blend. In the present context, it was 50 °C based on the PE matrix. Prior to raw material loading, both the core and cavity of the two-piece mold should be cleaned with a suitable reagent followed by usage of a heavy-duty mold release silicone spray for easy part ejection. During molding, an appropriate amount of holding time/residence time (~20–30 sec) should be provided to the molten composition to allow its uniform distribution throughout the core and cavity as well as for its gradual cooling.

12.6 DIMENSIONAL TOLERANCE AND 3D MICROSTRUCTURAL ANALYSIS

Figure 12.3 Panel B illustrates the injection-molded finished HU AL prototype with carefully measured dimensional indices, ID, OD, and thickness. A closer assessment illustrated that a range of material compositions (both HU and HUmGO) and dimensions can be processed using injection molding. We observed slight deviations (<1%) from the CAD model in different orthogonal projections of the molded AL. The significance of the dimensional analysis for THR is also emphasized by Schwartsmann et al. (2013), who evaluated a range of commercially available cemented and uncemented acetabular liners; the authors found that the uncemented acetabular liners exhibited higher dimensional accuracy in terms of OD, ID, and thickness than did the cemented liners. Furthermore, to justify dimensional limits of the molded prototypes, the dimensions of the finished AL (Ø 28 mm) can be compared with those of the medically used UHMWPE AL (Ø 28 mm) using a coordinate measuring machine.

BOX 12.5

The dimensional features of any shape/prototype can be measured using a coordinate measuring machine (CMM). A CMM is a measuring tool that establishes discrete points on a physical surface using a contact probe to quantify an object's geometry. CMMs provide three-dimensional coordinate systems with the displacement from the probe's origin point along XYZ axes. A CMM can accurately measure crucial 3D dimensions, record the measured data, and extract intricate details. Non-contact models employ additional tools like cameras and lasers.

To demonstrate product conformity as well as dimensional stability, it is necessary for the finished ALs to meet important quality indices (roughness and sphericity), in accordance with ISO standard 7206–2:2011 (Table 12.3). For instance, the surface roughness of the finished injection-molded AL prototype is < 2 µm, which is within ISO 7206–2:011 standards and is better than the machined UHMWPE AL (Table 12.3).

TABLE 12.3
Clinically Relevant Geometrical Features of Finished Acetabular Liners (UHMWPE (GUR 1050) was a Clinically Used Product from Orthotech India Pvt Ltd.)

	Dimensions	
Geometrical Features	**UHMWPE**	**HU**
Inner diameter (ID)	28.3 mm	28.4 ± 0.35 mm
Sphericity	33.2 μm	7.0 ± 2.83 μm
Roughness (R_a)	0.71 μm	0.12 ± 0.37μm

However, customized fixtures can be deployed to perform a little finishing to further enhance the conformity of the prototype with the FH counterface. Similarly, another essential feature is the AL sphericity. In accordance with ISO 7206–2:2011, the deviation of the sphericity, especially inner sphericity, should not be greater than 100 μm for AL. In the present context, the sphericity of the injection-molded AL was better than that of the conventionally manufactured AL. It is worth mentioning that in addition to sphericity and roughness, complete 3D rendered volume and microstructure can be investigated, using 3D micro-computed tomography (micro-CT) to inspect possible inner defects in a prototype.

BOX 12.6

Micro-CT is an effective tool to capture and visualize 3D-rendered volume of any complicated geometry. It works on the principle of x-ray attenuation. In this, X-rays from a source are passed through the mounted sample. After absorption, the attenuated X-rays are detected using the various detectors (0.39, 1, 4, 20 and 40×). The sample rotates 360° to capture 3D-rendered volume.

Figure 12.7 reveals perspective and bottom views of 3D-rendered micro-CT images of the HU and UHMWPE ALs. Throughout the molded prototype, we observed no processing defects like major cracks or porosity, and these findings were the same for the 2D XY, YZ, and XZ orthoslices (Figure 12.7(a-c)), indicating that UHMWPE-blend AL prototypes can be fabricated using injection molding.

Although the overall design is different for the two liners, it is worth mentioning that we compared the manufacturing strategies and resulting dimensional conformity. In addition to dimensional features and manufacturability, we also noticed that both HU and HUmGO exhibited comparable properties to those of the clinically used UHMWPE AL. These properties mainly include the clinically relevant performance-limiting mechanical and wear properties, summarized in Tables 12.2 and 12.4 (Bhusari et al., 2019; Dumbleton et al., 2009).

In addition to assessing the dimensional features, the articulating surface of the prototype should also allow suitable rotational motion in a commercial zirconia-toughened alumina (ZTA) FH, resulting in excellent geometrical conformity. The injection-molded liner abides with the stated ISO guideline. Overall, the measured dimensional tolerances for the injection-molded ALs appear to also be well suited for clinical usage.

BOX 12.7

Another requirement for accelerating the bench-to-bedside translation of new-generation articulating-joint materials is evaluating their capacity to withstand load and cyclic damage, especially when new manufacturing strategies are implemented.

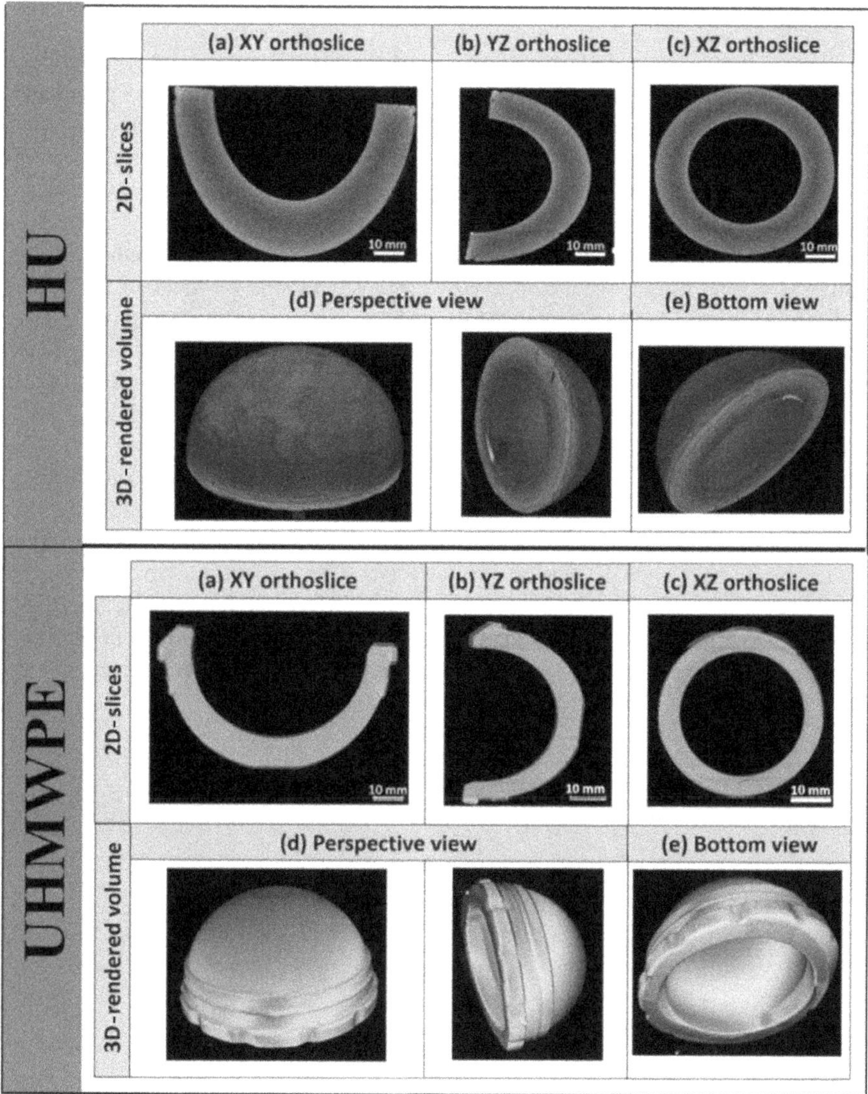

FIGURE 12.7 3D microstructural analysis is significant for a more realistic understanding of complex prototypes. 2D-reconstructed orthoslices: (a) XY; (b) YZ; (c) ZX and perspective views of 3D-rendered volume: (d) HU and (e) UHMWPE (Orthotech India, Pvt Ltd, India) acetabular liner. The area of the cubic ROI: 46372 × 46372 × 46372 μm³.

TABLE 12.4
Influence of Wear Rate and Acetabular Liner Radius on Femoral Head Penetration Depth for UHMWPE (GUR 1050) and HU Acetabular Liners

Acetabular liner (composition)	Wear rate (mm^3/Nm)	Acetabular liner radius (mm)	Wear depth (mm)
UHMWPE (GUR 1050)	1.93×10^{-6}	14.14	0.111
HU (60 wt.% HDPE/40 wt. %UHMWPE)	1.39×10^{-6}	13.62	0.128

12.7 WEAR AND FATIGUE

Prior to clinical studies, it is desirable to examine the functional capability of new-generation implant prototypes in joint simulators. In joint simulators, dynamic loading cycles and articulations are applied to the implant prototypes, especially to simulate physiological conditions. For instance, hip joint simulator studies benchmark new-generation liner material prototypes against ASTM 1714 guidelines and evaluate the interplay of material properties with manufacturing approaches.

Herein, we tested both HU and UHMWPE AL against a ceramic (ZTA) FH with ID-Ø 28 mm) in a ceramic-on-polymer (CoP) configuration. We selected the CoP configuration owing to its reduced *in vivo* wear rates, ~50%, compared with those of metal-on-metal or metal-on-polymer. The specifications for all the components of the tribocouple should be maintained in accordance with ISO 21535:2010 and ISO 7206–2:011. In the present context, the tribocouples possess an average clearance of 0.26 mm. In general, hip simulator tests are conducted at 37 ± 2 °C, at a frequency of 1.0 Hz in level walking mode in wet conditions. The lubricant is composed of 25 g/L fetal bovine calf serum in distilled (DI) water with 0.2 wt% sodium azide.

Before the test, both the test and control implants should be soaked in lubricant for 48 h at maintained temperature and humid conditions. After 48 h, both AL and FH should be cleaned sequentially while ultrasonication in DI water, antiseptic (Dettol), and again with DI, followed by drying. The samples should be weighed, and the axis of rotation for articulation must be marked before loading the tribocouple. During testing, the FH/AL assembly should be completely immersed in the lubricant (with maintained pH). Additionally, the pH of the lubricant should be checked periodically after each intermittent stop and the wear debris particles should be collected carefully every time for further analysis.

BOX 12.8

It is necessary to be very cautious while preparing AL and FH for articulation in the hip simulator as it is likely to have a significant effect on the tribological behavior of the bearing, especially polymeric AL.

The outcomes of a hip-simulator study are in general captured in terms of gravimetric weight loss as a function of time, measured in million cycles (MC). In this chapter, we compared the tribological performance of UHMWPE AL and HU AL when articulated against ZTA FH and captured weight loss after every 0.5 MC. On average, the amount of wear with the UHMWPE AL was ~30% higher than that with the HU AL (Figure 12.8(a)). For both the UHMWPE and HU liners, the amount of wear decreased drastically from 1 MC to 2 MC, and we observed similar trends in the case of the wear rate. Figure 12.8(a) reflects that the wear decreased linearly throughout the testing period.

The average wear rate after 2 MC was 42.1 mg/MC for HU AL and 50.7 mg/MC for UHMWPE AL. The linear regression showed that the steady-state wear rates calculated between 1 MC and 1.5 MC and between 1.5 MC and 2 MC were 79.2 and 22.3 mg/MC, respectively, for UHMWPE AL. On the other hand, in the case of HU AL, the wear rates were 63.6 and 20.5 mg/MC, respectively. In the run-in-phase as well, the wear rate was in the same range as the average wear rate: 72.3 mg/MC for UHMWPE AL and 44.8 mg/MC for HU AL. Notably, the observed differences in the wear rates in the present context with every 0.5 MC were not statistically significant.

The wear performance of ALs can be further understood by investigating the worn surfaces post-articulation. The worn surfaces of both the UHMWPE and HU ALs appeared smooth macroscopically (see Figure 12.9). However, changes in surface roughness are inevitable

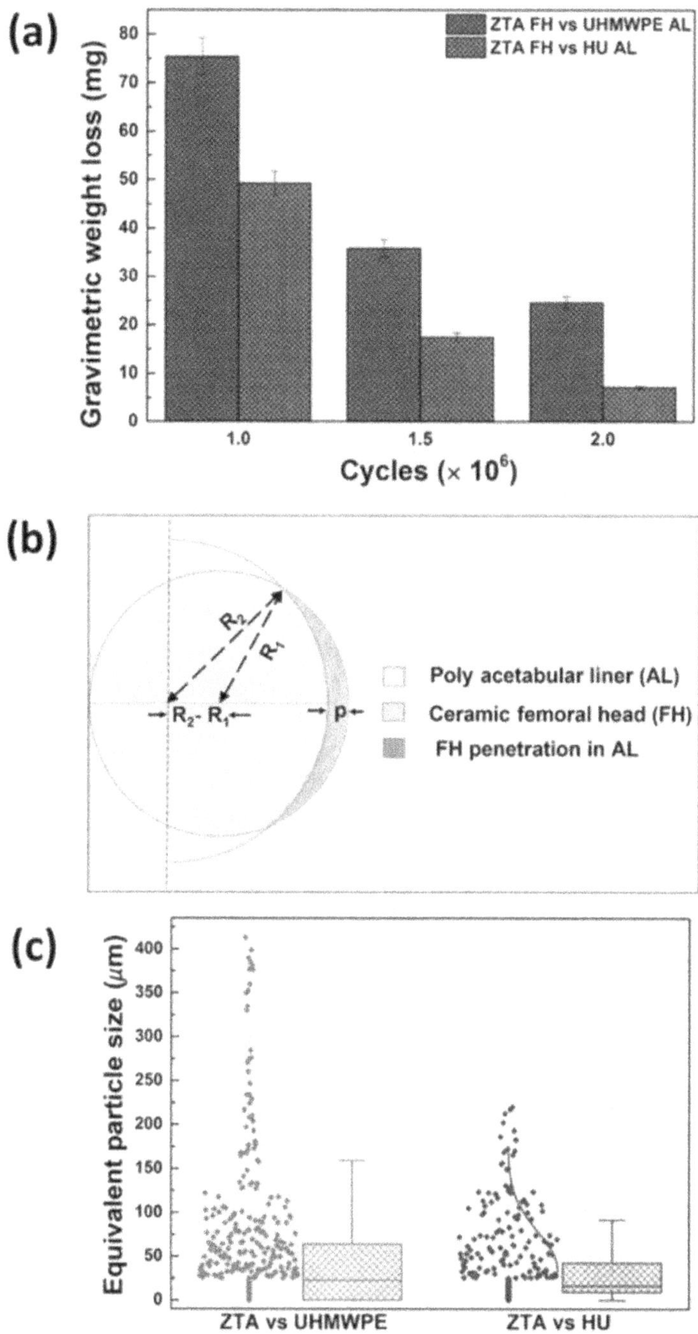

FIGURE 12.8 Hip simulators are one of the reliable screening devices for assessing the tribological performance of new-generation biomaterials: (a) gravimetric wear loss as a function of 2 MC loading cycles for ZTA FH vs. UHMWPE AL and ZTA FH vs. HU AL; (b) schematic diagram depicting penetration of spherical FH into a polymeric AL. p, R_1, and R_2 refer to the FH penetration in AL, radius of FH, and radius of AL, respectively. (c) Box plot showing wear particle size distribution generated from UHMWPE and HU against ZTA FH. ZTA FH OD is commercially procured Ø 28 mm from Stryker Orthopedics, USA. UHMWPE AL is a commercially procured Ø 28 mm (ID) GUR 1050 AL from Orthotech Pvt India Ltd, and HU is an indigenous injection-molded Ø 28 mm (ID) AL composed of HDPE/UHMWPE blend.

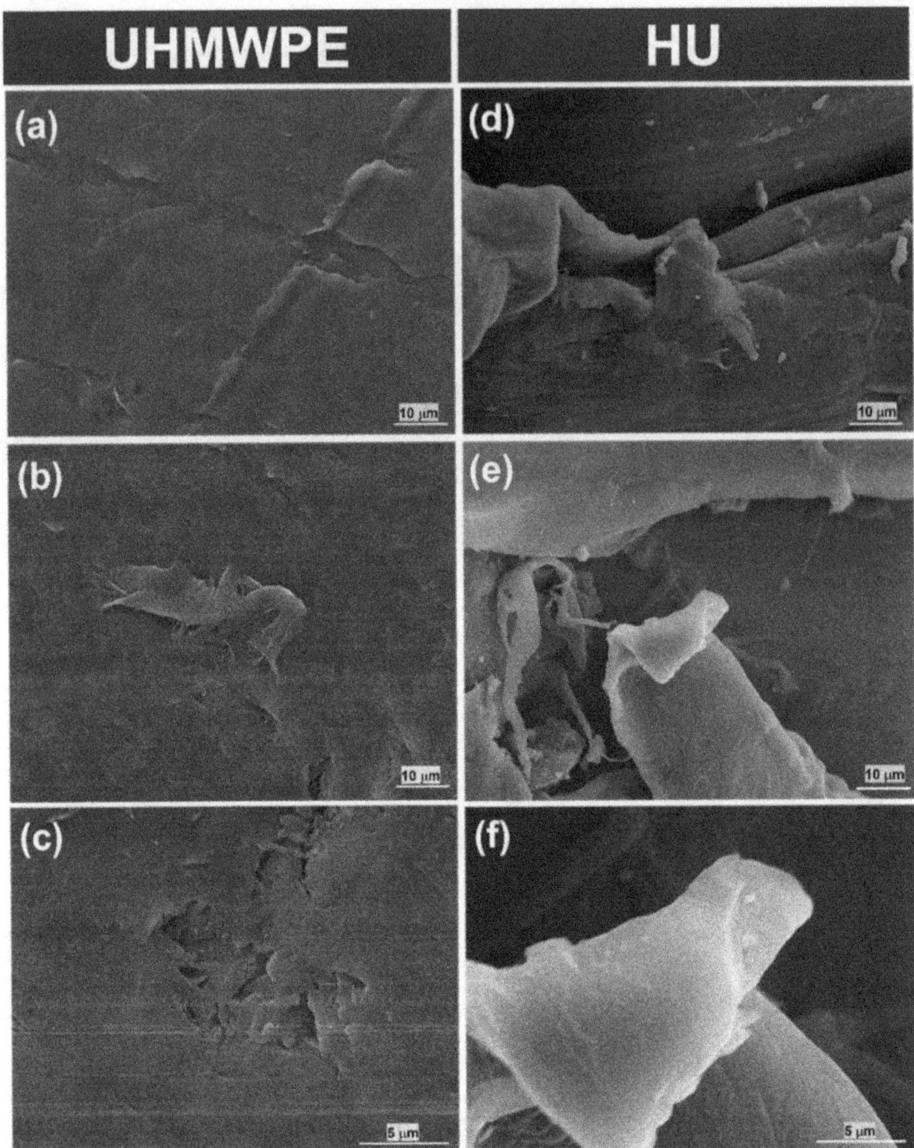

FIGURE 12.9 For THR, a deeper understanding of the wear mechanism allows for more accurate estimates of implant lifespan. The morphologies of the ALs post-articulation: (a), (b), (c) UHMWPE AL articulated against ZTA FH; (d), (e), (f) HU AL articulated against ZTA FH.

post-articulation and are associated with the surface morphology as well as with possible wear mechanisms exhibited by the two tribocouples. Figure 12.9(a) reveals the worn surfaces of medically used commercial UHMWPE AL; the figure shows that the parallel arrays of cracks, oriented both parallel and perpendicular to the wear direction, are formed post-articulation. In general, these microcracks coalesced to form longer cracks. The UHMWPE lamellae, when ploughed by ceramic asperities, resulted in small flakes and fine polymeric debris (Figure 12.10), and these particles resulted in third-body abrasion, as indicated by the embedded polymer debris on polymer debris (Figure 12.9(c)).

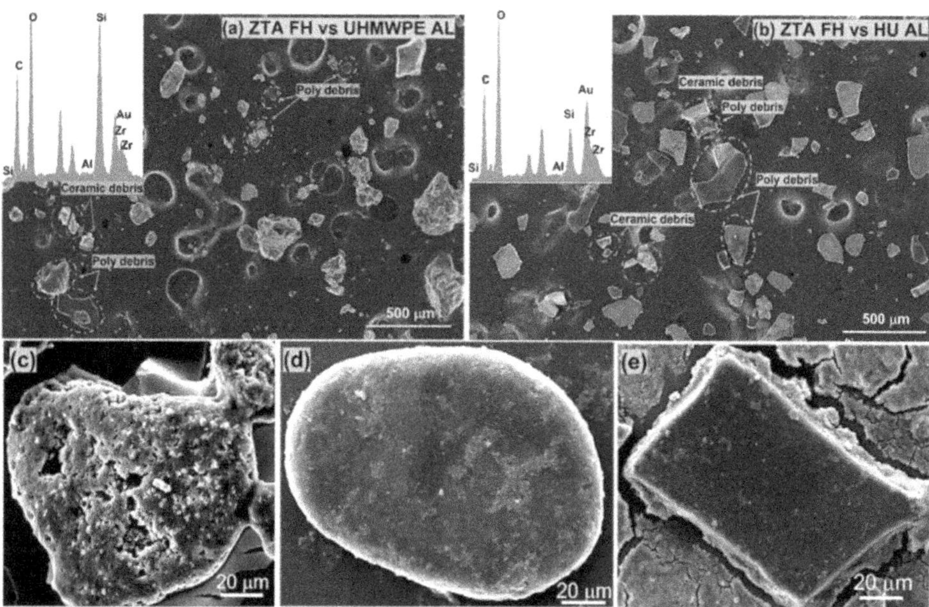

FIGURE 12.10 The size, form, and amount of the wear debris generated during articulation are directly correlated to specific osteolysis thresholds and play a critical role in implant lifespan assessment. Scanning electron micrographs along with elemental analysis revealing the morphology, shape, and size of the wear debris generated from the hip simulator: (a) ZTA FH vs. UHMWPE AL; (b) ZTA FH vs. HU AL; morphology of polymer from (c) ZTA-UHWMPE tribocouple, (d,e) ZTA-HU tribocouple. ZTA FH is commercially procured Ø 28 mm (OD) from Stryker Orthopedics, USA, UHMWPE AL is a commercially procured Ø 28 mm (ID) GUR 1050 AL from OrthoTech Pvt India Ltd, and HU is an indigenous injection-molded Ø 28 mm (ID) AL composed of HDPE/UHMWPE blend.

However, after assessing EDS compositional outcomes (Figure 12.10(a,b)), strong peaks pertaining to the constituents of the AL (i.e., C) and FH (i.e., Zr, Al, O) can be observed indicating the absence of any tribochemical layer on the implant's surface. Severe wear damage on the surface of HU AL can be noticed in the forms of polymeric ribbons, longer abrasions, and detached polymer fibrils that clung to the abraded grooves (Figure 12.9(d–f)). In contrast, for UHMWPE AL, the damage severity was found to be lesser and can be perceived as pitting (Figure 12.9(a–c)).

For the HU matrix, the polyethylene blend is ploughed by hard counterbody asperities during articulation, resulting in abrasive wear leading to the excessive detachment of bundles of polymer fibrils (Figure 12.9(d,e)). It can be anticipated that the polymer matrix is mechanically pulled by the ceramic counterface and withdrawn as continuous thin polymer layers/ribbons. On the contrary, no such behavior can be observed in the case of UHMWPE AL apart from the deep abrasive grooves (Figure 12.9(a,b)).

The wear life of the polymeric AL with specified dimensions can be effectively determined in terms of FH penetration into the AL. Although FH penetration is correlated with both wear and creep, wear has a crucial influence on artificial implant lifespan (Figure 12.8(b)). The wear depth (or penetration) of AL can be examined using the Dowson and Jabson equation:

$$p = \frac{0.001186}{\pi}\left(\frac{kBN}{R_1}\right)\left[1+\sqrt{1+\frac{1686\pi R_1\left(R_2 - R_1\right)}{kBN}}\right] \tag{12.6}$$

TABLE 12.4
Influence of Wear Rate and Acetabular Liner Radius on Femoral Head Penetration Depth for UHMWPE and HU Acetabular Liners

Acetabular liner (composition)	Wear rate (mm^3/Nm)	Acetabular liner radius (mm)	Wear depth (mm)
UHMWPE (GUR 1050)	1.93×10^{-6}	14.14	0.111
HU (60 wt.% HDPE/40 wt. %UHMWPE)	1.39×10^{-6}	13.62	0.128

where p is the wear depth; k is the wear rate (mm^3/Nm); B is the body weight in Newton (N); N is the number of cycles; R_1 is the outer radius of the femoral head (14 mm), and R_2 is the inner radius of the acetabular liner (mm). The wear rates for both HU and UHMWPE ALs are adapted from the literature (Sharma et al., 2020; Suner et al., 2015). Table 12.4 summarizes the wear depths for the different ALs; the table shows that FH penetrated the HU liner up to 0.128 mm depth, which is similar to the wear depth of UHMWPE AL (0.11).

In these findings, HU AL exhibited equivalent and even superior tribological performance to that of medical-grade UHMWPE. When coupled with the findings of the microscopic examination, these findings represent improved tribological performance. Interestingly, the wear rate recorded for injection-molded UHMWPE-blend AL (HU) matches the *in vivo* wear rate requirements in the literature. For instance, Livermore et al. (1990) reported a mean wear rate of 48.4 mg/MC when UHMWPE was articulated against CoCrMo FH in an *in vivo* radiographic study. In another radiographic study, mean wear rates were found to be between 48.2 mg/MC and 61.6 mg/MC against Ti FH (Cates et al., 1993).

Later, McKellop et al. (1995) reported wear rates of 55 mg/MC, 39 mg/MC, and 50 mg/MC against stainless steel (316L), Ti, and explanted Ti femoral heads. Structurally, UHMWPE showed a higher wear rate and severity attributed to intermolecular failure, in accordance with the orientation softening theory (Wang et al., 1997, 1998a). According to this theory, the UHMWPE polymeric chains preferentially align in the frictional force direction, and as a result, the material is strain hardened in one direction but weakened in the transverse, depending on the biaxial wear routes (abduction/adduction and flexion/extension).

However, in the case of HU, the easy alignment of chains might be impaired owing to the possible structural reorganization that has happened due to blending with HDPE (Figure 12.9). Lim et al. (2005) attributed the significant changes in the various properties of the HDPE/UHMWPE blend to a number of possible causes, for instance the effective fusion/incorporation of UHMWPE in HDPE matrix to form a single-melt-phase HU blend, as demonstrated in the stabilized force profile shown in Figure 12.1(a,b) (Kurtz et al., 1999).

BOX 12.9

Wear rate depends on several factors both *in vitro* (hip simulators, lubricants, and laboratory conditions) and *in vivo* (patient activity, weight, bone quality, and the position of acetabular implantation). The present findings should not be directly compared with those from other studies that used a complete pelvic endoprosthesis simulator as well as cycle time, in accordance with ISO 14172 guidelines.

Another important guiding factor to be considered in predicting the lifespans of ALs is the size, shape, and volume of the wear debris generated during articulation. In general, wear debris generation is dependent on various considerations, such as the types of joints, bearing geometry, material combination/counterbody, and lubricant. However, the characterization of implant wear debris is essential for estimating wear rate and comprehending implant wear mechanisms.

We observed that HU exhibited less wear debris than did UHMWPE (see Figure 12.8 (c)). The box plot shown in Figure 12.8(c) shows the particle size distribution for both HU and UHMWPE. Figure 12.10 shows the qualitative and quantitative SEM-EDS assessment of the wear particles (morphology, shape, and size) retrieved from the hip simulator specimen chamber. EDS compositional analysis reveals that the wear particles shown in Figure 12.10(a,b) are a combination of both ceramic (ZTA) and polymer (UHMWPE and HU). The wear particles obtained from UHMWPE and HU ALs exhibit both regular and irregular shapes, with considerable variations in size, as shown in Figure 12.10(a,b). For both the tribocouples, most of the wear particles appeared to be predominantly submicron in size (Figure 12.8(c)), although we observed some larger fragments (>50 μm in size) for both tribocouples (ZTA-UHMWPE and ZTA-HU). These larger fragments resembled flakes, slice/blocky shards, slices, polygonal pieces, and radially broken wear particles (Figure 12.10).

In the case of UHMWPE AL, the size range of the debris varied up to 400 μm (Figure 12.8(c)), while the maximum wear size was less than 220 μm. Furthermore, after close assessment (at 500 μm), the wear debris morphology for the polymeric counterface appeared to be irregular or spherical, while the ceramic wear particles were coarser. The present observations can be validated based on the varying hardness of the hardness differences between UHMWPE and HU, in accordance with the following equation (Sharma et al., 2020):

$$d \geq 6 \times 10^4 \left(\frac{W}{H} \right) \tag{12.7}$$

where d is the minimum equivalent diameter of wear debris, W is the work of adhesion of the contacting materials, and H is the substrate's hardness. It is interesting to note that the minimal wear particle diameter (d) produced by adhesive-abrasive type wear (Figure 12.8(c)) is inversely proportional to the hardness of UHMWPE and HU. These findings pertaining to the equivalent diameter of various wear debris align with the hardness of the various substrates (e.g., $H_{UHMWPE} < H_{HU}$; Sharma et al., 2020). Overall, the results we have summarized here establish good tribological properties for both HU and HUmGO w.r.t. UHMWPE.

CONCLUSION

This chapter unravels the translational potential of UHMWPE derivatives, specifically a UHMWPE blend (HU) and a composite (HUmGO), for THR applications. As a concluding note, the results discussed in this chapter explicitly highlight several important aspects.

Firstly, it is necessary to comprehensively understand thermophysical properties specific to polymer injection molding. Our detailed assessment indicated comparable behavior for HU and HUmGO. The addition of HDPE to UHMWPE, however, facilitated melt mixing and injection moldability for both HU and HUmGO. The presence of UHMWPE and the effect of its higher melt viscosity were reflected in terms of a lower melt-flow index (0.14). Additionally, the volumetric shrinkage was 2.15% for HU and 1.17% for HUmGO. These properties play a significant role in establishing the manufacturability of the UHMWPE-based acetabular liner.

Secondly, FEA evaluation of periprosthetic biomechanical response revealed similar responses in terms of von Mises stress, distribution, and magnitude of periprosthetic bone strain (max and min principal strains) around HU and HUmGO implant in the acetabulum w.r.t. medical grade UHMWPE AL (GUR 1050).

Importantly, injection molding enabled clinically acceptable dimensional parameters, especially sphericity (7 μm) and roughness (0.38 μm) in the case of HU AL prototypes, when compared with medical grade UHMWPE.

The injection-molded HUmGO acetabular liners demonstrated better wear and fatigue performance, when articulated against ceramic femoral head, under simulated physiological walking conditions (in accordance with ASTM F1714 guidelines). Specifically, HU-based acetabular liner exhibited a better wear rate of 42.1 mg/0.5 million cycles, which is ~17% less than medical grade UHMWPE liners (50.7 mg/0.5 million cycles).

Taken together, the research results presented in this chapter establish an end-to-end understanding of material properties, biomechanical responses, manufacturing processes, geometrical features, dimensional tolerances, and wear performance of UHMWPE blend with HDPE and many of these properties were benchmarked against medically used UHMWPE. More details of the results summarized in this chapter can be found elsewhere (Sharma et al., 2020; Bhusari et al., 2019; Sharma et al., 2022b, 2015).

ACKNOWLEDGEMENTS

The authors duly acknowledge the Department of Biotechnology (DBT), and the Science and Engineering Research Board (SERB). We would also like to acknowledge the Centre of Excellence's Programme support on translational research on biomaterials for orthopedic and dental applications (No. BT/PR13466/COE/34/26/2015) and IMPRINT (IMP/2018/000622). We are also thankful to Central Manufacturing Technology Institute (CMTI), Bangalore, India, for their help finishing the molded prototypes and CMM measurements and Mr. Nihal Kottam (Project Assistant, IISc, Bangalore) and Dr. Sanotsh Kumar (Research Associate, IISc, Bangalore) for assisting us with this process. We are also grateful to Mr. Sachin Hiremani, Mr. Abhilash T, Mr. Biswajit, Mr. Niranjan, Ms. Preethi, and Mr. Sachin, INDO-MIM Pvt. Ltd, Bangalore, India, for their consistent guidance on technical aspects related to injection molding and implant design.

LIST OF ABBREVIATIONS

AL	Acetabular liner
CAD	Computer-aided design
CT	Computed tomography
FEA	Finite element analysis
GO	Graphene oxide
HDPE	High-density polyethylene
OA	Osteoarthritis
SA	Shoulder Arthroplasty
SEM	Scanning electron microscope
TAR	Total ankle replacement
TDR	Total disc replacement
TEA	Total elbow arthroplasty
THR	Total hip joint replacement
TKA	Total knee Arthroplasty
UHMWPE	Ultra-high molecular weight polyethylene
XL-UHMWPE	Crosslinked UHMWPE

REFERENCES

Anderson, D. E., & Madigan, M. L. (2013). Effects of age-related differences in femoral loading and bone mineral density on strains in the proximal femur during controlled walking. *J. Appl. Biomech.* 29: 505–516.

Barnetson, A., & Hornsby, P. R. (1995). Observations on the sintering of Ultra-High Molecular Weight Polyethylene (UHMWPE) powders. *J. Mater. Sci. Lett.* 14: 80–84.

Basu, B., & Ghosh, S. (2017). *Biomaterials for Musculoskeletal Regeneration.* Singapore: Springer.

Bellare, A., & Cohen, R. E. (1996). Morphology of rod stock and compression-moulded sheets of ultra-high-molecular-weight polyethylene used in orthopaedic implants. *Biomaterials*. 17: 2325–2333.

Bhusari, S. A., Sharma, V., Bose, S., & Basu, B. (2019). HDPE/UHMWPE hybrid nanocomposites with surface functionalized graphene oxide towards improved strength and cytocompatibility. *J. R. Soc. Interface*. 16: 20180273.

Bitar, D., & Parvizi, J. (2015). Biological response to prosthetic debris. *World J. Orthop*. 6: 172.

Brach del Prever, E. M., Bistolfi, A., Bracco, P., & Costa, L. (2009). UHMWPE for arthroplasty: Past or future? *J. Orthop. Trauma*. 10: 1–8.

Callaghan, J. J., Albright, J. C., Goetz, D. D., Olejniczak, J. P., & Johnston, R. C. (2000). Charnley total hip arthroplasty with cement: Minimum twenty-five-year follow-up. *J. Bone Joint Surg. Am*. 82: 487.

Cates, H. E., Faris, P. M., Keating, E. M., & Ritter, M. A. (1993). Polyethylene wear in cemented metal-backed acetabular cups. *J. Bone Joint Surg. Br*. 75: 249–253.

Chang, R. Y., & Tsaur, B. D. (1995). Experimental and theoretical studies of shrinkage, warpage, and sink marks of crystalline polymer injection molded parts. *Polym. Eng. Sci*. 35: 1222–1230.

Chang, T. C., & Faison III, E. (2001). Shrinkage behavior and optimization of injection molded parts studied by the Taguchi method. *Polym. Eng. Sci*. 41: 703–710.

Chatterjee, S., Kobylinski, S., & Basu, B. (2018). Finite element analysis to probe the influence of acetabular shell design, liner material, and subject parameters on biomechanical response in periprosthetic bone. *J. Biomech. Eng*. 140: 101014.

Chen, H. T., Yao, C. H., Chao, P. D. L., Hou, Y. C., Chiang, H. M., Hsieh, C. C., Ke, C. J., & Chen, Y. S. (2008). Effect of serum metabolites of Pueraria lobata in rats on peripheral nerve regeneration: *In vitro* and *in vivo* studies. *J. Biomed. Mater. Res. Part B*. 84: 256–262.

Clarke, S. G., Phillips, A. T. M., & Bull, A. M. J. (2013). Evaluating a suitable level of model complexity for finite element analysis of the intact acetabulum. *Comput. Methods Biomech. Biomed. Eng*. 16: 717–724.

Cubillos, P. O., Dos Santos, V. O., Pizzolatti, A. L. A., da Rosa, E., & Roesler, C. R. (2018). Evaluation of surface finish and dimensional control of tribological metal-ultra high molecular weight polyethylene pair of commercially available hip implants. *J. Arthroplasty*. 33: 939–944.

Dalstra, M., & Huiskes, R. (1995). Load transfer across the pelvic bone. *J. Biomech*. 28: 715–724.

Dostal, W. F., & Andrews, J. G. (1981). A three-dimensional biomechanical model of hip musculature. *J. Biomech*. 14: 803–812.

Dumbleton, J. H., Wang, A., Sutton, K., & Manley, M. T. (2009). Highly crosslinked and annealed UHMWPE. In *UHMWPE Biomaterials Handbook*. S. M. Kurtz, Ed. MA: Elsevier, pp. 205–219.

Feng, J., Wang, L., Zhang, R. Y., Wu, J. J., Wang, C. Y., Yang, M. B., & Fu, X. R. (2014). Formation of double skin-core orientated structure in injection-molded Polyethylene parts: Effects of ultra-high molecular weight Polyethylene and temperature field. *J. Polym. Res*. 21: 1–14.

Fisher, J. (1994). Wear of ultra high molecular weight polyethylene in total artificial joints. *Curr. Orthop*. 8: 164–169.

Gallo, J., Goodman, S. B., Konttinen, Y. T., & Raska, M. (2013). Particle disease: Biologic mechanisms of periprosthetic osteolysis in total hip arthroplasty. *Innate Immun*. 19: 213–224.

Ghosh, R., & Gupta, S. (2014). Bone remodelling around cementless composite acetabular components: The effects of implant geometry and implant—Bone interfacial conditions. *J. Mech. Behav. Biomed. Mater*. 32: 257–269.

Ghosh, R., Pal, B., Ghosh, D., & Gupta, S. (2015). Finite element analysis of a hemi-pelvis: The effect of inclusion of cartilage layer on acetabular stresses and strain. *Comput. Methods Biomech. Biomed. Eng*. 18: 697–710.

Gispert, M. P., Serro, A. P., Colaco, R., & Saramago, B. (2006). Friction and wear mechanisms in hip prosthesis: Comparison of joint materials behaviour in several lubricants. *Wear*. 260: 149–158.

Glyn-Jones, S., Palmer, A., Agricola, R., Price, A., Vincent, T., Weinans, H., & Carr, A. (2015). Osteoarthritis. *Lancet*. 386: 376–387.

Grupp, T. M., Holderied, M., Mulliez, M. A., Streller, R., Jäger, M., Blömer, W., & Utzschneider, S. (2014). Biotribology of a vitamin E-stabilized polyethylene for hip arthroplasty—Influence of artificial ageing and third-body particles on wear. *Acta Biomater*. 10: 3068–3078.

Gul, R. M., & McGarry, F. J. (2004). Processing of ultra-high molecular weight polyethylene by hot isostatic pressing, and the effect of processing parameters on its microstructure. *Polym. Eng. Sci*. 44: 1848–1857.

Hall, R. M., Siney, P., Unsworth, A., & Wroblewski, B. M. (1997). The effect of surface topography of retrieved femoral heads on the wear of UHMWPE sockets. *Med. Eng. Phys.* 19: 711–719.

Han, K. S., Wallace, J. F., Truss, R. W., & Geil, P. H. (1981). Powder compaction, sintering, and rolling of ultra high molecular weight polyethylene and its composites. *J. Macromol. Sci. Part B: Phys.* 19: 313–349.

Harris, W. H. (1994). Osteolysis and particle disease in hip replacement: A review. *Acta Orthop. Scand.* 65: 113–123.

Hu, M., Yu, D., & Wei, J. (2007). Thermal conductivity determination of small polymer samples by differential scanning calorimetry. *Polym. Test.* 26: 333–337.

Hua, X., Wang, L., Al-Hajjar, M., Jin, Z., Wilcox, R. K., & Fisher, J. (2014). Experimental validation of finite element modelling of a modular metal-on-polyethylene total hip replacement. *Proc. Inst. Mech. Eng. Part H.* 228: 682–692.

Huang, C., Qian, X., & Yang, R. (2018). Thermal conductivity of polymers and polymer nanocomposites. *Mater. Sci. Eng. R Rep.* 132: 1–22.

Hussain, M., Naqvi, R. A., Abbas, N., Khan, S. M., Nawaz, S., Hussain, A., Zahra, N., & Khalid, M. W. (2020). Ultra-High-Molecular-Weight-Polyethylene (UHMWPE) as a promising polymer material for biomedical applications: A concise review. *Polymers.* 12: 323.

Ito, H., Minami, A., Matsuno, T., Tanino, H., Yuhta, T., & Nishimura, I. (2001). The sphericity of the bearing surface in total hip arthroplasty. *J. Arthroplasty.* 16: 1024–1029.

Izmin, N. A. N., Hazwani, F., Todo, M., & Abdullah, A. H. (2021). Computational analysis on bone adaptation in resurfacing hip arthroplasty with valgus-varus placement. In *Recent Trends in Manufacturing and Materials Towards Industry 4.0.* M. N. O. Zahid, A. S. A. Sani, M. R. M. Yasin, Z. Ismail, N. A. C. Lah, and F. M. Turan, Eds. Singapore: Springer, pp. 179–189.

Jasty, M., Goetz, D. D., Bragdon, C. R., Lee, K. R., Hanson, A. E., Elder, J. R., & Harris, W. H. (1997). Wear of polyethylene acetabular components in total hip arthroplasty: An analysis of one hundred and twenty-eight components retrieved at autopsy or revision operations. *J. Bone Joint Surg.* 79: 349–358.

Jedenmalm, A., Affatato, S., Taddei, P., Leardini, W., Gedde, U. W., Fagnano, C., & Viceconti, M. (2009). Effect of head surface roughness and sterilization on wear of UHMWPE acetabular cups. *J. Biomed. Mater. Res. Part A.* 90: 1032–1042.

Jonkers, I., Sauwen, N., Lenaerts, G., Mulier, M., Van der Perre, G., & Jaecques, S. (2008). Relation between subject-specific hip joint loading, stress distribution in the proximal femur and bone mineral density changes after total hip replacement. *J. Biomech.* 41: 3405–3413.

Kashyap, S., & Datta, D. (2015). Process parameter optimization of plastic injection molding: A review. *Int. J. Plast. Technol.* 19: 1–18.

Knight, S. R., Aujla, R., & Biswas, S. P. (2011). Total hip arthroplasty-over 100 years of operative history. *Orthop. Rev.* 3: e16.

Kurtz, S. M., Edidin, A. A., & Bartel, D. L. (1997). The role of backside polishing, cup angle, and polyethylene thickness on the contact stresses in metal-backed acetabular components. *J. Biomech.* 30: 639–642.

Kurtz, S. M., Muratoglu, O. K., Evans, M., & Edidin, A. A. (1999). Advances in the processing, sterilization, and crosslinking of ultra-high molecular weight polyethylene for total joint arthroplasty. *Biomaterials.* 20: 1659–1688.

Larsen, B. M., Borgwardt, A., Ribel-Madsen, S., & Zerahn, B. (2021). False profile view is independently associated with serum metal levels in patients with metal-on-metal hip arthroplasty. *Eur. J. Orthop. Surg. Traumatol.* 31: 1029–1036.

Lee, P. C., Shih, C. H., Chen, W. J., Tu, Y. K., & Tai, C. L. (1999). Early polyethylene wear and osteolysis in cementless total hip arthroplasty: The influence of femoral head size and polyethylene thickness. *J. Arthroplasty.* 14: 976–981.

Lestari, W. D., Nugroho, A., Ismail, R., Jamari, J., & Bayuseno, A. P. (2021). Study of wear performance of crosslinking UHMWPE acetabular liner for artificial hip joint made from CNC milling. *IOP Conf. Ser. Mater. Sci. Eng.* 1078: 012009.

Li, S., & Burstein, A. H. (1994). Ultra-high molecular weight polyethylene: The material and its use in total joint implants. *J. Bone Joint Surg.* 76: 1080–1090.

Lim, K. L. K., Ishak, Z. M., Ishiaku, U. S., Fuad, A. M. Y., Yusof, A. H., Czigany, T., Pukanszky, B., & Ogunniyi, D. S. (2005). High-density polyethylene/ultrahigh-molecular-weight polyethylene blend. I: The processing, thermal, and mechanical properties. *J. Appl. Polym. Sci.* 97: 413–425.

Liphardt, A. M., Windahl, S. H., Sehic, E., Hannemann, N., Gustafsson, K. L., Bozec, A., Schett, G., & Engdahl, C. (2020). Changes in mechanical loading affect arthritis-induced bone loss in mice. *Bone*. 131: 115149.

Livermore, J., Ilstrup, D., & Morrey, B. (1990). Effect of femoral head size on wear of the polyethylene acetabular component. *J. Bone Joint Surg*. 72: 518–528.

Mak, M. M., Besong, A. A., Jin, Z. M., & Fisher, J. (2002). Effect of microseparation on contact mechanics in ceramic-on-ceramic hip joint replacements. *Proc. Inst. Mech. Eng. H*. 216: 403–408.

McKellop, H., Ebramzadeh, E., Lu, B., & Sarmiento, A. (1995). Effect of ball material, diameter and surface roughness on the wear of polyethylene acetabular cups. *21st Annual Meeting of the Society for Biomaterials*. San Francisco, CA, 18–22 March 1995, Vol. XVIII, p. 46.Milošev, I., Levašič, V., Kovač, S., Sillat, T., Virtanen, S., Tiainen, V. M., & Trebše, R. (2021). Metals for joint replacement. In *Joint Replacement Technology*. P. Revell, Ed. United States: Woodhead Publishing, pp. 65–122.National Science and Technology Council (US). (2011). Materials genome initiative for global competitiveness. *Executive Office of the President, National Science and Technology Council*. www.mgi.gov/sites/default/files/documents/materials_genome_initiative-final.pdf

Nine, M. J., Choudhury, D., Hee, A. C., Mootanah, R., & Osman, N. A. A. (2014). Wear debris characterization and corresponding biological response: Artificial hip and knee joints. *Materials*. 7: 980–1016.

Oral, E., Christensen, S. D., Malhi, A. S., Wannomae, K. K., & Muratoglu, O. K. (2006). Wear resistance and mechanical properties of highly cross-linked, ultrahigh—Molecular weight polyethylene doped with vitamin E. *J. Arthroplasty*. 21: 580–591.

Patil, N. A., Njuguna, J., & Kandasubramanian, B. (2020). UHMWPE for biomedical applications: Performance and functionalization. *Eur. Polym. J*. 125: 109529.

Pietrzak, W. S. (2021). Ultra-high molecular weight polyethylene for total hip acetabular liners: A brief review of current status. *J. Invest. Surg*. 34: 321–323.

Pramanik, S., Agarwal, A. K., & Rai, K. N. (2005). Chronology of total hip joint replacement and materials development. *Trends Biomater. Artif. Organs*. 19: 15–26.

Ramani, K., & Parasnis, N. C. (1998). Process-induced effects in compression molding of Ultra-High Molecular Weight Polyethylene (UHMWPE). *ASTM Spec. Tech. Publ*. 1307: 5–23.

Rumpf, H. (1990). The characteristics of systems and their changes of state disperse. In *Particle Technology*. Berlin: Springer, pp. 8–55.

Saikko, V. O. (1995). Wear of the polyethylene acetabular cup: The effect of head material, head diameter, and cup thickness studied with a hip simulator. *Acta Orthop. Scand*. 66: 501–506.

Saikko, V. O. (2016). Effect of increased load on the wear of a large diameter metal-on-metal modular hip prosthesis with a high inclination angle of the acetabular cup. *Tribol. Int*. 96: 149–154.

Sánchez, R., Aisa, J., Martinez, A., & Mercado, D. (2012). On the relationship between cooling setup and warpage in injection molding. *Meas*. 45: 1051–1056.

Sarkar, D., Sambi Reddy, B., Mandal, S., RaviSankar, M., & Basu, B. (2016). Uniaxial compaction-based manufacturing strategy and 3D microstructural evaluation of near-net-shaped ZrO2-toughened Al2O3 acetabular socket. *Adv. Eng. Mater*. 18: 1634–1644.

Scholes, S. C., Unsworth, A., Hall, R. M., & Scott, R. (2000). The effects of material combination and lubricant on the friction of total hip prostheses. *Wear*. 241: 209–213.

Schwartsmann, C. R., Spinelli, L. D. F., Boschin, L. C., Gonçalves, R. Z., Yépez, A. K., Strohaecker, T. R., & Souza, R. W. D. (2013). Dimensional analysis of total hip arthroplasty polyethylenes. *Rev. Bras. Ortop*. 48: 500–504.

Sharma, M., Madras, G., & Bose, S. (2015). Contrasting effects of graphene oxide and poly (ethylenimine) on the polymorphism in poly (vinylidene fluoride). *Cryst. Growth Des*. 15: 3345–3355.

Sharma, V., Bose, S., Kundu, B., Bodhak, S., Mitun, D., Balla, V. K., & Basu, B. (2020). Probing the influence of γ-sterilization on the oxidation, crystallization, sliding wear resistance, and cytocompatibility of chemically modified graphene-oxide-reinforced HDPE/UHMWPE nanocomposites and wear debris. *ACS Biomater. Sci. Eng*. 6: 1462–1475.

Sharma, V., Chowdhury, S., Keshavan, N., & Basu, B. (2022a). Six decades of UHMWPE in reconstructive surgery. *Int. Mater. Rev*. 68: 46–81.

Sharma, V., Gupta, R. K., Kailas, S. V., & Basu, B. (2022b). Probing lubricated sliding wear properties of HDPE/UHMWPE hybrid bionanocomposite. *J. Biomater. Appl*. 37: 204–218.

Singh, J. A. (2011). Epidemiology of knee and hip arthroplasty: A systematic review. *Open J. Orthop*. 5: 80–85.

Spiegelberg, S., Kozak, A., & Braithwaite, G. (2016). Characterization of physical, chemical, and mechanical properties of UHMWPE. In *UHMWPE Biomaterials Handbook*. S. M. Kurtz, Ed. Norwich: Elsevier, pp. 531–552.

Stops, A., Wilcox, R., & Jin, Z. (2012). Computational modelling of the natural hip: A review of finite element and multibody simulations. *Comput. Methods Biomech. Biomed. Eng.* 15: 963–979.

Suner, S., Joffe, R., Tipper, J. L., & Emami, N. (2015). Ultra high molecular weight polyethylene/graphene oxide nanocomposites: Thermal, mechanical and wettability characterisation. *Compos. B.* 78: 185–191.

Taddei, F., Pancanti, A., & Viceconti, M. (2004). An improved method for the automatic mapping of computed tomography numbers onto finite element models. *Med. Eng. Phys.* 26: 61–69.

Tanem, B. S., & Stori, A. (2000). Thermal analysis of single-site polymers in binary blends of low-molecular-weight linear polyethylene and high-molecular-weight branched polyethylene. *Thermochim. Acta.* 345: 73–80.

Tanem, B. S., & Stori, A. (2001). Blends of single-site linear and branched polyethylene. II: Morphology characterisation. *Polymer.* 42: 6609–6618.

Tanner, M. G., Whiteside, L. A., & White, S. E. (1995). Effect of polyethylene quality on wear in total knee arthroplasty. *Clin. Orthop. Relat. Res.* 317: 83–88.

Thompson, M. S., Northmore-Ball, M. D., & Tanner, K. E. (2002). Effects of acetabular resurfacing component material and fixation on the strain distribution in the pelvis. *Proc. Inst. Mech. Eng. Part H.* 216: 237–245.

Truss, R. W., Han, K. S., Wallace, J. F., & Geil, P. H. (1980). Cold compaction molding and sintering of ultra high molecular weight polyethylene. *Polym. Eng. Sci.* 20: 747–755.

Vallés, G., & Vilaboa, N. (2019). Osteolysis after total hip arthroplasty: Basic science. In *Acetabular Revision Surgery in Major Bone Defects*. E. García-Rey, and E. García-Cimbrelo, Eds. Cham: Springer, pp. 1–31.

Wang, A., Edwards, B., Yau, S. S., Polineni, V. K., Essner, A., Klein, R., Sun, D. C., Stark, C., & Dumbleton, J. H. (1998a). Orientation softening as a mechanism of Ultra-High Molecular Weight Polyethylene (UHMWPE) wear in artificial hip and knee joints. *ASTM Spec. Tech. Publ.* 1307: 56–76.

Wang, A., Polineni, V. K., Stark, C., & Dumbleton, J. H. (1998b). Effect of femoral head surface roughness on the wear of ultrahigh molecular weight polyethylene acetabular cups. *J. Arthroplasty.* 13: 615–620.

Wang, A., Sun, D. C., Yau, S. S., Edwards, B., Sokol, M., Essner, A., Polineni, V. K., Stark, C., & Dumbleton, J. H. (1997). Orientation softening in the deformation and wear of ultra-high molecular weight polyethylene. *Wear.* 203: 230–241.

Yamako, G., Chosa, E., Zhao, X., Totoribe, K., Watanabe, S., Sakamoto, T., & Nakane, N. (2014). Load-transfer analysis after insertion of cementless anatomical femoral stem using pre-and post-operative CT images based patient-specific finite element analysis. *Med. Eng. Phys.* 36: 694–700.

Yamamoto, K., Tateiwa, T., & Takahashi, Y. (2017). Vitamin E-stabilized highly crosslinked polyethylenes: The role and effectiveness in total hip arthroplasty. *J. Orthop. Sci.* 22: 384–390.

Zachariades, A. E., & Kanamoto, T. (1986). The effect of initial morphology on the mechanical properties of ultra-high molecular weight polyethylene. *Polym. Eng. Sci.* 26: 658–661.

13 The Physiology of Bone Homeostasis to Aid Experimental Therapeutics in Disease Conditions

Konica Porwal and Naibedya Chattopadhyay

13.1 INTRODUCTION

Deposition of bone matrix and minerals is achieved by bone modeling and remodeling. Modeling-based bone formation does not require prior bone resorption, which occurs during growth and fracture healing. Bone remodeling consists of five sequential phases: resting, resorption, reversal, formation, and mineralization. During the resorption phase, osteoclasts break down damaged bones. In the reversal phase, mononuclear cells and preosteoblasts appear in the resorbed area. In the formation and mineralization phases, osteoblasts first form osteoids (unmineralized bones) at the resorbed area, and then the osteoids undergo primary mineralization (to form osteons).

Following the mineralization process, osteoblasts transform, becoming flattened and aligning themselves with the surface, where they are called lining cells. The majority of these lining cells then transform into osteocytes, which are embedded within the bone (Sharma et al., 2022). After the completion of mineralization, bones enter the resting phase once again (Figure 13.1).

The bone-forming cells, osteoblasts, originate from mesenchymal stem cells (MSCs) and express Runt-related transcription factor 2 (Runx2). Osteoblast differentiation from MSCs occurs in response to many physiologic stimuli, of which the most potent are bone morphogenic proteins (BMPs), parathyroid hormone (PTH), and prostaglandins. Differentiated osteoblasts typically express matrix proteins consisting of collagen type I (Col 1) and a minor amount of noncollagenous proteins, including osteocalcin (OCN), osteopontin (OPN), matrix Gla protein, and bone sialoprotein (BSP). Moreover, these cells abundantly express alkaline phosphatase (ALP), an enzyme that is critically required for the mineralization of the matrix (Donsante et al., 2021).

Bone formation during remodeling, on the other hand, occurs in response to prior resorption of bone on a given bone surface. Remodeling is a maintenance process that takes place in response to microdamage and occurs predominantly in adult weight-bearing bones, including the lumbar spine, femur, tibia, and distal radius. Osteoclasts, differentiated from hematopoietic stem cells in response to receptor activator of nuclear factor kappa-B ligand (RANKL), the most potent osteoclastogenic cytokine produced by differentiated osteoblasts and osteocytes, initiate the remodeling process.

In addition to RANKL, osteoblasts produce a macrophage colony-stimulating factor (M-CSF) that supports the colony formation of monocytes that coalesce to form multinucleated osteoclasts by the action of RANKL. Bone-marrow-resident macrophages and endothelial cells of blood vessels that supply bones are also M-CSF sources (Asagiri & Takayanagi, 2007). Differentiated osteoclasts express genes required for bone resorption, including matrix metalloproteinases (MMPs), cathepsin K, chloride channel-7 (ClC7), vacuolar-type ATPase (V-ATPase), and tartrate-resistant acid phosphatase (TRAP) in addition to receptor activator of nuclear factor κB (RANK) and tumor necrosis

DOI: 10.1201/9781003307310-16

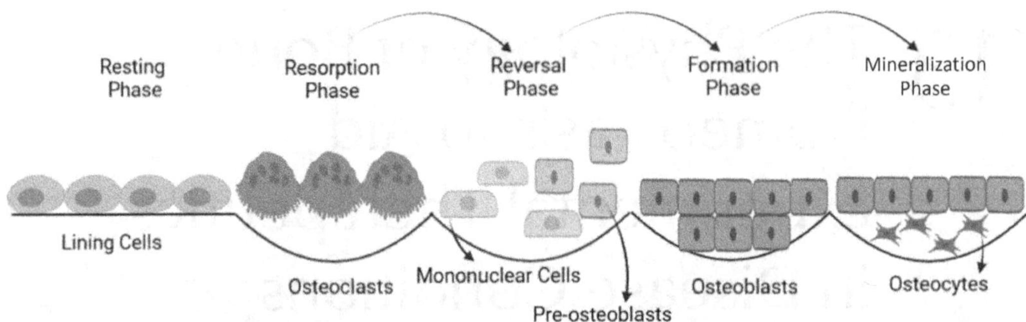

FIGURE 13.1 Physiology of bone remodeling. The bone remodeling process begins with the resorption phase, during which osteoclasts gather at the bone surface and begin the digestion of damaged bone tissue. The reversal phase succeeds this phase, where mononuclear and preosteoblast cells are recruited. In the formation phase, differentiated osteoblasts fill the resorbed area with collagen and minerals to deposit new bone. After the completion of mineralized bones, osteoblasts become flattened and transform into lining cells, which become embedded in the bone as osteocytes and remain in a resting phase until a new remodeling cycle begins. The image is generated by Biorender.

factor receptor-associated factor 6. Cathepsin K and MMPs are matrix-degrading proteases that have collagenolytic effects. The mineral component of bone is dissolved at the resorption lacuna by acidic pH caused by the actions of V-ATPase and ClC7 (Boyce et al., 2009; Florencio-Silva et al., 2015).

Remodeling is a tightly coupled process in which the amount of bone resorbed is replaced by the newly formed bone first as osteoid or unmineralized bones that are then mineralized. The osteoblasts involved in the process have three fates: a) most undergo apoptosis, b) some become terminally differentiated and reside in the mineralized matrix and are termed osteocytes, and c) the rest reside as surface epithelial cells that could be differentiated to osteoblasts by anabolic agents (Allen & Burr, 2014). Microdamage is caused by fatigue that results in the loss of osteocyte integrity by initiating osteocyte apoptosis. The dying osteocytes then set remodeling in motion by the increased production of RANKL. Aging is accompanied by microdamage accumulation, and the decline in gonadal hormones results in increased remodeling. Increased remodeling leads to a net loss of bone mass as the resorption phase of the remodeling cycle is much shorter than the formation phase (Langdahl et al., 2016).

Aging is also accompanied by the increased adipogenic differentiation of MSCs over osteogenic differentiation. As adipocytes express high levels of monocyte chemoattractant protein-1 that promote monocyte and macrophage accumulation, osteoclastogenesis is favored, leading to enhanced bone resorption (Ferland-McCollough et al., 2018). Moreover, increased marrow adipose tissue (MAT) induces local reactive oxygen species (ROS) production that further favors osteoclastogenesis and concomitantly inhibits the function of osteoblasts (Atashi et al., 2015). Higher MAT also reduces blood flow by constricting the nutrient arteries and their branches, causing osteonecrosis (Porwal et al., 2019).

13.2 CELLULAR AND MOLECULAR EVENTS DURING SKELETAL HOMEOSTASIS

Among the hormones and cytokines that promote bone formation, BMP-2, -4, -6, -7, and -9 are the most potent. BMPs belong to the transforming growth factor-β (TGF-β) superfamily and for transmembrane signaling require two BMP receptors: BMP-RI and BMP-RII (Lademann et al., 2020).

Binding of BMPs forms a dimeric complex of the serine–threonine kinase receptors to start the signaling cascade. The activated receptor kinase then phosphorylates the transcription factor SMAD, which acting in conjunction with other coactivators stimulates the transcription of genes including Runx2, ALP, Col1, BSP, OCN, and OPN (Gomez-Puerto et al., 2019).

Of the five BMPs, recombinant forms of BMP-2 and BMP-7 are available and are used for open tibial fracture and critical-sized long bone defects (Zhu et al., 2022). The skeletal effects of hormones including PTH, estradiol, and growth hormone (GH) are mediated by BMPs (Yamamoto et al., 2002; Nakao et al., 2009). For example, we have shown that both BMP-2 and BMP-4 are required for maintaining bone mass in the adult skeleton and further that these BMPs mediated the osteogenic effect of PTH in ovariectomized (OVX) mice (Khan et al., 2016).

GH has also been shown to induce BMP-2 and BMP-4 in dental pulp cells and the effect was independent of insulin-like growth factor 1 (IGF-1), which predominantly mediated the osteogenic effect of this hormone (Kim et al., 2012). Estrogens including phytoestrogens activate BMP-2 in MSC through estrogen receptors alpha (ERα) and beta (ERβ) and promote osteogenic differentiation of MSCs (Zhou et al., 2003; Dai et al., 2013). That is, in addition to directly promoting osteogenic differentiation, BMPs mediate the effects of major osteogenic hormones.

BMP signaling stimulates osteoblast differentiation and survival in addition to stimulating osteoclastogenesis mediated by RANKL as BMP inhibitors, twisted gastrulation protein homolog 1, and noggin abolished the osteoclastogenic effect of BMPs (Sotillo Rodriguez et al., 2009; Huntley et al., 2015). Conditional deletions of BMPRIa and BMPRIIa in osteoclasts in mice resulted in increased bone mass (Bordukalo-Nikšić et al., 2022; Okamoto et al., 2011).

Among the BMPs, BMP-2 has the most potent effect in inhibiting osteoclastogenesis followed by BMP-4 and BMP-6 (Huntley et al., 2019). The lack of BMPRIa in osteoclasts increased the expression of the abundant gap junction protein connexin 43 that is known to promote osteoclastogenesis and bone resorption. BMPRIa-null osteoclasts when cocultured with osteoblasts led to increased osteoblast differentiation, which suggested that BMP signaling is required for osteoclast-osteoblast communication (Shi et al., 2017).

Increased osteoblast function in mice with osteoclastic deletion of BMPRIa resulted in increased bone mass. Conversely, deletion of BMPRIa in osteoblasts increased osteoclastogenesis, albeit indirectly, likely through the downregulation of sclerostin, a Wnt (wingless-related integration site) antagonist that upregulates RANKL (Kamiya et al., 2008; Okamoto et al., 2011). These reports indicate that BMPRIa participates in osteoclast function via osteoblastic regulation. BMPs have direct effects on osteoclastogenesis, which is mediated by the canonical receptor-regulated SMAD (smad1/5/8), and co-SMAD (SMAD4) as well. BMPs also signal through noncanonical (SMAD-independent) pathways such as mitogen-activated protein kinase–extracellular signal-regulated kinase, c-Jun N-terminal kinase, and p38 pathways (Greenblatt et al., 2022; Wu et al., 2016).

Wnt proteins elicit crucial signaling pathways in skeletal homeostasis. This pathway consists of a canonical Wnt-β-catenin and the noncanonical Wnt signaling events. In hematopoietic niches of bone marrow, the canonical Wnt signaling regulates stem cell self-renewal and fate decisions of progenitor cells. Findings show that loss-of-function mutations in low-density lipoprotein receptor-related protein-5 (LRP5), a coreceptor for Wnt-catenin signaling, cause osteoporosis and that sclerostin, the osteocyte-derived inhibitor of Wnt-catenin signaling, reduces bone formation highlight the significance of Wnt-β-catenin signaling in osteogenesis.

Among the several Wnt ligands, Wnt3a regulates osteoblast differentiation at the early rather than late stages (Morsczeck et al., 2017). Undifferentiated MSCs treated with Wnt3 and/or expressed with constitutively activated β-catenin are inhibited from undergoing osteogenic differentiation, but treatment with dominant negative transcription factor 4 and/or secreted frizzled related protein 1 enhances osteogenic differentiation. Treatment with Wnt3a also reduces osteogenesis in a dose-dependent manner in young calvarial osteoblasts. On the other hand, Wnt3a treatment substantially and dose-dependently stimulates osteogenesis in mature calvarial osteoblasts (Quarto et al., 2010). However, in a calvarial defect model in juvenile mice, low-dose Wnt3a promotes bone regeneration but high doses impair it. Thus, it appears that the differentiation state of the cells and the levels of Wnt3a are key determinants of the regulation of osteogenic response of Wnt3a.

Wnt 10B increases osteogenic differentiation and suppresses adipogenic differentiation. The preferential stimulation of osteogenic fate of MSCs by Wnt 10B is achieved by inducing the osteoblastogenic transcription factors Runx2, distal-less homeobox 5 gene (Dlx5), and osterix, and adipogenic suppression is achieved by downregulating C/EBP and PPARγ. Wnt 10B as an important regulator of bone formation has been demonstrated in Wnt 10b-/- mice that suffer lower trabecular bone mass and circulating osteocalcin than that in WT mice. T-cell-produced Wnt 10B mediates the anabolic effect of teriparatide (Li et al., 2014) as it increases the levels of Wnt 10B in osteoporotic patients (D'Amelio et al., 2015).

Wnt5a is a noncanonical Wnt ligand that mediates its action through Ror2, a receptor protein tyrosine kinase. Wnt5a-Ror2 signaling is responsible for the upregulation of RANK on osteoclast progenitor cells, which in turn amplifies RANKL action, leading to increased osteoclast formation (Maeda et al., 2012). Moreover, Wnt5a-Ror2 signaling also upregulates RANKL in the subchondral trabecular bones of temporomandibular joints, leading to bone loss (Yang et al., 2015). It thus appears that Wnt ligands regulate bone remodeling by positive regulation of osteoblast function (Wnt 3a and Wnt 10b) and promoting osteoclast function via the osteoblasts (Wnt 5a).

Of the Wnt signaling pathways regulating skeletal homeostasis, a *SOST* gene product called sclerostin has been clinically targeted. Sclerostin is a Wnt inhibitor that is expressed in osteoblastic cells with high expression in osteocytes. Sclerostin is also expressed in vascular smooth muscle cells (VSMCs), arteries, and aorta. Sclerostin levels are increased under bone loss conditions such as postmenopausal osteoporosis, advanced stages of CKD, and high-dose corticosteroids.

Sclerosteosis (OMIM 269500) and van Buchem disease (OMIM 239 100) are rare diseases caused by the mutation of *SOST* that gives rise to sclerostin protein (Balemans et al., 2002; Wergedal et al., 2003). Sclerosteosis is caused by the loss-of-function mutation of *SOST*, and van Buchem disease is caused by a 52-kb deletion from about 35 kb downstream of *SOST*, resulting in low levels of sclerostin. Consequently, both diseases present with high bone mass due to increased osteoblast function from increased serum osteogenic markers such as procollagen type I N-terminal propeptide (P1NP) and osteocalcin, and sclerostin level is negatively correlated with serum P1NP (Garnero et al., 2013).

At the cellular levels, sclerostin induces RANKL production from osteocytes to stimulate osteoclastogenesis in addition to inhibiting osteoblast differentiation (Wijenayaka et al., 2011). Moreover, sclerostin stimulates the osteocytic osteolysis of the bone matrix by inducing the expression of bone-matrix-degrading enzymes such as cathepsin K, TRAP, and carbonic anhydrase-2 in osteocytes, and in the process, it produces the characteristic lacuno-canalicular structures that surround osteocytes (Kogawa et al., 2013). Because sclerostin levels increase with aging and are higher in postmenopausal women (Mödder et al., 2011), a humanized neutralizing antibody was approved by the U.S. FDA for treating postmenopausal osteoporosis (Ominsky et al., 2017; Cosman et al., 2016; Bhattacharyya et al., 2018). Given the expression of sclerostin in VSMCs and arteries (Nsengiyumva et al., 2020; He et al., 2020; Krishna et al., 2017; Zhu et al., 2011), and given that the deficiency of aortic sclerostin expression in a mouse model of abdominal aortic aneurysm induced by subcutaneous angiotensin II infusion (Krishna et al., 2017) implicated the protein in cardiovascular disease, the safety aspects of romosozumab warrant more investigation (Figure 13.2). In vitro assays measuring the differentiation and activities of osteoblasts, osteoclasts, and adipocytes are discussed in detail in the supplementary file.

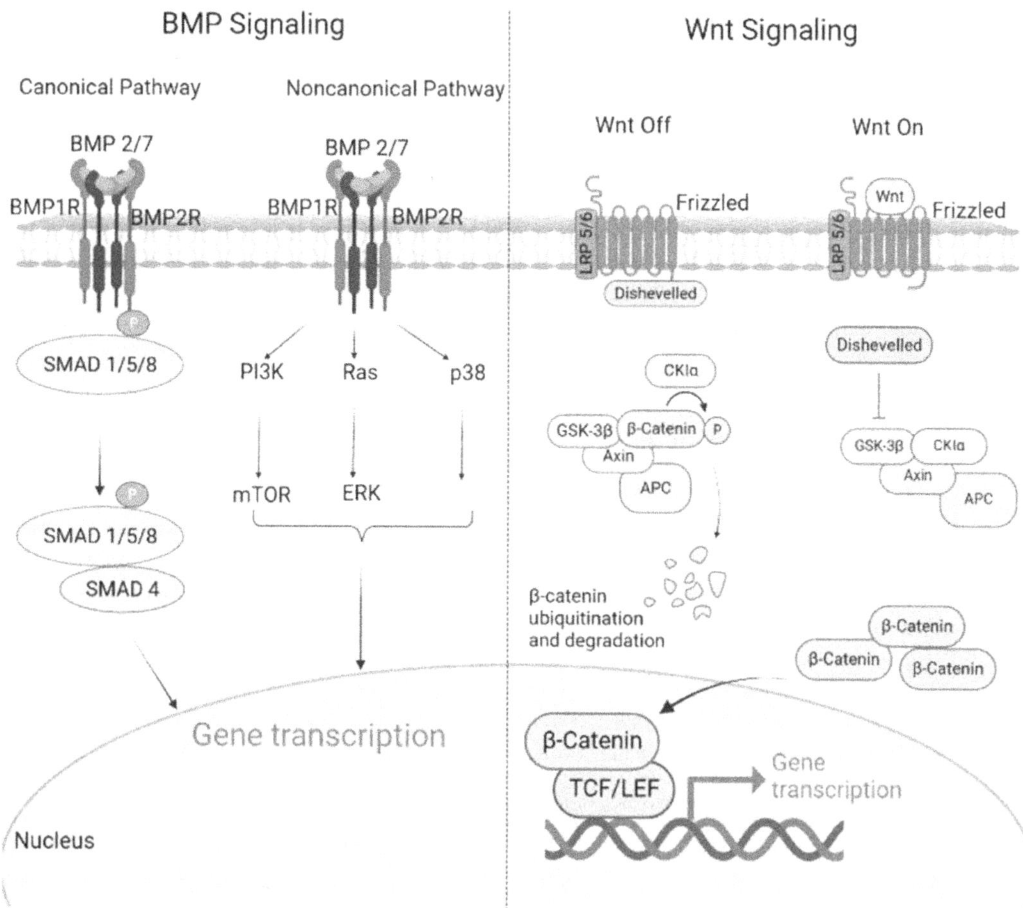

FIGURE 13.2 Canonical and noncanonical signaling pathways in BMP and Wnt/β-catenin signaling for osteogenic differentiation. The left panel demonstrates the canonical and noncanonical signaling pathways of BMP. BMP 2/7 binds to BMP receptors (BMP-R) 1 and 2 in the canonical pathway, forming a heteromeric complex. This leads to the activation of the BMP-R1 by BMP-R2, resulting in the phosphorylation of SMAD 1/5/8. The phosphorylated SMAD 1/5/8 then forms a complex with SMAD 4 and translocates into the nucleus, initiating the gene transcription necessary for osteogenic differentiation. On the other hand, the noncanonical BMP signaling pathway is independent of SMAD proteins and involves the activation of MAPKs (PI3K, Ras, p38). The activated MAPKs translocate to the nucleus and phosphorylate various transcription factors. The right panel illustrates the Wnt/β-catenin signaling pathway. In the absence of Wnt, Axin and APC facilitate the interaction of β-catenin with GSK-3β and CKIα, leading to β-catenin phosphorylation at serine/threonine residues. Phosphorylated β-catenin is subsequently targeted for ubiquitination and degradation (Wnt off). In the presence of Wnt, it binds to LRP5/6 and frizzled receptors, initiating the Wnt/β-catenin signaling pathway. Axin interacts with dishevelled, preventing β-catenin phosphorylation and degradation. As a result, β-catenin accumulates in the cytoplasm and translocates into the nucleus. In the nucleus, β-catenin partners with TCF/LEF and initiates the transcription of target genes involved in osteoblast differentiation. BMP: bone morphogenic protein; BMPR 1/2—BMP receptors 1 and 2; PI3K: phosphoinositide 3-kinase; ERK: extracellular signal-regulated kinases; Ras: small GTPase; mTOR: mammalian target of rapamycin; SMAD—small mothers against decapentaplegic; LRP—low-density lipoprotein receptor-related protein; GSK—glycogen synthase kinase; CKIα—casein kinase Iα; APC—adenomatous polyposis coli; TCF/LEF—T-cell factor/lymphoid enhancer-binding factor. The image is generated by Biorender.

13.3 PRECLINICAL MODELS FOR OSTEOPOROSIS AND FRACTURE HEALING

Osteoporosis is a metabolic bone disease that is the leading cause of fracture, and it has primary and secondary causes. Primary osteoporosis is bone loss that occurs as a natural part of normal aging; secondary osteoporosis is defined as bone loss induced by preexisting clinical conditions. In patients with low BMD, secondary causes of bone loss are commonly overlooked. Secondary osteoporosis can be caused by a variety of medical conditions, such as endocrine disorders, adverse effects of drugs, immobilization, gastrointestinal or biliary system disorders, renal disease, and cancer. It is crucial to establish the etiology of bone loss before making therapeutic recommendations. Various well-established animal models are available for studying the effects of experimental drugs for the treatment of osteoporosis along with discussions of their advantages over their disadvantages.

13.3.1 Models for Metabolic Bone Disorders

13.3.1.1 Ovariectomy

This is a widely used model of bone loss that mimics estrogen deficiency that mimics the postmenopausal state. In laboratory rodents, similar to postmenopausal humans, bilateral ovariectomy (OVX) results in bone resorption that exceeds bone formation due to increased osteoclast activity, and concomitant decrease in osteoblast activity, resulting in osteopenia (Liu et al., 2015; Permuy et al., 2019). Osteopenia develops 90 days after OVX in rats (Bhattacharyya et al., 2019a) or rabbits (Pal et al., 2019) and 45 days in mice (Pal et al., 2020). In these animals, bone resorption markers (serum CTX-1 or urinary pyridinoline and deoxypyridinoline crosslinks) are elevated, and volumetric BMD (vBMD) is decreased at the trabecular sites when assessed by μCT scanning of live animals.

The trabecular site typically assessed in vivo is the proximal femur. After the end of the study period, when animals are killed, μCT scanning of the fifth lumbar vertebra (L5) provides vBMD data. Histological examinations of the proximal femur, distal tibia, and L5 yield bone volume data indicative of bone loss.

Rats attain sexual maturity at six to eight weeks but are considered skeletally mature around 36–38 weeks (age ~ nine months), when the peak bone mass has been achieved (Jee & Yao, 2001; Liu et al., 2015; Jiang et al., 2018). The U.S. FDA recommends that OVX be conducted in rats aged ≥6 months to assess the efficacy of an investigational drug (Thompson et al., 1995). This is because the rate of longitudinal bone growth slows in rats after six months, making them more susceptible to OVX-induced bone loss than younger rats. Moreover, at ≥6 months, the bone turnover markers are stable in serum and urine (Yousefzadeh et al., 2020).

After 90 days post-OVX, trabecular bone in the proximal tibia is reduced by 80% and by 99% after 540 days (18 months). In the femur, this reduction is ~25% after 30–90 days and ~50% after 180 days (6 months) and remains at this level until 360 days post-OVX. The trabecular bone in lumbar vertebrae is decreased by ~25% after 180 days and by ~50% after 180–270 days post-OVX (Wronski et al., 1989). The cortical bone loss is characterized by increased marrow cavity and decreased cortical thickness. Compared with the trabecular bones, the loss of cortical bone due to OVX is much less: a ~10% decrease in endocortical bone surface after 180 days of OVX (Danielsen et al., 1993; Kimmel & Wronski, 1990; Ke et al., 1993; Komori, 2015; Zhang et al., 2007).

There are some limitations with the OVX model. First, it causes a sudden drop in estrogen level, whereas estrogen in humans depletes slowly during menopause. Second, the bone loss in OVX is not uniform across the skeletal sites; BMD losses in the tibia, femur, and lumbar vertebra were 75%, 70.4%, and 36.6%, respectively, after 36 weeks of OVX (Yousefzadeh et al., 2020; Liu et al., 2015). Moreover, rats/mice lack a Haversian system of intracortical remodeling (Turner et al., 2001), unlike larger mammals such as rabbits, dogs, and primates (Lelovas et al., 2008).

However, since the trabecular bone loss is much higher than cortical bone loss, the study of bone in OVX rats/mice is not affected by the absence of a Haversian system (Lelovas et al., 2008; Yousefzadeh et al., 2020).

13.3.1.2 Senile Osteoporosis

A good model of senile osteoporosis in rat or mouse must undergo bone loss as a function of age. Unlike postmenopausal osteoporosis, senile osteoporosis is not accompanied by high-turnover bone loss, and it leads to an increased risk of hip fracture, morbidity, and mortality. The age-related bone mass decline in both sexes starts in humans in their mid-70s.

In laboratory conditions, rats live for two to three years and attain peak bone mass by nine months, after which bone mass begins to decline. Therefore, rats aged 20–22 months are suitable for the senile osteoporosis model (Ma et al., 2020; Pietschmann et al., 2007). Between the ages of 6 and 24 months, C57BL/6J mice had 60% trabecular and a 10% cortical bone loss (Ferguson et al., 2003). CW-1 mice represent a spontaneous senile osteoporosis model that displays ~60% reduction in bone mass (both trabecular and cortical sites) from the peak values due to age. Senescence-accelerated mouse-prone 6 is claimed to be the first mouse model for senile osteoporosis, having morphological and molecular features similar to those of human aging bone (Matsushita et al., 1986). Therefore, these mice strains are suitable choices for studying senile osteoporosis.

13.3.1.3 Orchiectomy

Men do not experience menopause; they experience osteoporosis following lowered testosterone levels caused by hypogonadism or castration due to diseases like prostate cancer. The male rodent orchiectomy (ORX) model is the best-known model for bone loss that mimics male osteoporosis. ORX reduces ~20% and ~50% trabecular bones after four weeks in rats (Gunness & Orwoll, 1995) and mice (Wang et al., 2005), respectively. Similar to OVX, greater bone remodeling is linked to the loss of trabecular bone in ORX. Resorption markers including CTX-1 and TRAcP and formation markers such as PINP and osteocalcin can be used to quantify this increased bone remodeling. The major drawback of the male rat ORX models is that the rat skeleton continues grow throughout life because their epiphyseal growth plate remains open till 30 months (Jee & Yao, 2001; Turner, 2001); therefore, the rat model fails to mimic the clinical osteoporotic conditions in human men.

13.3.1.4 Chronic Kidney Disease-Induced Mineral and Bone Disorder

Chronic kidney disease-induced mineral and bone disorder (CKD-MBD) is a metabolic disorder that is characterized by hyperphosphatemia, low 1,25 $(OH)_2D_3$, and hypocalcemia leading to increased parathyroid hormone (PTH) secretion and secondary hyperparathyroidism (SHPT). Bone loss and vascular calcification are two major pathological manifestations of SHPT. In studies of CKD-MBD-induced bone loss, the 5/6 nephrectomy (5/6 Nx) model, electrocautery models, and adenine diet and obstructive nephropathy models are well established.

One widely used model for inducing CKD is 5/6Nx. This model displays progressive changes in serum calcium and phosphorus depending on the CKD stage. The pathological features include increased serum PTH and total or bone-specific ALP, PINP, TRAB-5b, FGF23, osteocalcin, osteoprotegerin, SOST, and various uremic toxins. Additionally, serum 1,25 $(OH)_2D_3$ and αKlotho are decreased in advanced stages of CKD induced by 5/6Nx (Drüeke & Massy, 2016).

The increases in FGF23 and estimated glomerular filtration rate are directly proportional to the severity of disease and lead to bone loss and fractures (Kim et al., 2021). To advance the progression of CKD-MBD-induced bone loss equivalent to human CKD stages 4–5, high-phosphate diet (1.2–1.8% phosphate) is fed to 5/6Nx rats that induces hyperphosphatemia and SHPT. The affected sites include the distal and proximal metaphysis along with diaphysis regions of the long bone. Cortical porosity is observed near the endosteal surface of diaphysis that progresses with the disease severity (McNerny et al., 2019). Though the pathophysiological conditions in

5/6Nx are similar to those in humans, it is difficult to induce vascular calcification in this model. Furthermore, ureteral injury leading to excessive bleeding increases the mortality rate up to 50% (Wang et al., 2017).

Another model of chronic renal failure with metabolic characteristics similar to those seen in humans can be obtained by feeding chronic adenine to rats; 2,8-dihydroxyadenine is an adenine metabolite that causes tubular injury, inflammation, tubular atrophy, and fibrosis by crystalizing within renal tubules (Klinkhammer et al., 2020). When comparing 5/6Nx- and adenine induced-CKD models, the authors of one study found no differences in serum phosphate, ionized calcium, intact parathyroid hormone, or FGF23 after nine weeks (Ferrari et al., 2014). However, the bone effect varies between male and female animals; therefore, care should be taken when choosing CKD-MBD models. Bone effects also vary depending upon the duration of model induction and the percentage of high-phosphate diet.

13.3.1.5 Nutrition Deficiency

Nutritional deficiencies including low-calorie diet, low calcium, and protein intake disrupt the metabolic processes (Flanagan et al., 2020). The rat model of calorie restriction showed delayed aging and aging-related bone loss (Masoro, 2005) via the suppression of serum PTH (Kalu et al., 1984). However, the impact on bone depends entirely on the experimental duration and animal species.

Researchers who combined vitamin D (Melhus et al., 2007) and calcium restriction (Costa et al., 2011) with OVX did not find any significant impact on bone loss. However, the combined dietary deficiency of vitamin D, vitamin K, calcium, and phosphorus in OVX rats caused bone loss (El Khassawna et al., 2013). Therefore, this model might be useful in studying the effects of nutrition deficiencies postmenopause. Acute or moderate calcium deficiency (Yadav et al., 2021, 2020; Viguet-Carrin et al., 2014) during peak bone mass could serve as a good model for studying the efficacy of a putative osteogenic agent.

13.3.2 Iatrogenic Osteoporosis Models

Recurrent or long-term medications including corticosteroids, retinoids, heparin, and antidepressant drugs cause bone loss. These drugs cause increased osteoclastogenesis and decreased osteoblastogenesis, leading to high turnover rates and/or the inhibition of osteoid calcification (Sewell, 1995). Among these drugs, the most prevalent form of osteoporosis is caused by corticosteroids/glucocorticoids.

13.3.2.1 Glucocorticoid-Induced Model

Rats and mice are routinely used for creating glucocorticoid (GC)-induced osteoporosis (GIOP). The choice of GCs and their dose, duration of treatment and route of administration have varying effects on bone loss. The most frequently used GCs for GIOP models in order of their potency to impact bone are dexamethasone (DEX) > methylprednisolone (MP)> prednisolone/prednisone>hydrocortisone/corticosterone.

In addition to small rodents, rabbits, sheep, and dogs can be used to make the GIOP model. In a comparative study in the same rat strain of two GCs, DEX and MP, at doses of 0.6 mg/kg twice weekly and 1 mg/kg once daily, respectively, for the same duration (12 weeks) and route of administration, DEX caused greater bone loss at vertebrae L1–L3 than MP (Ren et al., 2015). Morbidity and mortality in small rodents were higher when 200 μg/kg DEX or 5 mg/kg MP was given for 5 days/week by parenteral routes (Khan et al., 2013).

In addition to causing mortality, high doses of GCs are associated with side effects including sarcopenia, hypertension, and insulin resistance that could secondarily confound skeletal homeostasis. For example, osteonecrosis (ON) is frequently caused by long-term use of GCs, particularly at the femur head. Increased adipogenic differentiation of bone marrow MSCs by GCs is the cause of ON as these drugs cause excessive accumulation of marrow adipose tissue, impairing bone marrow vasculature.

Clofazimine (CFZ) is a drug used to treat lepromatous leprosy and has been reported to cause ON in rats. CFZ acts on bone-marrow-derived MSCs to induce adipogenic differentiation, resulting in impaired fracture healing, osteopenia, and ON at 1/3rd human equivalent dose without metabolic or hematologic adverse effects (Porwal et al., 2019). Therefore, CFZ treatment in adult rats provides a simple and reproducible way to make an ON model.

13.3.2.2 Immobilization Model of Bone Loss

Immobilization (IM) models involve the local or systemic IM of bone by either surgical or conventional methods. The surgical method includes nerve, tendon, and spinal cord resection, and conventional methods include casting, suspension, and limb bandaging. The bone loss in surgical methods occurs more rapidly than it does in conventional methods due to regional acceleration (Frost, 1983).

The IM triggers transient remodeling marked by increased resorption and decreased formation, resulting in trabecular bone loss adjacent to marrow. After a lag time, bone loss reaches a steady state, and cellular activity returns to normal. The loss mostly affects trabecular rather than cortical bones (Ijiri et al., 1995).

The load-bearing hind limbs are the target sites for IM-induced bone loss. In rats after IM, the loss takes around 14–30 days, and it takes ~70 days for significant bone loss to occur in the proximal-distal tibia metaphysis and diaphysis. The steady state is reached around 70–126 days for trabecular bones and ~180 days for cortical bone in rats (Jaworski & Uhthoff, 1986). The low bone turnover rate in the IM model makes it suitable for studying the effect of osteogenic agents.

13.3.2.3 Alcohol-Induced Bone Loss Model

Researchers have found a positive correlation between alcohol consumption and osteoporosis (Cheraghi et al., 2019; Jang et al., 2017). However, we observed that individuals who already had normal body mass index when alcohol use disorder (AUD) commenced in their 30s or 40s and whose AUD had already lasted for a decade may not experience significant changes in BMD (Balhara et al., 2022). Researchers have studied an ethyl alcohol-induced osteoporosis model and developed a better understanding of the pathogenesis of bone loss. The underlying mechanisms include modulation of Wnt and mTOR signaling, which leads to bone loss via the increased adipogenic differentiation of stromal cells, increased osteoclast activity, and reduced osteoblast activity (Luo et al., 2017; Chakkalakal, 2005).

13.3.3 Preclinical Models for Fracture Healing

The mechanism and rate of bone healing differ between species. Small rodents (rats and mice) have faster bone-healing rates than those larger animals. Moreover, the age of the animal is also important; older animals show delayed callus formation (Clark et al., 2017). The two mechanisms involved in fracture healing are intramembranous and endochondral ossification.

Intramembranous ossification is the predominant mechanism of healing at the distal and proximal ends of critical-sized tibial and calvarial defects, whereas endochondral ossification occurs in osteotomy fractures (Gao et al., 2023). Stable femoral fractures in mice and rats takes four weeks for fracture healing (Meyer et al., 2003), whereas in rabbits, dogs, and nonhuman primates, they require more medullary healing and take longer to heal (Chen et al., 2015; Zhang et al., 2016; Pozzi et al., 2012).

The histomorphometry of bone also differs between the species. Rodents do not have a Haversian system, whereas the long bones of nonhuman primates are avascular with irregular Haversian systems. On the other hand, dogs have vascular bone combined with a Haversian system similar to that in humans. Therefore, the dog fracture model is more appropriate than the nonhuman primate and murine species for studying the effects of osteogenic agents (Brits et al., 2014). Animal models for fracture healing mostly use the femur and tibia and include both open and closed fractures.

13.3.3.1 Closed Fractures

This fracture is defined as a break in the bone's continuity without rupturing the skin (Rude, 1985). A closed fracture model is accomplished by delivering three-point stress to an animal's long bone stem using a particular fracture-producing apparatus (Histing et al., 2011; Sun et al., 2015). The preferred animals for this model are small animals like mice or rats. Compared with open fractures, closed fractures are less iatrogenic and comminuted. Close fracture models are easier to operate and have less impact on the surrounding soft tissues and blood flow conditions. However, the fracture angle and line and direction of force cannot be precisely controlled and therefore may have inconsistent fracture points and different fracture healing effects in different animals.

13.3.3.2 Open Fracture Model

In an open fracture model, a wound is created by traumatizing the surrounding skin and/or soft tissues exposing the broken bone and/or fracture hematoma to the outside environment (Sop & Sop, 2023). Briefly, muscles are separated to expose the femur or tibia, and osteotomy is performed at a particular angle and position using wire saws, electric swing saws, a drill, or other suitable equipment. Rabbit, rat, and mice are preferably used for this model. The advantage of the open fracture model is the ability to control the angle and position of the fracture. However, due to destruction of the periosteum and marrow cavity, blood flow is reduced, and this leads to slow fracture healing.

13.3.3.3 Critical-Sized Defect Model

There is no universal definition of a critical-sized defect. One research group has described it as the smallest intra-osseous wound in a bone that does not heal spontaneously during the animal's life (Schmitz & Hollinger, 1986). Rats, rabbits, dogs, pigs, goats, and sheep are the preferred choice for this model, and long bones are the preferred site for creating the defects. This model is widely used for studies on bone tissue engineering and the development of degradable and nondegradable scaffolds (McGovern et al., 2018). It is noteworthy that a critical-size defect differs from a nonunion, which has impaired cellular and molecular signaling and/or biomechanical instability (Nauth et al., 2018).

13.3.3.4 Calvarial Defect Model

This model is preferably created in rats or mice. A standardized circular bone defect spanning the entire depth of the bone is created, and the bone disk is removed. Calvarial defect models are useful for evaluating the efficacy of biomaterials, progenitor cells, growth factors, and epigenetic medications (McGovern et al., 2018) (Figure 13.3).

13.3.4 Osteoporosis Therapies

According to clinicians' guidelines for pharmacologic intervention, osteoporosis therapy should be initiated in patients with a T-score of –2.5 or lower in the spine and femoral neck and a history of fragility fracture in hip or spine (Cosman et al., 2014). The FDA-approved pharmacological interventions are antiresorptive drugs including bisphosphonates (alendronate, ibandronate, risedronate, and zoledronic acid), denosumab (RANKL inhibitor), SERMs (raloxifene, conjugated estrogens, bazedoxifene, and lasofoxifene), calcitonin, and strontium ranelate and anabolic drugs including teriparatide, abaloparatide, and anti-SOST antibody (romosozumab) (Table 13.1).

BMD: bone mineral density; RANK: receptor activator of nuclear factor κB; RANKL: receptor activator of nuclear factor κ B ligand; PTH1R: parathyroid hormone 1 receptor; cAMP: cyclic adenosine monophosphate; PKA: protein kinase A; CREB: cAMP-response element binding protein

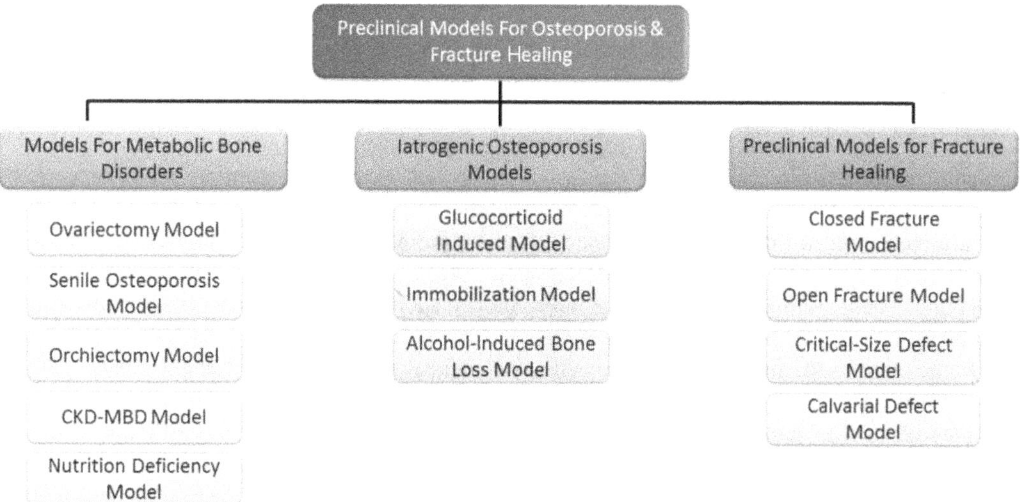

FIGURE 13.3 Preclinical models for osteoporosis and fracture healing for assessment of therapeutic efficacy of putative compounds/peptides.

TABLE 13.1
Pharmacologic Interventions for Osteoporosis and Their Modes of Actions

Drug Name	Mode of Action
Antiresorptive drugs	
Bisphosphonates	Inhibit mevalonate pathway and protein prenylation required for osteoclast survival and function; reduce bone remodeling; increase BMD and decrease bone turnover markers; reduce fracture risk.
Denosumab	Human antibody against RANKL that acts like OPG; induces osteoclast apoptosis; increases BMD and decreases bone turnover markers; reduces fracture risk.
Selective estrogen receptor modulators	Act like estrogen in osteoclast; inhibit osteoclast proliferation and differentiation; increase BMD and decrease bone turnover markers; reduce fracture risk.
Calcitonin	Binds to calcitonin receptors and suppresses osteoclast migration and function; increases BMD to decrease fracture risk.
Anabolic drugs	
Teriparatide (TPTD: 1–34 PTH)	TPTD binds to PTH1R and activates cAMP-PKA-CREB signaling to increase RunX2; promotes MSC differentiation to osteoblasts and survival; increases BMD to decrease fracture risk.
Abaloparatide (1–36 PTHRP)	Acts similar to TPTD; shorter cAMP pulse; enhances bone formation and increases BMD; decreases fracture risk.
Romosozumab	Humanized antibody against sclerostin; inhibits sclerostin function to activate Wnt pathway; stimulates osteoblast function; increases BMD to decrease fracture risk.

13.3.4.1 Antiresorptive Drugs

13.3.4.1.1 Bisphosphonates

Bisphosphonates (BPs) are the first-line therapy for the treatment of osteoporosis. They are derivatives of pyrophosphate with high binding affinity to hydroxyapatite crystals. Their binding affinity is due to R1 and R2 groups attached to the central carbon backbone. The binding affinity of BPs to hydroxyapatite in the order of potency is zoledronate > pamidronate > alendronate > ibandronate > risedronate > etidronate > clodronate (Miki & Naka, 2005). High binding affinity of BPs to hydroxyapatite allows their rapid incorporation into active bone remodeling sites with high skeletal turnover.

BPs are categorized into two classes: first-generation non-nitrogen-containing (etidronate, clodronate, and tiludronate) and second- and third-generation nitrogen-containing (alendronate, risedronate, and zoledronate). The two classes differ in their modes of action. Non-nitrogen-containing BPs are incorporated into ATP by aminoacyl-transfer RNA synthetases and convert to nonhydrolyzable analogs of ATP after osteoclast-mediated uptake of bone mineral and matrix following resorption. These nonhydrolyzable ATP analogs induce apoptosis of the osteoclasts that are actively resorbing bones, reducing the extent of resorption.

On the other hand, nitrogen-containing BPs specifically inhibit farnesyl pyrophosphate synthase (FPPS), a key regulatory enzyme of the mevalonate pathway involved in the synthesis of cholesterol, other sterols, and isoprenoid lipids. Inhibition of FPPS blocks the production of FPP and its downstream metabolite, geranylgeranyl pyrophosphate (GGPP). GGPP is a critical regulator of function and survival of osteoclasts as it is necessary for the prenylation of small GTPases like the Rab, Rac, and Rho family proteins.

Inhibiting prenylation results in loss of ruffled borders of osteoclasts, essential for bone resorption (Lewiecki, 2010). Thus, inhibiting osteoclast activity reduces bone remodeling, leading to increased BMD. However, the long-term use of BPs is thought to alter bone material properties as these drugs suppress bone formation and result in increased crystallinity (homogenous crystals or crystals of equal size), microdamage, and nonenzymatic crosslinking of collagen (Farlay et al., 2021; Ma et al., 2017; Allen & Burr, 2007). These changes produce brittleness in bones with the long-term use of BPs manifested by atypical femur fracture, although the incidence is very low (Saita et al., 2015).

In addition to osteoporosis, BPs are recommended for the treatment of early-stage osteonecrosis of femur head (ONFH), but meta-analysis of seven clinical trials failed to find significant efficacy of BPs in ONFH (Li et al., 2018). The other adverse effects of BPs include nausea, dyspepsia, abdominal pain, gastritis, severe musculoskeletal pain, esophageal cancer, and ocular inflammation (Kennel & Drake, 2009). These adverse events could be reasons that 50% of all patients discontinue BP therapy within one to two years (Park et al., 2019).

13.3.4.1.2 Denosumab

Denosumab is the human monoclonal antibody against RANKL that effectively blocks the interaction between RANK and RANKL, thus inhibiting osteoclastogenesis. The resulting outcome in patients suffering from osteoporosis is increased BMD and significantly decreased bone turnover markers (i.e., CTX-1 and P1NP) (Eastell et al., 2011; Bone et al., 2011). The decrease in CTX-1 is more rapid than that of P1NP, confirming the efficacy of denosumab in suppressing resorption.

In a study consisting of 7868 postmenopausal women, denosumab treatment lasting from 6 to 36 months resulted in a 68% reduction in new radiographic vertebral fracture, a 40% reduction in hip fracture risk, and a 20% reduction in nonvertebral fracture risk compared with placebo (Cummings et al., 2009). In another clinical trial performed on postmenopausal women (n = 28 denosumab, n = 22 placebo), denosumab reduced cortical porosity in the proximal femur and enhanced hip joint strength by 7.9% (Zebaze et al., 2016). As antiosteoporosis treatment is expected to run a long duration, the safety of denosumab was assessed. Denosumab treatment for up to 10 years was associated with low rates of adverse events, a low fracture incidence relative to the original FREEDOM clinical trial, and continuous gains in BMD without plateauing (Bone et al., 2017).

Since the RANKL signals promotes the survival of dendritic cells by regulating T-lymphocytes (Loser et al., 2006), the inhibition of RANKL may generate immunological tolerance through increasing Treg formation in autoimmune conditions (Walsh & Choi, 2014). RANKL is required for regulatory T cells to suppress cytotoxic destruction of pancreatic beta islet cells in a mouse type 1 diabetes model (Green et al., 2002), as well as for Treg-mediated regulation of a colitis model

(Totsuka et al., 2009). In adult mice, blocking RANKL signaling impaired dendritic cell activity and the survival of intestinal M cell populations (Akiyama et al., 2012; Knoop et al., 2009). These findings have implications for the use of human anti-RANKL antibodies for a variety of applications.

For example, in a prospective community-based Bruneck study, serum RANKL was strongly associated with type 2 diabetes mellitus (T2DM) manifestation, and hepatic or systemic blockage of RANKL signaling in a mouse model of T2DM markedly improved hepatic insulin sensitivity and ameliorated or even normalized plasma glucose concentrations and glucose tolerance (Kiechl et al., 2013). These data imply that denosumab treatment of osteoporosis patients who have T2DM might benefit both conditions. Regarding the skeletal effect, BMD is reversible upon cessation of denosumab, and this is accompanied by increased bone turnover and reduced osteocyte viability, which may increase fracture risk and bone loss (Tay & Tay, 2022; Jähn-Rickert et al., 2020). The treatment also elevates bone hardness and the number of micropetrotic osteocyte lacunae that are features of aging bone (Jähn-Rickert et al., 2020).

13.3.4.1.3 Selective Estrogen Receptor Modulators

Selective estrogen receptor modulators (SERMs) belong to the class of nonsteroidal compounds that interact with estrogen receptors ERα and/or ERβ depending upon the tissue type. In bone, ERα is predominantly expressed in developing cancellous bone, whereas ERβ is expressed in cortical bone (Bord et al., 2001). SERMs exert a similar mechanism to that of estrogen without having any adverse effect on breast or endometrium. The most commonly used SERMs for postmenopausal osteoporosis are raloxifene, equine estradiol, lasofoxifene, and bazedoxifene.

Until now, the most-prescribed SERM for postmenopausal osteoporosis has been raloxifene, a second-generation SERM. A raloxifene clinical trial on 601 postmenopausal women found a relative increase in lumbar spine, hip, and total body BMD over the placebo group without altering the endometrium (Delmas et al., 1997). A multicenter, randomized, blinded, placebo-controlled study, Multiple Outcomes of Raloxifene Evaluation, of 7705 women aged 31–80 years in 25 countries for 36 months concluded that raloxifene reduced vertebral fracture risk by 30%, but it did not affect nonvertebral fracture. The adverse effects included vaginal bleeding, hot flashes, worsening of pre-existing hypertriglyceridemia, venous thromboembolism, death due to stroke in history of coronary heart disease, and cardiovascular disease. In another long-term raloxifene study on women, Continuing Outcomes Relevant to Evista, raloxifene showed no significant changes in nonvertebral fracture but decreased bone turnover markers by 30–40%; it also increased BMD at the lumbar spine by up to 50%, with major side effects including hot flushes, leg cramps, peripheral edema, and gallbladder disease (Siris et al., 2005).

Lasofoxifene is a third-generation SERM that is structurally different from raloxifene. There have so far been 23 clinical pharmacological studies and 17 phase II/III clinical trials to evaluate the efficacy of lasofoxifene. The key findings come from two phase III trials, a randomized controlled clinical trial postmenopausal evaluation and risk reduction with lasofoxifene (Goldstein et al., 2011) and one on osteoporosis prevention and lipid lowering (Lewiecki, 2009) in postmenopausal women. Lasofoxifene reduced vertebral fracture risk by 42%, but benign changes in endometrium were observed. It also increased BMD at the femur, lumbar spine, and hip and reduced bone turnover markers. Unlike raloxifene, lasofoxifene reduced the nonvertebral fractures; its adverse effects were similar to those of raloxifene including venous thromboembolism, hot flushes, muscle spasm, and vaginal bleeding (Gennari et al., 2010).

Bazedoxifene is an indole-based SERM with structural similarities to raloxifene and tamoxifen. It binds with both ERα and Erβ, with higher affinity for ERα. It can be given alone or in combination with equine estrogen for postmenopausal osteoporosis (Gruber & Gruber, 2004). Based on the clinical data, bazedoxifene prevents bone loss in healthy postmenopausal women at all skeletal sites and improves BMD. Furthermore, it reduces serum bone turnover markers and prevents vertebral and non-vertebral fractures (Komm & Chines, 2012; Genant, 2011). The adverse effects of bazedoxifene include headache, infection, arthralgia, pain, hot flush, and back pain (Miller et al., 2008). When given in combination with equine estradiol to postmenopausal women, bazedoxifene improved BMD and efficiently helped in managing the vasomotor symptoms (hot flushes) (Umland et al., 2016).

13.3.4.1.4 Calcitonin

This short-peptide hormone (32 amino acid) is produced in parafollicular C-cells, and an analog of human calcitonin is used for treatment of postmenopausal osteoporosis. Calcitonin is not approved by the European Medicine Agency for osteoporosis treatment. However, FDA has approved it as a second-line therapy to the patients having menopause for more than five years and when first-line therapy is infective or intolerable (Pavone et al., 2017; Tabatabaei-Malazy et al., 2017; Bandeira et al., 2016; McLaughlin et al., 2024). The action of calcitonin is opposite to PTH as it decreases the calcium concentration in blood. In the kidney, calcitonin inhibits calcium reuptake. In bone, it suppresses the osteoclast migration and action (Xie et al., 2020). Calcitonin signals through the calcitonin receptor to activate protein kinase C pathway (McLaughlin et al., 2024). Data from phase 3 trials of a study on oral calcitonin in postmenopausal osteoporosis (Binkley et al., 2012) and from the Prevent Recurrence of Osteoporotic Fractures study (Chesnut et al., 2000) showed the efficacy of calcitonin in improving trochanteric and total proximal femur BMD and significant reductions in bone resorption markers compared with the placebo group. Calcitonin delivery by parenteral and nasal routes causes pain and discomfort, as well as epistaxis and nasal ulcers (Hamza & Şaramet, 2020). As a result, there is a need to develop an oral formulation of calcitonin, which is challenging.

13.3.4.2 Anabolic Drugs

13.3.4.2.1 Teriparatide

Teriparatide (TPTD) is the N-terminal segment of human parathyroid hormone (PTH 1–34). Like the full-length PTH, TPTD has binding affinity with the PTH type 1R receptor (PTH1R). PTH1R is a G-protein-coupled receptor and is expressed on the surfaces of osteoblasts and precursors. PTH1R activation by TPTD induces cAMP signaling by activating membrane-bound adenylyl cyclase that converts ATP to cAMP, and it activates protein kinase A (PKA), which subsequently phosphorylates cAMP response element-binding protein (CREB). The activation of cAMP-PKA-CREB pathway induces RUNX2 and BMP2/4 signaling in a MAP kinase-dependent manner. Moreover, TPDT also functions via noncanonical endosomal cAMP signaling (Bhattacharyya et al., 2019b; Porwal et al., 2021).

The osteogenic effect of TPDT results in the formation of new bone, leading to increased BMD and improvements in bone microarchitecture in osteoporotic individuals. Consequently, TPTD reduces the risk of vertebral and nonvertebral fractures. It also increases serum levels of the bone formation markers that precede the resorption markers. In a clinical study with 1637 postmenopausal women with a history of vertebral fracture, TPTD increased the BMD of lumbar vertebrae, femur neck, and total hip by, respectively, 13.7%, 2.8%, and 5.1% (Neer et al., 2001).

TPTD had superior efficacy over risedronate when given to postmenopausal women with severe osteoporosis and prior history of fracture in a study on vertebral fracture treatment comparisons in osteoporotic women. In this study, TPDT reduced vertebral fracture by 69% and nonvertebral fracture by 54% compared with the placebo (Geusens et al., 2018). TPDT is also effective in GIOP treatment; when given for 18 months, it decreased the incidences of vertebral and nonvertebral fractures (Saag et al., 2007).

The bone anabolic effect of TPTD is transient. This is because the exuberant bone formation effect of TPTD exceeds bone resorption, which lasts two years. Beyond this time, bone resorption catches up with formation and the "anabolic window" of TPTD is lost. Subsequently, bone resorption becomes the dominant effect (Bilezikian, 2007).

In an attempt to extend the anabolic window of TPTD, antiresorptive drugs including alendronate, zoledronic acid (Zol), and raloxifene were used in combination, and the presence of alendronate reduced the osteogenic effect of TPTD in postmenopausal women (Finkelstein et al., 2010). This finding was consistent with the theory that functional remodeling is required for TPTD to exert its osteogenic effect; however, the presence of Zol did not impair the osteogenic effect of TPTD (Cosman et al., 2011).

Combining Zol with TPTD enhanced lumbar spine BMD more than TPTD during the first 13 weeks, suggesting an additive effect of the combination. At 52 weeks, spine BMD increase by the combination was similar to the increase with TPTD alone but higher than that with Zol. When elevation of BMD at both spine and hip was considered, the combination of TPTD and Zol had more rapid effects than either drug. Furthermore, when compared with TPTD alone, the combination improved BMD at total hip, trochanter, and femoral neck faster and in a more sustained manner. The combination group was more effective at increasing total-hip BMD than Zol at 13 weeks (Cosman et al., 2011).

From these data, it appears that remodeling suppression by BPs does not interfere with the anabolic action of TPTD. Indeed, in postmenopausal women, when TPTD was combined with raloxifene, the bone-forming effect of the hormone was found to be intact. Moreover, the combination of raloxifene and TPTD increased total-hip BMD more than TPTD alone (Deal et al., 2005). Denosumab in combination with TPTD fully blocks TPTD-induced bone resorption while allowing for continuing TPTD-induced bone formation, resulting in greater improvements in hip and spine BMD than with either medication alone (Tsai et al., 2013). From the available data, it appears that TPTD in combination with Zol, raloxifene, or denosumab is useful for treating patients at high risk of fracture.

13.3.4.2.2 Abaloparatide

Abaloparatide is the second generation of osteoanabolic drugs. It is an analog of human parathyroid hormone-related protein (PTHrP). Structurally, it has 76% homology with PTHrP (1–34) and 41% with teriparatide. In abaloparatide, Ala-29 substitution with α-aminoisobutyric acid (Aib, α-methylalanine) stabilizes its helical conformation. Both TPTD and abaloparatide signal via parathyroid hormone receptor type 1 (PTHR1); however, the downstream signaling varies between the two ligands.

PTH1R exists in two distinct conformations based on their sensitivities to the nonhydrolyzable GTP analog GTPγS. The R^G conformation is sensitive to GTPγS and is coupled to the heterotrimeric G protein; the second R^0 conformation is insensitive to GTPγS and is functionally uncoupled from G protein. The R^0 selectivity is associated with longer signaling response than with R^G conformation and is associated with shorter signaling responses. TPTD has a four-fold higher affinity for R^0 (GTPγS-insensitive) than that of PTHrP, resulting in extended cAMP signaling (Dean et al., 2008). Abaloparatide has a greater selectivity for R^G conformation, which is responsible for the shorter cAMP pulse than that of TPTD, resulting in enhanced bone formation and reduced bone resorption (Bhattacharyya et al., 2019b).

A randomized, double-blind, phase-3 clinical trial with abaloparatide showed increased BMD at the total hip, femur neck, and lumbar spine in postmenopausal women. It also decreased the vertebral and nonvertebral fracture risk. However, there were adverse effects of abaloparatide including nausea (1.6%), dizziness (1.2%), headache (1.2%), and palpitations (0.9%) (Miller et al., 2016). Other adverse effects of abaloparatide are orthostatic hypotension, hypercalcemia, hypercalciuria, and urolithiasis. Head-to-head clinical trials are required to establish the beneficial effects of abaloparatide over TPTD in osteoporosis patients.

13.3.4.2.3 Romosozumab

Romosozumab is a humanized monoclonal antibody against sclerostin, a glycoprotein secreted by osteocytes; sclerostin is a Wnt inhibitor. The canonical Wnt signaling involves the interaction of

Wnt ligands with their receptor complex including frizzled receptor protein and a low-density lipoprotein receptor-related protein LRP5/6. Activating this pathway stimulates osteoblast proliferation and differentiation.

Sclerostin binds to LRP5/6 and suppresses the formation of the LRP5/6-frizzled-Wnt complex, as well as inhibiting osteoblastogenesis and bone production. Moreover, Wnt signaling increases β-catenin accumulation that in-turn increases osteoprotegerin (OPG) expression. OPG binds to RANKL, a decoy receptor, preventing the RANKL–RANK interaction, necessary for osteoclast activation and differentiation. The serum levels of sclerostin are raised in bone loss conditions such as in postmenopausal osteoporosis and GIOP (Vasiliadis et al., 2022), and PTH and estradiol suppress sclerostin levels (Fujita et al., 2014; Drake et al., 2010). These findings suggest that sclerostin is an attractive therapeutic target for preventing bone loss.

Neutralization of sclerostin by romosozumab allows the Wnt signaling pathway to be activated and stimulate osteoblast function and suppress osteoclastogenesis. In phase 2 clinical trial with 419 postmenopausal women, romosozumab for 12 months significantly increased BMD at the lumbar spine, total hip and femoral neck compared with placebo, and this increase was also significantly greater compared with alendronate and TPTD (McClung et al., 2014). In postmenopausal women with osteoporosis, one year of romosozumab treatment resulted in a decreased risk of vertebral and clinical fractures compared with placebo, likely due to the increase in bone formation and inhibition of bone resorption (Cosman et al., 2016). The effect of romosozumab is reversible, and a second course of romosozumab after its discontinuation for a year led to rapid and significant gains in BMD. Romosozumab protects BMD in patients who switched over from denosumab (Kendler et al., 2019).

In an extension study, the women received romosozumab (12 months) and then denosumab (12 months) showed continuous accrual of bone mass, whereas BMD in the placebo group returned to close to baseline. In continuation of this, a second extension study was performed on the subjects who received the first course of romosozumab (12 months) followed by placebo (12 months) and a second course of romosozumab or denosumab (12 months). After 12 months off-treatment, a second romosozumab course led to rapid and large BMD gains whereas with denosumab, BMD were smaller than the initial treatment compared with those with romosozumab (Kendler et al., 2019).

In phase III FRAME (Fracture Study in Postmenopausal Women with Osteoporosis), a study of romosozumab, 12 months of treatment decreased new vertebral fracture risk by 73%. However, no significant effect was observed for nonvertebral fractures (Cosman et al., 2016). The interesting finding came with the comparison of BMD T-score from the FRAME trial with FREEDOM trial of denosumab: The effect of one year of romosozumab treatment at the lumbar spine and total hip was equal to the effects of 4.5 and 3 years of denosumab, respectively. Moreover, one year treatment of romosozumab followed by one year of denosumab was equal to seven years of denosumab treatment at both sites (Cosman et al., 2018).

A recent recommendation by the International Osteoporosis Foundation and European Society for Clinical and Economic Aspects of Osteoporosis and Osteoarthritis to use romosozumab followed by an antiresorptive agent or teriparatide in combination with denosumab produced the most rapid and robust changes in BMD in patients at very high risk of fracture (Kanis et al., 2020). However, in another one-year double-blind clinical study (ARCH) concern regarding a potential risk of cardiovascular disease was raised (Saag et al., 2017). Therefore, on the basis of ARCH study findings, the FDA-approved romosozumab with a boxed warning indicating potential risk of myocardial infarction, stroke, and cardiovascular death (Rauner et al., 2021).

13.3.5 Potential of Botanicals/Herbal Medicines with Antiosteoporosis Effects

The first line of osteoporosis therapy is BPs, and alendronate is the most widely prescribed BP. It is noteworthy that except for oral BPs, all currently used antiosteoporosis therapies are biologics that have parenteral mode of administration. Even the most recent BP, Zol, is injectable.

Furthermore, the current pharmacological repertoire either suppresses bone resorption, which suppresses bone formation, or stimulates bone formation, which stimulates bone resorption. SERMs do not have this limitation, although they are no longer the preferred medication for osteoporosis treatment.

Romosozumab was thought to have a dual effect of stimulating bone formation and preventing bone resorption, but in clinical trials, the drug performed similarly to TPTD; that is, it stimulated both bone formation and resorption. The concurrent use of an anabolic drug with an antiresorptive drug as described before is used experimentally and is not approved by regulators. One drug with the dual beneficial effect that is orally active is an unmet clinical need for osteoporosis therapy.

In this regard, phytochemicals hold potential given the vast body of preclinical data supporting their roles in affording dual effects in bone metabolism. There are low-quality clinical data showing bone-conserving effects of various classes of phytochemicals that support their favorable roles in bone metabolism. In this regard, phytoestrogens that are structurally similar to estrogen including isoflavones, flavonoids, lignans, coumestans, and stilbenes have been widely studied in preclinical disease models as well as their mechanisms of action (Table S13.2). They are classified into two groups: flavonoids and non-flavonoids. Flavonoids include isoflavonoids, coumestans, and prenylflavonoids, while non-flavonoids include lignans.

13.3.5.1 Isoflavonoids

The majority of isoflavonoids that have been studied in bone metabolism are derived from Fabaceae legumes, including soybean (*Glycine max*), red clover (*Trifolium pratense*), Sheesham (*Dalbergia sissoo*), and palas or Bastard teak (*Butea monosperma*). Soyabean is a rich source of genistein, daidzein, and glycitein; red clover for biochanin A and formononetin; Sheesham for genstein, biochanin A, pratensein, kaempferol, and quercetin; and Bastard teak for cajanin, cladrin, formononetin, isoformononetin, prunetin, a pterocarpan, and medicarpin. Other isoflavonoid-containing plants include alfalfa (*Medicago saltiva L.*), beans (green bean, mung bean), Psoralea (*Psoralea corylifolia*), and kudzu root (*Pueraria lobata L.*).

Isoflavones are activated by the removal of glucose moiety (aglycon) in the gastrointestinal flora before absorption. Thus, the efficacy and bioavailability of phytoestrogen depend on the bacterial flora of individuals (Lagari & Levis, 2014). Isoflavones act by two mechanisms: activating the ER-mediated signaling and activating intracellular protein tyrosine kinase, phospholipase C, and MAPK pathway. Due to their selectivity for ER like the way SERMs act, they target bone cells without adversely affecting other estrogen-sensitive organs.

13.3.5.1.1 Soy Isoflavonoids

Numerous clinical studies, systematic reviews, and meta-analyses have been performed on soy flavonoids. In a clinical study, the dietary inclusion of 60 mg/day of isoflavones for 12 weeks on 42 postmenopausal women significantly increased serum levels of phytoestrogens and reduced several clinical risk factors for osteoporosis in normal postmenopausal women (Scheiber et al., 2001). Soy isoflavone supplementation for two meals twice a week increased serum osteocalcin, the osteogenic marker in postmenopausal women (Chiechi et al., 2002).

In a double-blind, randomized, controlled study on postmenopausal women, soy isoflavone supplementation for 12 months preserved hip bone mineral content in later postmenopausal women (>4 years after menopause) in women with lower body weight (≤median, 55.5 kg) and women with low calcium intake (≤median, 1095 mg/d) (Chen et al., 2004). In nonobese postmenopausal women, soy isoflavones dose-dependently inhibited bone loss at the spine and femoral neck by inhibiting bone resorption evident from reduced urinary deoxypyridinoline levels compared with the placebo group (Ye et al., 2006). In another study, isoflavones for three years increased vBMD in postmenopausal women (Shedd-Wise et al., 2011). Isoflavone supplementation on perimenopausal women for six months significantly reduced bone turnover markers CTX and PINP. This also significantly improved cardiovascular risk markers. However, a significant increase in TSH and reduced free thyroxine indicated a detrimental effect on thyroid function (Sathyapalan et al., 2017).

A meta-analysis of 26 randomized controlled trials on 2652 postmenopausal women found that isoflavones moderately reduced estrogen-deficient bone loss in the lumbar spine, femoral neck, and distal radius. Moreover, this beneficial effect against bone loss may be enhanced for isoflavone aglycones (Lambert et al., 2017a, 2017b). A recent meta-analysis of 52 controlled trials (5313 patients) also showed the protective effect of soy isoflavones on osteoporosis-related bone loss and BMD in the femur, neck, lumbar spine, and hip (Akhlaghi et al., 2020). These findings imply that soy phytoestrogens significantly affect bone metabolism and prevent osteoporosis in postmenopausal women. However, several meta-analyses of data suggest that the effect of isoflavones on the prevention of bone loss is negligible (Arcoraci et al., 2017; Liu et al., 2009; Jin et al., 2017).

In multiple clinical trials, the phytoestrogen genistein positively affected bone formation and prevented osteopenia in postmenopausal women (Marini et al., 2007, 2008; Atteritano et al., 2008, 2009). In a randomized, placebo-controlled, double-blind study, genistein given for six months prevented osteoporosis and reduced fracture risk (Lappe et al., 2013). Genistein in the form of aglycone tablets for two years had positive benefits on women with osteoporosis and postmenopausal osteopenia (Arcoraci et al., 2017).

13.3.5.1.2 Red Clover (Trifolium Pratense)

Red clover (RC) is rich in isoflavones, including formononetin, biochanin A, genistein, and daidzein. RC interacts with ER receptors and elicits a weak agonist, antagonist, or partial agonist-antagonist response depending upon the target tissue. A RC preparation (Rimostil) containing genistein, daidzein, formononetin, and biochanin was administered to 46 postmenopausal women in a double-blind protocol after a single-blind placebo phase followed by a single-blind washout phase. The Rimostil increased BMD in the radius and ulna in postmenopausal women (Thorup et al., 2015).

RC-derived isoflavone supplementation including biochanin A, formononetin, genistein, and daidzein for one year not only improved bone formation markers BALP and PINP but also ameliorated the decreases in BMC and BMD in lumbar spine in pre-, peri-, and postmenopausal women (Atkinson et al., 2004). In a double-blind, parallel design, placebo-controlled randomized controlled trial with 78 postmenopausal osteopenic women, RC extract in combination with calcium, magnesium, and calcitriol was given for 12 months. The combined RC extract was more effective than supplementation alone. Moreover, twice-daily intake of RC extract over one year prevented menopause-induced BMD loss, improved bone turnover markers, promoted a favorable estrogen metabolite profile (2-OH:16α-OH), and stimulated equal production in postmenopausal women with osteopenia (Lambert et al., 2017a, 2017b). Despite the limited evidence, it appears that RC isoflavones are beneficial for improving BMD in peri- and postmenopausal women.

13.3.5.1.3 Sheesham

D. sissoo, also known as Indian rosewood and Sheesham, has been used in traditional medicine to treat a variety of ailments. Ethanolic extracts of *D. sissoo* leaves are rich in 16 isoflavones and flavonols along with glucosides and an itaconic derivative. Of these, genstein, biochanin A, pratensein, biochanin 7-O-glucoside, and caviunin 7-O-[β-D-apiofuranosyl- (1$\rightarrow$6)-β-D-glucopyranoside] (CAFG) showed osteogenic effect (Dixit et al., 2012).

The standardized butanolic extract of *D. Sissoo* leaves accelerated new bone generation at osteotomy sites in rat femur, imitating improved fracture healing (Khedgikar et al., 2017). In a rat OVX model of postmenopausal osteoporosis, Sheesham leaves improved the trabecular microarchitecture of the long bones, increased the biomechanical strength of the vertebrae and femur, decreased bone turnover markers and osteoclastogenic genes expression, and increased osteogenic gene expression and new bone formation in the femur compared with vehicle (Khedgikar et al., 2012). It also prevented monosodium iodoacetate-induced osteoarthritis in rats and maintained the articular cartilage structure, morphology, and architecture at affected joints as well as the integrity of subchondral bone (Kothari et al., 2022).

Heartwood extract of *D. sissoo* stimulated new bone formation and accelerated callus formation at the osteotomy site. It not only improved trabecular parameters of the femur and L5, but it also restored femur-bending strength in an OVX-induced postmenopausal osteoporosis rat model. *D. sissoo* heartwood extract was also free of uterine and hepatic toxicity (Karvande et al., 2017). In a single-arm, pilot clinical study of adults (age 18–60 years) of both sexes, *D. sissoo* leaf extract (CAFG, 0.67%; biochanin 7-O-glucoside, 1.5%; genistein, 0.75%; pratensein, 0.2%, and biochanin-A, 1%) was given. The facture sites were humerus, ulna, fibula, radius, and tibia. After eight weeks, 300 mg b.d. *D. sissoo* extract, all fractures were healed and functional mobility was restored. The extract was well tolerated and posed no safety concerns (Raut et al., 2019).

13.3.5.1.4 Palas

Palas, also known as Bastard teak, has been known as a source of isoflavonoid and pterocarpan constitutive osteogenic agents. In a preclinical OVX model of osteoporosis, ethanolic extract from stem bark of *B. monosperma* prevented OVX-induced bone loss and the deterioration of bone microarchitecture and strength (Pandey et al., 2010). The stem bark extract of *B. monosperma* was found to be rich in 10 isoflavones, four coumestans, two pterocarpans, one flavanonol, two triterpenes, and three fatty esters (Maurya et al., 2009).

Of these, the skeletal effects and action mechanisms of isoflavones including cajanin (Bhargavan et al., 2009), cladrin (Khan et al., 2013; Gautam et al., 2011), formononetin (Gautam et al., 2011; Tyagi et al., 2012), isoformononetin (Srivastava et al., 2013), prunetin (Khan et al., 2015), and medicarpin (Dixit et al., 2015) have been extensively studied in preclinical models. All of these compounds showed osteogenic efficacy by increasing osteoblast survival and differentiation. In a preclinical rat model of OVX-induced bone loss, all of these prevented the deterioration of bone microarchitecture and strength and promoted new bone formation.

13.3.5.2 Other Isoflavonoid-Containing Plants

13.3.5.2.1 Alfalfa

Like red clover, alfalfa (*Medicago sativa*) is a member of the legume family. It is a well-known source of phytoestrogens such as coumestan, spinasterol, and ipriflavone. In a systematic review and meta-analysis of randomized controlled trials on 6427 postmenopausal women, ipriflavone showed efficacy for preventing and treating postmenopausal osteoporosis (Sansai et al., 2020).

13.3.5.2.2 Kasamadra

Cassia occidentalis is a common weed belonging to the family *Ceasalpiniaceae. C. occidentalis* is a rich source of apigenin-6 C-glucoside. The ethanolic extract of the leaf and stem of *C. occidentalis* has osteogenic effects and mitigates glucocorticoid-induced osteoporosis (Pal et al., 2019). The preclinical safety and toxicity of this extract showed no mortality and no adverse effects on the central nervous, cardiovascular, or respiratory systems at a 10 times higher dose. Moreover, the extract was not mutagenic and did not cause clastogenicity (Mugale et al., 2021).

13.3.5.2.3 Kudzu Root

Pueraria mirifica is a rich source of the isoflavones puerarin, daidzein, daidzin, mirficin, and salvianolic acid. In a randomized, double-blind, placebo-controlled study, after 24 weeks, *Pueraria mirifica* demonstrated an estrogen-like effect on bone turnover without affecting endometrial thickness and endometrial histology (Manonai et al., 2008).

SUMMARY AND CONCLUSION

Adult bone is maintained by remodeling that begins with bone resorption and culminates with the formation of new bone at the resorption site. The major cell types involved in bone remodeling are osteoclasts, osteoblasts, their progenitor cells, and adipocytes. Normal remodeling is characterized by the deposition of the same amount of bone following resorption to the site that underwent remodeling. An imbalance in remodeling in which resorption exceeds formation gives rise to osteoporosis that subsequently increases the risk of fracture. Hypogonadism, senility, imbalance of corticosteroid and thyroid hormones, CKD, and certain drugs are the major causes of osteoporosis.

In vitro and animal models for specific diseases of bone loss are routinely used for the discovery and development of osteoporosis therapies, and biologics dominate the therapeutic landscape of this most common bone disease. The current clinically used antiosteoporosis therapies are either antiresorptive or osteoanabolic. The fracture reduction efficacy of both classes of drugs has significant scope for improvement, particularly when hip fracture risk reduction is considered. This can be accomplished with a medication that will inhibit bone resorption while stimulating bone formation, by altering the bone remodeling cycle so that the balance in the coupled process of bone resorption and formation is restored.

The molecular targets that have been used so far include ERs, FPPS, RANKL, PTH1R, and Wnt pathway. In vitro assays measuring the differentiation and activities of osteoblasts, osteoclasts, and adipocytes provide initial screening tools for identifying the dual agent. The cellular effects are confirmed by measuring the expression of marker genes of these cell types. The in vivo efficacy of the lead compounds could be determined in at least two of the preclinical disease models that we have discussed in this chapter.

Phytochemicals have the dual function of promoting osteoblast function while diminishing osteoclast function, which is attributed to their pleiotropic effects, targeting the multiple molecular pathways involved in bone metabolism. Unlike traditional antiosteoporosis drugs, which typically target a specific pathway, the multifaceted actions of phytochemicals enable wide control of bone remodeling processes. However, their low bioavailability makes their clinical application challenging. To maximize their therapeutic potential, strategies are needed to improve their bioavailability such as nanoformulations or combination therapies.

ACKNOWLEDGEMENTS

Naibedya Chattopadhyay acknowledges grant-in-aid support from CSIR, project no: MLP2035.

CONFLICTS OF INTEREST

Naibedya Chattopadhyay has received a speaking fee from Eris Life Sciences, Ahmedabad; a sitting fee from Alkem Laboratories, Bengaluru; consultancy fees from Glaxo-Smith-Kline Consumer Health, Gurugram; Glenmark Pharmaceuticals, Mumbai; and Kinemora Biosciences, Mumbai, India; and sponsored research grants from Eurofins Advinus, Bengaluru; Sphaera Pharma, Gurugram; Tata Chemicals Limited, Pune; and Glaxo-Smith-Kline Consumer Health, Gurugram, India.

Konica Porwal has no conflicts of interest to declare.

LIST OF ABBREVIATIONS

5/6Nx	5/6 nephrectomy
ACTIVE	Abaloparatide comparator trial in vertebral endpoints
ALP	Alkaline phosphatase
BMP	Bone morphogenic proteins

BMSC	Bone marrow stromal cells
BPs	Bisphosphonates
C/EBP	CCAAT/enhancer-binding proteins
cAMP	Cyclic adenosine 3′,5′-monophosphate
CaP	Calcium phosphate
CKD-MBD	Chronic kidney disease-induced mineral and bone disorder
CPC	Cetylpyridinium chloride
CTX-1	C-terminal end of the telopeptide of type I collagen
DEX	Dexamethasone
ERα	Estrogen receptors alpha
ERβ	Estrogen receptors beta
FGF23	Fibroblast growth factor 23
GIOP	Glucocorticoid-induced osteoporosis
LRP5	Receptor related protein-5
M-CSF	Macrophage colony-stimulating factor
MP	Methylprednisolone
MSCs	Mesenchymal stem cells
NFATc1	Nuclear factor of activated T cells-1
ON	Osteonecrosis
OPN	Osteopontin
OVX	Ovariectomized
P1NP	Procollagen type I N-terminal propeptide
p-NPP	Para-nitrophenyl phosphate
PPARγ	Peroxisome proliferator-activated receptor gamma
PTH	Parathyroid hormone
PTH	Parathyroid hormone
PTH1R	PTH type 1R receptor
PTHrP	Parathyroid hormone-related protein
RANK	Receptor activator of nuclear factor κ B
RANKL	Receptor activator of nuclear factor kappa-B ligand
RC	Red clovers
Runx2	Runt-related transcription factor 2
SCD1	Stearoyl-coa desaturase
SERMs	Selective estrogen receptor modulators
SOST	Sclerostin
TGF-	β Transforming Growth Factor-β
TPTD	Teriparatide
TRAB-5b	Tartrate-resistant acid phosphatase-5b
Wnt	Wingless-related integration
Zol	Zoledronic acid

REFERENCES

Akhlaghi, M., Ghasemi Nasab, M., Riasatian, M., & Sadeghi, F. (2020). Soy isoflavones prevent bone resorption and loss, a systematic review and meta-analysis of randomized controlled trials. *Crit. Rev. Food Sci. Nutr.* 60: 2327–2341.

Akiyama, T., Shinzawa, M., & Akiyama, N. (2012). RANKL-RANK interaction in immune regulatory systems. *World J. Orthop.* 3: 142–150.

Allen, M. R., & Burr, D. B. (2007). Mineralization, microdamage, and matrix: How bisphosphonates influence material properties of bone. *IBMS BoneKEy*. 4: 49–60.

Allen, M. R., & Burr, D. B. (2014). Bone modeling and remodeling. In *Basic Appl. Bone Biol.* D. B. Burr, and M. R. Allen, Eds. Cambridge: Elsevier, pp. 75–90.

Arcoraci, V., Atteritano, M., Squadrito, F., D'Anna, R., Marini, H., Santoro, D., Minutoli, L., Messina, S., Altavilla, D., & Bitto, A. (2017). Antiosteoporotic activity of genistein aglycone in postmenopausal women: Evidence from a post-hoc analysis of a multicenter randomized controlled trial. *Nutrients*. 9: 179.

Asagiri, M., & Takayanagi, H. (2007). The molecular understanding of osteoclast differentiation. *Bone*. 40: 251–264.

Atashi, F., Modarressi, A., & Pepper, M. S. (2015). The role of reactive oxygen species in mesenchymal stem cell adipogenic and osteogenic differentiation: A review. *Stem Cells Dev*. 24: 1150–1163.

Atkinson, C., Compston, J. E., Day, N. E., Dowsett, M., & Bingham, S. A. (2004). The effects of phytoestrogen isoflavones on bone density in women: A double-blind, randomized, placebo-controlled trial. *Am. J. Clin. Nutr*. 79: 326–333.

Atteritano, M., Mazzaferro, S., Frisina, A., Cannata, M. L., Bitto, A., D'Anna, R., Squadrito, F., Macrì, I., Frisina, N., & Buemi, M. (2009). Genistein effects on quantitative ultrasound parameters and bone mineral density in osteopenic postmenopausal women. *Osteoporosis Int*. 20: 1947–1954.

Atteritano, M., Pernice, F., Mazzaferro, S., Mantuano, S., Frisina, A., D'Anna, R., Cannata, M. L., Bitto, A., Squadrito, F., Frisina, N., & Buemi, M. (2008). Effects of phytoestrogen genistein on cytogenetic biomarkers in postmenopausal women: 1 year randomized, placebo-controlled study. *Eur. J. Pharmacol*. 589: 22–26.

Balemans, W., Patel, N., Ebeling, M., Van Hul, E., Wuyts, W., Lacza, C., Dioszegi, M., Dikkers, F. G., Hildering, P., Willems, P. J., & Verheij, J. B. G. M. (2002). Identification of a 52 Kb deletion downstream of the SOST gene in patients with van buchem disease. *J. Med. Genet*. 39: 91–97.

Balhara, Y. P. S., Narang, P., Saha, S., Kandasamy, D., Chattopadhyay, N., & Goswami, R. (2022). Bone mineral density, bone microarchitecture and vertebral fractures in male patients with alcohol use disorders. *Alcohol Alcohol*. 57: 552–558.

Bandeira, L., Lewiecki, E. M., & Bilezikian, J. P. (2016). Pharmacodynamics and pharmacokinetics of oral salmon calcitonin in the treatment of osteoporosis. *Expert Opin. Drug Metab. Toxicol*. 12: 681–689.

Bhargavan, B., Gautam, A. K., Singh, D., Kumar, A., Chaurasia, S., Tyagi, A. M., Yadav, D. K., Mishra, J. S., Singh, A. B., Sanyal, S., & Chattopadhyay, N. (2009). Methoxylated isoflavones, cajanin and isoformononetin, have non-estrogenic bone forming effect via differential Mitogen Activated Protein Kinase (MAPK) signaling. *J. Cell. Biochem*. 108: 388–399.

Bhattacharyya, S., Pal, S., & Chattopadhyay, N. (2018). Targeted inhibition of sclerostin for post-menopausal osteoporosis therapy: A critical assessment of the mechanism of action. *Eur. J. Pharmacol*. 826: 39–47.

Bhattacharyya, S., Pal, S., & Chattopadhyay, N. (2019b). Abaloparatide, the second generation osteoanabolic drug: Molecular mechanisms underlying its advantages over the first-in-class teriparatide. *Biochem. Pharmacol*. 166: 185–191.

Bhattacharyya, S., Pal, S., Mohamed, R., Singh, P., Chattopadhyay, S., China, S. P., Porwal, K., Sanyal, S., Gayen, J. R., & Chattopadhyay, N. (2019a). A nutraceutical composition containing diosmin and hesperidin has osteogenic and anti-resorptive effects and expands the anabolic window of teriparatide. *Biomed. Pharmacother*. 118: 109207.

Bilezikian, J. P. (2007). Anabolic therapy for osteoporosis. *Women's Health*. 3: 243–253.

Binkley, N., Michael, B., Anna, S., Tasneem, V., Richard, T., Colin, M., Christine, E. B., James, P. G., & David, S. K. (2012). A phase 3 trial of the efficacy and safety of oral recombinant calcitonin: The oral alcitonin in postmenopausal osteoporosis (ORACAL) trial. *J. Bone Miner. Res*. 27: 1821–1829.

Bone, H. G., Bolognese, M. A., Yuen, C. K., Kendler, D. L., Miller, P. D., Yang, Y. C., Grazette, L., San Martin, J., & Gallagher, J. C. (2011). Effects of denosumab treatment and discontinuation on bone mineral density and bone turnover markers in postmenopausal women with low bone mass. *J. Clin. Endocrinol. Metab*. 96: 972–980.

Bone, H. G., Wagman, R. B., Brandi, M. L., Brown, J. P., Chapurlat, R., Cummings, S. R., Czerwiński, E., Fahrleitner-Pammer, A., Kendler, D. L., Lippuner, K., & Papapoulos, S. (2017). 10 years of denosumab treatment in postmenopausal women with osteoporosis: Results from the phase 3 randomised FREEDOM trial and open-label extension. *Lancet Diabetes Endocrinol*. 5: 513–523.

Bord, S., Horner, A., Beavan, S., & Compston, J. (2001). Estrogen receptors alpha and beta are differentially expressed in developing human bone. *J. Clin. Endocrinol. Metab*. 86: 2309–2314.

Bordukalo-Nikšić, T., Kufner, V., & Vukičević, S. (2022). The role of BMPs in the regulation of osteoclasts resorption and bone remodeling: From experimental models to clinical applications. *Front. Immunol.* 13: 869422.

Boyce, B., Yao, Z., & Xing, L. (2009). Osteoclasts have multiple roles in bone in addition to bone resorption. *Crit. Rev. Eukaryot. Gene Expr.* 19: 171–180.

Brits, D., Steyn, M., & L´ Abbé, E. N. (2014). A Histomorphological analysis of human and non-human femora. *Int. J. Leg. Med.* 128: 369–377.

Chakkalakal, D. A. (2005). Alcohol-induced bone loss and deficient bone repair. *Alcohol Clin. Exp.* 29: 2077–2090.

Chen, W. T., Han, D. C., Zhang, P. X., Han, N., Kou, Y. H., Yin, X. F., & Jiang, B. G. (2015). A special healing pattern in stable metaphyseal fractures. *Acta Orthop.* 86: 238–242.

Chen, Y. M., Ho, S. C., Lam, S. S., Ho, S. S., & Woo, J. L. (2004). Beneficial effect of soy isoflavones on bone mineral content was modified by years since menopause, body weight, and calcium intake: A double-blind, randomized, controlled trial. *Menopause.* 11: 246–254.

Cheraghi, Z., Doosti-Irani, A., Almasi-Hashiani, A., Baigi, V., Mansournia, N., Etminan, M., & Mansournia, M. A. (2019). The effect of alcohol on osteoporosis: A systematic review and meta-analysis. *Drug Alcohol Depend.* 197: 197–202.

Chesnut III, C. H., Silverman, S., Andriano, K., Genant, H., Gimona, A., Harris, S., Kiel, D., LeBoff, M., Maricic, M., Miller, P., & Moniz, C. (2000). A randomized trial of nasal spray salmon calcitonin in postmenopausal women with established osteoporosis: The prevent recurrence of osteoporotic fractures study. *Am. J. Med.* 109: 267–276.

Chiechi, L. M., Secreto, G., D'amore, M., Fanelli, M., Venturelli, E., Cantatore, F., Valerio, T., Laselva, G., & Loizzi, P. (2002). Efficacy of a soy rich diet in preventing postmenopausal osteoporosis: The menfis randomized trial. *Maturitas.* 42: 295–300.

Clark, D., Nakamura, M., Miclau, T., & Marcucio, R. (2017). Effects of aging on fracture healing. *Curr. Osteoporos. Rep.* 15: 601–608.

Cosman, F., Crittenden, D. B., Adachi, J. D., Binkley, N., Czerwinski, E., Ferrari, S., Hofbauer, L. C., Lau, E., Lewiecki, E. M., Miyauchi, A., & Grauer, A. (2016). Romosozumab treatment in postmenopausal women with osteoporosis. *N. Engl. J. Med.* 375: 1532–1543.

Cosman, F., Crittenden, D. B., Ferrari, S., Khan, A., Lane, N. E., Lippuner, K., Matsumoto, T., Milmont, C. E., Libanati, C., & Grauer, A. (2018). FRAME study: The foundation effect of building bone with 1 year of romosozumab leads to continued lower fracture risk after transition to denosumab. *J. Bone Miner. Res.* 33: 1219–1226.

Cosman, F., de Beur, S. J., LeBoff, M. S., Lewiecki, E. M., Tanner, B., Randall, S., & Lindsay, R. (2014). Clinician's guide to prevention and treatment of osteoporosis. *Osteoporosis Int.* 25: 2359–2381.

Cosman, F., Eriksen, E. F., Recknor, C., Miller, P. D., Guañabens, N., Kasperk, C., Papanastasiou, P., Readie, A., Rao, H., Gasser, J. A., & Boonen, S. (2011). Effects of intravenous zoledronic acid plus subcutaneous teriparatide [RhPTH(1–34)] in postmenopausal osteoporosis. *J. Bone Miner. Res.* 26: 503–511.

Costa, G. P., Leite, D. S., Prado, R. F. D., Silveira, V. Á. S., & Carvalho, Y. R. (2011). Effect of low-calcium diet and grind diet on bone turnover of ovariectomized female rats. *Oral med. pathol.* 16: 497–502.

Cummings, S. R., Martin, J. S., McClung, M. R., Siris, E. S., Eastell, R., Reid, I. R., Delmas, P., Zoog, H. B., Austin, M., Wang, A., & Kutilek, S. (2009). Denosumab for prevention of fractures in postmenopausal women with osteoporosis. *N. Engl. J. Med.* 361: 756–765.

Dai, J., Li, Y., Zhou, H., Chen, J., Chen, M., & Xiao, Z. (2013). Genistein promotion of osteogenic differentiation through BMP2/SMAD5/RUNX2 signaling. *Int. J. Biol. Sci.* 9: 1089–1098.

D'Amelio, P., Sassi, F., Buondonno, I., Fornelli, G., Spertino, E., D'Amico, L., Marchetti, M., Lucchiari, M., Roato, I., & Isaia, G. C. (2015). Treatment with intermittent PTH increases Wnt10b production by T cells in osteoporotic patients. *Osteoporosis Int.* 26: 2785–2791.

Danielsen, C. C., Mosekilde, L., & Svenstrup, B. (1993). Cortical bone mass, composition, and mechanical properties in female rats in relation to age, long-term ovariectomy, and estrogen substitution. *Calcif. Tissue Int.* 52: 26–33.

Deal, C., Omizo, M., Schwartz, E. N., Eriksen, E. F., Cantor, P., Wang, J., Glass, E. V., Myers, S. L., & Krege, J. H. (2005). Combination teriparatide and raloxifene therapy for postmenopausal osteoporosis: Results from a 6-month double-blind placebo-controlled trial. *J. Bone Miner. Res.* 20: 1905–1911.

Dean, T., Vilardaga, J. P., Potts Jr., J. T., & Gardella, T. J. (2008). Altered selectivity of Parathyroid Hormone (PTH) and PTH-related Protein (PTHrP) for distinct conformations of the PTH/PTHrP receptor. *Mol. Endocrinol.* 22: 156–166.

Delmas, P. D., Bjarnason, N. H., Mitlak, B. H., Ravoux, A. C., Shah, A. S., Huster, W. J., Draper, M., & Christiansen, C. (1997). Effects of raloxifene on bone mineral density, serum cholesterol concentrations, and uterine endometrium in postmenopausal women. *N. Engl. J. Med.* 337: 1641–1647.

Dixit, M., Raghuvanshi, A., Gupta, C. P., Kureel, J., Mansoori, M. N., Shukla, P., John, A. A., Singh, K., & Purohit, D. (2015). Medicarpin, a natural pterocarpan, heals cortical bone defect by activation of notch and Wnt canonical signaling pathways. *PLoS One*. 10: e0144541.

Dixit, P., Chillara, R., Khedgikar, V., Gautam, J., Kushwaha, P., Kumar, A., Lavanya, A., Pushpavalli, S. N. C. V. L., & Maurya, R. (2012). Constituents of dalbergia sissoo roxb. leaves with osteogenic activity. *Bioorganic Med. Chem. Lett.* 22: 890–897.

Donsante, S., Palmisano, B., Serafini, M., Robey, P. G., Corsi, A., & Riminucci, M. (2021). From stem cells to bone-forming cells. *Int. J. Mol. Sci.* 22: 3989.

Drake, M. T., Srinivasan, B., Mödder, U. I., Peterson, J. M., McCready, L. K., Riggs, B. L., Dwyer, D., Stolina, M., Kostenuik, P., & Khosla, S. (2010). Effects of parathyroid hormone treatment on circulating sclerostin levels in postmenopausal women. *J. Clin. Endocrinol. Metab.* 95: 5056–5062.

Drüeke, T. B., & Massy, Z. A. (2016). Changing bone patterns with progression of chronic kidney disease. *Kidney Int.* 89: 289–302.

Eastell, R., Christiansen, C., Grauer, A., Kutilek, S., Libanati, C., McClung, M. R., Reid, I. R., Resch, H., Siris, E., Uebelhart, D., Wang, A., Weryha, G., & Cummings, S. R. (2011). Effects of denosumab on bone turnover markers in postmenopausal osteoporosis. *J. Bone Miner. Res.* 26: 530–537.

El Khassawna, T., Böcker, W., Govindarajan, P., Schliefke, N., Hürter, B., Kampschulte, M., Schlewitz, G., Alt, V., Lips, K. S., Faulenbach, Möllmann, H., M., Zahner, D., Dürselen, L., Ignatius, A., Bauer, N., Wenisch, A. C. L., Schnettler, R., & Heiss, C. (2013). Effects of multi-deficiencies-diet on bone parameters of peripheral bone in ovariectomized mature rat. *PLoS One*. 8: e71665.

Farlay, D., Rizzo, S., Ste-Marie, L. G., Michou, L., Morin, S. N., Qiu, S., Chavassieux, P., Chapurlat, R. D., Rao, S. D., Brown, J. P., & Boivin, G. (2021). Duration-dependent increase of human bone matrix mineralization in long-term bisphosphonate users with atypical femur fracture. *J. Bone Miner. Res.* 36: 1031–1041.

Ferguson, V. L., Ayers, R. A., Bateman, T. A., & Simske, S. J. (2003). Bone development and age-related bone loss in male C57BL/6J mice. *Bone*. 33: 387–398.

Ferland-McCollough, D., Maselli, D., Spinetti, G., Sambataro, M., Sullivan, N., Blom, A., & Madeddu, P. (2018). MCP-1 feedback loop between adipocytes and mesenchymal stromal cells causes fat accumulation and contributes to hematopoietic stem cell rarefaction in the bone marrow of patients with diabetes. *Diabetes*. 67: 1380–1394.

Ferrari, G. O., Ferreira, J. C., Cavallari, R. T., Neves, K. R., dos Reis, L. M., Dominguez, W. V., Oliveira, E. C., Graciolli, F. G., Passlick-Deetjen, J., Jorgetti, V., & Moyses, R. (2014). Mineral bone disorder in chronic kidney disease: Head-to-head comparison of the 5/6 nephrectomy and adenine models. *BMC Nephrol.* 15: 1–7.

Finkelstein, J. S., Wyland, J. J., Lee, H., & Neer, R. M. (2010). Effects of teriparatide, alendronate, or both in women with postmenopausal osteoporosis. *J. Clin. Endocrinol. Metab.* 95: 1838–1845.

Flanagan, E. W., Most, J., Mey, J. T., & Redman, L. M. (2020). Calorie restriction and aging in humans. *Annu. Rev. Nutr.* 40: 105–133.

Florencio-Silva, R., Sasso, G. R. D. S., Sasso-Cerri, E., Simões, M. J., & Cerri, P. S. (2015). Biology of bone tissue: Structure, function, and factors that influence bone cells. *Biomed Res. Int.* 2015: 1–18.

Frost, H. M. (1983). The regional acceleratory phenomenon: A review. *Henry Ford Hosp. Med. J.* 31: 3–9.

Fujita, K., Roforth, M. M., Demaray, S., McGregor, U., Kirmani, S., McCready, L. K., Peterson, J. M., Drake, M. T., Monroe, D. G., & Khosla, S. (2014). Effects of estrogen on bone MRNA levels of sclerostin and other genes relevant to bone metabolism in postmenopausal women. *J. Clin. Endocrinol. Metab.* 99: E81.

Gao, H., Huang, J., Wei, Q., & He, C. (2023). Advances in animal models for studying bone fracture healing. *Bioengineering*. 10: 201.

Garnero, P., Sornay-Rendu, E., Munoz, F., Borel, O., & Chapurlat, R. D. (2013). Association of serum sclerostin with bone mineral density, bone turnover, steroid and parathyroid hormones, and fracture risk in postmenopausal women: The OFELY study. *Osteoporosis Int.* 24: 489–494.

Gautam, A. K., Bhargavan, B., Tyagi, A. M., Srivastava, K., Yadav, D. K., Kumar, M., Singh, A., Mishra, J. S., Singh, A. B., Sanyal, S., Maurya, R., Manickavasagam, L., Singh, S. P., Wahajuddin, W., Jain, G. K., Chattopadhyay, N., & Singh, D. (2011). Differential effects of formononetin and cladrin on osteoblast function, peak bone mass achievement and bioavailability in rats. *J. Nutr. Biochem.* 22: 318–327.

Genant, H. K. (2011). Bazedoxifene: A new selective estrogen receptor modulator for postmenopausal osteoporosis. *Menopause Int.* 17: 44–49.

Gennari, L., Merlotti, D., De Paola, V., & Nuti, R. (2010). Lasofoxifene: Evidence of its therapeutic value in osteoporosis. *Core Evid.* 4: 113–129.

Geusens, P., Marin, F., Kendler, D. L., Russo, L. A., Zerbini, C. A., Minisola, S., & Fahrleitner-Pammer, A. (2018). Effects of teriparatide compared with risedronate on the risk of fractures in subgroups of postmenopausal women with severe osteoporosis: The VERO trial. *J. Bone Miner. Res.* 33: 783–794.

Goldstein, S. R., Neven, P., Cummings, S., Colgan, T., Runowicz, C. D., Krpan, D., Proulx, J., Johnson, M., Thompson, D., Thompson, J., & Sriram, U. (2011). Postmenopausal evaluation and risk reduction with lasofoxifene (PEARL) trial: 5-year gynecological outcomes. *Menopause.* 18: 17–22.

Gomez-Puerto, M. C., Iyengar, P. V., García de Vinuesa, A., Ten Dijke, P., & Sanchez-Duffhues, G. (2019). Bone morphogenetic protein receptor signal transduction in human disease. *J. Pathol.* 247: 9–20.

Green, E. A., Choi, Y., & Flavell, R. A. (2002). Pancreatic lymph node-derived CD4(+)CD25(+) treg cells: Highly potent regulators of diabetes that require TRANCE-RANK signals. *Immunity.* 16: 183–191.

Greenblatt, M. B., Shim, J. H., Bok, S., & Kim, J. M. (2022). The extracellular signal-regulated kinase mitogen-activated protein kinase pathway in osteoblasts. *J. Bone Metab.* 29: 1–15.

Gruber, C., & Gruber, D. (2004). Bazedoxifene (Wyeth). *Curr. Opin. Investig. Drugs.* 5: 1086–1093.

Gunness, M., & Orwoll, E. (1995). Early induction of alterations in cancellous and cortical bone histology after orchiectomy in mature rats. *J. Bone Miner. Res.* 10: 1735–1744.

Hamza, A., & Şaramet, G. (2020). Actualities in endocrine pharmacology: Advances in the development of oral formulations for calcitonin and semaglutide. *Acta Endocrinol.* 16: 383–387.

He, F., Li, L., Li, P. P., Deng, Y., Yang, Y. Y., Deng, Y. X., Luo, H. H., Yao, X. T., Su, Y. X., Gan, H., & He, B. C. (2020). Cyclooxygenase-2/Sclerostin mediates TGF-B1-induced calcification in vascular smooth muscle cells and rats undergoing renal failure. *Aging.* 12: 21220–21235.

Histing, T., Garcia, P., Holstein, J. H., Klein, M., Matthys, R., Nuetzi, R., Steck, R., Laschke, M. W., Wehner, T., Bindl, R., Recknagel, S., Stuermer, E. K., Vollmar, B., Wildemann, B., Lienau, J., Willie, B., Peters, A., Ignatius, A., Pohlemann. T., Claes, L., & Menger, M. D. (2011). Small animal bone healing models: Standards, tips, and pitfalls results of a consensus meeting. *Bone.* 49: 591–599.

Huntley, R., Davydova, J., Petryk, A., Billington Jr., C. J., Jensen, E. D., Mansky, K. C., & Gopalakrishnan, R. (2015). The function of twisted gastrulation in regulating osteoclast differentiation is dependent on BMP binding. *J. Cell. Biochem.* 116: 2239–2246.

Huntley, R., Jensen, E., Gopalakrishnan, R., & Mansky, K. C. (2019). Bone morphogenetic proteins: Their role in regulating osteoclast differentiation. *Bone Rep.* 10: 100207.

Ijiri, K., Ma, Y. F., Jee, W. S. S., Akamine, T., & Liang, X. (1995). Adaptation of non-growing former epiphysis and metaphyseal trabecular bones to aging and immobilization in rat. *Bone.* 17: S207–S212.

Jähn-Rickert, K., Wölfel, E. M., Jobke, B., Riedel, C., Hellmich, M., Werner, M., McDonald, M. M., & Busse, B. (2020). Elevated bone hardness under denosumab treatment, with persisting lower osteocyte viability during discontinuation. *Front. Endocrinol.* 11: 250.

Jang, H. D., Hong, J. Y., Han, K., Lee, J. C., Shin, B. J., Choi, S. W., Suh, S. W., Yang, J. H., Park, S. Y., & Bang, C. (2017). Relationship between bone mineral density and alcohol intake: A nationwide health survey analysis of postmenopausal women. *PLoS One.* 12: e0180132.

Jaworski, Z. F. G., & Uhthoff, H. K. L. (1986). Disuse osteoporosis: Current status and problems. In *Curr. Concep. Bone Frag.* Z. F. G. Jaworski, and H. K. L. Uhthoff, Eds. Berlin: Springer, pp. 181–194.

Jee, W. S., & Yao, W. (2001). Overview: Animal models of osteopenia and osteoporosis. *J. Musculoskeletal Neuronal Interact.* 1: 193–207.

Jiang, Z., Li, Z., Zhang, W., Yang, Y., Han, B., Liu, W., & Peng, Y. (2018). Dietary natural N-Acetyl-d-Glucosamine prevents bone loss in ovariectomized rat model of postmenopausal osteoporosis. *Molecules.* 23: 2302.

Jin, Y. X., Wu, P., Mao, Y. F., Wang, B., Zhang, J. F., Chen, W. L., Liu, Z., & Shi, X. L. (2017). Chinese herbal medicine for osteoporosis: A meta-analysis of randomized controlled trials. *J. Clin. Densitom.* 20: 516–525.

Kalu, D. N., Hardin, R. H., Cockerham, R., & Yu, B. P. (1984). Aging and dietary modulation of rat skeleton and parathyroid hormone. *Endocrinology*. 115: 1239–1247.

Kamiya, N., Ye, L., Kobayashi, T., Mochida, Y., Yamauchi, M., Kronenberg, H. M., Feng, J. Q., & Mishina, Y. (2008). BMP signaling negatively regulates bone mass through sclerostin by inhibiting the canonical Wnt pathway. *Development*. 135: 3801–3811.

Kanis, J. A., Harvey, N. C., McCloskey, E., Bruyère, O., Veronese, N., Lorentzon, M., Cooper, C., Rizzoli, R., Adib, G., Al-Daghri, N., Campusano, C., Chandran, M., Dawson-Hughes, B., Javaid, K., Jiwa, F., Johansson, H., Lee, J. K., Liu, E., Messina, D., Mkinsi, O., Pinto, D., Prieto-Alhambra, D., Saag, K., Xia, W., & Reginster, J. Y. (2020). Algorithm for the management of patients at low, high and very high risk of osteoporotic fractures. *Osteoporosis Int*. 31: 1–12.

Karvande, A., Khedgikar, V., Kushwaha, P., Ahmad, N., Kothari, P., Verma, A., Kumar, P., Nagar, G. K., Mishra, P. R., Maurya, R., & Trivedi, R. (2017). Heartwood extract from Dalbergia Sissoo promotes fracture healing and its application in ovariectomy-induced osteoporotic rats. *J. Pharm. Pharmacol*. 69: 1381–1397.

Ke, H. Z., Jee, W. S., Zeng, Q. Q., Li, M., & Lin, B. Y. (1993). Prostaglandin E2 increased rat cortical bone mass when administered immediately following ovariectomy. *Bone Miner*. 21: 189–201.

Kendler, D. L., Bone, H. G., Massari, F., Gielen, E., Palacios, S., Maddox, J., Yan, C., Yue, S., Dinavahi, R. V., Libanati, C., & Grauer, A. (2019). Bone mineral density gains with a second 12-month course of romosozumab therapy following placebo or denosumab. *Osteoporos. Int*. 30: 2437–2448.

Kennel, K. A., & Drake, M. T. (2009). Adverse effects of bisphosphonates: Implications for osteoporosis management. *Mayo. Clin. Proc*. 84: 632–638.

Khan, K., Pal, S., Yadav, M., Maurya, R., Trivedi, A. K., Sanyal, S., & Chattopadhyay, N. (2015). Prunetin signals via G-protein-coupled receptor, GPR30(GPER1): Stimulation of adenylyl cyclase and CAMP-mediated activation of MAPK signaling induces Runx2 expression in osteoblasts to promote bone regeneration. *J. Nutr. Biochem*. 26: 1491–1501.

Khan, K., Sharan, K., Swarnkar, G., Chakravarti, B., Mittal, M., Barbhuyan, T. K., China, S. P., Khan, M. P., Nagar, G. K., Yadav, D., Dixit, P., Maurya, R., & Chattopadhyay, N. (2013). Positive skeletal effects of cladrin, a naturally occurring dimethoxydaidzein, in osteopenic rats that were maintained after treatment discontinuation. *Osteoporos. Int*. 24: 1455–1470.

Khan, M. P., Khan, K., Yadav, P. S., Singh, A. K., Nag, A., Prasahar, P., Mittal, M., China, S. P., Tewari, M. C., Nagar, G. K., Tewari, D., Trivedi, A. K., Sanyal, S., Bandyopadhyay, A., & Chattopadhyay, N. (2016). BMP signaling is required for adult skeletal homeostasis and mediates bone anabolic action of parathyroid hormone. *Bone*. 92: 132–144.

Khedgikar, V., Gautam, J., Kushwaha, P., Kumar, A., Nagar, G. K., Dixit, P., Chillara, R., Voruganti, S., Singh, S. P., Uddin, W., & Jain, G. K. (2012). A standardized phytopreparation from an Indian medicinal plant (Dalbergia Sissoo) has antiresorptive and bone-forming effects on a postmenopausal osteoporosis model of rat. *Menopause*. 19: 1336–1346.

Khedgikar, V., Kushwaha, P., Ahmad, N., Gautam, J., Kumar, P., Maurya, R., & Trivedi, R. (2017). Ethanolic extract of dalbergia sissoo promotes rapid regeneration of cortical bone in drill-hole defect model of rat. *Biomed. Pharmacother*. 86: 16–22.

Kiechl, S., Wittmann, J., Giaccari, A., Knoflach, M., Willeit, P., Bozec, A., Moschen, A. R., Muscogiuri, G., Sorice, G. P., Kireva, T., & Summerer, M. (2013). Blockade of Receptor Activator of Nuclear Factor-KB (RANKL) signaling improves hepatic insulin resistance and prevents development of diabetes mellitus. *Nat. Med*. 19: 358–363.

Kim, K., Anderson, E. M., Thome, T., Lu, G., Salyers, Z. R., Cort, T. A., O'Malley, K. A., Scali, S. T., & Ryan, T. E. (2021). Skeletal myopathy in CKD: A comparison of adenine-induced nephropathy and 5/6 nephrectomy models in mice. *Am. J. Physiol.—Ren. Physiol*. 321: F106–F119.

Kim, S. G., Zhou, J., Solomon, C., Zheng, Y., Suzuki, T., Chen, M., Song, S., Jiang, N., Cho, S., & Mao, J. J. (2012). Effects of growth factors on dental stem/progenitor cells. *Dent. Clin. N. Am*. 56: 563–575.

Kimmel, D. B., & Wronski, T. J. (1990). Nondestructive measurement of bone mineral in femurs from ovariectomized rats. *Calcif. Tissue Int*. 46: 101–110.

Klinkhammer, B. M., Djudjaj, S., Kunter, U., Palsson, R., Edvardsson, V. O., Wiech, T., Thorsteinsdottir, M., Hardarson, S., Foresto-Neto, O., Mulay, S. R., & Moeller, M. J. (2020). Cellular and molecular mechanisms of kidney injury in 2,8-dihydroxyadenine mephropathy. *J. Am. Soc. Nephrol*. 31: 799–816.

Knoop, K. A., Kumar, N., Butler, B. R., Sakthivel, S. K., Taylor, R. T., Nochi, T., Akiba, H., Yagita, H., Kiyono, H., & Williams, I. R. (2009). RANKL is necessary and sufficient to initiate development of antigen-sampling M cells in the intestinal epithelium. *J. Immun*. 183: 5738–5747.

Kogawa, M., Wijenayaka, A. R., Ormsby, R. T., Thomas, G. P., Anderson, P. H., Bonewald, L. F., Findlay, D. M., & Atkins, G. J. (2013). Sclerostin regulates release of bone mineral by osteocytes by induction of carbonic anhydrase 2. *J. Bone Miner. Res.* 28: 2436–2448.

Komm, B. S., & Chines, A. A. (2012). Bazedoxifene: The evolving role of third-generation selective estrogen-receptor modulators in the management of postmenopausal osteoporosis. *Ther. Adv. Musculoskelet. Dis.* 4: 21–34.

Komori, T. (2015). Animal models for osteoporosis. *Eur. J. Pharmacol.* 759: 287–294.

Kothari, P., Tripathi, A. K., Girme, A., Rai, D., Singh, R., Sinha, S., Choudhary, D., Nagar, G. K., Maurya, R., Hingorani, L., & Trivedi, R. (2022). Caviunin glycoside (CAFG) from dalbergia sissoo attenuates osteoarthritis by modulating chondrogenic and matrix regulating proteins. *J. Ethnopharmacol.* 282: 114315.

Krishna, S. M., Seto, S. W., Jose, R. J., Li, J., Morton, S. K., Biros, E., Wang, Y., Nsengiyumva, V., Lindeman, J. H., Loots, G. G., & Rush, C. M. (2017). Wnt signaling pathway inhibitor sclerostin inhibits angiotensin II-induced aortic aneurysm and atherosclerosis. *Arterioscler. Thromb. Vasc. Biol.* 37: 553–566.

Lademann, F., Hofbauer, L. C., & Rauner, M. (2020). The bone morphogenetic protein pathway: The osteoclastic perspective. *Front. Cell Dev. Biol.* 8: 586031.

Lagari, V. S., & Levis, S. (2014). Phytoestrogens for menopausal bone loss and climacteric symptoms. *J. Steroid Biochem. Mol. Biol.* 139: 294–301.

Lambert, M. N. T., Hu, L. M., & Jeppesen, P. B. (2017a). A systematic review and meta-analysis of the effects of isoflavone formulations against estrogen-deficient bone resorption in peri- and postmenopausal women. *Am. J. Clin. Nutr.* 106: 801–811.

Lambert, M. N. T., Thybo, C. B., Lykkeboe, S., Rasmussen, L. M., Frette, X., Christensen, L. P., & Jeppesen, P. B. (2017b). Combined bioavailable isoflavones and probiotics improve bone status and estrogen metabolism in postmenopausal osteopenic women: A randomized controlled trial. *Am. J. Clin. Nutr.* 106: 909–920.

Langdahl, B., Ferrari, S., & Dempster, D. W. (2016). Bone modeling and remodeling: Potential as therapeutic targets for the treatment of osteoporosis. *Ther. Adv. Musculoskelet. Dis.* 8: 225–235.

Lappe, J., Kunz, I., Bendik, I., Prudence, K., Weber, P., Recker, R., & Heaney, R. P. (2013). Effect of a combination of genistein, polyunsaturated fatty acids and vitamins D3 and K1 on bone mineral density in postmenopausal women: A randomized, placebo-controlled, double-blind pilot study. *Eur. J. Nutr.* 52: 203–215.

Lelovas, P. P., Xanthos, T. T., Thoma, S. E., Lyritis, G. P., & Dontas, I. A. (2008). The laboratory rat as an animal model for osteoporosis research. *Comp. Med.* 58: 424–430.

Lewiecki, E. M. (2009). Lasofoxifene for the prevention and treatment of postmenopausal osteoporosis. *Ther. Clin. Risk Manag.* 5: 817–827.

Lewiecki, E. M. (2010). Bisphosphonates for the treatment of osteoporosis: Insights for clinicians. *Ther. Adv. Chronic Dis.* 1: 115–128.

Li, D., Yang, Z., Wei, Z., & Kang, P. (2018). Efficacy of bisphosphonates in the treatment of femoral head osteonecrosis: A PRISMA-compliant meta-analysis of animal studies and clinical trials. *Sci. Rep.* 8: 1450.

Li, J. Y., Walker, L. D., Tyagi, A. M., Adams, J., Weitzmann, M. N., & Pacifici, R. (2014). The sclerostin-independent bone anabolic activity of intermittent PTH treatment is mediated by T-cell-produced Wnt10b. *J. Bone Miner. Res.* 29: 43–54.

Liu, J., Ho, S. C., Su, Y. X., Chen, W. Q., Zhang, C. X., & Chen, Y. M. (2009). Effect of long-term intervention of soy isoflavones on bone mineral density in women: A meta-analysis of randomized controlled trials. *Bone*. 44: 948–953.

Liu, X. L., Li, C. L., Lu, W. W., Cai, W. X., & Zheng, L. W. (2015). Skeletal site-specific response to ovariectomy in a rat model: Change in bone density and microarchitecture. *Clin. Oral Implants Res.* 26: 392–398.

Loser, K., Mehling, A., Loeser, S., Apelt, J., Kuhn, A., Grabbe, S., Schwarz, T., Penninger, J. M., & Beissert, S. (2006). Epidermal RANKL controls regulatory T-cell numbers via activation of dendritic cells. *Nat. Med.* 12: 1372–1379.

Luo, Z., Liu, Y., Liu, Y., Chen, H., Shi, S., & Liu, Y. (2017). Cellular and molecular mechanisms of alcohol-induced osteopenia. *Cell. Mol. Life Sci.* 74: 4443–4453.

Ma, S., Goh, E. L., Jin, A., Bhattacharya, R., Boughton, O. R., Patel, B., Karunaratne, A., Vo, N. T., Atwood, R., Cobb, J. P., & Hansen, U. (2017). Long-term effects of bisphosphonate therapy: Perforations, microcracks and mechanical properties. *Sci. Rep.* 7: 43399.

Ma, S., Qin, J., Hao, Y., & Fu, L. (2020). Association of gut microbiota composition and function with an aged rat model of senile osteoporosis using 16S RRNA and metagenomic sequencing analysis. *Aging*. 12: 10795–10808.

Maeda, K., Kobayashi, Y., Udagawa, N., Uehara, S., Ishihara, A., Mizoguchi, T., Kikuchi, Y., Takada, I., Kato, S., Kani, S., & Nishita, M. (2012). Wnt5a-Ror2 signaling between osteoblast-lineage cells and osteoclast precursors enhances osteoclastogenesis. *Nat. Med.* 18: 405–412.

Manonai, J., Apichart, C., Umaporn, U., Hathai, T., & Urusa, T. (2008). Effects and safety of *Pueraria mirifica* on lipid profiles and biochemical markers of bone turnover rates in healthy postmenopausal women. *Menopause.* 3: 530–35.

Marini, H., Bitto, A., Altavilla, D., Burnett, B. P., Polito, F., Di Stefano, V., Minutoli, L., Atteritano, M., Levy, R. M., D'Anna, R., Frisina, N., Mazzaferro, S., Cancellieri, F., Cannata, M. L., Corrado, F., Frisina, A., Adamo, V., Lubrano, C., Sansotta, C., Marini, R., Adamo, E. B., & Squadrito, F. (2008). Breast safety and efficacy of genistein aglycone for postmenopausal bone loss: A follow-up study. *J. Clin. Endocrinol. Metab.* 12: 4787–4796.

Marini, H., Minutoli, L., Polito, F., Bitto, A., Altavilla, D., Atteritano, M., Gaudio, A., Mazzaferro, S., Frisina, A., Frisina, N., Lubrano, C., Bonaiuto, M., D'Anna, R., Cannata, M. L., Corrado, F., Adamo, E. B., Wilson, S., & Squadrito, F. (2007). Effects of the phytoestrogen genistein on bone metabolism in osteopenic postmenopausal women: A randomized trial. *Ann. Intern. Med.* 12: 839–847.

Masoro, E. J. (2005). Overview of caloric restriction and ageing. *Mech. Ageing Dev.* 126: 913–922.

Matsushita, M., Tsuboyama, T., Kasai, R., Okumura, H., Yamamuro, T., Higuchi, K., Higuchi, K., Kohno, A., Yonezu, T., Utani, A., & Umezawa, M. (1986). Age-related changes in bone mass in the Senescence-Accelerated Mouse (SAM): SAM-R/3 and SAM-P/6 as new murine models for senile osteoporosis. *Am. J. Pathol.* 125: 276–286.

Maurya, R., Yadav, D. K., Singh, G., Bhargavan, B., Murthy, P. N., Sahai, M., & Singh, M. M. (2009). Osteogenic activity of constituents from butea monosperma. *Bioorganic Med. Chem. Lett.* 19: 610–613.

McClung, M. R., Grauer, A., Boonen, S., Bolognese, M. A., Brown, J. P., Diez-Perez, A., Langdahl, B. L., Reginster, J. Y., Zanchetta, J. R., Wasserman, S. M., & Katz, L. (2014). Romosozumab in postmenopausal women with low bone mineral density. *N. Engl. J. Med.* 370: 248–259.

McGovern, J. A., Griffin, M., & Hutmacher, D. W. (2018). Animal models for bone tissue engineering and modelling disease. *Dis. Model Mech.* 11: dmm033084.

McLaughlin, M. B., Awosika, A. O., & Jialal, I. (2024). *Calcitonin*. StatPearls Publishing. Treasure Island, Florida, United States.

McNerny, E. M., Buening, D. T., Aref, M. W., Chen, N. X., Moe, S. M., & Allen, M. R. (2019). Time course of rapid bone loss and cortical porosity formation observed by longitudinal MCT in a rat model of CKD. *Bone*. 125: 16–24.

Melhus, G., Solberg, L. B., Dimmen, S., E Madsen, J., Nordsletten, L., & P Reinholt, F. (2007). Experimental osteoporosis induced by ovariectomy and vitamin D deficiency does not markedly affect fracture healing in rats. *Acta Orthop*. 78: 393–403.

Meyer Jr., R. A., Meyer, M. H., Tenholder, M., Wondracek, S., Wasserman, R., & Garges, P. (2003). Gene expression in older rats with delayed union of femoral fractures. *J. Bone Joint Surg. Am.* 85: 1243–1254.

Miki, T., & Naka, H. (2005). Bisphosphonates and bone quality. *Clin. Calcium*. 15: 1020–1025.

Miller, P. D., Chines, A. A., Christiansen, C., Hoeck, H. C., Kendler, D. L., Lewiecki, E. M., Woodson, G., Levine, A. B., Constantine, G., & Delmas, P. D. (2008). Effects of bazedoxifene on BMD and bone turnover in postmenopausal women: 2-yr results of a randomized, double-blind, placebo-, and active-controlled study. *J. Bone Miner. Res.* 23: 525–535.

Miller, P. D., Hattersley, G., Riis, B. J., Williams, G. C., Lau, E., Russo, L. A., Alexandersen, P., Zerbini, C. A., Hu, M. Y., Harris, A. G., & Fitzpatrick, L. A. (2016). Effect of abaloparatide vs placebo on new vertebral fractures in postmenopausal women with osteoporosis: A randomized clinical trial. *JAMA*. 316: 722–733.

Mödder, U. I., Hoey, K. A., Amin, S., McCready, L. K., Achenbach, S. J., Riggs, B. L., Melton III, L. J., & Khosla, S. (2011). Relation of age, gender, and bone mass to circulating sclerostin levels in women and men. *J. Bone Miner. Res.* 26: 373–379.

Morsczeck, C., Reck, A., & Reichert, T. E. (2017). WNT3A and the induction of the osteogenic differentiation in adipose tissue derived mesenchymal stem cells. *Tissue Cell*. 49: 489–494.

Mugale, M. N., Shukla, S., Chourasia, M. K., Hanif, K., Nazir, A., Singh, S., Gayen, J. R., Kumaravelu, J., Tripathi, R. K., Mohrana, B., & Kumar, A. (2021). Regulatory safety pharmacology and toxicity assessments of a standardized stem extract of cassia occidentalis linn. in rodents. *Regul. Toxicol. Pharmacol.* 123: 104960.

Nakao, Y., Koike, T., Ohta, Y., Manaka, T., Imai, Y., & Takaoka, K. (2009). Parathyroid hormone enhances bone morphogenetic protein activity by increasing intracellular 3', 5'-cyclic adenosine monophosphate accumulation in osteoblastic MC3T3-E1 cells. *Bone*. 44: 872–877.

Nauth, A., Schemitsch, E., Norris, B., Nollin, Z., & Watson, J. T. (2018). Critical-size bone defects: Is there a consensus for diagnosis and treatment? *J. Orthop. Trauma*. 32: S7–S11.

Neer, R. M., Arnaud, C. D., Zanchetta, J. R., Prince, R., Gaich, G. A., Reginster, J. Y., Hodsman, A. B., Eriksen, E. F., Ish-Shalom, S., Genant, H. K., & Wang, O. (2001). Effect of parathyroid hormone (1–34) on fractures and bone mineral density in postmenopausal women with osteoporosis. *N. Engl. J. Med*. 344: 1434–1441.

Nsengiyumva, V., Krishna, S. M., Moran, C. S., Moxon, J. V., Morton, S. K., Clarke, M. W., Seto, S. W., & Golledge, J. (2020). Vitamin D deficiency promotes large rupture-prone abdominal aortic aneurysms and cholecalciferol supplementation limits progression of aneurysms in a mouse model. *Clin. Sci*. 134: 2521–2534.

Okamoto, M., Murai, J., Imai, Y., Ikegami, D., Kamiya, N., Kato, S., Mishina, Y., Yoshikawa, H., & Tsumaki, N. (2011). Conditional deletion of Bmpr1a in differentiated osteoclasts increases osteoblastic bone formation, increasing volume of remodeling bone in mice. *J. Bone Miner. Res*. 26: 2511–2522.

Ominsky, M. S., Boyd, S. K., Varela, A., Jolette, J., Felx, M., Doyle, N., Mellal, N., Smith, S. Y., Locher, K., Buntich, S., & Pyrah, I. (2017). Romosozumab improves bone mass and strength while maintaining bone quality in ovariectomized cynomolgus monkeys. *J. Bone Miner. Res*. 32: 788–801.

Pal, S., Porwal, K., Khanna, K., Gautam, M. K., Malik, M. Y., Rashid, M., Macleod, R. J., Wahajuddin, M., Parameswaran, V., Bellare, J. R., & Chattopadhyay, N. (2019). Oral dosing of pentoxifylline, a pan-phosphodiesterase inhibitor restores bone mass and quality in osteopenic rabbits by an osteogenic mechanism: A comparative study with human parathyroid hormone. *Bone*. 123: 28–38.

Pal, S., Rashid, M., Singh, S. K., Porwal, K., Singh, P., Mohamed, R., Gayen, J. R., Wahajuddin, M., & Chattopadhyay, N. (2020). Skeletal restoration by phosphodiesterase 5 inhibitors in osteopenic mice: Evidence of osteoanabolic and osteoangiogenic effects of the drugs. *Bone*. 135: 115305.

Pandey, R., Gautam, A. K., Bhargavan, B., Trivedi, R., Swarnkar, G., Nagar, G. K., Yadav, D. K., Kumar, M., Rawat, P., Manickavasagam, L., & Kumar, A. (2010). Total extract and standardized fraction from the stem bark of butea monosperma have osteoprotective action: Evidence for the nonestrogenic osteogenic effect of the standardized fraction. *Menopause*. 17: 602–610.

Park, C. H., Jung, K. J., Nho, J. H., Kim, J. H., Won, S. H., Chun, D. I., & Byun, D. W. (2019). Impact on bisphosphonate persistence and compliance: Daily postprandial administration. *J. Bone Metab*. 26: 39–44.

Pavone, V., Testa, G., Giardina, S. M., Vescio, A., Restivo, D. A., & Sessa, G. (2017). Pharmacological therapy of osteoporosis: A systematic current review of literature. *Front. Pharmacol*. 8: 803.

Permuy, M., López-Peña, M., Muñoz, F., & González-Cantalapiedra, A. (2019). Rabbit as model for osteoporosis research. *J. Bone Miner. Metab*. 37: 573–583.

Pietschmann, P., Skalicky, M., Kneissel, M., Rauner, M., Hofbauer, G., Stupphann, D., & Viidik, A. (2007). Bone structure and metabolism in a rodent model of male senile osteoporosis. *Exp. Gerontol*. 42: 1099–1108.

Porwal, K., Pal, S., Bhagwati, S., Siddiqi, M. I., & Chattopadhyay, N. (2021). Therapeutic potential of phosphodiesterase inhibitors in the treatment of osteoporosis: Scopes for therapeutic repurposing and discovery of new oral osteoanabolic drugs. *Eur. J. Pharmacol*. 899: 174015.

Porwal, K., Pal, S., Tewari, D., Pal China, S., Singh, P., Chandra Tewari, M., Prajapati, G., Singh, P., Cheruvu, S., Khan, Y. A., & Sanyal, S. (2019). Increased bone marrow-specific adipogenesis by clofazimine causes impaired fracture healing, osteopenia and osteonecrosis without extra-skeletal effects in rats. *Toxicol. Sci*. 172: 167–180.

Pozzi, A., Risselada, M., & Winter, M. D. (2012). Assessment of fracture healing after minimally invasive plate osteosynthesis or open reduction and internal fixation of coexisting radius and ulna fractures in dogs via ultrasonography and radiography. *J. Am. Vet. Med*. 241: 744–753.

Quarto, N., Behr, B., & Longaker, M. T. (2010). Opposite spectrum of activity of canonical Wnt signaling in the osteogenic context of undifferentiated and differentiated mesenchymal cells: Implications for tissue engineering. *Tissue Eng. A*. 16: 3185–3197.

Rauner, M., Taipaleenmäki, H., Tsourdi, E., & Winter, E. M. (2021). Osteoporosis treatment with anti-sclerostin antibodies-mechanisms of action and clinical application. *J. Clin. Med*. 10: 1–21.

Raut, A. A., Agashe, S. V., Wajahat, A., Sarada, C. V., Vaidya, A. D., & Vaidya, R. A. (2019). A clinical study of a standardized extract of leaves of dalbergia sissoo (Roxb Ex DC) in postmenopausal osteoporosis. *J. Mid-Life Health*. 10: 37–42.

Ren, H., Liang, D., Jiang, X., Tang, J., Cui, J., Wei, Q., & Lin, S. (2015). Variance of spinal osteoporosis induced by dexamethasone and methylprednisolone and its associated mechanism. *Steroids*. 102: 65–75.

Rude, C. (1985). Management of closed fractures. *Clin Podiatry*. 2: 199–216.

Saag, K. G., Petersen, J., Brandi, M. L., Karaplis, A. C., Lorentzon, M., Thomas, T., Maddox, J., Fan, M., Meisner, P. D., & Grauer, A. (2017). Romosozumab or alendronate for fracture prevention in women with osteoporosis. *N. Engl. J. Med*. 377: 1417–1427.

Saag, K. G., Shane, E., Boonen, S., Marín, F., Donley, D. W., Taylor, K. A., Dalsky, G. P., & Marcus, R. (2007). Teriparatide or alendronate in glucocorticoid-induced osteoporosis. *N. Engl. J. Med*. 357: 2028–2039.

Saita, Y., Ishijima, M., & Kaneko, K. (2015). Atypical femoral fractures and bisphosphonate use: Current evidence and clinical implications. *Ther. Adv. Chronic Dis*. 6: 185–193.

Sansai, K., Na Takuathung, M., Khatsri, R., Teekachunhatean, S., Hanprasertpong, N., & Koonrungsesomboon, N. (2020). Effects of isoflavone interventions on bone mineral density in postmenopausal women: A systematic review and meta-analysis of randomized controlled trials. *Osteoporos. Int*. 31: 1853–1864.

Sathyapalan, T., Aye, M., Rigby, A. S., Fraser, W. D., Thatcher, N. J., Kilpatrick, E. S., & Atkin, S. L. (2017). Soy reduces bone turnover markers in women during early menopause: A randomized controlled trial. *Bone Miner. Res*. 32: 157–164.

Scheiber, M. D., Liu, J. H., Subbiah, M. T. R., Rebar, R. W., & Setchell, K. D. (2001). Dietary inclusion of whole soy foods results in significant reductions in clinical risk factors for osteoporosis and cardiovascular disease in normal postmenopausal women. *Menopause*. 8: 384–392.

Schmitz, J. P., & Hollinger, J. O. (1986). The critical size defect as an experimental model for craniomandibulofacial nonunions. *Clin. Orthop. Relat. Res*. 205: 299–308.

Sewell, K. L. (1995). Iatrogenic osteoporosis. *Arch. Dermatol*. 131: 1321–1322.

Sharma, K., Awasthi, P., Prakash, R., Khanka, S., Bajpai, R., Sahasrabuddhe, A. A., Goel, A., & Singh, D. (2022). Maintenance of increased bone mass after PTH withdrawal by sequential medicarpin treatment via augmentation of CAMP-PKA pathway. *J. Cell. Biochem*. 123: 1762–1779.

Shedd-Wise, K. M., Alekel, D. L., Hofmann, H., Hanson, K. B., Schiferl, D. J., Hanson, L. N., & Van Loan, M. D. (2011). The soy isoflavones for reducing bone loss study: 3-yr effects on PQCT bone mineral density and strength measures in postmenopausal women. *J. Clin. Densitom*. 14: 47–57.

Shi, C., Zhang, H., Louie, K. A., Mishina, Y., & Sun, H. (2017). BMP signaling mediated by BMPR1A in osteoclasts negatively regulates osteoblast mineralization through suppression of Cx43. *J. Cell. Biochem*. 118: 605–614.

Siris, E. S., Harris, S. T., Eastell, R., Zanchetta, J. R., Goemaere, S., Diez-Perez, A., Stock, J. L., Song, J., Qu, Y., Kulkarni, P. M., & Siddhanti, S. R. (2005). Skeletal effects of raloxifene after 8 years: Results from the continuing outcomes relevant to Evista (CORE) study. *J. Bone Miner. Res*. 20: 1514–1524.

Sop, J. L., & Sop, A. (2023). *Open Fracture Management*. StatPearls Publishing. Treasure Island, Florida, United States.

Sotillo Rodriguez, J. E., Mansky, K. C., Jensen, E. D., Carlson, A. E., Schwarz, T., Pham, L., MacKenzie, B., Prasad, H., Rohrer, M. D., Petryk, A., & Gopalakrishnan, R. (2009). Enhanced osteoclastogenesis causes osteopenia in twisted gastrulation-deficient mice through increased BMP signaling. *J. Bone Miner. Res*. 24: 1917–1926.

Srivastava, K., Tyagi, A. M., Khan, K., Dixit, M., Lahiri, S., Kumar, A., Changkija, B., Khan, M. P., Nagar, G. K., Yadav, D. K., & Maurya, R. (2013). Isoformononetin, a methoxydaidzein present in medicinal plants, reverses bone loss in osteopenic rats and exerts bone anabolic action by preventing osteoblast apoptosis. *Phytomedicine*. 20: 470–480.

Sun, Y., Xu, L., Huang, S., Hou, Y., Liu, Y., Chan, K. M., Pan, X. H., & Li, G. (2015). Mir-21 overexpressing mesenchymal stem cells accelerate fracture healing in a rat closed femur fracture model. *Biomed Res. Int*. 2015: 412327.

Tabatabaei-Malazy, O., Salari, P., Khashayar, P., & Larijani, B. (2017). New horizons in treatment of osteoporosis. *DARU J. Pharm. Sci*. 25: 1–16.

Tay, W. L., & Tay, D. (2022). Discontinuing denosumab: Can it be done safely? A review of the literature. *Endocrinol Metab*. 37: 183–194.

Thompson, D. D., Simmons, H. A., Pirie, C. M., & Ke, H. Z. (1995). FDA guidelines and animal models for osteoporosis. *Bone*. 17: S125–S133.

Thorup, A. C., Lambert, M. N., Kahr, H. S., Bjerre, M., & Jeppesen, P. B. (2015). Intake of novel red clover supplementation for 12 weeks improves bone status in healthy menopausal women. *Evid. Based Complementary Altern. Med.* 2015: 689138.

Totsuka, T., Kanai, T., Nemoto, Y., Tomita, T., Okamoto, R., Tsuchiya, K., Nakamura, T., Sakamoto, N., Akiba, H., Okumura, K., & Yagita, H. (2009). RANK-RANKL signaling pathway is critically involved in the function of CD4+CD25+ regulatory T cells in chronic colitis. *J. Immun.* 182: 6079–6087.

Tsai, J. N., Uihlein, A. V., Lee, H., Kumbhani, R., Siwila-Sackman, E., McKay, E. A., Burnett-Bowie, S. A. M., Neer, R. M., & Leder, B. Z. (2013). Teriparatide and denosumab, alone or combined, in women with postmenopausal osteoporosis: The DATA study randomised trial. *Lancet.* 382: 50–56.

Turner, A. S. (2001). Animal models of osteoporosis—necessity and limitations. *Eur. Cells Mater.* 1: 66–81.

Turner, R. T., Maran, A., Lotinun, S., Hefferan, T., Evans, G. L., Zhang, M., & Sibonga, J. D. (2001). Animal models for osteoporosis. *Rev. Endocr. Metab. Disord.* 2: 117–127.

Tyagi, A. M., Srivastava, K., Singh, A. K., Kumar, A., Changkija, B., Pandey, R., Lahiri, S., Nagar, G. K., Yadav, D. K., Maurya, R., & Trivedi, R. (2012). Formononetin reverses established osteopenia in adult ovariectomized rats. *Menopause.* 19: 856–863.

Umland, E. M., Karel, L., & Santoro, N. (2016). Bazedoxifene and conjugated equine estrogen: A combination product for the management of vasomotor symptoms and osteoporosis rrevention associated with menopause. *Pharmacotherapy.* 36: 548–561.

Vasiliadis, E. S., Evangelopoulos, D. S., Kaspiris, A., Benetos, I. S., Vlachos, C., & Pneumaticos, S. G. (2022). The role of sclerostin in bone diseases. *J. Clin. Med.* 11: 806.

Viguet-Carrin, S., Hoppler, M., Scalfo, F. M., Vuichoud, J., Vigo, M., Offord, E. A., & Ammann, P. (2014). Peak bone strength is influenced by calcium intake in growing rats. *Bone.* 68: 85–91.

Walsh, M. C., & Choi, Y. (2014). Biology of the RANKL-RANK-OPG system in immunity, bone, and beyond. *Front. Immunol.* 5: 511.

Wang, X., Chaudhry, M. A., Nie, Y., Xie, Z., Shapiro, J. I., & Liu, J. (2017). A mouse 5/6th nephrectomy model that induces experimental uremic cardiomyopathy. *J. Vis. Exp.* 129: e55825.

Wang, X., Wu, J., Chiba, H., Yamada, K., & Ishimi, Y. (2005). Puerariae radix prevents bone loss in castrated malc micc. *Metab. Clin. Exp.* 54: 1536–1541.

Wergedal, J. E., Veskovic, K., Hellan, M., Nyght, C., Balemans, W., Libanati, C., Vanhoenacker, F. M., Tan, J., Baylink, D. J., & Van Hul, W. (2003). Patients with Van Buchem disease, an osteosclerotic genetic disease, have elevated bone formation markers, higher bone density, and greater derived polar moment of inertia than normal. *J. Clin. Endocr.* 88: 5778–5783.

Wijenayaka, A. R., Kogawa, M., Lim, H. P., Bonewald, L. F., Findlay, D. M., & Atkins, G. J. (2011). Sclerostin stimulates osteocyte support of osteoclast activity by a RANKL-dependent pathway. *PLoS One.* 6: e25900.

Wronski, T. J., Dann, L. M., & Horner, S. L. (1989). Time course of vertebral osteopenia in ovariectomized rats. *Bone.* 10: 295–301.

Wu, M., Chen, G., & Li, Y. P. (2016). TGF-β and BMP signaling in osteoblast, skeletal development, and bone formation, homeostasis and disease. *Bone Res.* 4: 16009.

Xie, J., Guo, J., Kanwal, Z., Wu, M., Lv, X., Ibrahim, N. A., Li, P., Buabeid, M. A., Arafa, E. A., & Sun, Q. (2020). Calcitonin and bone physiology: In vitro, in vivo, and clinical investigations. *Int. J. Endocrinol.* 2020: 3236828.

Yadav, S., Pal, S., Singh, P., Porwal, K., Sinha, R. A., Kumari, N., Chattopadhyay, N., & Gupta, S. K. (2020). Calcium repletion to rats with calcipenic rickets fails to recover bone quality: A calcipenic "memory". *Bone.* 141: 115562.

Yadav, S., Porwal, K., Sinha, R. A., Chattopadhyay, N., & Gupta, S. K. (2021). Moderate/subclinical calcium deficiency attenuates trabecular mass, microarchitecture and bone growth in growing rats. *Biochem. Biophys. Rep.* 26: 101033.

Yamamoto, T., Saatcioglu, F., & Matsuda, T. (2002). Cross-talk between bone morphogenic proteins and estrogen receptor signaling. *Endocrinology.* 143: 2635–2642.

Yang, T., Zhang, J., Cao, Y., Zhang, M., Jing, L., Jiao, K., Yu, S., Chang, W., Chen, D., & Wang, M. (2015). Wnt5a/Ror2 mediates temporomandibular joint subchondral bone remodeling. *J. Dent. Res.* 94: 803–812.

Ye, Y. B., Tang, X. Y., Verbruggen, M. A., & Su, Y. X. (2006). Soy isoflavones attenuate bone loss in early postmenopausal Chinese women : A single-blind randomized, placebo-controlled trial. *Eur. J. Nutr.* 45: 327–334.

Yousefzadeh, N., Kashfi, K., Jeddi, S., & Ghasemi, A. (2020). Ovariectomized rat model of osteoporosis: A practical guide. *EXCLI J.* 19: 89–107.

Zebaze, R., Libanati, C., McClung, M. R., Zanchetta, J. R., Kendler, D. L., Høiseth, A., Wang, A., Ghasem-Zadeh, A., & Seeman, E. (2016). Denosumab reduces cortical porosity of the proximal femoral shaft in postmenopausal women with osteoporosis. *J. Bone Miner. Res.* 31: 1827–1834.

Zhang, Y., Lai, W. P., Leung, P. C., Wu, C. F., & Wong, M. S. (2007). Short- to mid-term effects of ovariectomy on bone turnover, bone mass and bone strength in rats. *Biol. Pharm. Bull.* 30: 898–903.

Zhang, Y., Xu, J., Ruan, Y. C., Yu, M. K., O'Laughlin, M., Wise, H., Chen, D., Tian, L., Shi, D., Wang, J., Chen, S., Feng, J. Q., Chow, D. H. K., Xie, X., Zheng, L., Huang, L., Huang, S., Leung, K., Lu, N., Zhao, L., Li, H., Zhao, D., Guo, X., Chan, K., Witte, F., Chan, H. C., Zheng, Y., & Qin, L. (2016). Implant-derived magnesium induces local neuronal production of CGRP to improve bone-fracture healing in rats. *Nat. Med.* 22: 1160–1169.

Zhou, S., Turgeman, G., Harris, S. E., Leitman, D. C., Komm, B. S., Bodine, P. V., & Gazit, D. (2003). Estrogens activate bone morphogenetic protein-2 gene transcription in mouse mesenchymal stem cells. *Mol. Endocrinol.* 17: 56–66.

Zhu, D., Mackenzie, N. C. W., Millan, J. L., Farquharson, C., & MacRae, V. E. (2011). The appearance and modulation of osteocyte marker expression during calcification of vascular smooth muscle cells. *PLoS One.* 6: e19595.

Zhu, L., Liu, Y., Wang, A., Zhu, Z., Li, Y., Zhu, C., Che, Z., Liu, T., Liu, H., & Huang, L. (2022). Application of BMP in bone tissue engineering. *Front. Bioeng. Biotech.* 10: 810880.

14 Biomimetic Bone Models in Advancing Bone Regeneration and Repair

Tanjot Kaur, Sandhya Natesan, Mayank Singh, and Greeshma Thrivikraman

14.1 INTRODUCTION

Although in vivo systems are established as well-defined models for representing biological conditions, they are associated with many challenges such as species-specific variations, ethical concerns, and limited prediction power in animal models, particularly for large screening approaches. As a consequence, basic biological and medical research always commences with in vitro models; bioengineered organs and tissues such as bone, blood vessels, bladder, skin, cartilage, and cornea are applied as models in regenerative medicine, diagnostics, drug discovery/screening, and toxicological studies.

Moreover, bioengineered models in vivo can act as platforms for predicting cellular functions and their underlying mechanisms that are involved in aging processes and disease onset and progression in transplantation research. Bone is a connective tissue that is viscoelastic in nature in which the resident cells are cemented within a densely mineralized extracellular matrix (ECM) that confers substantial strength and rigidity. In addition to a rich supply of vasculature and innervation, dynamic equilibrium between the bone formation and bone resorption is tightly regulated.

With the increasing burden of bone diseases, it became pertinent to understand the organizational, biomechanical and remodelling attributes of both healthy and diseased native bone. However, accurately modelling the hierarchical osseous tissue embedded with multiple cell types, each with specialized functions, is still an ongoing challenge. In the macroscopic view, bone possesses two structures: trabecular and cortical; the former is porous, and the latter one is a compact shell.

The porosity of trabecular bone is one of its important features in engineering bone structures in vitro, as it defines properties such as toughness, elastic modulus, and high impact load resistance. Moreover, the cortical bone is anisotropic in nature since the strength is greater along the axis than the radial direction. Another key attribute is the highly dynamic nature of bone, as it continuously replenishes itself with new bones to ensure skeletal stability.

The process of remodelling is highly complicated and is triggered by several factors including nutritional status, hormonal factors, and biomechanical stress. Bone remodelling stages consist of resorption by osteoclasts; changeover from resorption to the new bone formation by osteoblasts via an integrated functioning of osteoclasts, osteoblasts, and osteocytes; and bone lining cells, known as basic multicellular units (BMUs). In addition to BMUs, the bone marrow cells adjacent to remodelling areas also have a central part in bone homeostasis. Indeed, several bone-related disorders such as osteosarcoma, osteoporosis, osteoarthritis, and osteomyelitis in both women and men are mainly because of imbalance in bone homeostasis associated with age, menopause-associated hormonal changes, changes in physical activity, and secondary diseases.

Researchers also have discovered that persons with type 1 diabetes have a higher risk of osteoporosis, osteopenia, and fragility fractures, whereas bone mineral density is high in type 2 diabetes (Blakytny et al., 2011; Hamann et al., 2012). According to the latest estimate released by the

DOI: 10.1201/9781003307310-17

International Osteoporosis Foundation, one-third of women and one-fifth of men over 50 years old may be affected by bone disorders over their lifespan. Therefore, studying the pathogenesis mechanisms and developing new treatment techniques for these conditions have been realized as critical. Consequently, in vitro, ex vivo, and in vivo bone models have all evolved.

One major challenge identified with in vivo models is the rigor in understanding various mechanisms since the bone niche is intricate in nature. For instance, researchers have studied angiogenesis and bone matrix mineralization using in vivo animal models with the combined action of osteogenic and endothelial precursors, but the development processes are still poorly understood due to the complex bone niche (Pirosa et al., 2018). Moreover, there is a severe paucity of suitable animal models for mimicking osteoporotic fracture healing. Choosing the right animal model requires considering the research question and an in-depth understanding of the advantages and disadvantages of each model (Haffner-Luntzer et al., 2019).

Since bone is a very rigid and complex tissue that is so dynamic and metabolically active and considering the many factors affecting its structure and mechanical properties, it is always challenging to mimic the bone tissue microenvironment in vitro. The various criteria one should integrate while designing an efficient biomimetic in vitro model are provided in Figure 14.1 (Fernandez-Yague

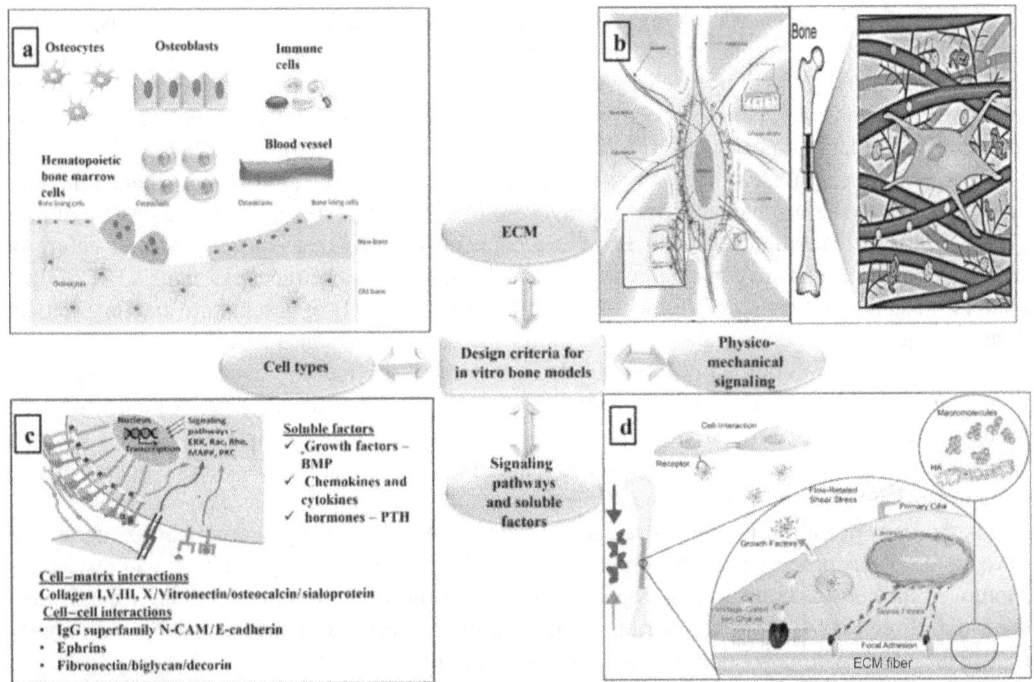

FIGURE 14.1 Design criteria for an efficient biomimetic in vitro model: (a) schematic of a bone cell niche; (b) ECM components and molecules (reproduced with permission from Gaharwar, A. K., Arpanaei, A., Andresen, T. L., & Dolatshahi-Pirouz, A.: 3D Biomaterial Microarrays for Regenerative Medicine: Current State-of-the-Art, Emerging Directions and Future Trends. Adv. Mater. 2016. 28. 771–781. Copyright 2016 John Wiley and Sons; reproduced under the terms of CC-BY 4.0 (https://creativecommons.org/licenses/by/4.0/) International License from Garg, P., Strigini, M., Peurière, L., Vico, L., & Iandolo, D.: The Skeletal Cellular and Molecular Underpinning of the Murine Hindlimb Unloading Model. Front Physiol. 2021. 12. 1798. Copyright 2021 Garg et al., published by Frontiers); (c) signaling pathways and growth factors (reproduced with permission from Shekaran, A., & García, A. J.: Extracellular matrix-mimetic adhesive biomaterials for bone repair. J. Biomed. Mater. Res. Part A. 2010. 96. 261–272. Copyright 2010 John Wiley and Sons); (d) mechano-transduction (reproduced with permission from Fernandez-Yague, M. A., Abbah, S. A., McNamara, L., Zeugolis, D. I., Pandit, A., & Biggs, M. J.: Biomimetic approaches in bone tissue engineering: Integrating biological and physicomechanical strategies. Adv. Drug Delivery Rev. 2015. 84. 1–29. Copyright 2015 Elsevier).

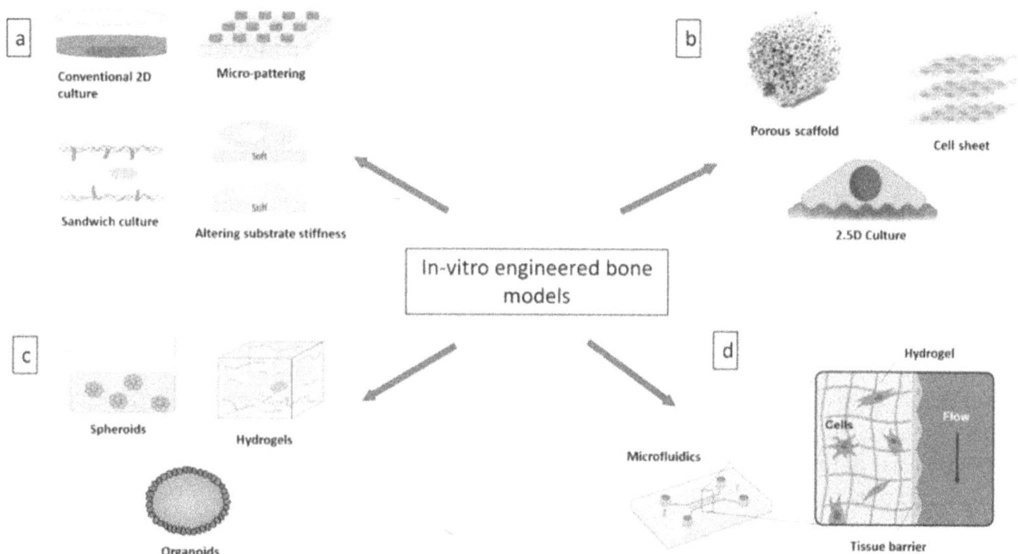

FIGURE 14.2 Existing in vitro bone models for understanding diseases, drug development, and toxicity screening: (a) 2D cell culture methods (reproduced with permission from Yuste, I., Luciano, F. C., González-Burgos, E., Lalatsa, A., & Serrano, D. R.: Mimicking bone microenvironment: 2D and 3D in vitro models of human osteoblasts. Pharmacol. Res. 2021. 169. 105626. Copyright 2021 Elsevier); (b) 2.5D culture, porous scaffold and cell sheets (reproduced with permission from De La Zerda, A., Kratochvil, M. J., Suhar, N. A., & Heilshorn, S. C.: Review: Bioengineering strategies to probe T cell mechanobiology. APL Bioeng. 2018. 2. 021501. Copyright 2018 AIP Publishing; reproduced under the terms of CC-BY 4.0 (https://creativecommons.org/licenses/by/4.0/) International License Ghouse, S., Reznikov, N., Boughton, O. R., Babu, S., Ng, K. G., Blunn, G., Cobb, J. P., Stevens, M. M. & Jeffers, J. R.: The design and in vivo testing of a locally stiffness-matched porous scaffold. Appl. Mater. Today. 2019. 15. 377–388. Copyright 2019 Ghouse et al., published by Elsevier; reproduced with permission from Yuste, I., Luciano, F. C., González-Burgos, E., Lalatsa, A., & Serrano, D. R.: Mimicking bone microenvironment: 2D and 3D in vitro models of human osteoblasts. Pharmacol. Res. 2021. 169. 105626. Copyright 2021 Elsevier); (c) 3D models (reproduced under the terms of CC-BY 4.0 (https://creativecommons.org/licenses/by/4.0/) International License from Akkerman, N., & Defize, L. H. K.: Dawn of the organoid era: 3D tissue and organ cultures revolutionize the study of development, disease, and regeneration. BioEssays. 2017. 39. 1600244. Copyright 2017 Akkerman and Defize, published by John Wiley & Sons; reproduced under the terms of CC-BY 4.0 (https://creativecommons.org/licenses/by/4.0/) International License from Ghouse, S., Reznikov, N., Boughton, O. R., Babu, S., Ng, K. C. G., Blunn, G., Cobb, J. P., Stevens, M. M., & Jeffers, J. R. T.: The design and in vivo testing of a locally stiffness-matched porous scaffold. Appl. Mater. Today. 2019. 15. 377–388. Copyright 2019 Ghouse et al., published by Elsevier; reproduced with permission from Yuste, I., Luciano, F. C., González-Burgos, E., Lalatsa, A., & Serrano, D. R.: Mimicking bone microenvironment: 2D and 3D in vitro models of human osteoblasts. Pharmacol. Res. 2021. 169. 105626. Copyright 2021 Elsevier); (d) microfluidics (reproduced with permission from Vera, D., García-Díaz, M., Torras, N., Álvarez, M., Villa, R., & Martinez, E.: Engineering Tissue Barrier Models on Hydrogel Microfluidic Platforms. ACS Appl. Mater. Interfaces. 2021. 13. 13920–13933. Copyright 2021 American Chemical Society).

et al., 2015; Gaharwar et al., 2016; Garg et al., 2021; Shekaran & García, 2010). In literature, there exists a range of strategies for studying bone by using in vitro models (Figure 14.2) like 2D, 3D, dynamic models and on-chip bone-mimetic systems.

However, the majority of the existing in vitro bone models are based on single cell types such as osteoblasts or their precursor cells, thus ignoring the key players in bone remodelling (osteoclasts), nutrient transport (vasculature), and sensory/sympathetic/parasympathetic actions (skeletal innervations). Due to the lack of cellular complexity, in vitro osseous models have been ineffective for studying bone disorders and bone density loss due to aging, such as osteoporosis, osteoarthritis, and osteomyelitis. Likewise, the low predictive power associated with these simplistic in vitro models also hampers their application in drug toxicity assessments in bone malignancies such as osteosarcoma. In this chapter, we summarize the evidence on all the available in vitro preclinical bone models and their benefits and inadequacies for the precise modelling of bone tissue. We also address how the field should advance in terms of complexity, predictability, personalized testing and high throughput formats.

14.2 DESIRED PROPERTIES FOR A BONE MIMETIC CONSTRUCT

The first important component involved in developing in vitro models is formulating a suitable construct that can replicate the native physiological microenvironment. Bone differs from other nonmineralized tissues due to its stiffness, which is measured in gigapascals and is considerably greater than the stiffness in the soft tissues, which are measured in kilopascals (Guelcher & Sterling, 2011). Because of this stiffness, tissue-engineered constructs (TECs) with high mechanical qualities are required (Ghouse et al., 2019). On the other hand, materials utilized in bone disease models such as for bone-targeting cancers vary greatly depending on the tumour fate and origin along with its ability to induce angiogenesis (Fischbach et al., 2007; Yamada & Cukierman, 2007). Engineers use a variety of materials and production processes to construct biomimetic matrices with encapsulated cell populations to develop TECs for suitable purposes. When selecting material to construct TECs for cancer and bone modelling, mechanical qualities, bioactivity, remodelling capacity, and chemical composition must be considered. The four major classes of biomaterials employed for bone mimetic materials owing to the strong mechanical capabilities essential for bone recapitulation are metals, ceramics, polymers, and composites, although each one is associated with some limitations (Kwakwa et al., 2017).

14.3 2D MODELS

Most 2D studies related to bone focus on establishing monolayer cultures using osteoblasts, osteocytes, and mesenchymal stem cells (MSCs) that are obtained in vitro from primary cultures, immortalized and cancerous cell lines, or induced osteoblasts derived from pluripotent stem cells. Such overly simplified in vitro models are completely different from what is present in native bone, thereby causing many clinical trials to fail.

In vivo, cells typically exist within a complex network consisting of a dense array of blood vessels, ECM, and various other cell types. This intricate system facilitates the delivery of oxygen and nutrients to cells. Despite the fact that 2D cell culture is widely and commonly used based on its simple operation procedure and high-throughput screening, 2D-bone models are generally developed on flat surfaces like petri dishes under a controlled environment. Furthermore, they are inexpensive to maintain and do not require sophisticated laboratory equipment.

Cells cultured on petri dishes do not have the same tissue-specific structure or interaction with extracellular stromal components as those cultivated in vivo, which is crucial for their growth, communication, signal transduction, and proper balance between cell survival and death during tissue formation such as in bones and bone marrow (Bicho et al., 2018). Increasing evidence indicates that 2D models are inadequate for replicating in vivo conditions consistently and accurately. However, despite this fact, 2D models are still extensively employed for preliminary assessments in developing diseases and conducting toxicity experiments.

The classification of these models is static, as they involve cultivating cells without any mechanical stimulation or flow. As a result, these models may not accurately replicate the dynamics present in the human body in vivo, which can result in inaccurate results pertaining to cellular proliferation, growth factor release, gene expression, protein expression, differentiation, and survival.

Advancements in recent research have enhanced 2D culture in several ways. For example, sandwich culture is sometimes classified as a 3D model, albeit with some ambiguity, since the cells are not entirely enclosed within the surrounding matrix. Therefore, it can be more accurately referred to as a 2.5D system (De La Zerda et al., 2018).

14.3.1 Monolayers

Monocultures of osteoblasts and their precursor cells are the most common culture models employed to evaluate drug treatment response, especially for conditions like osteoporosis, osteosarcoma, and osteonecrosis, as well as to test novel biomaterials for their osteoinductive properties. Chang et al. (2014) used a 2D cell culture of MG-63 osteosarcoma cells and healthy human osteoblasts to compare the cytotoxicity of curcumin at varying concentrations. Maugg et al. (2015) screened 25,000 small molecules to identify novel molecules that would specifically target osteosarcoma cells using U2OS and HOS cell lines grown in a 2D culture model.

Researchers used a similar monolayer culture model to assess the short- and long-term effects of high temperatures on bone tissue during surgical and orthopaedic procedures (Dolan et al., 2012). Likewise, the minimal effective concentrations of drug payloads (alendronate and zoledronic acid) required to inhibit osteoclastogenesis were tested using various monolayer cultures of osteoclast precursor cells (Lee et al., 2016; Li et al., 2018). However, this in vitro testing demonstrated that a very low concentration of therapeutics (in the micromolar range) was adequate to achieve the desired effects; this could possibly drastically underestimate the dose required to achieve therapeutic inhibitory response in vivo.

Researchers have 2D modelled a range of primary or immortalized osteoblastic, osteocytic, osteoclastic, and mesenchymal cell types (Yuste et al., 2021). Especially for bone remodelling studies, various types of cells from the osteoclastic lineage are frequently utilized in 2D model systems, including peripheral blood mononuclear cells (PBMCs), monocytes separated from PBMCs, monocyte osteoclast precursor cells, RAW264.7, and THP-1. The RAW264.7 cell line, derived from mice and characterized by leukemic monocyte macrophages, has the ability to transform into osteoclastic cells when stimulated with RANKL alone without requiring M-CSF costimulation (Collin-Osdoby & Osdoby, 2012). The proportion of RANKL, a cytokine that promotes the formation of osteoclasts, to its inhibitor, osteoprotegerin (OPG), is a significant factor in osteoclast remodelling and growth.

In contrast, THP-1 is a monocytic human cell line that came from the blood of a youthful adult who had acute monocytic leukaemia. Establishing a robust in vitro model for bone remodelling requires a reliable cell source capable of synthesizing RANKL, as established in studies that highlight the importance of accounting for biological factors such as hormones (especially oestrogen) and mechanical stimulation in future research on bone remodelling, as these factors influence the resorption process in vivo (Owen & Reilly, 2018).

Osteoblasts coexist with other resident cells such as osteocytes and osteoclasts that aid in the constant cycling of bone formation and resorption, but the traditional planar surfaces of cell monolayers fail to represent the dynamic remodelling microenvironment of bone and its associated disorders. As a consequence, the outcomes of experiments conducted on such 2D bone models greatly differs from the findings from cells residing in the native microenvironment, leading to poor translation efficiency (Yuste et al., 2021). Various osteoblastic cell types are utilized in vitro, including primary osteoblasts, MSCs, and osteoblast precursor cells that are immortalized and obtained from human bone marrow stroma, as well as ST-2 (murine stromal cells obtained from BC8 mice), MC3T3-E, and human periodontal ligament cells located between the tooth root and alveolar bone.

In addition, MLO-Y4 (murine osteocyte-like cells), an osteocyte cell line that was cloned from mouse long bone cells, is also used widely (Kato et al., 1997). A cell line derived from SV-40-immortalized mouse osteocytes has also been employed to evaluate the tumorigenic potential of osteocytes. MLO-A5 is another commonly utilized cell line in the field. Altogether, the development of cell lines that imitate osteocytes and display comparable characteristics has significantly contributed to identifying the molecular and cellular mechanisms underlying bone biology (Sottnik et al., 2014).

14.3.2 Cocultures

Cocultures of osteoblast and osteoclasts are commonly used as a 2D system to mimic the phenotypic traits of the bone remodelling process. For instance, Hayden and his colleagues conducted research on bone remodelling, metabolic activity, and calcium deposition in cultures of these two bone-specific cells alone and their cocultures when these are seeded on silk–hydroxyapatite (HA) films (Hayden et al., 2014). In some instances, rather than directly culturing subpopulations of cells together, they are cultured alone, and the culture medium extracted from one cell population containing suitable factors is used to condition the other cell populations.

However, this method is not ideal for studying the bidirectional communication that exists between metastatic cancer cells and bone cells. For this purpose, a transwell approach was utilized in which the cancer cells retrieved from breast tumours and bone cells were compartmentalized and connected only via porous membrane to be cultured in the same medium. This approach was ideal for monitoring the cell migration from one compartment to another (Arrigoni et al., 2016).

Authors of another study used the same coculturing technique to decipher the process of bone differentiation by employing human peripheral blood monocytes and bone marrow stem cells (hBMSCs) to differentiate them from bone-forming cells. The researchers established that coculturing cells induced differentiation without the use of any external supplementation in the media that could cause side effects. Moreover, the authors were able to successfully demonstrate the influence of osteoclastogenesis on hBMSCs (Bicho et al., 2018).

In general, cocultures have demonstrated their usefulness in studying the communication between different types of cells in laboratory settings, but special attention should be paid to the conditions in which they are cultured. This is important because various cells have unique requirements for growth, and deviations from the natural in vivo environment could lead to changes in cellular behaviour. Kulkarni et al. (2010) demonstrated another example of using cocultures: They employed a coculture model of mouse bone marrow cells and MLO-Y4 osteocytes and observed that coculturing enhanced the osteocytes' capacity to stimulate osteoclast development in RAW264.7. However, the osteoclastogenic potential of the osteocytes diminished as a result of mechanical loading.

Kulkarni et al. (2010) also showed that MEPE (matrix extracellular phosphoglycoprotein) is a signalling molecule generated by osteocytes due to mechanical loading that can inhibit osteoclastogenesis by tuning the RANKL/OPG ratio. Osteocytes secrete the molecules OPG and RANKL, which control osteoclastogenesis. Monitoring of the RANKL/OPG ratio showed a significant decrease in osteocytes undergoing mechanical loading compared with the nonloaded controls, suggesting a vital role of MEPE in regulating osteoclastogenesis (Kulkarni et al., 2010).

Recently, there has been a trend of developing more complex 2D cell culture models to enhance and more accurately mimic the bone environment found in vivo. Among the techniques utilized in pharmacokinetic research, the sandwich culture method has been identified, and some experts consider it a 3D model. The process involves placing cells within a layer of ECM made from either polyacrylamide or collagen, with another layer of matrix on top.

Sandwich culture has been shown to be particularly useful when working with cells that are surrounded by complex extracellular matrices, but there are very few studies on human osteoblasts cell culture (Yuste et al., 2021). Bernhardt et al. (2021) established an in vitro triple culture system in a 3D microenvironment that maintained the typical morphological features of osteoclasts, human primary osteocytes, and osteoblasts. This system allowed for examining cell–cell interactions among all three cell types simultaneously, as well as the separate analysis of each individual cell population. Additionally, triculture model (osteoblasts, osteoclasts, and endothelial cells [ECs]) developed by Grémare et al. (2019) maintained cell culture homeostasis in addition to cell phenotype and activity. Because the proliferation, morphology, and differentiation of bone cells are influenced by significant factors such as surface topography and charge, stiffness, hardness, surface ligands, pore sizes, and substrate wettability, biomaterials with varying substrate properties have also been utilized as 2D microenvironments (Yuste et al., 2021; Yang et al., 2009; Soon et al., 2017).

14.4 EX VIVO BONE MODELS

As we have described, in vitro studies are straightforward and cost-effective since they use conventional culture vessels with 2D single-cell cultures or cocultures on tissue-culture-treated flasks. Alterations in cell shape and protein expression in 2D cultures may occur since they lack the native ECM structures and organization found in vivo. Therefore, explant models are developed to make a connection between in vivo and in vitro studies in preclinical evaluation.

Explant models are made by culturing the organ's explants in vitro, which paves the way for studying cellular and matrix interactions, similar to in vivo but conserving the native ECM structure. Usually, explants from laboratory animal bone such as mice or rat or juvenile bones are used for ex vivo studies, which makes them somewhat ineffective in translational research. Conversely, using mature explants in static conditions reduces the viability of bone cells in ex vivo cultures, which has allowed for investigating methods of enhancing cell viability and incorporating mechanical stimulation such as loading, compression, and tension (Cramer et al., 2021).

In one study, the authors developed human femoral head osteochondral explants treated with inflammatory cytokines such as IL-1β and TNF-α that functioned as ex vivo bone models for testing novel drugs for OA treatment and understanding the detailed disease mechanisms (Li et al., 2021). Researchers also examined explant culture as a model to determine the role of exosomes secreted by canine osteosarcoma tumour tissues (Luu et al., 2018). Marino et al. (2016) studied multiple applications of bone ex vivo models, especially for cancer-induced bone diseases, using the rodent calvaria explant culture model and determined that the soluble factors secreted by the cancer cells induced proliferation, ultimately affecting the bone formation and resorption leading to bone metastasis.

Researchers have also developed a 3D trabecular explant coculture prototype to study osseous mechanobiology using osteocyte and osteoblast coculture. Osteoblasts were seeded onto the trabecular bone cores procured from juvenile tarsal-metatarsal joint explants, the osteogenic medium was sent through a perfusion system, and the system was mechanically stimulated using dynamic uniaxial deformational loading. This study demonstrated the intercellular communication between osteocytes and the seeded osteoblasts. One intriguing finding was that under dynamic uniaxial deformational loading, the elastic moduli of the explant changed, which stimulated the bone cells to release significantly more prostaglandin E_2 (Chan et al., 2009).

Osseon acts as a primitive site for the metastasis of prostate and breast cancer (Choudhary et al., 2018), and researchers have focussed on creating an explant culture to find the signalling between cancer and resident bone cells. For example, Choudhary et al. (2018) developed a human ex vivo bone model to figure out the interactions between prostate cancer cells and the bone cells in tumour formation and illustrated the key cellular responses exerted by the prostate cancer cells in the osteocytes, such as imbalanced elucidation of Wnt inhibitors, higher secretion of fibroblast growth factor 23, and more mineralization stimulated the alkaline phosphatase activity.

Apart from osteosarcoma, chronic osteomyelitis is another debilitating bone disorder, caused mostly by the bioluminescent pathogenic bacterium *Staphylococcus aureus*, that is difficult to cure. Therefore, Sweeney et al. (2019) established an in vitro antibiotic screening model to prevent biofilm formation in osteomyelitis infection caused by *S. aureus* using bovine femur bone block explants. Bone explant models have also been advantageous for testing bone damage or necrosis when the local temperature surpasses a threshold of 47 °C in orthopaedic surgery.

During cutting and bone drilling in orthopaedic surgery, temperatures can increase that can lead to bone injury or implant failure, and it is unclear how temperature impacts bone cells and tissue. Numerous investigations on enhanced temperature distribution prediction algorithms across bone tissues have been performed (Akhbar & Yusoff, 2018; Dolan et al., 2012; Lee et al., 2016). Notably, Akhbar and Yusoff (2018) used the DEFORM-3D software to predict the temperature distribution in bone while drilling with varied bits and estimated the reduction in drilling temperature and thermal osteonecrosis at angles from 110° to 140°, 5 to 40% web thickness and helix angles from 5° to 30° and validated their simulation findings with explant bone models.

Kniha et al. (2020) reported the bone necrosis temperature thresholds for dental implants. In knee arthroplasty, Tawy et al. (2016) studied bovine femur bone thermal damage due to burring and sawing. Similarly, Robles-Linares et al. (2020) studied the effects of machining on cortical bovine femur bones using histology and micro-pillar compression tests. Under low-temperature drilling, micromechanical damage was negligible, and only necrotic damage occurred.

Additionally, it is crucial to understand how the three main bone-graft-integrating mechanisms, osteoinduction, osteoconduction, and osteogenesis, affect transplanted bone material in the presence or absence of bone cells in creating a successful bone graft and combatting clinical challenges such as large bone defects. Since it is difficult to interpret the definitive responses of the transplanted bone material without bone matrix control, Jähn et al. (2010) generated uniform acellular bone explants from Swiss Alpine sheep iliac crest bone by exposing cancellous bone to UV and X-ray as a reliable control to identify the effects of the active bone cells in comparison with the bone matrix alone during transplantation studies. Explant cultures and 3D bone mimetic constructs serve as useful model systems for evaluating the micromechanical damage induced by high-temperature bone drilling during bone transplantation studies.

14.5 SHIFT FROM 2D TO 3D BONE MODELS

Bone tissue engineering has typically strived to develop constructs for regenerating bone. However, there is limited success in constructing biomimetic in vitro models for understanding the underlying biological aspects of bone disease progression, and drug screening in a high-throughput manner. This calls for a continuous hunt among tissue engineers to develop TECs that possess not only structural qualities but also physicochemical and mechanical attributes. Such TECs may be very helpful in investigating how these parameters impact disease development and medication response.

Beyond doubt, animal models have played a key role in understanding the origins, mechanisms, and progressions of many human diseases for designing new therapeutic targets. Many animal models, like mice, rats, hamsters, pigs, and sheep, have been employed for such studies, among which the most commonly used model is mouse. Although these studies are helpful, they sometimes give false results due to large species boundaries. In fact, they are often incapable of entirely mimicking human disease pathophysiology, making them unreliable for studying disease pathology and progression.

Another approach is to use primary human cells, but the 2D cultures are often unable to replicate the in vivo complex microenvironment and the necessary cues. In response, 3D in vitro bone models have bridged the gap between animal and 2D culture models and can provide valuable information for drug screening and toxicity testing. In response to the drawbacks associated with 2D models, researchers have developed 3D models such as cell sheets, spheroids, organoids, scaffolds, hydrogels, bioreactors and microfluidics, some of which we discuss here.

14.5.1 Spheroids and Organoids

A growing interest has arisen in 3D cell cultures, mostly spheroids and organoids, because they can closely replicate cell and tissue physiology and dynamics. In particular, when organoids are grown, their ECM is produced only by their cells, thus avoiding interference from a hydrogel, scaffold, or flask's plastic (Kronemberger et al., 2021). Contrary to the top-down 3D scaffold-based approach widely followed in tissue engineering, generating spheroids and organoids is a bottom-up process (Baptista et al., 2018).

Organoids are typically derived from adult, embryonic, or induced pluripotent stem cells (Davies, 2018); whereas spheroids are spherical aggregates of cells created from a single cell type or multicellular cells such as primary cells, fragments of human tissue, or immortalized cell lines. Cells are exposed to low adherent culture conditions to stimulate self-aggregation to form 3D spheres (Białkowska et al., 2020). In a nutshell, organoid development is driven by internal processes, while spheroids are mainly driven by cell-to-cell adhesion. The long-term viability of organoids is maintained by optimizing stem cell culture conditions, providing basement membranes in addition to agonists (Wnt, tyrosine kinase receptors) and inhibitors (BMP, TGF-β). Organoids are widely preferred over spheroids for mimicking the physiological properties of natural organs since they derive from stem cells that can maintain their self-renewal and differentiation potential under optimum conditions. In multiple drug discovery applications, organoids demonstrate long-term viability.

14.5.1.1 Spheroids

Cell spheroids have emerged as very attractive 3D models for studying cell-to-cell and cell-to-matrix interactions in high throughput, with the additional ability to mimic in vivo conditions that is superior to that of 2D models (Fennema et al., 2013; Souza et al., 2019). However, they are associated with low oxygen distribution and reproducibility. An optimum environment needs to be provided so that the cells in the spheroids stay viable and are produced quickly without any alteration in their phenotype (Restle et al., 2015). Spheroids can be generated employing a variety of techniques: embryoid bodies; microfluidics and microchips (Itel et al., 2018); liquid overlay, which entails arresting cell growth by adding a nonadherent material on the culture surface (Metzger et al., 2011); rotational culture; and hanging drop culture (Stahl et al., 2004).

Moritani et al. (2018) employed microwell chips to form human periodontal ligament MSC spheroids and analyzed their stemness and osteogenic potential. They established that the spheroids could be used for regeneration based on their stemness, in contrast with the monolayer culture. Authors of another study utilized hanging drop culture to monitor the osteogenic potential associated with human bone-derived MSCs. When entrapped in a collagen hydrogel, osteogenically generated MSCs had a more persistent osteoblastic phenotype than detached MSCs (Murphy et al., 2016).

In a different study, Tiaden et al. (2012) also employed hanging drop method to analyze the impact of recombinant mammalian high-temperature requirement serine protease A1 on matrix mineralization and MSC osteogenesis in humans. Likewise, researchers demonstrated that rotationally cultured scaffold-free 3D spheroids were better for forming preosteoblasts from adipose-derived stem cells than were 3D scaffolds and monolayers. On the contrary, adequate osteoblastic maturation occurs via cell attachment to the substrate (Rumiński et al., 2020).

Low attachment culture was used in a study that employed bone marrow stem cells to compare the antiregenerative potential of bone marrow-isolated rat MSC spheroids with that of rat MSC monolayers. In both in vivo and in vitro experiments, MSCs encapsulated in the spheroids had higher osteogenic efficiency than the MSCs that were grown in the monolayer culture (Yamaguchi et al., 2014). Another method, liquid overlay, was used to create SAOS2 spheroids, although in this instance, sterile ultrapure agarose was used to cover the culture surface. The authors of this study sought to examine the toxicity of titanium dioxide nanoparticles (TiO_2 NPs). Lower concentrations of the TiO_2 NPs caused increased collagen deposition via altering the cell cycle, but no concentrations altered cell viability (Souza et al., 2019).

To explore the angiogenesis process in vitro, Wenger et al. (2004) made co-spheres of human OB and human umbilical vein endothelial cells (HUVECs) using liquid overlay. These cells were then seeded in collagen gels such that the endothelial cells were mostly found in the shell and the osteoblastic cells were mostly confined in the core region. Upon treatment with vascular endothelial growth factor, the HUVEC spheroids formed tube-like structures. However, in co-spheroids of HUVECs and human osteoblasts (hOBs), this ability was lower, demonstrating hOBs' potential to limit angiogenesis. In contrast to HUVEC spheroids, which had more ordered cellular protrusions, hOB and HUVEC/hOB spheroids were more disordered (Wenger et al., 2004). For drug screening studies, osteosarcoma 3D spheroid models synthesized using hanging drop and low attachment showed significant resistance to anticancer drugs including doxorubicin, cisplatin, taxol, and taurolidine, in contrast with 2D models (Munoz-Garcia et al., 2021).

14.5.1.2 Organoids

Although spheroids have been considered a significant 3D bone model, organoids are preferred because they are derived from stem cells that have better self-renewal and differentiation ability (Akkerman & Defize, 2017). In vitro 3D-woven bone organoids of osteoblasts and osteoclasts were developed using bone marrow stromal cells for studying osteogenesis under physiological and pathological conditions (Akiva et al., 2021). The authors formed woven bone organoids by progressively embedding osteocytes within a collagen matrix produced by osteoblasts. They also observed bone mineralization, sclerostin-mediated communication, and network formation in the in vitro embedded bone organoid cultures (Akiva et al., 2021).

Similarly, researchers generated cartilage organoids using human pluripotent stem cells, hypothesizing that IL-1β would stimulate bone formation in cartilaginous organoids. Following four weeks of IL-1β treatment of the organoids after ectopic and orthotopic implantation on immunocompromised mice, cartilage reconstruction and bone formation were seen. Cartilage organoids could be used to repair prolonged bone damages without scaffolds and also could enable a bone mimetic model for various clinical studies (Tam et al., 2021).

In another interesting study, an artificial in vitro human bone organoid (osteosphere) model was created using primary human osteoblasts and tested for mechanical stiffness by treating it with adiponectin. The adiponectin-treated osteospheres reduced bone stiffness via increased proliferation and by higher expression of ECM proteins. To verify the results, adiponectin-treated organoids were compared with eight-week-old adiponectin knockout mice (APN-KO mice) (Naot et al., 2016). In APN-KO mice, cortical bone stiffness was found to be 15% higher than in adiponectin-treated organoids (Haugen et al., 2018).

However, performing mechanical testing in organoids is challenging due to irregular inner structure, geometry, and mineralization. Another area of research involving osseous tissue models is microgravity. Microgravity conditions (such as in space) cause bone resorption and bone formation decline at an accelerated rate 10 times that of osteoporosis (Baran et al., 2022). Therefore, understanding microgravity-induced bone loss is essential for creating therapeutic, dietary and exercise plans to mitigate bone atrophy in astronauts working in the International Space Station.

For instance, Iordachescu et al. (2021) created a structurally and functionally appropriate bone organoid similar to trabecular bone using a suspension of osteoclasts, osteoblasts alone, and a combination of both osteoclasts and osteoblasts obtained from thermally treated femoral head microtrabecular particles using hanging drop culture. These cell organoids were rich in actin and tubulin and created perforated bone loss patterns resembling pores and lacunae. Subsequently, the authors cultured bone organoids in the NASA Synthecon bioreactor to identify bone resorption in the microgravity environment; they observed the most resorption with the osteoclasts alone followed by the combined osteoclast–osteoblast organoids based on the secretion of PTHR1 and CX43 (found only in osteoclast organoid), sclerostin (in all three organoids), and RANKL (osteoclasts and combined construct). Trabecular organoids were encapsulated with fibrin to recapitulate into the biochemical environment, and in the new constructs, a new matrix formed that combined protein and inorganic components and indicated the possibility of quantitatively assessing the degree of ossification by measuring the elemental ratio (Iordachescu et al., 2021). Likewise, to study bone tissue development during endochondral ossification, a mesenchymal stem cell-derived in vitro 3D construct was fabricated and cultured under hypoxic condition (Sasaki et al., 2012).

Separately, bone marrow organoids (BMOs) were also produced using MSCs and ECs via embedding over polyethylene glycol microwells. The synthesized mesenchymal organoid model with a vascularization-like compartment because of endothelial cell morphogenesis triggered the homing and infiltration of hematopoietic stem and progenitor cells (HSPCs) and leukemic blast cells in BMOs, similar to the native process. In a 3D migration assay in BMOs, there was notably more HSPC homing in the vascular network than with BMOs without vascularization. HSPCs expressing CXCR4 were attracted to the BM niche through CXCL12 secretion in bone marrow stromal cells, mimicking their homing behaviour in vivo. BMOs were tested using carboxyfluorescein succinimidyl ester-labelled leukemic blast cells and suggested an active migration of leukemic blasts with an increased elucidation of CXCR4 similar to healthy HSPCs, which confirmed that BMOs can be used as an in vitro preclinical model to examine the toxicity of novel therapeutics as well as for analyzing their pharmacokinetic characteristics (Giger et al., 2022).

14.5.2 Scaffold-Based Systems

Osteoporosis, delayed or impaired bone repair, and osteoarthritis disease modelling have been quite a challenge to mimic in vitro, but scaffolds have emerged as an important model for mimicking them. In one study, planting optimized MSCs on a tricalcium phosphate (TCP) scaffold successfully produced 3D models of cancellous bone tissue which mimicked these disease conditions. Similarly, to elucidate the effects of osteomyelitis in a 3D in vitro model, HSPCs cultured along with MSCs on a macroporous material with cationized bovine serum albumin were created. This research focussed on deciphering the effects of bacteria that cause postoperative osteomyelitis on the bone marrow by testing biofilms formed on an implant. The bacteria affected the expression of MSC cytokines, the ability of MSCs to support HSPC maintenance, and the myeloid differentiation of HSPCs (Raic et al., 2018).

Authors of another study created a model for mimicking staphylococcal bone infection and examined the combinatorial effects of clindamycin and alginate/alginate-dialdehyde-gelatin hydrogels loaded on a TCP platform on treating the infection. They employed human tibia plateaus as the bone source during complete knee replacement surgery for this purpose (Kuehling et al., 2022). Researchers have also investigated developing a bone-mimetic model for physiological bone remodelling. The bone model used silk fibroin to serve as an organic matrix, poly-aspartic acid to serve as noncollagenous proteins, and a mineralization solution. This bone model elucidated the physiological sequence of bone remodelling by bone cells, osteoclasts and osteoblasts via nondestructive microcomputed tomography (de Wildt et al., 2022).

Along similar lines, 3D culture models involving hydrogels were also investigated owing to their high cell encapsulation, changeable biochemical and mechanical characteristics, and tissue biocompatibility with minimal immune reaction risk (Trojani et al., 2005; Jin et al., 2015). Although these hydrogels are well-established models for tissue regeneration, they have been less explored as biomimetic bone models, owing to their inability to match native bone's mechanical properties. In addition, 3D organotypic culture models cultivated with the aid of bioreactors can now be used to effectively create dynamic cell cultures, which further increases bone-like hallmarks (Sladkova & de Peppo, 2014) (Figure 14.3).

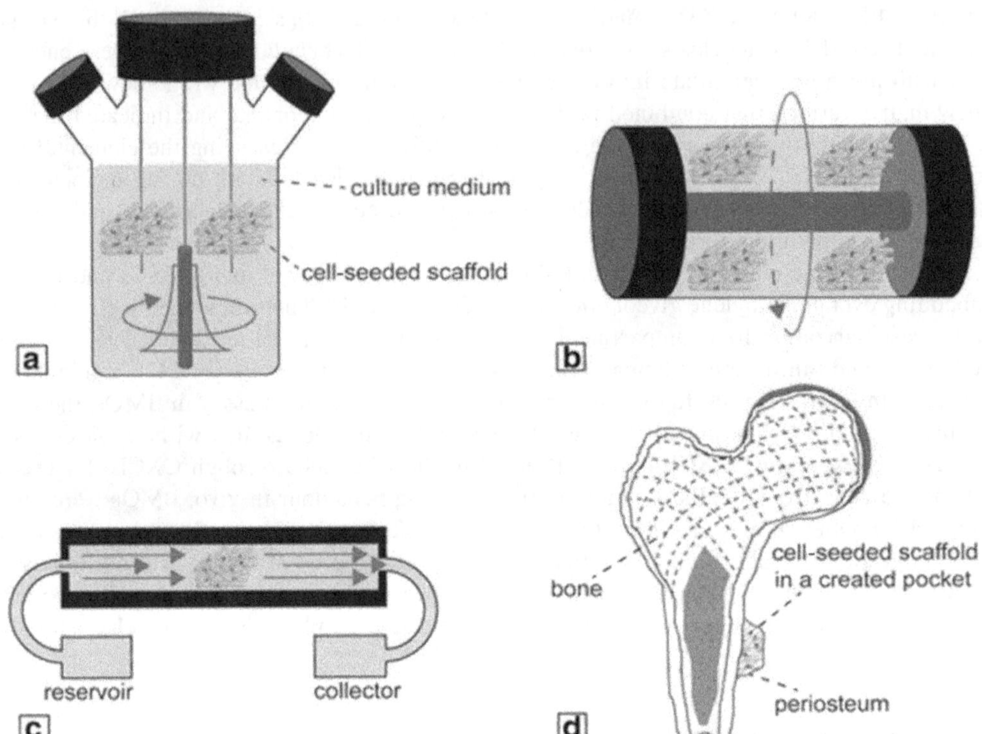

FIGURE 14.3 The main bioreactors for producing 3D bone tissue constructs for bone mimetic applications: (a) spinner flask, (b) rotating wall vessel, (c) perfusion, and d) in vivo bioreactor (reproduced under the terms of CC-BY 4.0 (https://creativecommons.org/licenses/by/4.0/) International License from Pirosa, A., Gottardi, R., Alexander, P. G., & Tuan, R. S.: Engineering in vitro stem cell-based vascularized bone models for drug screening and predictive toxicology. Stem Cell Res. Ther. 2018. 9. 112. Copyright 2018 Pirosa et al., published by Springer Nature).

14.6 MICROFLUIDICS AND ON-CHIP PLATFORMS

Microfluidic platforms are cutting-edge cell culture techniques that are similar to smaller versions of bioreactors, fabricating chips using micron and nanoscale manufacturing tools. Using microfluidics or lab-on-a-chip enables creating intricate structures at micron scale with precise features that closely resemble the dynamic nature of in vivo conditions and functions. We give detailed descriptions in the remainder of this chapter.

14.6.1 Bone-on-a-Chip Model

Scientists have recently discovered alternatives to animal models to reduce their usage in biomedical, pharmacological, and toxicological domains, such as in vitro models that mimic small organs with microfluidic channels (also known as organ-on-a-chip). Interestingly, these models overcome the constraints observed in in vitro 2D, 3D, and animal models by mimicking the human microenvironment. Furthermore, the major intention of the microfluidics platform is to develop therapeutics with a greater success rate that works better in humans.

Multiorgan chip models can be made by linking organs or cells via network connections (Vera et al., 2021). In this section, we focus on bone- and bone-marrow-on-a-chip models that have been designed and used in a wide range of clinical studies for bone-related illnesses. Various bone-on-a-chip systems have been introduced (Figure 14.4) as disease models for osteomyelitis, rheumatoid

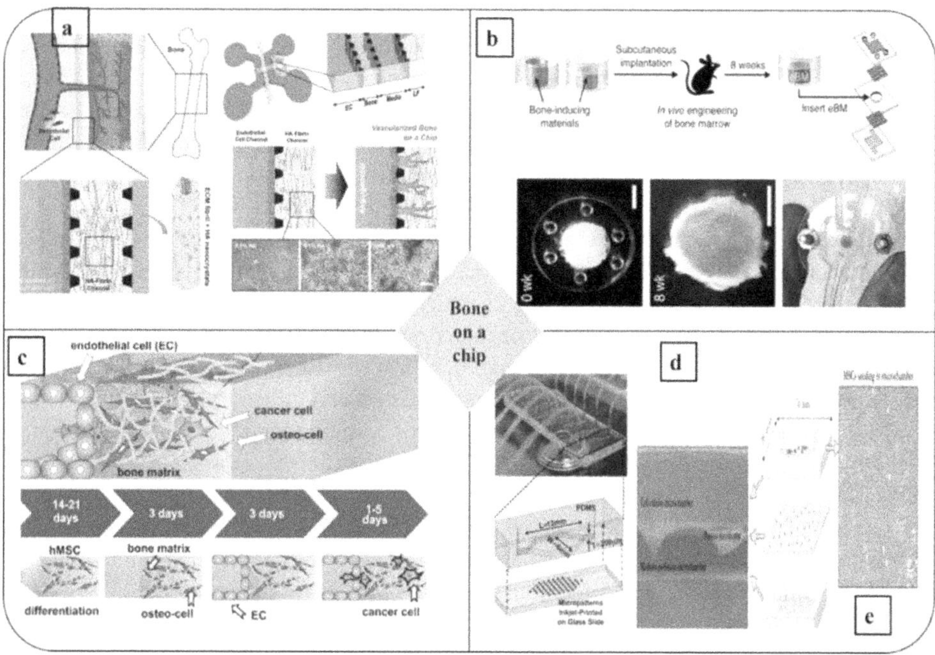

FIGURE 14.4 Bone and bone marrow on a microfluidic chip: (a) vascularized 3D bone on chip with ECM (reproduced with permission from Jusoh, N., Oh, S., Kim, S., Kim, J., & Jeon, N. L.: Microfluidic vascularized bone tissue model with the HA-incorporated extracellular matrix. Lab Chip. 2015. 15. 3984–3988. Copyright 2015 Royal Society of Chemistry); (b) hematopoietic niche on a chip (reproduced with permission from Torisawa, Y. S., Spina, C. S., Mammoto, T., Mammoto, A., Weaver, J. C., Tat, T., Collins, J. J., & Ingber, D. E.: Bone marrow-on-a-chip replicates hematopoietic niche physiology in vitro. Nat. Methods. 2014. 11. 663–669. Copyright 2014 Springer Nature); (c) in vitro 3D bone chip model to study breast cancer metastasis to the bone (Reproduced with permission from Bersini, S., Jeon, J. S., Dubini, G., Arrigoni, C., Chung, S., Charest, J. L., Moretti, M., & Kamm, R. D.: A microfluidic 3D in vitro model for the specificity of breast cancer metastasis to bone. Biomaterials. 2014. 35. 2454–2461. Copyright 2014 Elsevier); (d) microfluidic 3D bone tissue model for wound healing and biofilm prevention in biomaterials (reproduced with permission from Lee, J. H., Gu, Y., Wang, H., & Lee, W. Y.: Microfluidic 3D bone tissue model for high-throughput evaluation of wound-healing and infection-preventing biomaterials. Biomaterials. 2012. 33. 999–1006. Copyright 2012 Elsevier); (e) 3D bone marrow on a chip (Reproduced under the terms of CC-BY 4.0 (https://creativecommons.org/licenses/by/4.0/) International License from Kefallinou, D., Grigoriou, M., Boumpas, D. T., Gogolides, E., & Tserepi, A.: Fabrication of a 3D microfluidic cell culture device for bone marrow-on-a-chip. Micro Nano Eng. 2020. 9. 100075. Copyright 2020 Kefallinou et al., published by Elsevier).

arthritis (RA), and bone-targeting cancers and also as in vitro models for understanding osteoimmunology, human MSC osteogenic potential, and biomaterial efficacy in wound and infection healing (Lee et al., 2012).

For instance, citrullination, a process by which peptidyl arginine deiminase enzymes convert arginine to citrulline residues, is a significant contributor to the disease progression in RA. To study the effects of anticitrullinated protein antibodies (ACPAs) in bone remodelling that occurs in RA, Sethi et al. (2015) designed an in vitro bone-on-a-chip model using osteoclasts from bovine that were then grown on the chip and subsequently exposed to Fab and Fc fragments of IgG from RA patient-derived ACPAs. When the authors measured the bone turnover ratios, they were higher in the antibody-treated models than in the untreated osteoclasts. Although the antibody fragments significantly affected bone turnover ratios, the sample was too small to get robust statistical results, suggesting large sample requirements to validate conclusive outcomes.

Required cell quantity, cost, and process time are drastically reduced by using on-chip models, with the flexibility to incorporate multiple stimulation conditions in a highly efficient manner. Researchers examined hMSCs and human adipose-derived stem cells (hASCs) for their osteogenesis potential with mechanical stimuli on an integrated chip model (Park et al., 2012). Between the two stem cell types, hMSCs showed higher osteogenic differential potential than hASCs. The selective application of mechanical stimuli to human stem cells supports identifying the most suitable conditions to achieve osteogenesis (Park et al., 2012; Sim et al., 2007).

Several key studies adopted microfluidic devices to study the crosstalk between tumour cells and resident bone cells. For example, a 3D microfluidic bone model was developed by Bersini et al. (2014) to study cancer metastasis to the bone. The authors investigated cancer cell extravasation and micro-metastasis after three days of injection within the microfluidic device cocultured with endothelial cells and hMSCs. They found significant differences between the extravasation rates of tumour cells and their travelled distances in osteo-conditioned microenvironments compared with collagen matrix alone. In particular, the extravasation process of breast cancer cells is influenced by the bone-secreted chemokine CXCL5 and the cancer cell surface receptor CXCR2. The anti-CXCR2 molecule reduced the extravasation distance when added into the medium, and the rate significantly increased in the bone matrix niche after adding CXCL5 (Bersini et al., 2014). Therefore, microfluidic models are the best platforms for studying cancer invasion to bone, as they can emulate the microvascular and interstitial tissue components of native bone.

Mei et al. (2019) conducted one study to simulate breast cancer metastasis in a 3D microfluidic device using human mammary adenocarcinoma cells. The metastatic breast cancer cells were cocultured with HUVECs near a channel of osteocyte-like cells, that is, MLO-Y4. To mechanically excite the osteocytes, the authors used a physiologically comparable oscillating fluid flow. In the microfluidic device model with the integrated stimulatory bone fluid flow, the mechanically stimulated osteocytes showed less breast cancer extravasation than the static model (Mei et al., 2019).

Other strategies include a 3D microfluidic model based on perfusion designed to recapitulate the extravasation of cancer cells from breast and then intravasation into bone during metastasis by providing a suitable osteo-differentiation environment for MSCs (Jeon et al., 2015). The microfluidic device had a single channel filled with cancer cells, osteo-differentiated cells, and endothelial lining. The experimental results found that the cancer cell extravasation decreased while C2C12 myoblasts in the cancer cell compartment increased since the myoblasts have a higher permeability rate than cancer cells.

The authors also studied the role of adenosine in the bone-mimicking microenvironments and determined that the rates of extravasation and permeability were comparable to C2C12-conditioned matrices; this shows that the biomolecules can tune a specific milieu with antimetastatic properties. The authors also investigated the shear stress effect on cancer cell extravasation during fluid flow in on-chip platforms, and positing that the cancer cells would extravasate more slowly via the endothelium under flow circumstances than they would in static conditions. However, the extravasation distance was more significant in the flow condition than in the static environment (Jeon et al., 2015).

Jusoh et al. (2015) also showed enhanced angiogenesis in on-chip 3D bone models by incorporating various concentrations of HA into the fibrin ECM. Results confirmed that HA concentrations of ≤0.5% (0.2% HA) showed high-speed angiogenic sprout vessel growth, increased sprout length, a high number of sprouts, and increased lumen area. Altogether, these reported chip models that integrated endothelial microvasculature and 3D hydrogel systems were better models for toxicology, therapeutic screening, and cancer metastasis studies.

14.6.2 Bone-Marrow-on-a-Chip Model

In addition to the bone on-a-chip model for studying bone cell resorption and formation mechanisms in diseased conditions, Torisawa et al. (2014) designed an engineered bone marrow (eBM)-on-a-chip model that utilized a hollow cylindrical PDMS membrane containing type I collagen, demineralized bone matrix powder, and bone morphogenetic proteins. This model was implanted subcutaneously into a mouse. After eight weeks of implantation, the excised eBM was integrated into a microchip to serve as a prototype of a hematopoietic niche; the niche retained its properties completely and was supplied with a constant flow of culture medium through microchannels.

The cultured eBM was then transplanted into lethally irradiated mice, demonstrating similar functional potential with bone marrow from a mouse femur. However, it should be noted that this model cannot completely mimic the human bone marrow environment as it is derived from mice. Despite this limitation, the study authors concluded that human eBM on a chip can be developed in immunocompromised mice and can replace animal models to provide insights into bone marrow research (Torisawa et al., 2014).

Similarly, Sieber et al. (2018) developed multiorgan microfluidic chips utilizing HA-coated zirconium oxide scaffolds containing hMSCs and cord-blood-derived HSPCs. They created the chips to study breast cancer cells' colonization in bone during disease progression and drug resistance. For this purpose, they established a perivascular niche on a chip model using hMSCs that underwent phenotypic transformation into perivascular cell lineages. Capillary-like structures were generated surrounding the vascular lumen in this model. Furthermore, interstitial flow integrated perivascularly on a chip platform has been shown to promote the formation of stable vasculature as well as the colonization of breast cancer cells. The chip was equipped with a precisely controlled flow that allowed it to cultivate macroscopic tissues, enabling live monitoring of tissue growth and vascularization during extended culture periods (Marturano-Kruik et al., 2018).

Torisawa et al. (2014) created a microfluidic model for bone marrow to investigate continuous blood cell production and its response to radiation and radiation countermeasure drugs. The model showed an increase in the production of leukocytes and red blood cells under microfluidic flow conditions in the presence of erythropoietin. However, when exposed to gamma radiation, a sudden decrease in leukocyte production was observed. Treatment with hematopoietic growth factors and bactericidal proteins such as granulocyte-colony stimulating factor and bactericidal/permeability increasing protein followed by exposure to gamma radiation, resulted in an increase in blood stem cells and myeloid cells in the fluidic stream that was not observed in static models. These findings suggest that bone marrow on a chip has the potential to stimulate blood cell production, monitor the effects of hematopoietic modulators, and evaluate the effectiveness of radiation countermeasures.

Aleman et al. (2019) created a bone marrow microchip to investigate normal and malignant human hematopoietic stem/progenitor cell interactions in the hematopoietic niche, as well as the homing and engraftment of these cells into various niche components. The 3D chips were constructed using hyaluronic acid and gelatin-based hydrogel constructs containing all niche populations. This system allows for the real-time visualization, tracking, and quantification of interactions between fluorescently labelled HSPCs from normal human BMs, leukaemia cells (MOLM13), and lymphoma cells (U937). The results revealed different patterns of homing and lodging/retention in HSPC lines from leukaemia and lymphoma patients. Currently, bone marrow on-chip systems are limited to maintaining hematopoietic stem cells supported by 3D scaffolds.

Kefallinou et al. (2020) introduced an in vitro microfluidic device that is scaffold-free that can generate and maintain perivascular hematopoietic niches, with the aim of gaining insight into systemic lupus erythematosus. In a separate study on human bone marrow on a chip, Chou et al. (2020) utilized a fluidic vascular channel containing fibrin gel to cocultivate bone marrow $CD34^+$ and BM-derived stromal cells and then employed the human endothelial cells lining in alongside the channel to perfuse the culture medium, which improved $CD34^+$ cell maintenance for up to four weeks and facilitated the hematopoietic cells differentiation towards multiple blood cells. Furthermore, the chip mimicked BM injury, including myeloerythroid toxicity from chemotherapy and radiation, as well as BM recovery following myelosuppression.

Bruce et al. (2015) created a microfluidic chip that mimics in vivo 3D culture to investigate the mechanisms of acute lymphoblastic leukaemia. The authors evaluated the viability of tumour cells in response to the chemotherapy drug cytarabine, both in tumour cells alone and in tricultures made of osteoblasts and leukemic and stromal cells in 2D, 3D, and 3D microfluidic cultures. They found that the leukemic cells in the 3D triculture models were less responsive to chemotherapeutic drugs than were those in 2D static cultures. Additionally, the study demonstrated that the bone marrow niche plays a crucial role in maintaining tumour cell survival during drug treatment.

Zheng et al. (2016) developed a 3D biomimetic model of bone marrow angiogenesis that was induced by leukemic cells using microengineering. This model incorporated ECs, leukemic cells, and bone marrow stromal fibroblasts to effectively simulate early angiogenesis. The results from the experiments indicate that the proliferation and survival of leukemic cells are attributed to bone marrow angiogenesis.

CONCLUSION

Although investigators have used in vitro 2D and 3D models as models for bone diseases and drug testing, they still need to be validated in vivo in animal models. Biomaterial researchers throughout the world have come to a consensus that 3D bone models better replicate the microenvironment than 2D models. These 3D disease models ensure proper cell-to-cell communication along with the cell-to-matrix interaction that is observed in vivo and can be replicated ex vivo.

Fewer signals are available in 2D bone models than in 3D models due to the sheetlike morphology and abnormal phenotypes. This stressed microenvironment of cells in 2D results in altered cell growth and migration, which is less representative of the metastasis observed in vivo. Still, 2D cultures serve as a gold standard because of their ease of use and lower cost compared with animal studies and 3D models (Sitarski et al., 2018).

LIST OF ABBREVIATIONS

APN-KO	Adiponectin knockout mice
BCP	Biphasic Calcium Phosphate
BMMs	Bone marrow-derived macrophages
BMOs	Bone Marrow Organoids
BMP	Bone Morphogenetic Proteins
BMU	Basic Multicellular Unit
CX43	Connexin 43
CXCL12	C-X-C Motif Chemokine Ligand 12
CXCL5	C-X-C motif Chemokine 5
CXCR2	C-X-C Chemokine Receptor 2
CXCR4	C-X-C Chemokine Receptor 4
eBM	Engineered Bone Marrow
ECM	Extracellular matrix
ECs	Endothelial Cells
GNPs	Gold Nanoparticles
HA	Hydroxyapatite
HSPCs	Hematopoietic Stem and Progenitor Cells
HUVECs	Human Umbilical Vein Endothelial Cells
IL-1β	Interleukin-1-beta
MSCs	Mesenchymal Stem/Stromal Cells
OPG	Osteoprotegerin
RANKL	Receptor Activator of Nuclear Factor Kappa-B Ligand
TEC	Tissue Engineered Constructs

REFERENCES

Akhbar, M. F. A., & Yusoff, A. R. (2018). Optimization of drilling parameters for thermal bone necrosis prevention. *Technol. Health Care*. 26: 621–635.

Akiva, A., Melke, J., Ansari, S., Liv, N., van der Meijden, R., van Erp, M., Zhao, F., Stout, M., Nijhuis, W. H., de Heus, C., Muñiz Ortera, C., Fermie, J., Klumperman, J., Ito, K., Sommerdijk, N., & Hofmann, S. (2021). An organoid for woven bone. *Adv. Funct. Mater*. 31: 2010524.

Akkerman, N., & Defize, L. H. (2017). Dawn of the organoid era: 3D tissue and organ cultures revolutionize the study of development, disease, and regeneration. *Bioessays*. 39: 1600244.

Aleman, J., George, S. K., Herberg, S., Devarasetty, M., Porada, C. D., Skardal, A., & Almeida-Porada, G. (2019). Deconstructed microfluidic bone marrow on-A-chip to study normal and malignant hematopoietic cell—Niche interactions. *Small*. 15: 1902971.

Arrigoni, C., Bersini, S., Gilardi, M., & Moretti, M. (2016). *In vitro* co-culture models of breast cancer metastatic progression towards bone. *Int. J. Mol. Sci*. 17: 1405.

Baptista, L. S., Kronemberger, G. S., Côrtes, I., Charelli, L. E., Matsui, R. A. M., Palhares, T. N., Sohier, J., Rossi, A. M., & Granjeiro, J. M. (2018). Adult stem cells spheroids to optimize cell colonization in scaffolds for cartilage and bone tissue engineering. *Int. J. Mol. Sci*. 19: 1285.

Baran, R., Wehland, M., Schulz, H., Heer, M., Infanger, M., & Grimm, D. (2022). Microgravity-related changes in bone density and treatment options: A systematic review. *Int. J. Mol. Sci*. 23: 8650.

Bernhardt, A., Skottke, J., von Witzleben, M., & Gelinsky, M. (2021). Triple culture of primary human osteoblasts, osteoclasts and osteocytes as an *In vitro* bone model. *Int. J. Mol. Sci*. 22: 7316.

Bersini, S., Jeon, J. S., Dubini, G., Arrigoni, C., Chung, S., Charest, J. L., Moretti, M., & Kamm, R. D. (2014). A microfluidic 3D in vitro model for specificity of breast cancer metastasis to bone. *Biomaterials*. 35: 2454–2461.

Białkowska, K., Komorowski, P., Bryszewska, M., & Miłowska, K. (2020). Spheroids as a type of three-dimensional cell cultures—Examples of methods of preparation and the most important application. *Int. J. Mol. Sci*. 21: 1–17.

Bicho, D., Pina, S., Oliveira, J. M., & Reis, R. L. (2018). *In vitro* mimetic models for the bone-cartilage interface regeneration. *Adv. Exp. Med. Biol*. 1059: 373–394.

Blakytny, R., Spraul, M., & Jude, E. B. (2011). The diabetic bone: A cellular and molecular perspective. *Int. J. Low. Extrem. Wounds*. 10: 16–32.

Bruce, A., Evans, R., Mezan, R., Shi, L., Moses, B. S., Martin, K. H., Gibson, L. F., & Yang, Y. (2015). Three-dimensional microfluidic tri-culture model of the bone marrow microenvironment for study of acute lymphoblastic leukemia. *PLoS One*. 10: e0140506.

Chan, M. E., Lu, X. L., Huo, B., Baik, A. D., Chiang, V., Guldberg, R. E., Lu, H. H., & Guo, X. E. (2009). A trabecular bone explant model of osteocyte-osteoblast co-culture for bone mechanobiology. *Cell. Mol. Bioeng*. 2: 405–415.

Chang, R., Sun, L., & Webster, T. J. (2014). Short communication: Selective cytotoxicity of curcumin on osteosarcoma cells compared to healthy osteoblasts. *Int. J. Nanomed*. 9: 461.

Chou, D. B., Frismantas, V., Milton, Y., David, R., Pop-Damkov, P., Ferguson, D., MacDonald, A., Bölükbaşı, Ö. V., Joyce, C. E., Moreira Teixeira, L. S., Rech, A., Jiang, A., Calamari, E., Jalili-Firoozinezhad, S., Furlong, B. A., O'Sullivan, L. R., Ng, C. F., Choe, Y., Clauson, S., Myers, K. C., Weinberg, O. K., Hasserjian, R. P., Novak, R., Levy, O., Prantil-Baun, R., Novina, C. D., Shimamura, A., Ewart, L., & Ingber, D. E. (2020). On-chip recapitulation of clinical bone marrow toxicities and patient-specific pathophysiology. *Nat. Biomed. Eng*. 4: 394–406.

Choudhary, S., Ramasundaram, P., Dziopa, E., Mannion, C., Kissin, Y., Tricoli, L., Albanese, C., Lee, W., & Zilberberg, J. (2018). Human *ex vivo* 3D bone model recapitulates osteocyte response to metastatic prostate cancer. *Sci. Rep*. 8: 1–12.

Collin-Osdoby, P., & Osdoby, P. (2012). RANKL-mediated osteoclast formation from murine RAW 264.7 cells. *Methods Mol. Biol*. 816: 187–202.

Cramer, E. E. A., Ito, K., & Hofmann, S. (2021). *Ex vivo* bone models and their potential in preclinical evaluation. *Curr. Osteoporos. Rep*. 19: 75–87.

Davies, J. A. (2018). Organoids and mini-organs: Introduction, history, and potential. In *Organoids and Mini-Organs*. J. A. Davies, and M. L. Lawrence, Eds. Edinburgh: Elsevier, pp. 3–23.

De La Zerda, A., Kratochvil, M. J., Suhar, N. A., & Heilshorn, S. C. (2018). Review: Bioengineering strategies to probe T cell mechanobiology. *APL Bioeng*. 2: 021501.

de Wildt, B. W. M., van der Meijden, R., Bartels, P. A. A., Sommerdijk, N. A. J. M., Akiva, A., Ito, K., & Hofmann, S. (2022). Bioinspired silk fibroin mineralization for advanced *In vitro* bone remodelling models. *Adv. Funct. Mater.* 32: 2206992.

Dolan, E. B., Haugh, M. G., Tallon, D., Casey, C., & McNamara, L. M. (2012). Heat-shock-induced cellular responses to temperature elevations occurring during orthopaedic cutting. *J. R. Soc. Interface*. 9: 3503–3513.

Fennema, E., Rivron, N., Rouwkema, J., van Blitterswijk, C., & De Boer, J. (2013). Spheroid culture as a tool for creating 3D complex tissues. *Trends Biotechnol.* 31: 108–115.

Fernandez-Yague, M. A., Abbah, S. A., McNamara, L., Zeugolis, D. I., Pandit, A., & Biggs, M. J. (2015). Biomimetic approaches in bone tissue engineering: Integrating biological and physicomechanical strategies. *Adv. Drug Deliv. Rev.* 84: 1–29.

Fischbach, C., Chen, R., Matsumoto, T., Schmelzle, T., Brugge, J. S., Polverini, P. J., & Mooney, D. J. (2007). Engineering tumors with 3D scaffolds. *Nat. Methods*. 4: 855–860.

Gaharwar, A. K., Arpanaei, A., Andresen, T. L., & Dolatshahi-Pirouz, A. (2016). 3D biomaterial microarrays for regenerative medicine: Current state-of-the-art, emerging directions and future trends. *Adv. Mater.* 28: 771–781.

Garg, P., Strigini, M., Peurière, L., Vico, L., & Iandolo, D. (2021). The skeletal cellular and molecular underpinning of the murine hindlimb unloading model. *Front. Physiol.* 12: 1798.

Ghouse, S., Reznikov, N., Boughton, O. R., Babu, S., Ng, K. G., Blunn, G., Cobb, J. P., Stevens, M. M., & Jeffers, J. R. (2019). The design and in vivo testing of a locally stiffness-matched porous scaffold. *Appl. Mater. Today*. 15: 377–388.

Giger, S., Hofer, M., Miljkovic-Licina, M., Hoehnel, S., Brandenberg, N., Guiet, R., Ehrbar, M., Kleiner, E., Gegenschatz, K., Matthes, T., & Lutolf, M. P. (2022). Microarrayed human bone marrow organoids for modeling blood stem cell dynamics. *APL Bioeng*. 6: 036101.

Grémare, A., Aussel, A., Bareille, R., Paiva Dos Santos, B., Amédée, J., Thébaud, N. B., & Le Nihouannen, D. (2019). A unique triculture model to study osteoblasts, osteoclasts, and endothelial cells. *Tissue Eng., Part C*. 25: 421–432.

grTiaden, A. N., Breiden, M., Mirsaidi, A., Weber, F. A., Bahrenberg, G., Glanz, S., Cinelli, P., Ehrmann, M., & Richards, P. J. (2012). Human serine protease HTRA1 positively regulates osteogenesis of human bone marrow-derived mesenchymal stem cells and mineralization of differentiating bone-forming cells through the modulation of extracellular matrix protein. *Stem Cells*. 30: 2271–2282.

Guelcher, S. A., & Sterling, J. A. (2011). Contribution of bone tissue modulus to breast cancer metastasis to bone. *Cancer Microenviron.* 4: 247–259.

Haffner-Luntzer, M., Hankenson, K. D., Ignatius, A., Pfeifer, R., Khader, B. A., Hildebrand, F., van Griensven, M., Pape, H. C., & Lehmicke, M. (2019). Review of animal models of comorbidities in fracture-healing research. *J. Orthop. Res.* 37: 2491–2498.

Hamann, C., Kirschner, S., Günther, K. P., & Hofbauer, L. C. (2012). Bone, sweet bone—osteoporotic fractures in diabetes mellitus. *Nat. Rev. Endocrinol.* 8: 297–305.

Haugen, S., He, J., Sundaresan, A., Stunes, A. K., Aasarød, K. M., Tiainen, H., Syversen, U., Skallerud, B., & Reseland, J. E. (2018). Adiponectin reduces bone stiffness: Verified in a three-dimensional artificial human bone model *In vitro*. *Front. Endocrinol.* 9: 236.

Hayden, R. S., Vollrath, M., & Kaplan, D. L. (2014). Effects of clodronate and alendronate on osteoclast and osteoblast co-cultures on silk—hydroxyapatite films. *Acta Biomater.* 10: 486–493.

Iordachescu, A., Hughes, E. A., Joseph, S., Hill, E. J., Grover, L. M., & Metcalfe, A. D. (2021). Trabecular bone organoids: A micron-scale "humanised" prototype designed to study the effects of microgravity and degeneration. *NPJ Microgravity*. 7: 17.

Itel, F., Skovhus Thomsen, J., & Städler, B. (2018). Matrix vesicles-containing microreactors as support for bonelike osteoblasts to enhance biomineralization. *ACS Appl. Mater. Interfaces*. 10: 30180–30190.

Jähn, K., Braunstein, V., Furlong, P. I., Simpson, A. E., Richards, R. G., & Stoddart, M. J. (2010). A rapid method for the generation of uniform acellular bone explants: A technical note. *J. Orthop. Surg. Res.* 5: 1–4.

Jeon, J. S., Bersini, S., Gilardi, M., Dubini, G., Charest, J. L., Moretti, M., & Kamm, R. D. (2015). Human 3D vascularized organotypic microfluidic assays to study breast cancer cell extravasation. *Proc. Natl. Acad. Sci. U. S. A.* 112: 214–219.

Jin, Y., Kundu, B., Cai, Y., Kundu, S. C., & Yao, J. (2015). Bio-inspired mineralization of hydroxyapatite in 3D silk fibroin hydrogel for bone tissue engineering. *Colloids Surf. B*. 134: 339–345.

Jusoh, N., Oh, S., Kim, S., Kim, J., & Jeon, N. L. (2015). Microfluidic vascularized bone tissue model with hydroxyapatite-incorporated extracellular matrix. *Lab Chip*. 15: 3984–3988.

Kato, Y., Windle, J. J., Koop, B. A., Mundy, G. R., & Bonewald, L. F. (1997). Establishment of an osteocyte-like cell line, MLO-Y4. *J. Bone Miner. Res*. 12: 2014–2023.

Kefallinou, D., Grigoriou, M., Boumpas, D. T., Gogolides, E., & Tserepi, A. (2020). Fabrication of a 3D microfluidic cell culture device for bone marrow-on-a-chip. *Micro Nano Eng*. 9: 100075.

Kniha, K., Heussen, N., Weber, E., Möhlhenrich, S. C., Hölzle, F., & Modabber, A. (2020). Temperature threshold values of bone necrosis for thermo-explantation of dental implants—A systematic review on preclinical *In vivo* research. *Materials*. 13: 3461.

Kronemberger, G. S., Carneiro, F. A., Rezende, D. F., & Baptista, L. S. (2021). Spheroids and organoids as humanized 3D scaffold-free engineered tissues for SARS-CoV-2 viral infection and drug screening. *Artif. Organs*. 45: 548–558.

Kuehling, T., Schilling, P., Bernstein, A., Mayr, H. O., Serr, A., Wittmer, A., Bohner, M., & Seidenstuecker, M. (2022). A human bone infection organ model for biomaterial research. *Acta Biomater*. 144: 230–241.

Kulkarni, R. N., Bakker, A. D., Everts, V., & Klein-Nulend, J. (2010). Inhibition of osteoclastogenesis by mechanically loaded osteocytes: Involvement of MEPE. *Calcif. Tissue Int*. 87: 461.

Kwakwa, K. A., Vanderburgh, J. P., Guelcher, S. A., & Sterling, J. A. (2017). Engineering 3D models of tumors and bone to understand tumor-induced bone disease and improve treatments. *Curr. Osteoporos. Rep*. 15: 247.

Lee, D., Heo, D. N., Kim, H. J., Ko, W. K., Lee, S. J., Heo, M., Bang, J. B., Lee, J. B., Hwang, D. S., Do, S. H., & Kwon, I. K. (2016). Inhibition of osteoclast differentiation and bone resorption by bisphosphonate-conjugated gold nanoparticles. *Sci. Rep*. 6: 1–11.

Lee, J. H., Gu, Y., Wang, H., & Lee, W. Y. (2012). Microfluidic 3D bone tissue model for high-throughput evaluation of wound-healing and infection-preventing biomaterials. *Biomaterials*. 33: 999–1006.

Li, K., Zhang, P., Zhu, Y., Alini, M., Grad, S., & Li, Z. (2021). Establishment of an *Ex vivo* inflammatory osteoarthritis model with human osteochondral explants. *Front. Bioeng. Biotech*. 9: 1291.

Li, P., Zhao, Z., Wang, L., Jin, X., Shen, Y., Nan, C., & Liu, H. (2018). Minimally effective concentration of zoledronic acid to suppress osteoclasts *in vitro*. *Exp. Ther. Med*. 15: 5330–5336.

Luu, A., Macdonald, R., Oblak, M., Brisson, B., & Viloria-Petit, A. (2018). Optimization of an explant culture model to characterize cancerassociated exosomes in canine osteosarcoma. *J. Extracell. Vesicles*. 7: 47.

Marino, S., Staines, K. A., Brown, G., Howard-Jones, R. A., & Adamczyk, M. (2016). Models of *ex vivo* explant cultures: Applications in bone research. *BoneKEy Rep*. 5: 818.

Marturano-Kruik, A., Nava, M. M., Yeager, K., Chramiec, A., Hao, L., Robinson, S., Guo, E., Raimondi, M. T., & Vunjak-Novakovic, G. (2018). Human bone perivascular niche-on-a-chip for studying metastatic colonization. *Proc. Natl. Acad. Sci. U. S. A*. 115: 1256–1261.

Maugg, D., Rothenaigner, I., Schorpp, K., Potukuchi, H. K., Korsching, E., Baumhoer, D., Hadian, K., Smida, J., & Nathrath, M. (2015). New small molecules targeting apoptosis and cell viability in osteosarcoma. *PLoS One*. 10: e0129058.

Mei, X., Middleton, K., Shim, D., Wan, Q., Xu, L., Ma, Y. H. V., Devadas, D., Walji, N., Wang, L., Young, E. W. K., & You, L. (2019). Microfluidic platform for studying osteocyte mechanoregulation of breast cancer bone metastasis. *Integr. Biol*. 11: 119–129.

Metzger, W., Sossong, D., Bächle, A., Pütz, N., Wennemuth, G., Pohlemann, T., & Oberringer, M. (2011). The liquid overlay technique is the key to formation of co-culture spheroids consisting of primary osteoblasts, fibroblasts and endothelial cells. *Cytotherapy*. 13: 1000–1012.

Moritani, Y., Usui, M., Sano, K., Nakazawa, K., Hanatani, T., Nakatomi, M., Iwata, T., Sato, T., Ariyoshi, W., Nishihara, T., & Nakashima, K. (2018). Spheroid culture enhances osteogenic potential of periodontal ligament mesenchymal stem cells. *J. Periodontal Res*. 53: 870–882.

Munoz-Garcia, J., Jubelin, C., Loussouarn, A., Goumard, M., Griscom, L., Renodon-Cornière, A., Heymann, M. F., & Heymann, D. (2021). *In vitro* three-dimensional cell cultures for bone sarcomas. *J. Bone Oncol*. 30: 100379.

Murphy, K. C., Hoch, A. I., Harvestine, J. N., Zhou, D., & Leach, J. K. (2016). Mesenchymal stem cell spheroids retain osteogenic phenotype through $\alpha 2\beta 1$ signaling. *Stem Cells Transl. Med*. 5: 1229–1237.

Naot, D., Watson, M., Callon, K. E., Tuari, D., Musson, D. S., Choi, A. J., Sreenivasan, D., Fernandez, J., Tu, P. T., Dickinson, M., Gamble, G. D., Grey, A., & Cornish, J. (2016). Reduced bone density and cortical bone indices in female adiponectin-knockout Mice. *Endocrinology*. 157: 3550–3561.

Owen, R., & Reilly, G. C. (2018). In vitro models of bone remodelling and associated disorders. *Front. Bioeng. Biotech.* 6: 134.

Park, S. H., Sim, W. Y., Min, B. H., Yang, S. S., Khademhosseini, A., & Kaplan, D. L. (2012). Chip-based comparison of the osteogenesis of human bone marrow- and adipose tissue-derived mesenchymal stem cells under mechanical stimulation. *PLoS One.* 7: e46689.

Pirosa, A., Gottardi, R., Alexander, P. G., & Tuan, R. S. (2018). Engineering *in vitro* stem cell-based vascularized bone models for drug screening and predictive toxicology. *Stem Cell Res. Ther.* 9: 112.

Raic, A., Riedel, S., Kemmling, E., Bieback, K., Overhage, J., & Lee-Thedieck, C. (2018). Biomimetic 3D *in vitro* model of biofilm triggered osteomyelitis for investigating hematopoiesis during bone marrow infections. *Acta Biomater.* 73: 250–262.

Restle, L., Costa-Silva, D., Lourenço, E. S., Bachinski, R. F., Batista, A. C., Linhares, A. B. R., & Alves, G. G. (2015). A 3D osteoblast in vitro model for the evaluation of biomedical materials. *Adv. Mater. Sci. Eng.* 2015: 268930.

Robles-Linares, J. A., Axinte, D., Liao, Z., & Gameros, A. (2020). Machining-induced thermal damage in cortical bone: Necrosis and micro-mechanical integrity. *Mater. Des.* 197: 109215.

Rumiński, S., Kalaszczyńska, I., & Lewandowska-Szumieł, M. (2020). Effect of cAMP signaling regulation in osteogenic differentiation of adipose-derived mesenchymal stem cells. *Cells.* 9: 1587.

Sasaki, J. I., Matsumoto, T., Egusa, H., Matsusaki, M., Nishiguchi, A., Nakano, T., Akashi, M., Imazato, S., & Yatani, H. (2012). *In vitro* reproduction of endochondral ossification using a 3D mesenchymal stem cell construct. *Integr. Biol.* 4: 1207–1214.

Sethi, M. K., Dusad, A., Hollins, A., Hunter, C. D., Duryee, M. J., Mikuls, T. R., & Gravallese, E. M. (2015). An in vitro bovine bone chip model with micro-CT: A model for the assessment of autoantibody mediated bone resorption. *Arthritis Rheumatol.* 67: 2707.

Shekaran, A., & García, A. J. (2010). Extracellular matrix-mimetic adhesive biomaterials for bone repair. *J. Biomed. Mater. Res.* 96: 261–272.

Sieber, S., Wirth, L., Cavak, N., Koenigsmark, M., Marx, U., Lauster, R., & Rosowski, M. (2018). Bone marrow-on-a-chip: Long-term culture of human haematopoietic stem cells in a three-dimensional microfluidic environment. *J. Tissue Eng. Regener. Med.* 12: 479–489.

Sim, W. Y., Park, S. W., Park, S. H., Min, B. H., Park, S. R., & Yang, S. S. (2007). A pneumatic micro cell chip for the differentiation of human mesenchymal stem cells under mechanical stimulation. *Lab Chip.* 7: 1775–1782.

Sitarski, A. M., Fairfield, H., Falank, C., & Reagan, M. R. (2018). 3d tissue engineered *In vitro* models of cancer in bone. *ACS Biomater. Sci. Eng.* 4: 324–336.

Sladkova, M., & de Peppo, G. M. (2014). Bioreactor systems for human bone tissue engineering. *Processes.* 2: 494–525.

Soon, G., Pingguan-Murphy, B., & Akbar, S. A. (2017). Modulation of osteoblast behavior on nanopatterned yttria-stabilized zirconia surfaces. *J. Mech. Behav. Biomed. Mater.* 68: 26–31.

Sottnik, J. L., Campbell, B., Mehra, R., Behbahani-Nejad, O., Hall, C. L., & Keller, E. T. (2014). Osteocytes serve as a progenitor cell of osteosarcoma. *J. Cell. Biochem.* 115: 1420–1429.

Souza, W., Piperni, S. G., Laviola, P., Rossi, A. L., Rossi, M. I. D., Archanjo, B. S., Leite, P. E., Fernandes, M. H., Rocha, L. A., Granjeiro, J. M., & Ribeiro, A. R. (2019). The two faces of titanium dioxide nanoparticles bio-camouflage in 3D bone spheroids. *Sci. Rep.* 9: 9309.

Stahl, A., Wenger, A., Weber, H., Stark, G. B., Augustin, H. G., & Finkenzeller, G. (2004). Bi-directional cell contact-dependent regulation of gene expression between endothelial cells and osteoblasts in a three-dimensional spheroidal coculture model. *Biochem. Biophys. Res. Commun.* 322: 684–692.

Sweeney, E., Lovering, A. M., Bowker, K. E., MacGowan, A. P., & Nelson, S. M. (2019). An *in vitro* biofilm model of staphylococcus aureus infection of bone. *Lett. Appl. Microbiol.* 68: 294–302.

Tam, W. L., Freitas Mendes, L., Chen, X., Lesage, R., van Hoven, I., Leysen, E., Kerckhofs, G., Bosmans, K., Chai, Y. C., Yamashita, A., Tsumaki, N., Geris, L., Roberts, S. J., & Luyten, F. P. (2021). Human pluripotent stem cell-derived cartilaginous organoids promote scaffold-free healing of critical size long bone defects. *Stem Cell Res. Ther.* 12: 1–16.

Tawy, G. F., Rowe, P. J., & Riches, P. E. (2016). Thermal damage done to bone by burring and sawing with and without irrigation in knee arthroplasty. *J. Arthroplasty.* 31: 1102–1108.

Torisawa, Y. S., Spina, C. S., Mammoto, T., Mammoto, A., Weaver, J. C., Tat, T., Collins, J. J., & Ingber, D. E. (2014). Bone marrow-on-a-chip replicates hematopoietic niche physiology *in vitro*. *Nat. Methods.* 11: 663–669.

Trojani, C., Weiss, P., Michiels, J. F., Vinatier, C., Guicheux, J., Daculsi, G., Gaudray, P., Carle, G. F., & Rochet, N. (2005). Three-dimensional culture and differentiation of human osteogenic cells in an injectable hydroxypropylmethylcellulose hydrogel. *Biomaterials*. 26: 5509–5517.

Vera, D., Garcia-Diaz, M., Torras, N., Alvarez, M., Villa, R., & Martinez, E. (2021). Engineering tissue barrier models on hydrogel microfluidic platforms. *ACS Appl. Mater. Interfaces*. 13: 13920–13933.

Wenger, A., Stahl, A., Weber, H., Finkenzeller, G., Augustin, H. G., Stark, G. B., & Kneser, U. (2004). Modulation of *in vitro* angiogenesis in a three-dimensional spheroidal coculture model for bone tissue engineering. *Tissue Eng*. 10: 1536–1547.

Yamada, K. M., & Cukierman, E. (2007). Modeling tissue morphogenesis and cancer in 3D. *Cell*. 130: 601–610.

Yamaguchi, Y., Ohno, J., Sato, A., Kido, H., & Fukushima, T. (2014). Mesenchymal stem cell spheroids exhibit enhanced *in vitro* and *in vivo* osteoregenerative potential. *BMC Biotechnol*. 14: 1–10.

Yang, J. Y., Ting, Y. C., Lai, J. Y., Liu, H. L., Fang, H. W., & Tsai, W. B. (2009). Quantitative analysis of osteoblast-like cells (MG63) morphology on nanogrooved substrata with various groove and ridge dimensions. *J. Biomed. Mater. Res., Part A*. 90: 629–640.

Yuste, I., Luciano, F. C., González-Burgos, E., Lalatsa, A., & Serrano, D. R. (2021). Mimicking bone microenvironment: 2D and 3D *in vitro* models of human osteoblasts. *Pharmacol. Res*. 169: 105626.

Zheng, Y., Sun, Y., Yu, X., Shao, Y., Zhang, P., Dai, G., & Fu, J. (2016). Angiogenesis in liquid tumors: An *In vitro* assay for leukemic-cell-induced bone marrow angiogenesis. *Adv. Healthcare Mater*. 5: 1014–1024.

15 Biomaterials and Their Carriers for Managing Bone Disorders

Erdem Aras Sezgin

15.1 INTRODUCTION

Bone typically regenerates following minor injuries, but more critical injuries can require interventions, including surgical interventions. These generally encompass autologous bone grafting and conventional methods of delivery for pharmaceutical therapy. With recent breakthroughs in biomaterials and biomaterials as carriers, tissue engineering offers solid potential for mitigating the adverse effects of conventional treatments for bone disorders.

Critical-sized bone defects caused by trauma, infection, or tumors can be managed with traditional methods: autografting, allografting, distraction osteogenesis, induced membrane, or combinations of these. However, limitations regarding the quantity of bone available, persistent donor site pain, disease transmission, infection, and inadequate vascularization with these methods influenced the developments of synthetic biomaterials in clinical scenarios. The use of biomaterials in bone is not limited to critical-sized defects. They can also be utilized to enhance secondary bone healing in nonunions as an alternative to autologous bone grafts. Although methods for utilizing biomaterials to enhance osteogenesis, osteoinduction, and osteoconduction vary vastly and current evidence is not concrete, promising future research is likely to define the indications of tissue engineering in long bone nonunion treatment.

Joint replacement procedures are among the most successful surgeries in all medicine, with relatively high success and satisfaction rates (Learmonth et al., 2007). However, they typically come with limited lifespans due to their inorganic composition, and they are prone to loosening caused by periprosthetic osteolysis. To improve the stability and osteointegration, novel coating techniques are being studied that use biomaterials designed with the principles that govern physiological bone formation and regeneration (Critchley et al., 2020; Hoornenborg et al., 2023; Knudsen et al., 2022; Mosegaard et al., 2022; Valancius et al., 2013).

Aside from surface coatings that increase integration with inorganic and organic phases of bone, biomaterials can also be utilized to impede inflammation induced by wear particles, which can lead to loosening (Guo et al., 2019; Rothammer et al., 2021). There are also studies on surface modifications to suppress initial bacterial adhesion that led to biofilm formation and periprosthetic joint infections requiring revision arthroplasty (Fiore et al., 2021; Gahane et al., 2020; Qayoom et al., 2020; Romanò et al., 2016). In addition to arthroplasty implants, suture anchors used to restore enthesis in various orthopedic procedures can also be manufactured and/or augmented with tissue engineering principles (Pill et al., 2021; Raina et al., 2019a; Sugaya et al., 2019). The potential benefits of this approach are the promotion of peri-implant bone formation and the strength of the bone–implant interface, which can limit the enlargement of bone tunnels created in the index operation and increase pull-out resistance (Sugaya et al., 2019; von Recum et al., 2020).

Antibiotic-laden beads or spacers for the treatment of bone and implant infections have been in use since the 1970s (Schmitt et al., 2020; Wahlig et al., 1978). They are used as carriers to release antibiotics in the tissue and potentially surpass levels that can be achieved by parenteral

DOI: 10.1201/9781003307310-18

administration. However, contemporary techniques for antibiotic delivery using biomaterials are necessary, as traditional methods contribute to antimicrobial resistance caused by subtherapeutic antibiotic elution (Antoci et al., 2007; Güven, 2021; Qayoom et al., 2020, 2022; Romanò et al., 2016).

Biomaterials acting as scaffolds for critical-sized defects as well as vessels for the local introduction of therapeutics can ease the surgeon's burden in managing chronic osteomyelitis. Another developing controlled delivery method utilizing biomaterials is used to deliver the cytostatic agents used in bone cancer (Liu et al., 2021; Ma et al., 2015; Wang et al., 2020; Xie et al., 2022). Targeting high local concentrations of the agent to cancer cells may be the key to reducing off-target side effects and managing micro metastasis. Furthermore, nanoparticles can be used to recruit circulating agents to further increase the antitumor activity (Liu et al., 2022). In this chapter, we assess the current literature on biomaterials and biomaterial carriers used in bone-related disorders, focusing on their clinical applications.

15.2 BIOMATERIALS AS BONE GRAFT ALTERNATIVES

Natural pathways of regeneration may fail in critical-size bone defects, and in these cases, bone is typically the first option to bridge the gap and initiate regeneration. The gold standard in bone grafting is using the patient's own bone stock, typically the iliac crest, as it offers excellent histocompatibility as well as a high concentration of autologous progenitor cells. It also provides sufficient osteoconduction.

Despite these obvious advantages of autografts over other types of bone grafts, their limited supply and several donor-site complications including persistent pain, hematoma, inflammation and infection necessitating longer hospital stay are considerable setbacks related to their use (Attia et al., 2022; van de Wall et al., 2022). Bone grafts harvested from other humans or animals may be utilized as allografts and xenografts, respectively, after being subjected to several preparation procedures. Although these organic materials hold comparable osteoconductive and osteoinductive properties, the ability to induce new bone formation by altering pathways for regeneration, and progenitor cell recruitment, they lack cells themselves and are therefore not considered osteogenic (Miron et al., 2013). Furthermore, donor-originated bone grafts are associated with a risk of disease transmission and infection as well as immunogenicity (Giannoudis et al., 2005; Oryan et al., 2014).

Synthetic bone substitutes have been developed with the intention of designing a bone graft that mimics the natural bone structure, is neither immunogenic nor open to disease transmission, and can be available in large quantities, overcoming several problems associated with organic bone grafts (Bhattacharjee et al., 2017; Wu et al., 2014). Biomaterials used as first-generation bone grafts are inert materials such as poly-methyl-methacrylate (PMMA) bone cement, titanium or titanium alloys, carbon, and alumina that were developed to cause minimal host reaction. However, their bioinert nature did not allow for sufficient interaction with the surrounding tissue, and instead of forming bone and integration, their implantation typically resulted in fibrous tissue formation at the interface (Hench, 1998; Yu et al., 2015).

Next-generation biomaterials consisting of biodegradable polymers, biodegradable ceramics, bioactive glasses, and biodegradable metals were developed aiming to allow tissue growth into the material (Figure 15.1). These have far superior biocompatibility and biodegradability (Pérez et al., 2013; Ulery et al., 2011; Xynos et al., 2000; Yuan et al., 2001). Contemporary biomaterials influence cellular responses utilizing growth factors, structural properties, and external stimuli. Tailoring these cellular responses, third-generation biomaterials can be used to achieve the desired effects on bone healing in specific clinical scenarios. Although potential bone graft alternatives were developed in preclinical studies, current clinical research aims to find the optimal balance between mechanical properties and degradation rates that match the regeneration rate of bone tissue (Table 15.1).

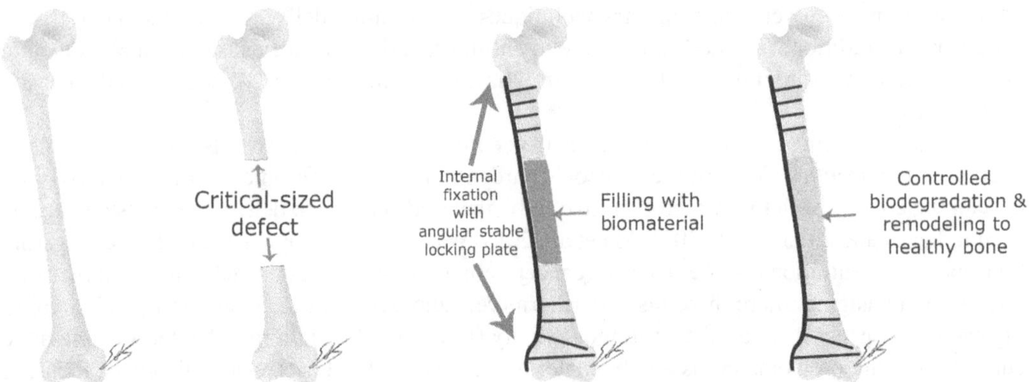

FIGURE 15.1 Biomaterial being used to fill a critical-sized defect. Controlled biodegradation allows tissue ingrowth and remodeling to healthy bone.

TABLE 15.1
Translational Stages for Biomaterials That Are in the Process of Clinical Translation

Bone Graft Alternatives	Translational Phase
Biodegradable polymers	
Collagen	T4
Chitosan	T2
Synthetic polymers	T3
Biodegradable ceramics	
CaS	T4
CaP	T4
Bioactive glasses	T3
Biodegradable metals	T3
Augmentation of implant anchorage	
CaP coating of orthopedic implants	T4
Biocomposite suture anchors	T4
Bio-active coating of dental implants	T3
Osteosynthesis augmentation with locally administered biomaterials	T2
Biomaterials in bone infections	
Surface coating for prophylaxis	
Defensive antibacterial coating	T3
Antibiotic loaded biodegradable cement	T2

T1: translation to humans, T2: translation to patients, T3: translation to practice, T4: translation to population health, CaS: calcium sulphate, CaP: calcium phosphate

15.2.1 Biodegradable Polymers

15.2.1.1 Collagen

Collagen is the dominant natural polymer found in the bone matrix, and therefore it has been widely studied as a biomaterial. On its own, collagen has a poor mechanical profile and is commonly included in composite materials (Brun et al., 2014; Feng et al., 2021; Tsai et al., 2020; Yu et al., 2020). It is also used as a barrier to cover autografts or allografts to guide cortical bone formation, especially in dental applications (Jung et al., 2009; Raina et al., 2019b).

In a 2018 randomized controlled trial (RCT) study of cystic maxillofacial bony defects, Vignesh et al. (2019) compared a composite collagen sponge supported by hydroxyapatite (HA) with bone marrow aspirate and HA alone; although follow-up was short, they reported earlier bone regeneration and faster wound healing. In another RCT on maxillofacial bone defects, Merli et al. (2018) showed that synthetic tricalcium phosphate (TCP) bone graft when combined with a natural collagen membrane produced similar results to natural bone graft. These methods of covering a collagen membrane on bone grafts may produce unpredictable results due to loss of augmented space due to the failure of collagen barrier membrane resistance to pressure (Thoma et al., 2019).

Soft-type blocks made of biphasic calcium phosphate (CaP) embedded in a collagen matrix were compared with the conventional aforementioned technique in a recent RCT aiming to provide an augmentation site with higher resistance, but even though the composite graft block scaffold had initial superior space-keeping ability, results at the six-month follow-up were similar in the two groups (Benic et al., 2022). Meanwhile, Cimatti et al. (2022) conducted a prospective observational study in the orthopedic field to explore using a commercially available collagen-HA composite scaffold in hip revision surgery. In two-year follow-ups of 29 patients, periacetabular scaffold integration and clinical outcome was good, there were no complications related to the scaffold, and the scaffold's survival rate was 100%.

Recombinant human bone morphogenetic protein-2 (rhBMP-2) is a bone-active molecule approved by the Food and Drug Administration for clinical use in filling bone defects. The approval was given for an absorbable collagen sponge (ACS) implant as the carrier to deliver this molecule. Several clinical trials evaluated the effectiveness of the rhBMP-2-soaked ACS in scenarios such as tibia fractures, vertebral fusion and alveolar ridge preservation (Arnold et al., 2016; Jo et al., 2019; Major Extremity Trauma Research Consortium (METRC), 2019).

In the RCT by the Major Extremity Trauma Research Consortium, its effectiveness was compared against autogenous iliac crest bone graft in tibia fractures with metaphyseal bone defects and results showed that both radiographic union and clinical healing were subpar in the ACS group within one year, while having a considerably higher cost of treatment (METRC, 2019). There are several other concerns raised over its use, namely its side effect profile including inflammation following implantation, heterotopic bone formation, and excessive bone resorption as a result of osteoclast activation (Arnold et al., 2016; James et al., 2016). Carriers of BMP-2 that allow a controlled and long-term release, such as synthetic calcium sulphate/HA cement instead of ACS, and adding bisphosphonates (BPs) as osteoclast deactivators overcame the side effects and increased bone regeneration in preclinical studies (Raina et al., 2020a).

15.2.1.2 Chitosan

Chitosan, another natural polymer has similar biologic properties to collagen (di Martino et al., 2005; Garric et al., 2017). Like collagen, it is also commonly combined with other polymers or bioceramics in scaffolds to achieve higher structural strength (Bharathi et al., 2022). The process of converting chitosan into three-dimensional (3D) scaffolds is common, and contemporary research focuses on their potential in drug delivery (Yadav et al., 2021). Despite many ongoing in vivo and in vitro studies, the clinical application of chitosan in bone defects is not yet widespread; clinical research is currently limited to preliminary studies and studies in joint cartilage regeneration (Babrawala et al., 2016; Boynueğri et al., 2009; Stanish et al., 2013).

15.2.1.3 Synthetic Biodegradable Polymers

Synthetic biodegradable polymers such as polylactic acid (PLA), poly(ε-caprolactone) (PCL), and polyglycolic acid (PGA) can be manufactured with adjusted porosity and physiochemical structure, which gives control over their shape, size, biodegradability, and biomechanical properties (Garric et al., 2017; Ogueri et al., 2021; Plantz et al., 2021). Instead of animal-sourced collagen membranes, some patients favor the use of synthetic polymers of nonanimal origins due to ethical or religious concerns (Bucchi et al., 2019). However, their mechanical properties, as other polymers can be insufficient and are also often combined with bioceramics as composite materials.

One of the limitations to their use is that the acidic degradation compounds cause an inflammatory foreign body reaction, altering the wound healing process and consequently accelerated absorption leading to mechanical failure, especially in load-bearing sites (Kohn et al., 2002). In a recent prospective study, the effectiveness of synthetic polymers was compared with natural collagen membranes in dental applications and significant bone regeneration and satisfactory density were achieved in either biomaterial (Kollek et al., 2022). Despite preliminary studies, further clinical research is needed to allow widespread acceptance in routine clinical practice.

Given the ability to modify their shape, size, and biodegradability, PLA and PGA were also used as early bioabsorbable fixation implants such as orthopedic interference screws and suture anchors. As PLA has a very long degradation rate, PLA and PGA were typically combined as copolymers (Nho et al., 2009). Despite favorable degradation rates in these implants, the degradation process did not include bone formation, often leaving bone tunnels at the implantation site and complicating revision surgical procedures. Combining these polymers with CaP-based ceramic biomaterials significantly promoted osteoconductive ability (Barber et al., 2017).

15.2.2 Biodegradable Ceramics

The most commonly used biodegradable ceramics in bone-related disorders are calcium sulphate (CaS) and various forms of CaP. Their biocompatibility and structural and compositional similarity to natural bone minerals and biological activity made them favored by many surgeons in treating bone defects and repairing fractures in the last few decades.

15.2.2.1 Calcium Sulphate

CaS is also known as plaster of Paris, and it has been used to fill void defects since the twentieth century (Amini et al., 2012) next to its conventional use in orthopedic casting. It has a fast resorption rate, mostly surpassing bone regeneration, and low mechanical strength making its implementation in the treatment of bone defects difficult. (Liodakis et al., 2022; Prins et al., 2016). These shortcomings may be overlooked in treating small bone defects when supported by rigid surgical fixation, but research is needed to widen the clinical scenarios where CaS can be used (Širka et al., 2018; Zampelis et al., 2013).

There are only a few clinical studies evaluating CaS as a bone graft substitute, but the indications are promising, and the number can be expected to increase. In a 2015 prospective study on proximal tibia fractures, Iundusi et al. (2015) reported that an injectable, biphasic HA and CaS ceramic bone substitute led to excellent bone regeneration 12 months after the operation, comparable with autografting. The authors suggested that with this biomaterial's injectable nature, it can be used to fill irregular defects, and its microporous structure allows an immediate flow of growth factors and cells, leading to early bone ingrowth.

Authors of an earlier prospective observational study examined the effectiveness of a commercially available, highly injectable, biphasic cement including CaS and HA to augment osteoporotic vertebral compression fractures and reported immediate and lasting pain relief, improved quality of life, and no device-related complications (Masala et al., 2012). Based on their results, its nontoxic character, and lower stiffness, this biphasic cement can be a valid and potentially better alternative to PMMA in vertebroplasty. In another study, the authors compared the effectiveness of injectable CaS with that of demineralized bone matrix-based grafts which are more expensive in filling contained bony defects created in tumor surgery (Kim et al., 2011). Radiological and clinical outcomes were similar between groups, and the success rate was over 85%. In the CaS group, cement was completely resorbed at three months in all but one patient who experienced a pathological fracture.

One of the articles with the highest level of evidence was published in 2020 by Hofmann et al. comparing autologous iliac bone graft with biphasic HA and CaS cement, in a clinical RCT on patients with tibia plateau fractures requiring reconstruction of the metaphyseal bone defect (Hofmann et al., 2020). Their results show that synthetic cement was as effective as the gold standard autologous iliac bone graft in filling the defect, with similar rates of fracture healing, defect remodeling, articular collapse, and similar patient-reported outcomes.

15.2.2.2 Calcium Phosphate and Hydroxyapatite

CaP ceramics are synthetic mineral crystals that are commonly used in implant coating to increase integration. On top of their common clinical use in implant coating, they are also widely adopted as bone grafts with their porous structure allowing ingrowth, higher resistance to compressive loads, and biocompatibility. They can be produced to mimic the microporous structure of bone tissue, which has advantages related to cell adhesion and proliferation (Putri et al., 2020).

HA is the naturally occurring mineral form of calcium apatite and makes up the majority of the weight of dry bone (Sheikh et al., 2015). Synthetic HA mimics cancellous bone with its low resistance to tension and shear stress as well as its macroporous structure. Although it combines with the new bone tissue fast and promotes vascular ingrowth, it has a high calcium-to-phosphate ratio, which slows the biodegradation (Brandt et al., 2010). Therefore, their use is mostly limited to implant coating, although many modifications are being studied to overcome these shortcomings (Kandasamy et al., 2020; Nie & Wang, 2007; Sheikh et al., 2015), such as nanocrystalline HA that allows for a significantly larger surface area to the volume, potentially increasing the resorption rate (Raina et al., 2020c).

Another molecule with history is TCP, which has a lower Ca/P ratio than HA and therefore faster degradation potential with lower mechanical strength (Campana et al., 2014). Among other biomaterials used in managing bone-related disorders, beta-tricalcium phosphate (β-TCP) is the most popular, especially in maxillofacial applications (Garcia et al., 2022). It has ideal clinical properties as a synthetic bone graft with its good absorption and regeneration profile.

However, even as the most popular option, calcium phosphates are also not fully resorbable; an amount of residual graft can still be detected at the implantation site years later despite bone regeneration (Abdullah et al., 2021; Okada et al., 2016; Putri et al., 2020) Despite this, most of the available clinical data show little to no complications observed with their use and high effectiveness (Garcia et al., 2022). In a 2019 RCT comparing allograft and β-TCP granules in an open-wedge high tibial osteotomy, authors showed that union rates and clinical outcomes were comparable between groups at the end of 12 months postoperative (Lee et al., 2019). More mild evidence from another observational study supports these results and expands the indications, suggesting that β-TCP granules can be used in the internal fixation of acute fractures of the proximal tibia to provide mechanical support and trabecular bone regeneration with high effectiveness (Oh et al., 2017).

Other options are combinations of β-TCP and HA in different concentrations to adjust absorption rates and mechanical properties. Biphasic calcium phosphate cement (BCP) should also be mentioned as another alternative that has been well studied in the last 30 years, BCP can be injected into bone voids and be used in various shapes, making it suitable for percutaneous vertebroplasty and kyphoplasty applications (Ishiguro et al., 2010; Kim & Park, 2020). Several contemporary studies also indicate that its uses can be expanded to numerous orthopedic and maxillofacial applications as a bone graft alternative.

In a 2018 RCT, Winge and Røkkum (2018) showed that an injectable CaP cement in distal radius fracture malunions can fill the voids in the corrective opening wedge osteotomy, with an effectiveness comparable with cortico-cancellous bone graft two years postoperative. A 2018 clinical trial showed that a BCP biomaterial consisting of 80% β-TCP and 20% HA can also be used as a scaffold for mesenchymal stem cells (MSCs) to fill maxillofacial bone defects, with high effectiveness that can challenge the gold standard, autologous grafting (Gjerde et al., 2018). Similarly, in an earlier observational study on posterior instrumentation surgery for adolescent idiopathic scoliosis, authors reported that silicate-substituted CaP (Si-CaP) can be enriched with bone marrow aspirate from vertebral bodies and lead to effective, easy, and safe posterior fusion (Lerner & Liljenqvist, 2013).

Silicate substitution prolongs the duration for complete resorption in conventional β-TCP biomaterials by enhancing bioactivity, speeding up angiogenesis, and triggering adaptive remodeling (Hing et al., 2006). Si-CaP was also recently tested as an alternative to autografting in an RCT on patients set to undergo two-step revision anterior cruciate ligament reconstruction to fill the bone tunnel defects originating from index surgery (von Recum et al., 2020). Results showed that at the end of three years, the Si-CaP group had similar clinical outcomes and knee laxity to the autologous iliac crest cancellous bone graft group while causing less perioperative hemoglobin drop and requiring half the surgical duration; making it a safe and effective alternative.

Synthetic PLA, PCL, and PGA are suitable polymers for suture anchor and interference screws used in orthopedic operations such as anterior cruciate ligament reconstruction, ligament repair, and rotator cuff repair. Combining these biodegradable implants with β-TCP to form hybrid scaffolds generates satisfactory bone regeneration in the implantation site instead of solely being absorbed (Barber et al., 2017). A systematic review of the clinical applications of these composite biomaterials used in the last 20 years showed excellent biocompatibility and good absorption and osseous regeneration three years after implantation (Barber et al., 2017). In a more recent study evaluating a commercially available composite suture anchor consisting of PLG, CaS, and β-TCP on 37 patients, 90% ossification was observed at the site of implantation two years after shoulder labral repair (Sugaya et al., 2019).

One of the contemporary approaches is utilizing CaP as a carrier of rhBMP-2 to provide a controlled release and further increase osteogenesis. Despite success reported in several preclinical studies, there are only a limited number of clinical studies published (Luo et al., 2017). In their 2018 RCT, Jo et al. (2019) compared the efficacy of rhBMP-2 loaded ACS with rhBMP-2-loaded CaP/HA biomaterial in alveolar ridge preservation and reported that both groups showed similar outcomes without severe adverse events four months after implantation.

In a more recent clinical trial also on maxillofacial surgery, authors evaluated a CaP cement system loaded with rhBMP-2 in repairing dental extraction sockets (Luo et al., 2022). Despite including a limited number of patients, these authors reported more bone formation than in the negative control at 12 months. In a similar approach, Šponer et al. (2018) used β-TCP as a scaffold carrier to deliver MSCs to fill femoral bone defects in revision hip arthroplasty. They found clinical and radiographic outcomes at one-year were similar to cancellous impaction allografting, while superior to β-TCP alone.

15.2.3 Bioactive Glasses

Synthetic Si-based ceramics, namely bioglass materials, have a history of 50 years and have been extensively studied in the clinical setting (Cook & Dalton, 1992). Upon implantation, bioglass typically gets covered with a HA layer, allowing integration with the host bone. However, Si-based bioglass has a slow degradation rate, which significantly reduces the integration. Borate- and phosphate-based bioglass was developed later to overcome these shortcomings (Dziadek et al., 2017; Lizzi et al., 2017).

There are several commercially available bioglasses in clinical use in the forms of coating, bone cement, and scaffolds (Drago et al., 2013; Sun et al., 2009). In an observational clinical study, al Malat et al. (2018) reported their experience with bioglass material to fill bone defects in patients with infected nonunions and found successful defect filling at one year in over 80% of patients, which can be regarded as a good rate in such clinical scenario. A similar study with more participants with chronic osteomyelitis in which bioactive glass material was used in one- or two-stage revisions, reported a success rate of 90% and effective defect filling (Lindfors et al., 2017).

Authors of a very recent RCT compared the efficacy of bioactive glass synthetic bone void filler and conventional bone grafting (autografting for small defects and allografting for large defects) in 49 adult patients with bone tumors (Aro et al., 2022). In this clinical study, Aro et al. reported over 80% treatment success at one year in either group, defined by no reoperation, no tumor recurrence, and no graft-related complications. Despite published clinical experiences with bioglass material in filling bone defects, available data are from a limited number of patients and is heterogeneous. Therefore, its widespread use is yet to be supported by further clinical trials also assessing its combinations with biological augmentation.

15.2.4 Biodegradable Metals

Bioinert metals such as stainless steel, titanium, and cobalt–chromium alloys are typically used in osteosynthesis, with their excellent corrosion resistance and loading characteristics (Sukotjo et al., 2020). However, they have also been used to fill bone defects despite their inert characteristics, which cause them to remain in the defect permanently. In addition, their elastic modulus and tensile strength are higher than bone, which is prone to stress shielding, which may lead to peri-implant fractures and implant loosening (Wang et al., 2022). Magnesium (Mg), zinc (Zn), iron (Fe), and their alloys are biodegradable alternatives that have good biocompatibility (Yang et al., 2021).

There is no evidence of toxicity or side effects of Mg, but its rapid degradation hinders its use as a bone graft alternative as well as an implant for osteosynthesis (Li et al., 2004; Wang et al., 2022). They also release hydrogen, which can lead to the separation of tissue layers, decreased vitality at the bone defect, and tissue necrosis (Sonnow et al., 2021). New techniques in manufacturing based on 3D printing may allow better corrosion resistance and biocompatibility. The majority of current animal studies on Mg-based implants investigate smaller defects instead of large defects, which are more common in orthopedic procedures and are more commonly associated with complications. Despite their potential, there currently is no evidence to support 3D-printed Mg-based implants used for large defects.

Pure Zn has low mechanical strength and fast biodegradation, although its alloys can improve these shortcomings; however, experience is currently limited to animal studies (Li et al., 2015; Zhang et al., 2018). Fe on the other hand has higher mechanical strength, similar to that of stainless steel. However, it has a very low degradation rate, which is associated with the same problems as conventional metal implants (Rabeeh & Hanas, 2022). Preclinical studies focus on optimizing the degradation rate with alloying, surface modification, and 3D printing (Li et al., 2019).

15.3 BIOMATERIALS TO AUGMENT IMPLANT ANCHORAGE

Prosthetic loosening and other failures of implants are the main cause of aseptic revisions in orthopedic and maxillofacial surgery leading to significant morbidity and cost (Raina et al., 2019a). Implant survival depends on initial mechanical strength and healthy integration that follows. Several orthobiologic techniques have been tried to enhance peri-implant bone formation utilizing bioactive molecules such as HA, growth factors, and BPs either by soaking, coating, or targeted local delivery (Raina et al., 2019b).

CaP-based coating of metallic implants (i.e., titanium, cobalt–chromium alloy) are widespread in arthroplasty applications (Hoornenborg et al., 2023). Stronger and faster secondary stability can be achieved by the osteoconductive properties of HA particles, which can increase implant life. Zweymuller-type femoral stems used in cementless hip arthroplasty are commonly coated with HA, and there are numerous clinical studies evaluating their effectiveness.

Although early reports show that HA-coated stems decrease stem migration and enhance implant longevity, recent reports show that this effect may be less apparent than previously thought (Furlong & Osborn, 1991; Hoornenborg et al., 2023). Recent RCTs show that noncoated stems demonstrate similar stability to that of coated stems in radiostereometric analyses and clinical evaluation

(Hoornenborg et al., 2023; van der Voort et al., 2020). Corail-type stems also portrayed similar characteristics in a 14-year follow-up study (Critchley et al., 2020).

On the other hand, another recent RCT compared two porous plasma-sprayed coated stems, one with an additional electrochemically applied HA coating, and the latter showed less early and mid-term migration (Knudsen et al., 2022). Similarly, HA-coated acetabular cups used without PMMA cement in total hip arthroplasty performed similarly in a recent RCT evaluating cup migration and polyethylene wear characteristics (Jørgensen et al., 2022; Valancius et al., 2013). In another contemporary study on coated acetabular cups, electrochemically applied HA did not show an advantage over a standard porous cup at five years (Mosegaard et al., 2022).

HA coating in total and unicondylar knee arthroplasty also allows for cementless designs (Pap et al., 2018). Available evidence from RCTs suggests that their overall migration is acceptable, and polyethylene wear and clinical results are similar (Horsager et al., 2019; van Hamersveld et al., 2018). Endosseous dental implants are also commonly treated with a similar HA coating with high rates of survival, even with early loading (Arghami et al., 2021).

Osseointegration is an important factor in tendinous and ligamentous healing as well as bone-to-bone integration. In orthopedic procedures of the joints, suture anchors are commonly used to repair or reconstruct tendon and ligament tears. Traditionally, these anchors are made of biocompatible metals, but with recent developments, biodegradable polymers and ceramics are now being used more extensively.

With the third generation of implants, efforts are focused on integrating the ability to influence cellular response with implementing growth factors and other bioactive materials as well as novel implant designs to increase peri-implant bone formation, which in return may help reduce early failure by reducing micro motion (Figure 15.2) (Raina et al., 2019b). I expect future orthobiologic applications to further enhance early integration and late bone formation in these clinical scenarios (Table 15.1).

Although clinical trials on these implants are limited, biodegradable implants coated or filled with various growth factors and BPs utilizing HA or CaS as carriers have been tested in numerous animal studies (Raina et al., 2016; Rodríguez-Évora et al., 2013; Yu et al., 2014). A recent case series evaluated the effectiveness of a rather new implant made from a combination of PGA, TCP, and CaS in shoulder labral repairs (Sugaya et al., 2019). Implanted in the glenoid, these biocomposite suture anchors demonstrated a high rate of osteoconductivity and good ossification quality at two years. In a more recent RCT, Pill et al. (2021) compared a similar composite suture anchor consisting of PLLA and PGA copolymer, TCP, and CaS with another PLLA and HA composite anchor in rotator cuff repairs and reported similar osteointegration, similar clinical outcomes, and good bone quality with both anchor types.

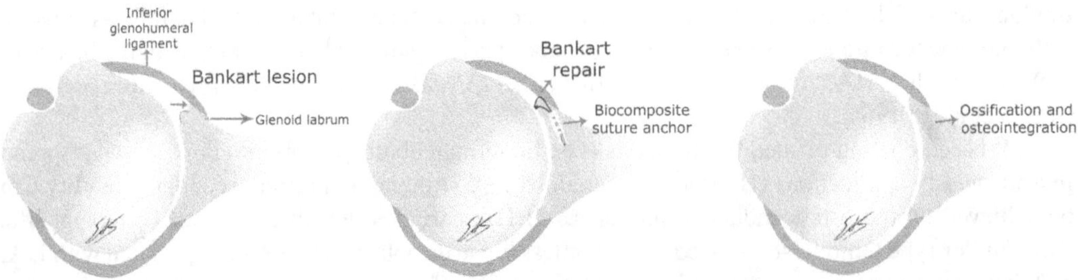

FIGURE 15.2 Biocomposite, degradable suture anchors made of polymers and ceramics can be used in arthroscopic Bankart repair surgery. The aim is to increase stability by peri-implant bone formation and achieving osteointegration in the long term, which allows preserving bone stock, beneficial for cases of revision.

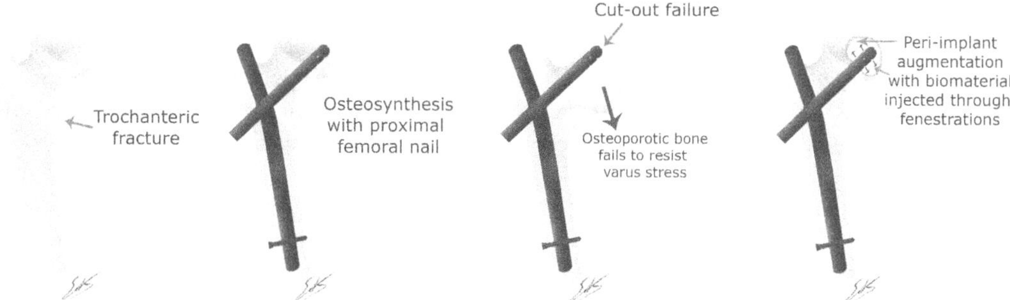

FIGURE 15.3 Fragility fractures observed in the trochanteric region of the osteoporotic femur are typically treated with osteosynthesis by proximal femoral nails. With low bone quality around the implant leading to reduced strength at the bone–implant interface, failure may occur with a cut-out mechanism. A biomaterial can be injected through the implant to increase initial resistance by spreading into the femoral head in the early period and influence bone formation in the midterm.

Another example where osseointegration is critical is in dental implants. With advances in technology, dental implants have gained delicate surface properties that enable rapid integration and high resistance (Jemat et al., 2015). In elderly patients with lower bone quality, biological augmentation is being studied to further strengthen the bone–implant interface (Palermo et al., 2019). In a preliminary clinical study, concentrated growth-factor-permeated titanium dental implants developed a biologically active dense network of fibrin rich with stem cells that was able to provide sustained release of growth factors (Palermo et al., 2022).

Fragility fractures of the hip in patients with osteoporosis are a significant burden with high morbidity rates and high revision rates despite the best available treatment (Sezgin et al., 2021). Therefore, it is one of the suitable targets for augmenting fracture fixation. Trochanteric fractures of the hip are commonly treated with osteosynthesis with a proximal femoral nail or dynamic hip plate. Augmenting the osteoporotic bone around the implant can increase the stability by strengthening the interface and thus reducing failures related to cut-out of the implant (Figure 15.3).

Previously described methods relying on contemporary biomaterials may be feasible instead of more established and conventional PMMA cement, which is associated with an increased risk of thermal damage and cement leakage leading to sudden blood pressure drop (Sezgin et al., 2020). Raina et al. (2022) reported that data from their preclinical research and preliminary clinical study shows a CaS/HA biomaterial can successfully be injected through a cannulated screw and used in the standard osteosynthesis device and can increase initial resistance by spreading into the femoral head, and has potential to increase bone formation in the midterm. With further biologic augmentation with BPs, recombinant human bone morphogenetic protein-2, or other growth factors, regeneration and integration can be further improved especially in the more fragile patients (Raina et al., 2020a, 2020b). Fractures, where cortical support is relatively low, are the other candidates for fixation augmentation. Fixation devices used in the proximal humerus, proximal tibia, vertebra and pelvic ring fractures, particularly in presence of low bone quality due to osteoporosis or other condition, are also commonly augmented with PMMA (Piccirilli et al., 2022). I expect that more biocompatible and regenerative biomaterials will be implemented for this purpose instead of the inert PMMA (Table 15.1).

15.4 BIOMATERIALS IN BONE INFECTIONS

15.4.1 Surface Coating for Infection Prophylaxis

Orthopedic implants in widespread use are typically manufactured from biocompatible metals with inert characteristics, and despite advanced technology, designs are still prone to microbial adhesion and biofilm formation that can cause devastating infective complications (Sebastian et al., 2021; Thompson et al., 2022). Novel approaches utilizing biomaterial coatings have been introduced recently and tested in a limited number of clinical studies. Anti-infective hydrogel coating was developed as an alternative to silver and gentamicin coatings, which are associated with cellular toxicity and limited applications, respectively (Fiore et al., 2021; Romanò et al., 2016).

Hydrogels are biocompatible and biodegradable, and they can release several anti-infective agents (Gahane et al., 2020; Qayoom et al., 2022). Defensive antibacterial coating (DAC; Novagenit Srl, Mezzolombardo, Italy) is the first commercially available antibacterial hydrogel; it mainly consists of hyaluronic acid and PLA. The idea is to introduce antibacterials and provide an antiadhesive effect in the early postoperative period when main bacterial colonization occurs (Antoci et al., 2008; Romanò et al., 2016).

DAC degrades completely within the first 72 h and can release various anti-infective agents in different concentrations. Despite numerous preclinical studies, there are only a handful of clinical findings on their use (Garg et al., 2021). In a 2016 clinical study on joint arthroplasty, DAC-coated implants were compared with conventional implants, and short-term results showed that surgical site infections were 10-fold lower with no apparent adverse effect (Romanò et al., 2016). In a case report, Ferry et al. (2020) shared their experience with DAC loaded with bacteriophages in the salvage treatment of an infected knee megaprosthesis; they showed that bacteriophages were released from the hydrogel, possibly reducing the infection rates in salvage procedures.

In a multicenter randomized controlled clinical trial, 256 patients undergoing osteosynthesis with DAC-coated implants versus uncoated implants were evaluated (Malizos et al., 2017). Either gentamicin, vancomycin, or a combination of vancomycin and meropenem was loaded to the DAC in the study group. The authors reported that in an average of 18 months after the operation, the DAC hydrogel-coated implant group had no surgical site infections, while this complication was encountered in six patients in the control group. Delayed wound healing and delayed union were observed at similar rates, and there were no complications.

Periprosthetic infection in arthroplasty typically requires revision procedures consisting of removing the implants, overcoming the infection, and reimplanting new prosthetics, which can be performed in one or two stages. With the use of a CaS/HA bone cement loaded with gentamicin or vancomycin as a coating for cementless joint prosthesis, Logoluso et al. (2016) showed high success in their preliminary report of 20 two-stage hip and knee arthroplasty revisions. Freischmidt et al. (2020) also reported their initial experiences with the same biomaterial loaded with the same antibiotics in a case series including a coated plate in an open tibia fracture, a coated femoral nail in infective femur nonunion, and a revision reverse shoulder arthroplasty due to an infected proximal humerus nonunion. During follow-up, the authors encountered no complications and observed good osseointegration of all the different implants. Overall, although limited evidence demonstrates encouraging outcomes, widespread use of these coatings still appears to be years away, and more clinical research is necessary to determine an optimal balance between effectiveness, cost, availability and adverse events such as interference with bone healing (Table 15.1).

15.4.2 Biomaterial Carriers to Deliver Antibiotics

There are many contemporary preclinical studies on utilizing biomaterials as drug carriers that can be activated with biological or physical stimuli to achieve the desired effect. Drugs to treat bone-related disorders consist primarily of antibiotics, growth factors, BPs and anticancer drugs.

Antibiotics in bone-related disorders typically have a localized target, which requires a high and sustained concentration; however, infected bone is a poorly vascularized target, which renders systemically administering antibiotics to achieve therapeutic doses challenging. Delivering antibiotics through biomaterial scaffolds has many potential advantages such as reducing systemic exposure to high doses and fluctuations in concentration. Traditionally, PMMA bone cements have been loaded with antibiotics and implanted into the infected area, expecting a passive release through surface diffusion. This technique cannot be regarded optimal as it uses an inert biomaterial that does not promote bone regeneration and requires to be removed and does not allow for a sustained antibiotic release.

Biphasic calcium sulphate ceramic carriers containing gentamicin or vancomycin have been approved for clinical use and more research is underway to extend the antibiotic options, such as rifampicin, isoniazid, tobramycin, or ciprofloxacin (Freischmidt et al., 2020; Logoluso et al., 2016; Lulu et al., 2018; McNally et al., 2016; Qayoom et al., 2020; Sebastian et al., 2022). This biomaterial can achieve the local and sustained delivery of desired concentrations of anti-infective agents, avoiding systemic toxic effects. As mentioned in previous sections of this chapter, with its regenerative properties, antibiotic-loaded CaS/HA bone void filler can also be used to treat small to medium-sized bone defects with a single-stage protocol in chronic osteomyelitis (McNally et al., 2016; Tian et al., 2021). Meanwhile, while many options for nanotechnology-based drug delivery systems were introduced in the preclinical setting, mostly in vitro, clinical trials are required to generalize and tailor their use for specific clinical scenarios as an alternative to conventional methods (Chen et al., 2023; Güven, 2021; Higino & França, 2022).

15.5 BIOMATERIAL CARRIERS FOR DELIVERING ANTICANCER DRUGS

Osteosarcoma is a devastating bone cancer that typically affects adolescents and young adults (Hernandez et al., 2020). Chemotherapy is commonly the initial approach in this aggressive cancer, followed by surgical resection and adjuvant chemotherapy and/or radiotherapy. The chemotherapeutic agents used are methotrexate, doxorubicin, cisplatin, ifosfamide, and etoposide, but these provide low five-year survival and high rates of adverse effects (Meazza et al., 2014). Research on developing alternative, targeted chemotherapy routes to increase survival and reduce side effects is underway, utilizing drug delivery with nano- and microparticle vehicles such as proteins, hyaluronic acid, BPs, and folate (Xie et al., 2022). Unfortunately, the majority of these are in the preclinical stage, and translation to clinical use may take years.

The literature holds remarkable approaches to limb-preserving osteosarcoma surgery that aim to fill the bone defects left from total resection with biomaterials that can kill osteosarcoma cells that are left over while influencing new bone formation (Fu et al., 2020; Ma et al., 2016). The mechanisms they use to target osteosarcoma cells are either photothermal impact or sustained drug delivery allowing local treatment (Fu et al., 2020; Liu et al., 2021; Ma et al., 2015; Wang et al., 2020; Zhou et al., 2015). With the implementation of 3D manufacturing techniques, multipurpose scaffolds can be developed to be used during resection surgery, allowing successful osteogenesis as well as a perfectly tailored, local chemotherapy.

In line with this vision, Liu et al. (2021) used a biodegradable CaS/HA bone cement currently in use to fill bone defects as a local delivery carrier for doxorubicin (DOX) in their in vitro and in vivo studies using human osteosarcoma xenograft models. They achieved the biphasic sustained release of DOX at a high local concentration for an impressive duration of 28 days, in contrast with the other delivery methods (Kamba et al., 2013; Ma et al., 2015; Zhou et al., 2017). In their animal model, they confirmed that by local delivery, in contrast with systemic, DOX could significantly inhibit tumor growth even with lower doses (Liu et al., 2021).

In another animal study by the same group, nanoparticles of HA, which can penetrate cell walls, were shown to be an effective target for circulating apatite-binding, cytostatic drugs, creating an alternative model of targeted chemotherapy directly into the mitochondria (Liu et al., 2022). Although the clinical application of this novel Trojan horse approach has not been tested, preclinical data appear to be promising. One concern is the risk of nanomaterials entering the circulation and creating adverse effects outside the intended region; however, the opposite has also been shown in animal models (Liu et al., 2022; Wang et al., 2021). Combining nanoparticles and microparticles of HA was suggested to be an effective method of reducing this risk; however, clinical data are necessary to assess the risk profiles of these nanomaterials with the ability to penetrate the cell membrane (Patra et al., 2018).

CONCLUSION

In conclusion, many scientifically thrilling advancements still appear to be several years away from routine clinical application. However, considering the rapid rate of development, approaches to difficult conditions related to bone regeneration, integration, infection, and carcinogenesis may begin to be more optimistic in the near future, for both the clinician and the patient.

LIST OF ABBREVIATIONS

ACS	Absorbable collagen sponge
BCP	Biphasic calcium phosphate cement
CaS	Calcium sulphate
CaP	Calcium phosphate
HA	Hydroxyapatite
PCL	Poly (ε-caprolactone)
PGA	Polyglycolic acid
PLA	Polylactic-acid
PLLA	Poly-l-lactic acid
PMMA	Poly-methyl-methacrylate
RCT	Randomized controlled trial
rhBMP-2	Recombinant human bone morphogenetic protein-2
Si-CaP	Silicate-substituted calcium phosphate
β-TCP	Beta-tricalcium phosphate

REFERENCES

Abdullah, A. A. B., Edrees, M. F., & Bakry, A. M. (2021). Clinical, radiographic, and histological assessment of socket preservation using melatonin with beta-tri-calcium phosphate for receiving dental implant. *Biomed Sci.* 7: 10.

al Malat, T., Glombitza, M., Dahmen, J., Hax, P. M., & Steinhausen, E. (2018). The use of bioactive glass S53P4 as bone graft substitute in the treatment of chronic osteomyelitis and infected non-unions—a retrospective study of 50 patients. *Z. fur Orthop. Unfallchirurgie.* 156: 152–159.

Amini, A. R., Adams, D. J., Laurencin, C. T., & Nukavarapu, S. P. (2012). Optimally porous and biomechanically compatible scaffolds for large-area bone regeneration. *Tissue Eng. Part A.* 18: 1376–1388.

Antoci, V., Adams, C. S., Hickok, N. J., Shapiro, I. M., & Parvizi, J. (2007). Antibiotics for local delivery systems cause skeletal cell toxicity in vitro. *Clin. Orthop. Relat. Res.* 462: 200–206.

Antoci, V., Adams, C. S., Parvizi, J., Davidson, H. M., Composto, R. J., Freeman, T. A., Wickstrom, E., Ducheyne, P., Jungkind, D., Shapiro, I. M., & Hickok, N. J. (2008). The inhibition of Staphylococcus epidermidis biofilm formation by vancomycin-modified titanium alloy and implications for the treatment of periprosthetic infection. *Biomaterials.* 29: 4684–4690.

Arghami, A., Simmons, D., Germain, J. st., & Maney, P. (2021). Immediate and early loading of hydrothermally treated, hydroxyapatite-coated dental implants: A 7-year prospective randomized clinical study. *Int. J. Implant Dent.* 7(1): 1–10.

Arnold, P. M., Anderson, K. K., Selim, A., Dryer, R. F., & Burkus, J. K. (2016). Heterotopic ossification following single-level anterior cervical discectomy and fusion: Results from the prospective, multicenter, historically controlled trial comparing allograft to an optimized dose of rhBMP-2. *J. Neurosurg. Spine.* 25: 292–302.

Aro, H. T., Välimäki, V. V., Strandberg, N., Lankinen, P., Löyttyniemi, E., Saunavaara, V., & Seppänen, M. (2022). Bioactive glass granules versus standard autologous and allogeneic bone grafts: A randomized trial of 49 adult bone tumor patients with a 10-year follow-up. *Acta Orthop.* 93: 519–527.

Attia, A. K., Mahmoud, K., ElSweify, K., Bariteau, J., & Labib, S. A. (2022). Donor site morbidity of calcaneal, distal tibial, and proximal tibial cancellous bone autografts in foot and ankle surgery: A systematic review and meta-analysis of 2296 bone grafts. *J. Foot Ankle Surg*. 28: 680–690.

Babrawala, I., Venkatesh, P. M. L., & Varadhan, K. B. (2016). A novel approach using 15% natural chitosan gel in the management of intrabony defects: A pilot study. *Chin. J. Dent. Res*. 19: 231–237.

Barber, F. A., Spenciner, D. B., Bhattacharyya, S., & Miller, L. E. (2017). Biocomposite implants composed of poly(Lactide-co-glycolide)/β-tricalcium phosphate: Systematic review of imaging, complication, and performance outcomes. *Arthroscopy*. 33: 683–689.

Benic, G. I., Bienz, S. P., Song, Y. W., Cha, J. K., Hämmerle, C. H. F., Jung, U. W., & Jung, R. E. (2022). Randomized controlled clinical trial comparing guided bone regeneration of peri-implant defects with soft-type block versus particulate bone substitutes: Six-month results of hard-tissue changes. *J. Clin. Periodontol*. 49: 480–495.

Bharathi, R., Ganesh, S. S., Harini, G., Vatsala, K., Anushikaa, R., Aravind, S., Abinaya, S., & Selvamurugan, N. (2022). Chitosan-based scaffolds as drug delivery systems in bone tissue engineering. *Int. J. Biol. Macromol*. 222: 132–153.

Bhattacharjee, P., Kundu, B., Naskar, D., Kim, H. W., Maiti, T. K., Bhattacharya, D., & Kundu, S. C. (2017). Silk scaffolds in bone tissue engineering: An overview. *Acta Biomater*. 63: 1–17.

Boynueğri, D., Özcan, G., Şenel, S., Uç, D., Uraz, A., Öğüş, E., Çakilci, B., & Karaduman, B. (2009). Clinical and radiographic evaluations of chitosan gel in periodontal intraosseous defects: A pilot study. *J. Biomed. Mater. Res. B Appl. Biomater*. 90: 461–466.

Brandt, J., Henning, S., Michler, G., Hein, W., Bernstein, A., & Schulz, M. (2010). Nanocrystalline hydroxyapatite for bone repair: An animal study. *J. Mater. Sci.: Mater. Med*. 21: 283–294.

Brun, V., Guillaume, C., Mechiche Alami, S., Josse, J., Jing, J., Draux, F., Bouthors, S., Laurent-Maquin, D., Gangloff, S. C., Kerdjoudj, H., & Velard, F. (2014). Chitosan/hydroxyapatite hybrid scaffold for bone tissue engineering. *Biomed. Mater. Eng*. 24: 63–73.

Bucchi, C., Del Fabbro, M., Arias, A., Fuentes, R., Mendes, J. M., Ordonneau, M., Orti, V., & Manzanares-Céspedes, M. C. (2019). Multicenter study of patients' preferences and concerns regarding the origin of bone grafts utilized in dentistry. *Patient Prefer. Adher*. 13: 179–185.

Campana, V., Milano, G., Pagano, E., Barba, M., Cicione, C., Salonna, G., Lattanzi, W., & Logroscino, G. (2014). Bone substitutes in orthopaedic surgery: From basic science to clinical practice. *J. Mater. Sci.: Mater. Med*. 25: 2445–2461.

Chen, Y., Zhu, M., Huang, B., Jiang, Y., & Su, J. (2023). Advances in cell membrane-coated nanoparticles and their applications for bone therapy. *Biomat. Adv*. 144: 213232.

Cimatti, P., Andreoli, I., Busacca, M., Govoni, M., Vivarelli, L., del Piccolo, N., Maso, A., Stagni, C., & Pignatti, G. (2022). An observational prospective clinical study for the evaluation of a collagen-hydroxyapatite composite scaffold in hip revision surgery. *J. Clin. Med*. 11: 6372.

Cook, S. D., & Dalton, J. E. (1992). Biocompatibility and biofunctionality of implanted materials. *Alpha Omegan*. 85: 41–47.

Critchley, O., Callary, S., Mercer, G., Campbell, D., & Wilson, C. (2020). Long-term migration characteristics of the Corail hydroxyapatite-coated femoral stem: A 14-year radiostereometric analysis follow-up study. *Arch. Orthop. Trauma Surg*. 140: 121–127.

di Martino, A., Sittinger, M., & Risbud, M. V. (2005). Chitosan: A versatile biopolymer for orthopaedic tissue-engineering. *Biomaterials*. 26: 5983–5990.

Drago, L., Romanò, D., de Vecchi, E., Vassena, C., Logoluso, N., Mattina, R., & Romanò, C. L. (2013). Bioactive glass bag-S53P4 for the adjunctive treatment of chronic osteomyelitis of the long bones: An in vitro and prospective clinical study. *BMC Infect. Dis*. 13: 1–8.

Dziadek, M., Stodolak-Zych, E., & Cholewa-Kowalska, K. (2017). Biodegradable ceramic-polymer composites for biomedical applications: A review. *Mater. Sci. Eng. C*. 71: 1175–1191.

Feng, C., Xue, J., Yu, X., Zhai, D., Lin, R., Zhang, M., Xia, L., Wang, X., Yao, Q., Chang, J., & Wu, C. (2021). Co-inspired hydroxyapatite-based scaffolds for vascularized bone regeneration. *Acta Biomater*. 119: 419–431.

Ferry, T., Batailler, C., Petitjean, C., Chateau, J., Fevre, C., Forestier, E., Brosset, S., Leboucher, G., Kolenda, C., Laurent, F., & Lustig, S. (2020). The potential innovative use of bacteriophages within the DAC® hydrogel to treat patients with knee megaprosthesis infection requiring "debridement antibiotics and implant retention" and soft tissue coverage as salvage therapy. *Front. Med*. 7: 342.

Fiore, M., Sambri, A., Zucchini, R., Giannini, C., Donati, D. M., & de Paolis, M. (2021). Silver-coated megaprosthesis in prevention and treatment of peri-prosthetic infections: A systematic review and meta-analysis about efficacy and toxicity in primary and revision surgery. *Eur. J. Orthop. Surg. Traumatol.* 31: 201–220.

Freischmidt, H., Armbruster, J., Reiter, G., Grützner, P. A., Helbig, L., & Guehring, T. (2020). Individualized techniques of implant coating with an antibiotic-loaded, hydroxyapatite/calcium sulphate bone graft substitute. *Ther. Clin. Risk Manag.* 16: 689–694.

Fu, S., Hu, H., Chen, J., Zhu, Y., & Zhao, S. (2020). Silicone resin derived larnite/C scaffolds via 3D printing for potential tumor therapy and bone regeneration. *J. Chem. Eng.* 382: 122928.

Furlong, R. J., & Osborn, J. F. (1991). Fixation of hip prostheses by hydroxyapatite ceramic coatings. *J. Bone Joint Surg. Br.* 73: 741–745.

Gahane, A. Y., Singh, V., Kumar, A., & Kumar Thakur, A. (2020). Development of mechanism-based antibacterial synergy between Fmoc-phenylalanine hydrogel and aztreonam. *Biomater. Sci.* 8: 1996–2006.

Garcia, D. C., Mingrone, L. E., & Sá, M. J. C. de. (2022). Evaluation of osseointegration and bone healing using pure-phase β—TCP ceramic implant in bone critical defects: A systematic review. *Front. Vet. Sci.* 9: 859920.

Garg, D., Matai, I., & Sachdev, A. (2021). Toward designing of anti-infective hydrogels for orthopedic implants: From lab to clinic. *ACS Biomater. Sci. Eng.* 7: 1933–1961.

Garric, X., Nottelet, B., Pinese, C., Leroy, A., & Coudane, J. (2017). Polymères synthétiques dégradables pour la conception de dispositifs médicaux implantables. *Med. Sci.* 33: 39–45.

Giannoudis, P. V., Dinopoulos, H., & Tsiridis, E. (2005). Bone substitutes: An update. *Injury.* 36: S20–S27.

Gjerde, C., Mustafa, K., Hellem, S., Rojewski, M., Gjengedal, H., Yassin, M. A., Feng, X., Skaale, S., Berge, T., Rosen, A., Shi, X. Q., Ahmed, A. B., Gjertsen, B. T., Schrezenmeier, H., & Layrolle, P. (2018). Cell therapy induced regeneration of severely atrophied mandibular bone in a clinical trial. *Stem Cell Res. Ther.* 9: 1–15.

Guo, X., Liu, Y., Bai, J., Yu, B., Xu, M., Sun, H., Shen, J., Lin, J., Zhang, H., Wang, D., Geng, D., & Pan, G. (2019). Efficient inhibition of wear-debris-induced osteolysis by surface biomimetic engineering of titanium implant with a mussel-derived integrin-targeting peptide. *Adv. Biosyst.* 3: 1800253.

Güven, E. (2021). Nanotechnology-based drug delivery systems in orthopedics. *Jt. Dis. Relat. Surg.* 32: 267–273.

Hench, L. L. (1998). Biomaterials: A forecast for the future. *Biomaterials.* 19: 1419–1423.

Hernandez, T. F. N., Zamudio, A., Marques-Piubelli, M. L., Cuglievan, B., & Harrison, D. (2020). Advances in the management of pediatric sarcomas. *Curr. Oncol. Rep.* 23: 1–9.

Higino, T., & França, R. (2022). Drug-delivery nanoparticles for bone-tissue and dental applications. *Biomed. Phys. Eng. Express.* 8: 042001.

Hing, K. A., Revell, P. A., Smith, N., & Buckland, T. (2006). Effect of silicon level on rate, quality and progression of bone healing within silicate-substituted porous hydroxyapatite scaffolds. *Biomaterials.* 27: 5014–5026.

Hofmann, A., Gorbulev, S., Guehring, T., Schulz, A. P., Schupfner, R., Raschke, M., Huber-Wagner, S., & Rommens, P. M. (2020). Autologous iliac bone graft compared with biphasic hydroxyapatite and calcium sulfate cement for the treatment of bone defects in tibial plateau fractures: A prospective, randomized, open-label, multicenter study. *J. Bone Joint Surg. Am.* 102: 179–193.

Hoornenborg, D., Schweden, A. M. C., Sierevelt, I. N., van der Vis, H. M., Kerkhoffs, G. M. M. J., & Haverkamp, D. (2023). The influence of hydroxyapatite coating on continuous migration of a Zweymuller-type hip stem: A double-blinded randomised RSA trial with 5-year follow-up. *Hip Int.* 33: 73–80.

Horsager, K., Madsen, F., Odgaard, A., Fink Jepsen, C., Rømer, L., Kristensen, P. W., Kaptein, B. L., Søballe, K., & Stilling, M. (2019). Similar polyethylene wear between cemented and cementless Oxford medial UKA: A 5-year follow-up randomized controlled trial on 79 patients using radiostereometry. *Acta Orthopaed.* 90: 67–73.

Ishiguro, S., Kasai, Y., Sudo, A., Iida, K., & Uchida, A. (2010). Percutaneous vertebroplasty for osteoporotic compression fractures using calcium phosphate cement. *Orthop. Surg.* 18: 346–351.

Iundusi, R., Gasbarra, E., D'Arienzo, M., Piccioli, A., & Tarantino, U. (2015). Augmentation of tibial plateau fractures with an injectable bone substitute: CERAMENT™: Three year follow-up from a prospective study. *BMC Musculoskelet. Disord.* 16: 1–5.

James, A. W., LaChaud, G., Shen, J., Asatrian, G., Nguyen, V., Zhang, X., Ting, K., & Soo, C. (2016). A review of the clinical side effects of bone morphogenetic protein-2. *Tissue Eng. Part B Rev*. 22: 284–297.

Jemat, A., Ghazali, M. J., Razali, M., & Otsuka, Y. (2015). Surface modifications and their effects on titanium dental implants. *Biomed. Res. Int.* 2015: 791725.

Jo, D. W., Cho, Y. D., Seol, Y. J., Lee, Y. M., Lee, H. J., & Kim, Y. K. (2019). A randomized controlled clinical trial evaluating efficacy and adverse events of different types of recombinant human bone morphogenetic protein-2 delivery systems for alveolar ridge preservation. *Clin. Oral Implants Res*. 30: 396–409.

Jørgensen, P. B., Tabori-Jensen, S., Mechlenburg, I., Humilius, M., Hansen, T. B., & Stilling, M. (2022). Cemented and cementless dual mobility cups show similar fixation, low polyethylene wear, and low serum cobalt-chromium in elderly patients: A randomized radiostereometry study with 6 years' follow-up. *Acta Orthopaed*. 93: 906.

Jung, R. E., Hälg, G. A., Thoma, D. S., & Hämmerle, C. H. F. (2009). A randomized, controlled clinical trial to evaluate a new membrane for guided bone regeneration around dental implants. *Clin. Oral Implants Res*. 20: 162–168.

Kamba, S. A., Ismail, M., Hussein-Al-Ali, S. H., Ibrahim, T. A. T., & Zakaria, Z. A. B. (2013). In vitro delivery and controlled release of doxorubicin for targeting osteosarcoma bone cancer. *Molecules*. 18: 10580–10598.

Kandasamy, S., Narayanan, V., & Sumathi, S. (2020). Zinc and manganese substituted hydroxyapatite/CMC/PVP electrospun composite for bone repair applications. *Int. J. Biol. Macromol*. 145: 1018–1030.

Kim, J. H., Oh, J. H., Han, I., Kim, H. S., & Chung, S. W. (2011). Grafting using injectable calcium sulfate in bone tumor surgery: Comparison with demineralized bone matrix-based grafting. *Clin. Orthop. Surg*. 3: 191–201.

Kim, S. E., & Park, K. (2020). Recent advances of biphasic calcium phosphate bioceramics for bone tissue regeneration. *Adv. Exp. Med. Biol*. 1250: 177–188.

Knudsen, M. B., Thillemann, J. K., Jørgensen, P. B., Jakobsen, S. S., Daugaard, H., Søballe, K., & Stilling, M. (2022). Electrochemically applied hydroxyapatite on the cementless porous surface of Bi-Metric stems reduces early migration and has a lasting effect: An efficacy trial of a randomized five-year follow-up radiostereometric study. *Bone Joint J*. 104-B: 647–656.

Kohn, D. H., Sarmadi, M., Helman, J. I., & Krebsbach, P. H. (2002). Effects of pH on human bone marrow stromal cells in vitro: Implications for tissue engineering of bone. *J. Biomed. Mater. Res*. 60: 292–299.

Kollek, N. J., Pérez-Albacete Martínez, C., Granero Marín, J. M., & Maté Sánchez De Val, J. E. (2022). Prospective clinical study with new materials for tissue regeneration: A study in humans. *Eur. J. Dent*. 17: 727–734.

Learmonth, I. D., Young, C., & Rorabeck, C. (2007). The operation of the century: Total hip replacement. *The Lancet*. 370: 1508–1519.

Lee, D. Y., Lee, M. C., Ha, C. W., Kyung, H. S., Kim, C. W., Chang, M. J., & Han, H. S. (2019). Comparable bone union progression after opening wedge high tibial osteotomy using allogenous bone chip or tri-calcium phosphate granule: A prospective randomized controlled trial. *Knee Surg. Sports Traumatol. Arthrosc*. 27: 2945–2950.

Lerner, T., & Liljenqvist, U. (2013). Silicate-substituted calcium phosphate as a bone graft substitute in surgery for adolescent idiopathic scoliosis. *Eur. Spine J*. 22: 185–194.

Li, H. F., Xie, X. H., Zheng, Y. F., Cong, Y., Zhou, F. Y., Qiu, K. J., Wang, X., Chen, S. H., Huang, L., Tian, L., & Qin, L. (2015). Development of biodegradable Zn-1X binary alloys with nutrient alloying elements Mg, Ca and Sr. *Sci. Rep*. 5: 10719.

Li, L., Gao, J., & Wang, Y. (2004). Evaluation of cyto-toxicity and corrosion behavior of alkali-heat-treated magnesium in simulated body fluid. *Surf. Coat. Technol*. 185: 92–98.

Li, Y., Jahr, H., Pavanram, P., Bobbert, F. S. L., Puggi, U., Zhang, X. Y., Pouran, B., Leeflang, M. A., Weinans, H., Zhou, J., & Zadpoor, A. A. (2019). Additively manufactured functionally graded biodegradable porous iron. *Acta Biomater*. 96: 646–661.

Lindfors, N., Geurts, J., Drago, L., Arts, J. J., Juutilainen, V., Hyvönen, P., Suda, A. J., Domenico, A., Artiaco, S., Alizadeh, C., Brychcy, A., Bialecki, J., & Romanò, C. L. (2017). Antibacterial bioactive glass, S53P4, for chronic bone infections—A multinational study. *Adv. Exp. Med. Biol*. 971: 81–92.

Liodakis, E., Giannoudis, V. P., Sehmisch, S., Jha, A., & Giannoudis, P. V. (2022). Bone defect treatment: Does the type and properties of the spacer affect the induction of Masquelet membrane? Evidence today. *Eur. J. Trauma Emerg. Surg*. 48: 440–4424.

Liu, Y., Nadeem, A., Sebastian, S., Olsson, M. A., Wai, S. N., Styring, E., Engellau, J., Isaksson, H., Tägil, M., Lidgren, L., & Raina, D. B. (2022). Bone mineral: A trojan horse for bone cancers: Efficient mitochondria targeted delivery and tumor eradication with nano hydroxyapatite containing doxorubicin. *Mater. Today*. 14: 100227.

Liu, Y., Raina, D. B., Sebastian, S., Nagesh, H., Isaksson, H., Engellau, J., Lidgren, L., & Tägil, M. (2021). Sustained and controlled delivery of doxorubicin from an in-situ setting biphasic hydroxyapatite carrier for local treatment of a highly proliferative human osteosarcoma. *Acta Biomatr*. 131: 555–571.

Lizzi, F., Villat, C., Attik, N., Jackson, P., Grosgogeat, B., & Goutaudier, C. (2017). Mechanical characteristic and biological behaviour of implanted and restorative bioglasses used in medicine and dentistry: A systematic review. *Dent. Mater*. 33: 702–712.

Logoluso, N., Drago, L., Gallazzi, E., George, D. A., Morelli, I., & Romanò, C. L. (2016). Calcium-based, antibiotic-loaded bone substitute as an implant coating: A pilot clinical study. *J. Bone Joint Infect*. 1: 59–64.

Lulu, G. A., Karunanidhi, A., Mohamad Yusof, L., Abba, Y., Mohd Fauzi, F., & Othman, F. (2018). In vivo efficacy of tobramycin-loaded synthetic calcium phosphate beads in a rabbit model of staphylococcal osteomyelitis. *Ann. Clin. Microbiol. Antimicrob*. 17: 1–11.

Luo, G., Huang, Y., & Gu, F. (2017). rhBMP2-loaded calcium phosphate cements combined with allogenic bone marrow mesenchymal stem cells for bone formation. *Biomed. Pharmacother*. 92: 536–543.

Luo, G., Huang, Y., & Gu, F. (2022). The osteogenesis effect of rhBMP2-loaded calcium phosphate cements in repairing dental extraction sockets. *Am. J. Transl. Res*. 14: 7172–7177.

Ma, H., He, C., Cheng, Y., Yang, Z., Zang, J., Liu, J., & Chen, X. (2015). Localized co-delivery of doxorubicin, cisplatin, and methotrexate by thermosensitive hydrogels for enhanced osteosarcoma treatment. *ACS Appl. Mater. Interfaces*. 7: 27040–27048.

Ma, H., Jiang, C., Zhai, D., Luo, Y., Chen, Y., Lv, F., Yi, Z., Deng, Y., Wang, J., Chang, J., & Wu, C. (2016). A bifunctional biomaterial with photothermal effect for tumor therapy and bone regeneration. *Adv. Funct. Mater*. 26: 1197–1208.

Major Extremity Trauma Research Consortium (METRC). (2019). A randomized controlled trial comparing rhBMP-2/Absorbable collagen sponge versus autograft for the treatment of tibia fractures with critical size defects. *J. Orthop. Trauma*. 33: 384–391.

Malizos, K., Blauth, M., Danita, A., Capuano, N., Mezzoprete, R., Logoluso, N., Drago, L., & Romanò, C. L. (2017). Fast-resorbable antibiotic-loaded hydrogel coating to reduce post-surgical infection after internal osteosynthesis: A multicenter randomized controlled trial. *J. Orthop. Trauma*. 18: 159–169.

Masala, S., Nano, G., Marcia, S., Muto, M., Fucci, F. P. M., & Simonetti, G. (2012). Osteoporotic vertebral compression fractures augmentation by injectable partly resorbable ceramic bone substitute (Cerament™|SPINE SUPPORT): A prospective nonrandomized study. *Neuroradiology*. 54: 589–596.

McNally, M. A., Ferguson, J. Y., Lau, A. C. K., Diefenbeck, M., Scarborough, M., Ramsden, A. J., & Atkins, B. L. (2016). Single-stage treatment of chronic osteomyelitis with a new absorbable, gentamicin-loaded, calcium sulphate/hydroxyapatite biocomposite: A prospective series of 100 cases. *Bone Joint J*. 98-B: 1289–1296.

Meazza, C., Luksch, R., Daolio, P., Podda, M., Luzzati, A., Gronchi, A., Parafioriti, A., Gandola, L., Collini, P., Ferrari, A., Casanova, M., Terenziani, M., Spreafico, F., Polastri, D., Biassoni, V., Schiavello, E., Pecori, E., & Massimino, M. (2014). Axial skeletal osteosarcoma: A 25-year monoinstitutional experience in children and adolescents. *Med. Oncol*. 31: 1–6.

Merli, M., Moscatelli, M., Mariotti, G., Pagliaro, U., Raffaelli, E., & Nieri, M. (2018). Comparing membranes and bone substitutes in a one-stage procedure for horizontal bone augmentation: Three-year post-loading results of a double-blind randomised controlled trial. *Eur. J. Oral Implantol*. 11: 441–452.

Miron, R. J., Gruber, R., Hedbom, E., Saulacic, N., Zhang, Y., Sculean, A., Bosshardt, D. D., & Buser, D. (2013). Impact of bone harvesting techniques on cell viability and the release of growth factors of autografts. *Clin. Implant Dent. Relat. Res*. 15: 481–489.

Mosegaard, S. B., Jørgensen, P. B., Jakobsen, S. S., Daugaard, H., Søballe, K., & Stilling, M. (2022). Larger 5-year migration but similar polyethylene wear of cementless hemispherical cups with electrochemically applied hydroxyapatite (BoneMaster) coating compared with porous plasma-spray titanium: A randomized 5-year RSA study. *Acta Orthop*. 93: 658–664.

Nho, S. J., Nam, D., Ala, O. L., Craig, E. V., Warren, R. F., & Wright, T. M. (2009). Observations on retrieved glenoid components from total shoulder arthroplasty. *J. Shoulder Elb. Surg*. 18: 371–378.

Nie, H., & Wang, C. H. (2007). Fabrication and characterization of PLGA/HAp composite scaffolds for delivery of BMP-2 plasmid DNA. *J. Control. Release*. 120: 111–121.

Ogueri, K. S., Ogueri, K. S., McClinton, A., Kan, H. M., Ude, C. C., Barajaa, M. A., Allcock, H. R., & Laurencin, C. T. (2021). In vivo evaluation of the regenerative capability of glycylglycine ethyl ester-substituted polyphosphazene and poly(lactic- co-glycolic acid) blends: A rabbit critical-sized bone defect model. *ACS Biomater. Sci. Eng*. 7: 1564–1572.

Oh, C. W., Park, K. C., & Jo, Y. H. (2017). Evaluating augmentation with calcium phosphate cement (chronOS Inject) for bone defects after internal fixation of proximal tibial fractures: A prospective, multicenter, observational study. *Orthop. Traumatol. Surg. Res*. 103: 105–109.

Okada, T., Kanai, T., Tachikawa, N., Munakata, M., & Kasugai, S. (2016). Long-term radiographic assessment of maxillary sinus floor augmentation using beta-tricalcium phosphate: Analysis by cone-beam computed tomography. *Int. J. Implant Dent*. 2: 1–9.

Oryan, A., Alidadi, S., Moshiri, A., & Maffulli, N. (2014). Bone regenerative medicine: Classic options, novel strategies, and future directions. *J. Orthop. Surg. Res*. 9: 1–27.

Palermo, A., Ferrante, F., Stanca, E., Damiano, F., Gnoni, A., Batani, T., Carluccio, M. A., Demitri, C., & Siculella, L. (2019). Release of VEGF from dental implant surface (IML® Implant) coated with Concentrated Growth Factors (CGF) and the Liquid Phase of CGF (LPCGF): In vitro results and future expectations. *Appl. Sci*. 9: 2114.

Palermo, A., Giannotti, L., di Chiara Stanca, B., Ferrante, F., Gnoni, A., Nitti, P., Calabriso, N., Demitri, C., Damiano, F., Batani, T., Lungherini, M., Carluccio, M. A., Rapone, B., Qorri, E., Scarano, A., Siculella, L., Stanca, E., & Rochira, A. (2022). Use of CGF in oral and implant surgery: From laboratory evidence to clinical evaluation. *Int. J. Mol. Sci*. 23: 15164.

Pap, K., Vasarhelyi, G., Gal, T., Nemeth, G., Abonyi, B., Hangody, L. R., Hangody, G. M., & Hangody, L. (2018). Evaluation of clinical outcomes of cemented vs uncemented knee prostheses covered with titanium plasma spray and hydroxyapatite: A minimum two years follow-up. *Jt. Dis. Relat. Surg*. 29: 65–70.

Patra, J. K., Das, G., Fraceto, L. F., Campos, E. V. R., Rodriguez-Torres, M. D. P., Acosta-Torres, L. S., Diaz-Torres, L. A., Grillo, R., Swamy, M. K., Sharma, S., Habtemariam, S., & Shin, H. S. (2018). Nano based drug delivery systems: Recent developments and future prospects. *J. Nanobiotechnol*. 16: 1–33.

Pérez, R. A., Won, J. E., Knowles, J. C., & Kim, H. W. (2013). Naturally and synthetic smart composite biomaterials for tissue regeneration. *Adv. Drug Deliv. Rev*. 65: 471–496.

Piccirilli, E., Cariati, I., Primavera, M., Triolo, R., Gasbarra, E., & Tarantino, U. (2022). Augmentation in fragility fractures, bone of contention: A systematic review. *BMC Musculoskelet. Disord*. 23: 1046.

Pill, S. G., McCallum, J., Tolan, S. J., Bynarowicz, T., Adams, K. J., Hutchinson, J., Alexander, R., Siffri, P. C., Brooks, J. M., Tokish, J. M., & Kissenberth, M. J. (2021). Regenesorb and polylactic acid hydroxyapatite anchors are associated with similar osseous integration and rotator cuff healing at 2 years. *J. Shoulder Elb. Surg*. 30: S27–S37.

Plantz, M. A., Minardi, S., Lyons, J. G., Greene, A. C., Ellenbogen, D. J., Hallman, M., Yamaguchi, J. T., Jeong, S., Yun, C., Jakus, A. E., Blank, K. R., Havey, R. M., Muriuki, M., Patwardhan, A. G., Shah, R. N., Hsu, W. K., Stock, S. R., & Hsu, E. L. (2021). Osteoinductivity and biomechanical assessment of a 3D printed demineralized bone matrix-ceramic composite in a rat spine fusion model. *Acta Biomatr*. 127: 146–158.

Prins, H.-J., Schulten, E. A. J. M., ten Bruggenkate, C. M., Klein-Nulend, J., & Helder, M. N. (2016). Bone regeneration using the freshly isolated autologous stromal vascular fraction of adipose tissue in combination with calcium phosphate ceramics. *Stem Cells Transl. Med*. 5: 1362–1374.

Putri, T. S., Hayashi, K., & Ishikawa, K. (2020). Bone regeneration using β-tricalcium phosphate (β-TCP) block with interconnected pores made by setting reaction of β-TCP granules. *J. Biomed. Mater. Res. A*. 108: 625–632.

Qayoom, I., Srivastava, E., & Kumar, A. (2022). Anti-infective composite cryogel scaffold treats osteomyelitis and augments bone healing in rat femoral condyle. *Biomat. Adv*. 142: 213133.

Qayoom, I., Verma, R., Murugan, P. A., Raina, D. B., Teotia, A. K., Matheshwaran, S., Nair, N. N., Tägil, M., Lidgren, L., & Kumar, A. (2020). A biphasic nanohydroxyapatite/calcium sulphate carrier containing Rifampicin and Isoniazid for local delivery gives sustained and effective antibiotic release and prevents biofilm formation. *Sci. Rep*. 10:1–14.

Rabeeh, V. P. M., & Hanas, T. (2022). Progress in manufacturing and processing of degradable Fe-based implants: A review. *Prog. Biomater*. 11: 163.

Raina, D. B., Isaksson, H., Hettwer, W., Kumar, A., Lidgren, L., & Tagil, M. (2016). A biphasic calcium sulphate/hydroxyapatite carrier containing bone morphogenic protein-2 and zoledronic acid generates bone. *Sci. Rep.* 6: 26033.

Raina, D. B., Larsson, D., Sezgin, E. A., Isaksson, H., Tägil, M., & Lidgren, L. (2019a). Biomodulation of an implant for enhanced bone-implant anchorage. *Acta Biomatr.* 96: 619–630.

Raina, D. B., Liu, Y., Isaksson, H., Tägil, M., & Lidgren, L. (2020a). Synthetic hydroxyapatite: A recruiting platform for biologically active molecules. *Acta Orthop.* 91: 126–132.

Raina, D. B., Markevičiūtė, V., Stravinskas, M., Kok, J., Jacobson, I., Liu, Y., Sezgin, E. A., Isaksson, H., Zwingenberger, S., Tägil, M., Tarasevičius, Š., & Lidgren, L. (2022). A new augmentation method for improved screw fixation in fragile bone. *Front. Bioeng. Biotech.* 10: 816250.

Raina, D. B., Matuszewski, L. M., Vater, C., Bolte, J., Isaksson, H., Lidgren, L., Tägil, M., & Zwingenberger, S. (2020b). A facile one-stage treatment of critical bone defects using a calcium sulfate/hydroxyapatite biomaterial providing spatiotemporal delivery of bone morphogenic protein—2 and zoledronic acid. *Sci. Adv.* 6: eabc1779.

Raina, D. B., Qayoom, I., Larsson, D., Zheng, M. H., Kumar, A., Isaksson, H., Lidgren, L., & Tägil, M. (2019b). Guided tissue engineering for healing of cancellous and cortical bone using a combination of biomaterial based scaffolding and local bone active molecule delivery. *Biomaterials.* 188: 38–49.

Raina, D. B., Širka, A., Qayoom, I., Teotia, A. K., Liu, Y., Tarasevicius, S., Tanner, K. E., Isaksson, H., Kumar, A., Tägil, M., & Lidgren, L. (2020c). Long-term response to a bioactive biphasic biomaterial in the femoral neck of osteoporotic rats. *Tissue Eng. Part A.* 26: 1042–1051.

Rodríguez-Évora, M., Delgado, A., Reyes, R., Hernández-Daranas, A., Soriano, I., San Román, J., & Évora, C. (2013). Osteogenic effect of local, long versus short term BMP-2 delivery from a novel SPU-PLGA-βTCP concentric system in a critical size defect in rats. *Eur. J. Pharm. Sci.* 49: 873–884.

Romanò, C. L., Malizos, K., Capuano, N., Mezzoprete, R., D'arienzo, M., Der, C. van, Scarponi, S., & Drago, L. (2016). Does an antibiotic-loaded hydrogel coating reduce early post-surgical infection after joint arthroplasty? *J. Bone Joint Infect.* 1: 34–41.

Rothammer, B., Marian, M., Neusser, K., Bartz, M., Böhm, T., Krauß, S., Schroeder, S., Uhler, M., Thiele, S., Merle, B., Kretzer, J. P., & Wartzack, S. (2021). Amorphous carbon coatings for total knee replacements-Part II: Tribological behavior. *Polymers.* 13: 1952.

Schmitt, D. R., Killen, C., Murphy, M., Perry, M., Romano, J., & Brown, N. (2020). The impact of antibiotic-loaded bone cement on antibiotic resistance in periprosthetic knee infections. *Clin. Orthop. Surg.* 12: 318–323.

Sebastian, S., Sezgin, E. A., Stučinskas, J., Tarasevičius, Š., Liu, Y., Raina, D. B., Tägil, M., Lidgren, L., & W-Dahl, A. (2021). Different microbial and resistance patterns in primary total knee arthroplasty infections—a report on 283 patients from Lithuania and Sweden. *BMC Musculoskelet. Disord.* 22: 1–10.

Sebastian, S., Tandberg, F., Liu, Y., Raina, D. B., Tägil, M., Collin, M., & Lidgren, L. (2022). Extended local release and improved bacterial eradication by adding rifampicin to a biphasic ceramic carrier containing gentamicin or vancomycin. *Bone Joint Res.* 11: 787–802.

Sezgin, E. A., Markevičiute, V., Širka, A., Tarasevičius, Š., Raina, D. B., Isaksson, H., Tägil, M., & Lidgren, L. (2020). Combined fracture and mortality risk evaluation for stratifying treatment in hip fracture patients: A feasibility study. *Jt. Dis. Relat. Surg.* 31: 163–168.

Sezgin, E. A., Tor, A. T., Markevičiūtė, V., Širka, A., Tarasevičius, Š., Raina, D. B., Liu, Y., Isaksson, H., Tägil, M., & Lidgren, L. (2021). A combined fracture and mortality risk index useful for treatment stratification in hip fragility fractures. *Jt. Dis. Relat. Surg.* 32: 583–589.

Sheikh, Z., Najeeb, S., Khurshid, Z., Verma, V., Rashid, H., & Glogauer, M. (2015). Biodegradable materials for bone repair and tissue engineering applications. *Materials.* 8: 5744–5794.

Širka, A., Raina, D. B., Isaksson, H., Tanner, K. E., Smailys, A., Kumar, A., Tarasevičius, Š., Tägil, M., & Lidgren, L. (2018). Calcium sulphate/hydroxyapatite carrier for bone formation in the femoral neck of osteoporotic rats. *Tissue Eng. Part A.* 24: 1753–1764.

Sonnow, L., Ziegler, A., Pöhler, G. H., Kirschner, M. H., Richter, M., Cetin, M., Unal, M., & Kose, O. (2021). Alterations in magnetic resonance imaging characteristics of bioabsorbable magnesium screws over time in humans: A retrospective single center study. *Innov. Surg. Sci.* 6: 105–113.

Šponer, P., Kučera, T., Brtková, J., Urban, K., Kočí, Z., Měřička, P., Bezrouk, A., Konrádová, Š., Filipová, A., & Filip, S. (2018). Comparative study on the application of mesenchymal stromal cells combined with tricalcium phosphate scaffold into femoral bone defects. *Cell Transplant.* 27: 1459–1468.

Stanish, W. D., McCormack, R., Forriol, F., Mohtadi, N., Pelet, S., Desnoyers, J., Restrepo, A., & Shive, M. S. (2013). Novel scaffold-based BST-CarGel treatment results in superior cartilage repair compared with microfracture in a randomized controlled trial. *J. Bone Joint Surg. Am.* 95: 1640–1650.

Sugaya, H., Suzuki, K., Yoshimura, H., Tanaka, M., Yamazaki, T., Watanabe, M., Iwaso, H., Inaoka, T., Sugimoto, H., Matsuki, K., & Mikasa, M. (2019). Osteointegration of a biocomposite suture anchor after arthroscopic shoulder labral repair. *Arthroscopy*. 35: 3173–3178.

Sukotjo, C., Lima-Neto, T. J., Júnior, J. F. S., Faverani, L. P., & Miloro, M. (2020). Is there a role for absorbable metals in surgery? A systematic review and meta-analysis of Mg/Mg alloy based implants. *Materials*. 13: 3914.

Sun, J. Y., Hao, S. C., Sun, R. B., & Yang, Y. S. (2009). Treatment of high-energy tibial shaft fractures with internal fixation and early prophylactic NovaBone grafting. *Orthop. Surg*. 1: 17–21.

Thoma, D. S., Bienz, S. P., Figuero, E., Jung, R. E., & Sanz-Martín, I. (2019). Efficacy of lateral bone augmentation performed simultaneously with dental implant placement: A systematic review and meta-analysis. *J. Clin. Periodontol.* 46: 257–276.

Thompson, O., W-Dahl, A., & Stefánsdóttir, A. (2022). Increased short- and long-term mortality amongst patients with early periprosthetic knee joint infection. *BMC Musculoskelet. Disord.* 23: 1–7.

Tian, Y., Liu, J., Hu, Y., Liu, L., Li, Y., Li, Z., Wang, X., Liu, Y., Feng, F., & Guo, J. (2021). Clinical study of calcium phosphate cement loaded with recombinant human bone morphogenetic protein 2 combined with calcium phosphate cement loaded with antibiotic for chronic osteomyelitis with bone defect. *CJPRS*. 35: 573–578.

Tsai, S. W., Huang, S. S., Yu, W. X., Hsu, Y. W., & Hsu, F. Y. (2020). Collagen scaffolds containing hydroxyapatite-CaO fiber fragments for bone tissue engineering. *Polymers*. 12: 1174.

Ulery, B. D., Nair, L. S., & Laurencin, C. T. (2011). Biomedical applications of biodegradable polymers. *J. Polym. Sci. Part B: Polym. Phys*. 49: 832–864.

Valancius, K., Soballe, K., Nielsen, P. T., & Laursen, M. B. (2013). No superior performance of hydroxyapatite-coated acetabular cups over porous-coated cups. *Acta Orthop*. 84: 544–548.

van der Voort, P., D Klein Nulent, M. L., Valstar, E. R., Kaptein, B. L., Fiocco, M., & GHH Nelissen, R. (2020). Long-term migration of a cementless stem with different bioactive coatings: Data from a "prime" RSA study: Lessons learned. *Acta Orthop*. 91: 660–668.

van de Wall, B. J. M., Beeres, F. J. P., Rompen, I. F., Link, B. C., Babst, R., Schoeneberg, C., Michelitsch, C., Nebelung, S., Pape, H. C., Gueorguiev, B., & Knobe, M. (2022). RIA versus iliac crest bone graft harvesting: A meta-analysis and systematic review. *Injury*. 53: 286–293.

van Hamersveld, K. T., Marang-Van De Mheen, P. J., Nelissen, R. G., & Toksvig-Larsen, S. (2018). Peri-apatite coating decreases uncemented tibial component migration: Long-term RSA results of a randomized controlled trial and limitations of short-term results. *Acta Orthop*. 89: 425–430.

Vignesh, U., Mehrotra, D., Howlader, D., Kumar, S., & Anand, V. (2019). Bone marrow aspirate in cystic maxillofacial bony defects. *J. Craniofac. Surg*. 30: E247–E251.

von Recum, J., Gehm, J., Guehring, T., Vetter, S. Y., von der Linden, P., Grützner, P. A., & Schnetzke, M. (2020). Autologous bone graft versus silicate-substituted calcium phosphate in the treatment of tunnel defects in 2-stage revision anterior cruciate ligament reconstruction: A prospective, randomized controlled study with a minimum follow-up of 2 years. *Arthroscopy*. 36: 178–185.

Wahlig, H., Dingeldein, E., Bergmann, R., & Reuss, K. (1978). The release of gentamicin from polymethylmethacrylate beads: An experimental and pharmacokinetic study. *J. Bone Joint Surg*. 60-B: 270–275.

Wang, X., Zhong, X., Li, J., Liu, Z., & Cheng, L. (2021). Inorganic nanomaterials with rapid clearance for biomedical applications. *Chem. Soc. Rev*. 50: 8669–8742.

Wang, Y., Sun, L., Mei, Z., Zhang, F., He, M., Fletcher, C., Wang, F., Yang, J., Bi, D., Jiang, Y., & Liu, P. (2020). 3D printed biodegradable implants as an individualized drug delivery system for local chemotherapy of osteosarcoma. *Mater. Des*. 186: 108336.

Wang, Z., Liu, B., Yin, B., Zheng, Y., Tian, Y., & Wen, P. (2022). Comprehensive review of additively manufactured biodegradable magnesium implants for repairing bone defects from biomechanical and biodegradable perspectives. *Front. Chem*. 10: 1066103.

Winge, M. I., & Røkkum, M. (2018). CaP cement is equivalent to iliac bone graft in filling of large metaphyseal defects: 2 year prospective randomised study on distal radius osteotomies. *Injury*. 49: 636–643.

Wu, S., Liu, X., Yeung, K. W. K., Liu, C., & Yang, X. (2014). Biomimetic porous scaffolds for bone tissue engineering. *Mater. Sci. Eng.: R: Rep*. 80: 1–36.

Xie, D., Wang, Z., Li, J., Guo, D. A., Lu, A., & Liang, C. (2022). Targeted delivery of chemotherapeutic agents for osteosarcoma treatment. *Front. Oncol.* 12: 843345.

Xynos, I. D., Hukkanen, M. V. J., Batten, J. J., Buttery, L. D., Hench, L. L., & Polak, J. M. (2000). Bioglass ®45S5 stimulates osteoblast turnover and enhances bone formation in vitro: Implications and applications for bone tissue engineering. *Calcif. Tissue Int.* 67: 321–329.

Yadav, L. R., Chandran, S. V., Lavanya, K., & Selvamurugan, N. (2021). Chitosan-based 3D-printed scaffolds for bone tissue engineering. *Int. J. Biol. Macromol.* 183: 1925–1938.

Yang, H., Lin, W., & Zheng, Y. (2021). Advances and perspective on the translational medicine of biodegradable metals. *Biomat. Translat.* 2: 177–187.

Yu, L., Rowe, D. W., Perera, I. P., Zhang, J., Suib, S. L., Xin, X., & Wei, M. (2020). Intrafibrillar mineralized collagen-hydroxyapatite-based scaffolds for bone regeneration. *ACS Appl. Mater. Interfaces.* 12: 18235–18249.

Yu, N. Y. C., Gdalevitch, M., Murphy, C. M., Mikulec, K., Peacock, L., Fitzpatrick, J., Cantrill, L. C., Ruys, A. J., Cooper-White, J. J., Little, D. G., & Schindeler, A. (2014). Spatial control of bone formation using a porous polymer scaffold co-delivering anabolic rhBMP-2 and anti-resorptive agents. *Eur. Cells Mater.* 27: 98–111.

Yu, X., Tang, X., Gohil, S. V., & Laurencin, C. T. (2015). Biomaterials for bone regenerative engineering. *Adv. Healthc. Mater.* 4: 1268–1285.

Yuan, H., Yang, Z., de Bruijn, J. D., de Groot, K., & Zhang, X. (2001). Material-dependent bone induction by calcium phosphate ceramics: A 2.5-year study in dog. *Biomaterials.* 22: 2617–2623.

Zampelis, V., Tägil, M., Lidgren, L., Isaksson, H., Atroshi, I., & Wang, J. S. (2013). The effect of a biphasic injectable bone substitute on the interface strength in a rabbit knee prosthesis model. *J. Orthop. Surg. Res.* 8: 1–7.

Zhang, N., Zhao, D., Liu, N., Wu, Y., Yang, J., Wang, Y., Xie, H., Ji, Y., Zhou, C., Zhuang, J., Wang, Y., & Yan, J. (2018). Assessment of the degradation rates and effectiveness of different coated Mg-Zn-Ca alloy scaffolds for in vivo repair of critical-size bone defects. *J. Mater. Sci.: Mater. Med.* 29: 1–11.

Zhou, H. F., Hernandez, C., Goss, M., Gawlik, A., & Exner, A. A. (2015). Biomedical imaging in implantable drug delivery systems. *Curr. Drug Targets.* 16: 672.

Zhou, Z. F., Sun, T. W., Chen, F., Zuo, D. Q., Wang, H. S., Hua, Y. Q., Cai, Z. D., & Tan, J. (2017). Calcium phosphate-phosphorylated adenosine hybrid microspheres for anti-osteosarcoma drug delivery and osteogenic differentiation. *Biomaterials.* 121: 1–14.

16 Next-Generation Theranostic Tools for Bone Repair and Skeletal Metabolism with Exosomes

Sneha Gupta, Prerna Singh, and Ashok Kumar

16.1 INTRODUCTION

Exosomes are released by cells in the extracellular spaces under both normal and disease conditions (Hu et al., 2012). They ferry proteins and nucleic acid from their host cells; their molecular composition represents their pathophysiological conditions, and therefore, they are pivotal biomarkers in clinical diagnostics (Yu et al., 2014). They also have an advantage over conventional methods as they can be taken up by the body for analysis using noninvasive procedures.

Exosomes are now being considered critical players in biomarker studies because major histocompatibility complex (MHC)-expressing exosomes present antigens via both direct and indirect pathways, they are composed of cell-specific surface markers, and they are highly stable under storage. Additionally, their content and the outer membranous layer are protected from extracellular proteases (Huda et al., 2021). The presence of exosomes in easily procurable biofluids such as urine, sweat, blood, milk, etc., have identified them as an attractive target for disease diagnostics. Especially in the case of cancer diagnosis wherein the presence of tumor specific RNAs can be identified in the exosomes released by tumor cells and thus can be used in early-stage diagnosis. Figure 16.1 presents some current therapeutic and diagnostic applications of exosomes.

16.2 EXOSOMES IN BONE DISEASE THERAPY AND METABOLISM

Bone comprises a mineral phase consisting of hydroxyapatite along with other ions, and the rest of the organic material: osteogenic cells, extracellular matrix (ECM) enriched in collagenous and non-collagenous proteins (Olszta et al., 2007). As mentioned, these cells are mainly osteoblasts, osteoclasts, osteocytes, and exosomes, and they influence bone metabolism and remodeling. Exosomes also play a crucial role in the synthesis of bone ECM (Marsell & Einhorn, 2011).

Researchers reported that the exosomal membrane, rich in phosphatidylserine, was involved in the synthesis of hydroxyapatite crystal for osteogenesis; additionally, the calcium deposited in the exosomal annexins enhances osteogenesis, and the phosphate formed by exosomal ATPases, pyrophosphatases and membrane transporters expedited the process of osteogenesis (Boyan et al., 2022). Bone metabolism and remodeling is a continuous process that involves the coordination of different cells and growth factors. The bone cells also produce exosomes to influence the metabolic cycle by acting through autocrine and paracrine mechanisms on target cells (Einhorn & Gerstenfeld, 2015).

For instance, osteocytes secrete exosomes throughout the course of bone remodeling to govern processes such as bone resorption mediated by osteoclasts and osteoblast-mediated bone formation, and they influence endothelial cells to achieve osteogenesis (Plotkin & Wallace, 2021). Exosomes derived from cells show considerable therapeutic potential; they are responsible for cellular communication,

DOI: 10.1201/9781003307310-19

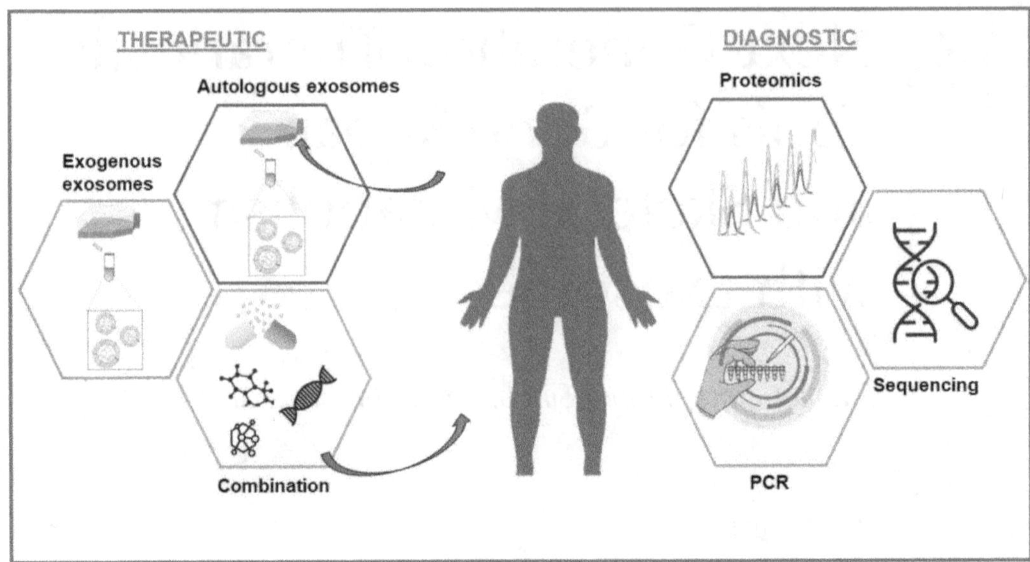

FIGURE 16.1 The diagnostic and therapeutic potential of exosomes. For therapy, the exogenous or autologous exosomes after the cell expansion can be isolated and can be delivered with chemotherapeutics, biomaterials and adjuvants. For diagnostics, biomarkers can be deciphered using various techniques from biological fluids. PCR = Polymerase chain reaction.

they can help in disease progression and they have been reported in many studies (Zhai et al., 2020). The therapeutic potential of exosomes is being employed in three main areas: for initiating tissue repair, modifying immune reactions, or conveying drugs/therapeutic molecules (Al-Sowayan et al., 2020). Exosomes, owing to their nanoscale vesicular structure, are used as drug carriers due to their effective osmotic retention, good biocompatibility and low immune response (Figure 16.2).

Bone is a highly vascularized tissue. In one study, the authors reported that MSC-derived exosomes isolated from human-induced pluripotent stem cells (hiPS) were able to promote bone formation and enhance vascularization in an ovariectomized rat model with a critical-sized bone defect (Qi et al., 2016). Exosomes released by MSCs that are already committed to the osteogenic phenotype, through the early activation of osteogenic genes, can reinforce the other MSCs toward osteoblastic differentiation, thus promoting bone formation (Yu et al., 2014). MSC exosomes can be easily assimilated by osteoblasts wherein they induce the synthesis of GLUT3 and MAPK pathway-related proteins, thus promoting their proliferation and differentiation (Masaoutis & Theocharis, 2019).

In an interesting study, BMSC-derived exosomes were conjugated with BMSC-targeting aptamer and were easily internalized by BMSCs in vitro; they also showed accumulation in bone marrow in vivo. The complex also showed enhanced bone formation and regeneration in postmenopausal osteoporotic and femur fracture mouse models. Still in its nascent stage, the application of exosomes derived from cell sources holds much promise in the field of bone regeneration (Luo et al., 2019).

Liu et al. (2021) showed efficient osteoinductive properties of BMSC-derived exosomes in bone regeneration in a rat cranial defect model. The osteoinductive property of the exosomes was accredited to miRNAs (let-7a-5p, let-7c-5p, miR-328a-5p and miR-31a-5p) through the Bmpr2/Acvr2b competitive receptor-activated Smad pathway. Wang et al. (2022a) investigated the role of miRNAs present in BMSC exosomes on bone degeneration in diabetic rat models. They found that miR-140–3p overexpressed exosomes mitigated bone degradation and enhanced bone healing by targeting Plxnb1. Another study proved the bone regeneration potential of BMSCs exosomes in acellular fish scale scaffolds in a mouse calvarial defect model (Wang et al., 2022b).

Although there are many reports on the experimental efficacy of exosomes derived from MSCs and different cell lines, the clinical studies are still limited. Osteoblasts and osteoclasts are bone-forming

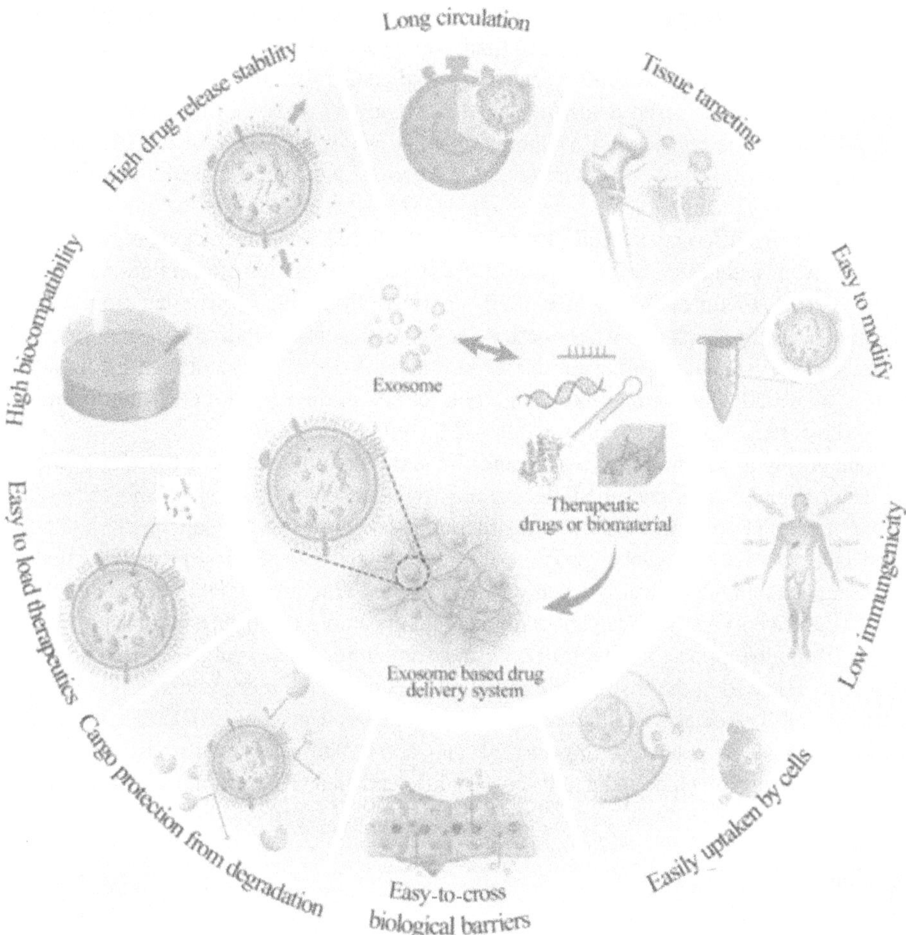

FIGURE 16.2 The role of MSC-derived exosomes as efficient delivery vehicles for tissue engineering applications (reproduced under the terms of CC-BY 4.0 (https://creativecommons.org/licenses/by/4.0/) International License from Lu, Y., Mai, Z., Cui, L. & Zhao, X.: Engineering exosomes and biomaterial-assisted exosomes as therapeutic carriers for bone regeneration. Stem Cell Res Ther. 2023. 14. 55. Copyright 2023 Lu et al., published by Springer Nature).

and bone-resorbing cells, and their exosomes might carry useful information for bone repair and regeneration. Proteomics analysis of the exosomes from mouse MC3T3 osteoblastic cells revealed many proteins involved in signaling pathways for osteogenesis such as eukaryotic initiation factor 2 signaling, integrin signaling and mTOR signaling (Liu et al., 2017a). Exosomes derived from mouse MC3T3 osteoblastic cells were also able to encourage osteoblastic differentiation of mouse bone-marrow-derived stromal ST2 cells due to the presence of osteogenic miRNAs (Cui et al., 2016).

In a study on mouse marrow cultures, osteoclast-precursor-derived exosomes promoted 1,25-dihydroxyvitamin D3-dependent osteoclast formation that was inhibited by mature osteoclast-derived exosomes. The exosomes from mature osteoclasts showed the presence of RANK, thereby competitively inhibiting the stimulation of RANK on osteoclast surfaces by RANKL (Huynh et al., 2016). It is also reported that exosomes derived from osteoclast precursor monocytes directed the osteogenic differentiation of MSCs, hinting at communication signals between osteoblasts and osteoclast precursors (Ekström et al., 2013). Exosomes from osteoclasts with miR-214–3p were able to inhibit bone formation when transferred to osteoblasts (Liu et al., 2017b).

It has been elucidated that interaction between osteoclasts exosomes and osteoblasts is through EphrinA2 and EphA2 (Sun et al., 2016), and Liang et al. (2021a) validated the potential of osteoclast-derived exosomes using decalcified bone matrix scaffold coated with the exosomes for pro-osteogenic regeneration in a mouse calvarial defect model; they found that exosomes that were rich in miR-324 showed the highest bone regeneration. Although there have not been many bone regeneration studies using osteoblasts and osteoclast-derived exosomes, the current data indicate that the exosomes from both cell types will have a potential role in bone remodeling (Liang et al., 2021a). The other bone cell type is osteocytes, terminally differentiated cells that are embedded in the bone matrix (Vig & Fernandes, 2022).

Exosomes from osteocytes are reported to cause the osteogenic differentiation of periodontal ligament stem cells by upregulating miR-181B-5P (Lv et al., 2020). Osteocytes are mechanosensitive cells, and a study reports that when these cells were subjected to fluid shear, they secreted extracellular vesicles (EVs), which enhanced the recruitment of stromal progenitor cells for osteogenesis (Eichholz et al., 2020). The immediate actin contractions in the regulation of smooth muscle cells resulted in the enhanced secretion of exosomes (Morrell et al., 2018).

The bone is highly vascularized tissue, and the endothelium cells form the major part of bone marrow. The exosomes from endothelial progenitor cells present in the bone reinforced osteogenesis through the upregulation of miR-126 in a distraction osteogenesis rat model (Jia et al., 2019). These exosomes have also been shown to promote the recruitment of osteoclast precursors that enhance neovascularization and bone healing when studied in a bone fracture model in mice (Cui et al., 2019). Dendritic cell-derived EVs (the resident immune cells) promote osteogenesis through various pathways such as through hippo signaling, miR-335, and immunoregulatory cargo (TGFB1 and IL-10) that is conditionally released in the case of inflammation to enhance the recruitment of regulatory T-cells; this in turn inhibits osteoclasts and thereby prevents bone loss (Cao et al., 2021; Elashiry et al., 2020).

Macrophages in their polarized, unpolarized, and anti-inflammatory states also release exosomes enriched in miRNA-5106, which induces osteoblast differentiation (Xiong et al., 2020). These exosomes

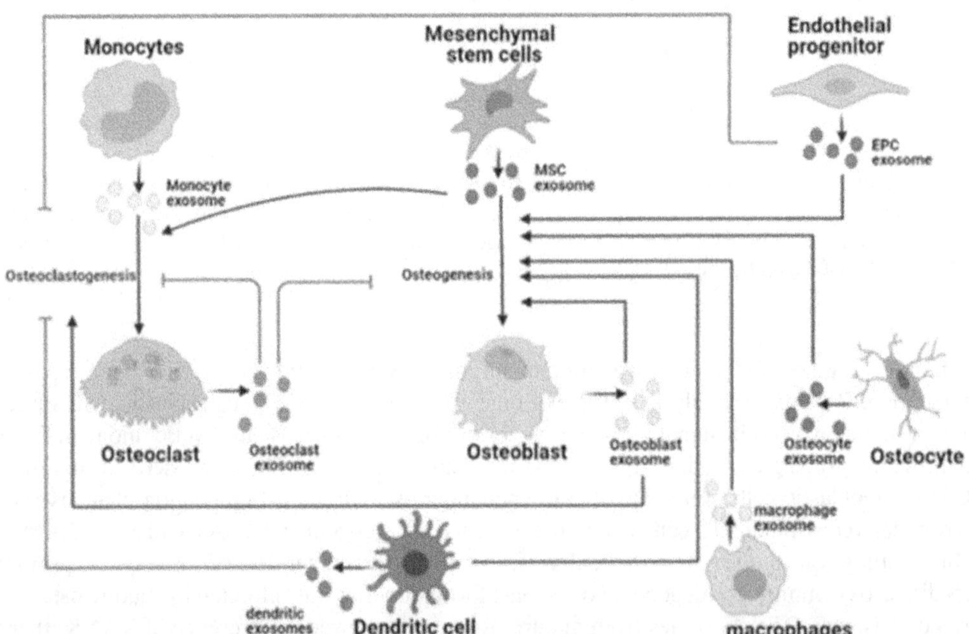

FIGURE 16.3 Roles of resident bone cells and microenvironment for influencing the bone remodeling through exosomes (reproduced under the terms of CC-BY 4.0 (https://creativecommons.org/licenses/by/4.0/) International License from Vig, S., & Fernandes, M. H.: Bone cell exosomes and emerging strategies in bone engineering. Biomedicines. 2022. 10(4).767. Copyright 2022 Vig & Fernandes, published by MDPI).

also have distinct osteogenic lineage specifications such as from bone marrow (Xia et al., 2020). Figure 16.3 sums up the overall mechanism of how the resident bone cells affect the bone metabolism and can be used in the regeneration of bone tissue.

16.2.1 Osteosarcoma

The key role of exosomes in the case of osteosarcoma (OS) opens new pathways to explore it as a therapeutic agent (Yang et al., 2021a). OS-derived exosomal biomarkers can be employed as therapeutic targets for the cells. OS therapy through exosomes is mainly due to derived RNAs or proteins or the use of exosomes as the drug delivery carriers.

A study shows that exosome-derived miR-101 had metastatic inhibitory properties and could potentially be used to stop OS progression (Zhang et al., 2020a). In another study, Wang et al. (2019) reported that through the downregulation of mRNA expression of SCAI, miR-1228 helped with OS invasion and migration, thus representing a possible therapeutic target. Exosomal miR-143 showed good internalization in OS cells and inhibited the migration of OS cell line 143B in vitro (Shimbo et al., 2014).

Some authors have reported that BMSC-derived exosomal LCP1 facilitated OS progression through the JAK2/STAT3 pathway and that miR-135a-5p inhibited OS tumorigenesis by acting downstream of LCP1 (Ge et al., 2020a). BMSC-derived exosomal miR-206 was also reported to suppress OS progression by targeting TRA2B, which is responsible for the development of OS (Zhang et al., 2020b). Exosomes can also be used as a carrier to deliver chemotherapy with fewer serious effects and long drug half-lives (Yang et al., 2021a).

MSC exosomes were combined with doxorubicin (chemotherapy drug) to functionalize nanocement, effectively regenerated bone and inhibited OS progression after debridement in in a rat tibia OS model (Gupta et al., 2023). They also have site specificity, as reported in an interesting study, wherein it was shown that after injecting human umbilical cord MSC exosomes in mice model of OS, the exosomes continuously accumulated in the tumors within 24–48 h and thus could be utilized in targeted therapy (Abello et al., 2019). A recent study reported that when doxorubicin was encapsulated in the exosomes, it was able to kill OS cells more effectively than free doxorubicin (Wei et al., 2019).

16.2.2 Osteoporosis

Current treatment of osteoporosis (OP) uses drug-based agents that stimulate apoptosis in osteoclasts, thus preventing bone resorption; however, they have certain limitations, such as osteonecrosis of the jaw and ectopic bone formation, etc. as reported (Khan et al., 2009; Canalis et al., 2004). In OP, exosomal treatment is mainly based on three approaches: maintaining equilibrium between osteoblasts and osteoclasts, modifying the exosomes structurally, and using exosomes as drug carriers (Masaoutis & Theocharis, 2019). Different cells with their enriched cargos have been reported for the treatment of OP.

In the postmenopausal OP, bone marrow MSC-derived exosomes with enhanced miR-186 expression were shown to promote YAP expression by regulating Mobl, resulting in enhanced osteogenesis (Masaoutis & Theocharis, 2019). Another study indicated the role of umbilical cord MSC-derived exosomes enriched in miR-1263 in inhibiting bone marrow MSC apoptosis by 1263/Mobl/Hippo signaling pathway, thus preventing the disused osteoporosis in rats (Masaoutis & Theocharis, 2019). Even the exosomes from cyclic mechanical-stretch-exposed bone marrow cells showed therapeutic effects in a disused OP model by inhibiting RANKL-induced osteoclast genesis through the NF-kB signaling pathway (Masaoutis & Theocharis, 2019).

Exosomes derived from young rat bone marrow highly enriched in miRNA-19b-3p significantly increased the expression of osteogenic genes such as type I collagen, alkaline phosphatase, and RUNX2, thus promoting the osteogenic differentiation of fatigue-loaded osteoporotic rat bone marrow MSCs (Masaoutis & Theocharis, 2019). Bone marrow stem-cell-derived exosomes were able to enhance the osteoblastic differentiation in vitro effectually; however, they failed to treat bilateral ovariectomy (OVX)-induced postmenopausal osteoporosis in a mouse model. Thus, the study authors conjugated those exosomes with the BMSC-targeting aptamer to form a complex. This complex was successfully internalized by BMSCs in vitro and promoted bone formation by enhancing the bone mass in the postmenopausal osteoporosis mouse model formed by OVX. This study establishes the role of aptamer conjugated exosomes as an innovative competent approach for the deterrence and treatment of osteoporosis and fracture (Masaoutis & Theocharis, 2019).

In another study, alendronate-conjugated extracellular vesicles were synthesized by click chemistry. Their efficacy was evaluated in an OVX-induced OP model and were shown to specifically target bone, thus representing a new therapeutic approach in OP treatment (Masaoutis & Theocharis, 2019). Even the progenitor cells of endothelial cells present in the blood vessels secrete exosomes and supported bone formation by stimulating angiogenesis or by facilitating the recruitment and differentiation of osteoclast precursors (Masaoutis & Theocharis, 2019). MSCs exosomes due to their rich repertoire helps to regenerate injured tissue. They act on various tissues by affecting the cells present on the site of the injury through various signaling pathways (Rudiyansh et al., 2022) (Figure 16.4).

Exosomes derived from endothelial cells have been shown to oppose glucocorticoid-induced osteoporosis by inhibiting the ferritinophagy of osteoblasts, offering potential for mitigating glucocorticoid-induced OP (Yang et al., 2021b). A study also reports that the exosomes from the supernatant of the cultured endothelial cells were more efficient in bone targeting as compared to the bone marrow derived exosomes or osteoblast derived exosomes. The authors were able to improve the OP recovery both in vitro and in vivo by the delivery of miR-155 (Song et al., 2019).

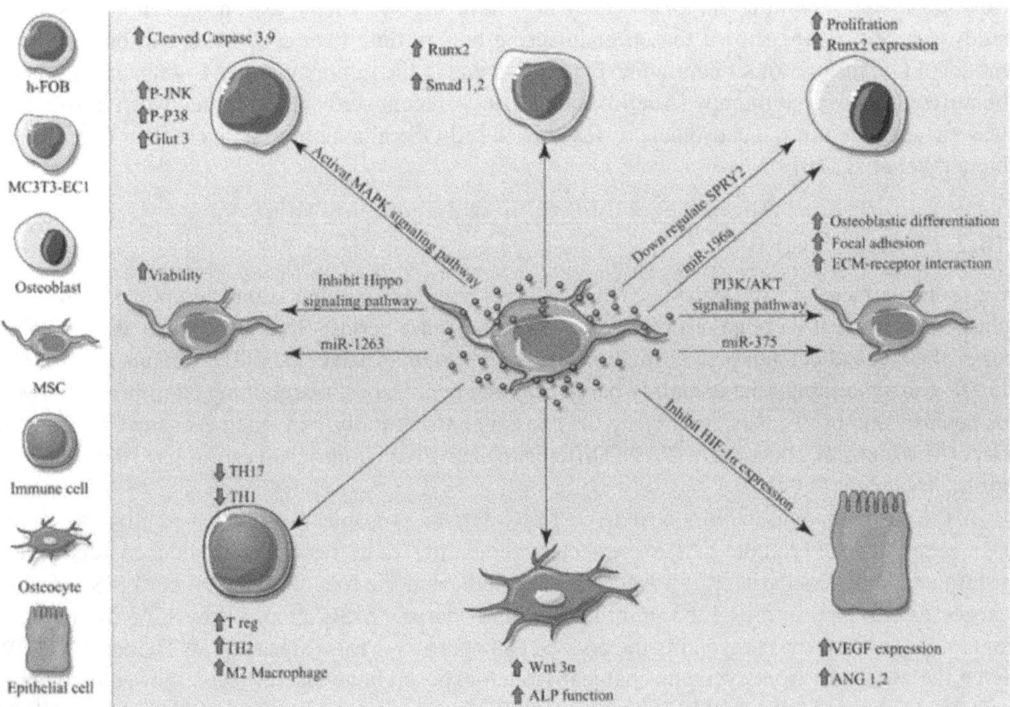

FIGURE 16.4 MSC-derived exosomes regulating different pathways for bone regeneration (reproduced with permission from Rudiansyah, M., El-Sehrawy, A. A., Ahmad, I., Terefe, E. M., Abdelbasset, W. K., Bokov, D. O., Salazar, A., Rizaev, J. A., Muthanna, F.M.S., & Shalaby, M. N.: Osteoporosis treatment by mesenchymal stromal/stem cells and their exosomes: Emphasis on signaling pathways and mechanisms. Life Sci. 2022. 306. 120717. Copyright 2022 Elsevier).

The exosomes derived from human umbilical cord cells were also analyzed for OP treatment in an estrogen-deficient mouse model and showed therapeutic and preventive effects (Ge & Wang, 2020). In a study by Sadat-Ali et al. (2021), the potency of autologous bone-marrow-derived MSCs, osteoblasts and the exosomes derived from the osteoblasts significantly reversed OVX-induced OP in the rabbit model. These authors described an alternative to conventional therapy for osteoporosis. mammalian exosomes, authors of a recent study used yam-derived nanovesicles to evaluate the exosomes' therapeutic potential in OVX-induced osteoporotic female mice, and the exosomes prevented OP by stimulating osteoblast formation (Hwang et al., 2023).

Similarly, altering specific exosome substances and using differing tissue engineering approaches to quantitatively densify exosomes has shown successful OP treatment outcomes in research. For instance, a nano-cement consisting of nano-hydroxyapatite and calcium sulphate was used as a local delivery carrier for BMP2 and zoledronic acid along with rat bone-marrow-derived MSC exosomes. This approach successfully enhanced bone formation in the rat osteoporotic model of femoral neck canal defect (Qayoom et al., 2019). In another study, the authors used a porous beta-TCP scaffold to deliver hiPSC–MSC exosomes for repairing cranial defect by improving the osteogenesis and angiogenesis in osteoporotic rats (Li et al., 2022a).

Authors of another study reported on the role of microRNA-935-modified bone marrow MSC-derived exosomes in enhancing osteoblast proliferation and differentiation by inhibiting the STAT1 level in osteoporotic rats (Zhang et al., 2021a). A few studies report on the roles of different RNAs as therapeutic targets for OP progression. For instance, some investigators showed the role of microRNA-5106 in M2 macrophage-derived exosomes in the induction of osteogenic differentiation of bone MSCs by targeting the SIK2 and SIK3 genes (Xie et al., 2020). The role of miR-31a-5p was also shown to play a significant role in the bone loss in the aged rats (Xu et al., 2018).

In a recent report, bovine-colostrum-derived exosomes were administered orally in a glucocorticoid-induced rat OP model to establish a treatment regime. The authors observed significant improvement in the bone density in the osteoporotic animal that was comparable with that in the sham control; the exosomes also altered the gut microbiota (Yun et al., 2020). Although these kinds of modified exosomes have shown significant clinical results, the main challenge is still preserving their biological function during their modification and applying the key findings from the basic research to the benefit of patients (Liang et al., 2021b).

Some researchers report on the use of exosomes isolated from adipose-derived MSCs to treat OP by inhibiting the activation of NLRP3 inflammasome in osteoclasts, further preventing the apoptosis of osteoblasts (Ren et al., 2019; Wang et al., 2021; Zhang et al., 2021b). The therapeutic potential of these exosomes was attributed to the presence of miR-130a-3p, which downregulated the expression of SIRT7 and upregulated Wnt signaling pathway proteins. Furthermore, their osteogenic potential can be enhanced by pretreating them with TNF-alpha or osteogenic media (Liu et al., 2017a; Zhu et al., 2021). Table 16.1 gives some examples of serum- and plasma-derived exosomes to treat OP.

16.2.3 Joint Diseases

Exosomes and their derivatives can be effectively delivered through intra-articular systemic injections, opening new directions in treating joint diseases (Li et al., 2018a). These exosomes contain specific information about the source cells, and many studies have shown that exosome miRNA plays a vital role in joint homeostasis. As mentioned earlier, due to site specificity, exosomes are efficient vehicles for delivering molecules to a particular organ or tissue, even those located distally.

TABLE 16.1
Serum- and Plasma-Derived Exosomal Content in Treating Osteoporosis (OP)

Sources	miRs	Functions	Model System	Application
Serum	-	Suppresses the integrin-mediated mechanosensation and activation of osteoblasts. Triggers the differentiation and resorption of osteoclasts.	Elderly OP patients' serum-derived exosomes	OP
Plasma	-	Promotes the proliferation and differentiation of osteoblasts.	Mouse tibia fracture with traumatic brain injury models	Bone fracture
Plasma	MiR-642a-3p	Contributes to the prediction and diagnosis of early postmenopausal OP.	Exosomes in early postmenopausal women	OP
Plasma	TRF-25, tRF-38, tRF-18	Diagnostic biomarkers for osteoporosis detection.	OP patients	OP
Plasma	-	Provides references for further investigations into the pathological mechanisms of OP.	Participants from the PLAGH Hip Fracture Database	OP
Serum	has_ circ_0006859	A potential biomarker for OP and enhances adipogenic versus osteogenic differentiation in BMSCs.	BMSCs	OP
Serum	LncRNAs	Potential diagnostic markers and therapeutic modules for OP.	OP patients	OP
Serum	-	Serum-derived exosomes from young rats improve the reduced osteogenic differentiation of BMSCs in aged rats with OP after fatigue loading.	Ovariectomized rats after fatigue-loading models	OP

Exosomal miRNAs, specifically miR-140, showed promising results with osteoarthritis of knee (OAK) therapy (Liu et al., 2022; Maehara et al., 2021). This miRNA is predominantly expressed in the articular cartilage and plays a vital role in the development of cartilage. It also helps in maintaining the metabolic balance of the cartilage matrix by inhibiting disintegrin and MMP13, an enzyme that works by the cleavage of type II collagen, which in turn helps break down the cartilage in osteoarthritis (Miyaki & Asahara, 2012).

Some miRNAs, such as miR-199a-3p, 193b, and 320c, have also been identified as markers to repress age-related cartilage metabolism (Ukai et al., 2012). The exosomal miRNAs are protected from endogenous RNase activity by the exosomal membrane and thus can be easily isolated and administered through the body fluids. Table 16.2 lists some studies on exosomal miRNA for maintaining chondrocyte function during intra-articular treatments (Maehara et al., 2021).

After identifying the specific miRNAs for their therapeutic potential, they can be effectively packaged in the exosomes and can be effectively delivered to the desired target (Tominaga et al., 2015).

16.2.4 Osteonecrosis of Femoral Head and Other Bone-Related Diseases

Exosomes derived from synovial MSCs facilitated proliferation and mitigated apoptotic effect in hBMSCs in vitro and helped reduce osteonecrosis of the femoral head (ONFH) in a rat model of steroid-induced ONFH (Guo et al., 2016). Kuang et al. (2019) isolated exosomes from the cells from the Wharton jelly of human umbilical cord-derived MSCs, and the exosomes inhibited the proliferation and resulted in apoptosis of osteocyte-like cells treated with steroids. Furthermore,

TABLE 16.2
Studies on Using Exosomal miRNA to Regulate Chondrocytes in Intra-Articular Treatment

Exosome Origin Cell Source	Study Design	Animal Models	miRNA	Result(s)	Target(s)
Human BMSCs	in vitro	–	miR-320c	Upregulates SOX9 and downregulates MMP13 expression in osteoarthritis (OA) chondrocytes.	Not mentioned
Human BMSCs	in vitro	–	miR-95–5p	Enhances histone H3 acetylation and maintains the function of articular chondrocytes. Promotes SOX9, COL2A1 and Aggrecan expression and enhances cartilage development.	HDAC2/8
Human chondrocytes	in vitro	–	miR-8485	Activates Wnt/β-catenin pathways. Promotes the chondrogenic differentiation of hBMSCs.	GSK3B, DACT1
Human BMSCs	in vitro and in vivo	Mice	miR-92a-3p	Promotes cartilage proliferation. In both MSCs and PHCs, promotes matrix gene expression and inhibits WNT5A expression.	WNT5A
Human BMSCs	in vitro and in vivo	Rats	miR-26a-5p	Suppresses damage to synovial fibroblasts in vitro and alleviates OA damage in vivo.	PTGS2
Human IPFP MSCs	in vitro and in vivo	Mice	miR-100–5p	Protects cartilage from damage and ameliorates gait patterns of DMM-induced OA mice.	mTOR
Human SMSCs	in vitro and in vivo	Rats	miR-140–5p	Enhances the proliferation and migration of ACs and the progression of early OA and prevents severe damage to knee articular cartilage in OA rats.	RalA

administration of this exosome led to the prevention of osteonecrosis and reversed bone loss in a rat model of steroid induced ONFH.

Exosomes improve ONFH by decreasing fatty deterioration of the bone marrow, reducing apoptosis, augmenting osteogenic and tube formation and neovascularization in vivo, etc. (Huber et al., 2022). Osteomyelitis, a bone infection caused by *Staphylococcus aureus*, is an inflammatory disease that eventually destroys bone; in addition to localizing extracellularly, it also colocalizes intracellularly with lysosomes, thus showing limited efficacy of antibiotic treatment (Birt et al., 2017). Yang et al. (2018) incorporated linezolid into macrophage-derived exosomes and augmented the efficiency of the antibiotic both in vitro and in vivo.

Researchers used BMSC-derived exosomes to treat the autoimmune disease systemic lupus erythematosus (SLE), in which the body's cells affect the joints, leading to osteopenia. The authors utilized the SLE-BMSCs both in vitro and in vivo and observed decreased miR-29b and Notch downregulation leading to enhanced osteogenic differentiation and bone formation. The authors proposed exosomes as a significant approach for treating osteopenia in SLE (Li et al., 2012).

Impaired fracture healing causes multiple bone pathologies, and MSC-derived exosomes have been shown to be an important regulator in the tissue regeneration process (Furuta et al., 2016). Even the exosomes derived from aged rat MSCs enriched in miRNA-128-3p regulate the osteogenesis and improved fracture healing by targeting Smad5 (Xu et al., 2020). Several studies have also shown the effect of hypoxic MSC-derived exosomes for promoting bone fracture healing through the transfer of miR-126 (Liu et al., 2020).

Radiation treatment for OP causes bone loss that is a major cause of fractures in cancer patients (Zuo et al., 2019). Radiation damages DNA and increases both reactive oxygen species and BMSC cell aging of BMSCs, reducing their proliferative and differentiative capacity. Studies on animal models describe that endothelial progenitor-cell-derived exosomes contain miR-155 that blocks osteoclast induction and thereby inhibits OP (Song et al., 2019). In another interesting study, Kim et al. (2005) showed the therapeutic efficacy of EVs derived from IL-10-treated bone-marrow-derived dendritic cells by suppressing the inflammatory and autoimmune responses in a murine model of collagen-induced arthritis, presenting a novel strategy for treating orthopedic complications.

Indoleamine 2,3-dioxygenase that overexpressed exosomes produced by dendritic cells showed anti-inflammatory and immune effects in a mouse model of collagen-induced rheumatoid arthritis. The exosomes also reversed arthritis due to the presence of markers such as CD80/86, CD81, Hsc70, MHC I and MHC II (Zakeri et al., 2019). In another study of collagen-induced mouse arthritis model, when MSCs exo transduced with miR-146a were used for the treatment, there was an upregulation in the expression of regulatory T cells, IL-10 and TGF-beta (Tavasolian et al., 2020).

Researchers have also explored using exosomes in oral tissue regeneration, mostly of the periodontium. In one study, the authors explored exosomes from PDLSCs, and they influenced angiogenesis by transferring the miR-17-5p that targets vascular endothelial growth factor A (Zhang et al., 2020c). Researchers explored the therapeutic efficacy of treating bone loss caused by periodontitis using SHEDs-derived exosomes that were enriched within the Wnt3a and BMP2; these influenced the osteogenic differentiation of cells (Wang et al., 2020a).

A pioneer animal study demonstrated the local use of adipose-derived stem cell (ADSC) exosomes, and the results showed new periodontal tissue formation in the ligature-induced periodontitis model; then, MSC exosomes were used to enhance periodontal regeneration by influencing the migration and proliferation of periodontal ligament cells (Mohammed et al., 2018; Chew et al., 2019). Findings are being reported from a human clinical trial involving ADSC exosomes to treat periodontitis (NCT04270006) conducted by an Egyptian researcher (Xing et al., 2020). The research on exosomes as therapeutic molecules for periodontal and dental regeneration is still in a novice state and needs further exploration.

16.3 EXOSOMES IN THE DIAGNOSIS OF BONE DISEASES

In the case of bone diseases, exosomes have been successfully utilized in the diagnosis of various diseases including osteosarcoma, rheumatoid arthritis (RA), OP, osteoarthritis (OA), femoral neck necrosis and various inflammatory diseases associated with bone (Meng et al., 2022; Hu et al., 2021). In this section, we discuss applications of exosomes specifically for diagnosing bone diseases.

16.3.1 Bone Cancer/Osteosarcoma

OS is a malignant tumor that generally occurs in the soft tissue along with the bone accompanied by lung metastasis and mortality (Otoukesh et al., 2018). The treatment includes preoperative chemotherapy followed by surgical debridement and postoperative chemotherapy. However, the prognosis is very poor for patients with nonresectable, metastasized tumors and in cases of relapsed disease (Otoukesh et al., 2018).

Therefore, it is necessary to diagnose OS early with suitable biomarkers that have high sensitivity for increasing the long-term survival of patients. Exosomes have been shown to be important agents in metastasis, tumorigenesis, and angiogenesis (Yang et al., 2021a). Garimella et al. (2014) reported initial findings of exosomes' role in OS; they detected the factors MMPs, RAKL, TGF beta, and CD-9 in the exosomal content of osteosarcoma cells and identified the exosomes' role in accelerating osteoclast-mediated bone resorption and thereby disrupting the bone remodeling homeostasis. This finding opened up new avenues for the role of exosomes in osteosarcoma.

For instance, the expression of two miRNAs that are normally increased during osteoclastogenesis, miR16 and miR378 were enhanced in mice under heavy bone tumor metastasis and thus can be used as a potential biomarker for the disease progression (Ell et al., 2013). In a clinical study of OS patients, patient serum miR-25-3p levels were elevated, which correlated with a poor prognosis (Al-Sowayan et al., 2020). The role of miR-25-3p in cancer was further elucidated when it was found to be overexpressed in the exosomes secreted by an established cell line; this finding confirmed that the exosomes in the patient's circulation had derived from tumors.

Another study reports the detection of significantly elevated levels of long noncoding RNAs (lncRNA) DANCR expression in the serum-derived exosomes of an OS patient, in contrast with healthy donor serum and serum from a patient with a benign tumor. The exosomes' membranous structure stabilized lncRNA DANCR, and the authors suggested them as more valid biomarkers for osteosarcoma than other tumor-related circulating lncRNAs described in the literature (Al-Sowayan et al., 2020). Ye et al. (2020) reported the upregulation of miR-92a-3p, miR-130a-3p, miR-195-3p, miR-335-5p, and let-7i-3p expression in the exosomal cargo of OS patients when compared with healthy patients.

Using high-throughput screening of microRNAs, miR-195-3p was identified to be upregulated significantly in OS patients and was also involved in the progression. Further, its overexpression was observed in 143B OS cells. When validated in vitro by stimulating 143B cells by the exosomes secreted from miR-195-3p-transfected OS cells, they showed enhanced invasive and proliferative capacities when compared with the cells stimulated by normal exosomes (Ye et al., 2020; Zhang et al., 2021c). The miRNA profile in the plasma exosome is also greatly influenced by tumor microenvironment, thus paving a way for diagnostic and therapeutic application (Ye et al., 2020).

Fujiwara et al. (2017) utilized miR-25-3p expression in serum exosomes as a noninvasive blood-based biomarker for monitoring tumors in OS patients. Exosomal cargo can be effectively used as not only diagnostic but also prognostic indicators by monitoring the variability in the miRNA and mRNA as a response to chemotherapy. In one study, Xu et al. (2017) found noteworthy decreases in miR-124, miR-133a, miR-199a-3p, and miR-385 and upregulated miR-135b, miR-148a, miR-27ax, and miR-9 in OS patients with adverse reactions to chemotherapy. Thus, these can be used as definitive biomarkers for OS with variable chemosensitivities.

In another study, miR-1258 expression was reduced in OS tissues and cell lines and associated with substandard clinical prognoses for OS patients (Liu et al., 2019). A negative correlation exists between OS cell imbalance and clinical prognosis; in contrast, Dkk3 correlated positively with clinical prognosis (Yoshida et al., 2018). The findings reported in this section demonstrate that certain miRNAs can be effective biomarkers for OS diagnosis. Table 16.3 summarizes the osteosarcoma diagnostic markers that have been reported on to date.

16.3.2 Rheumatoid Arthritis

RA is an autoimmune disease commonly identified by inflammation of the synovial tissue and infiltration of joints with leukocytes; it destroys bone and cartilage causing joint damage in the whole body (Al-Sowayan et al., 2020). MSC exosomes that overexpress miR-150-5p reduce RA markers, MMP-14, and VEGF in the synovial tissue, inhibiting synovial cell migration and invasion and thereby mitigating the extent of arthritis (Chen et al., 2018). Similarly, exosomes produced by

TABLE 16.3
Exosomes Extracted from Different Biofluids in the Diagnostic and Prognostic Markers of Osteosarcoma

Exosomal cargo	Existence	Extraction Method	Identification Method	Method	Clinical Value in Osteosarcoma (OS)
miR-675	Serum	Ultracentrifugation	TEM and Western blot	qRT-PCR	Biomarker for predicting the metastasis of OS
miR-148a, miR-27a, miR-9 and miR-199a-3p	Serum	Differential centrifugation	Not shown	qRT-PCR	Diagnostic biomarkers for differential chemotherapeutic response to OS
miR-25–3p	Extracellular fluid	Ultracentrifugation	SEM and Western blot	RT-PCR	Diagnostic biomarker and indicates poor prognosis in OS patients
miR-21–5p and miR-143–3p	Extracellular fluid	Ultracentrifugation	NTA	qRT-PCR	Elevated expression in OS and can be used as diagnostic biomarkers
miR-130a-3p and miR-195–3p	Plasma	Ultracentrifugation	TEM and Western blot	qRT-PCR	Elevated expression in OS and can be used as diagnostic biomarkers
miR-101	Plasma	Differential centrifugation	Scanning confocal microscope and Western blot	qRT-PCR	Circulating biomarker for OS detection
linc00852	Extracellular fluid	Differential centrifugation	TEM and Western blot	qRT-PCR	Biomarker for OS
circ-0000190	Plasma	Ultracentrifugation	TEM, Western blot, and fluorescence microscope	qRT-PCR	Potential biomarker for OS detection
Has-circ-103801	Serum	Ultracentrifugation	TEM and Western blot	qRT-PCR	Effective prognostic biomarker for OS

BMSCs with an overexpression of miR-192-5p halt the inflammatory response and the deterioration of joints. These analyses can be linked to treatment outcomes (Zheng et al., 2020).

In a clinical study of 60 RA patients, there was a positive correlation between serum C-reactive protein (CRP) and serum exo-amyloid A. In the non-remission group, the exosome–lymphatic vessel endothelial hyaluronic acid receptor-1 correlated positively with CRP, indicating its potential as a biomarker for RA activity (Zhou et al., 2022), although some reports offer contrasting findings. In one study, serum miR-548a-3p was significantly lower in the RA patients' exosomes, that is, negatively related to serum CRP, rheumatoid factor, and erythrocyte sedimentation rate in patients suffering from RA (Schioppo et al., 2021). This exosomal miRNA controls inflammation mediated by macrophages through the TLR4/NF-Kb signaling pathway (Liu et al., 2018). Song et al. (2015) found that the expression of Hotair, a lncRNA that can cause the migration of active macrophages, was significantly upregulated in the exosomal samples of 10 RA patients. In contrast, in non-RA patients, Hotair expression was lower with high CRP, identifying Hotair as a strong biomarker for the diagnosis of RA.

16.3.3 Femoral Head Necrosis and Other Bone-Related Diseases

Osteonecrosis of the femoral head, also known as avascular necrosis, is a metabolic bone disease that is mainly caused by disruptions in blood supply to the proximal femur due to ischemia. Long-term steroid usage, trauma, and osteoporosis lead to reduced blood supply, resulting in the collapse of the femoral head, joint pain, and bone dysfunction (Fang et al., 2020). The number of exosomes secreted by cells in ONFH changes in disease conditions and thus can be used as a parameter for diagnosing this disease. For instance, in steroid-induced femoral head necrosis, exosome levels in the blood are significantly lower in individuals with necrotic bone than in healthy individuals, indicating a possible marker for detecting ONFH (Li et al., 2018b; Zhu et al., 2020).

With the progress in proteomics and bioinformatics, several studies give insights into exosomal contents and their courses of action. In patients with myelodysplastic syndromes in which the immature blood cells in the bone marrow do not become mature, affecting the bone functionality, researchers observed overexpression of 21 miRNA (the highest being microR-10 and miR-15a) in BM–MSC-derived exosomes, potentiating their role in the diagnosis of this disease condition (Muntion et al., 2016). Exosomes are secreted by macrophages and dendritic cells composed of proteins without N-terminal signaling peptides and various inflammatory cytokines. These exosomal components influence the advancement of inflammatory bone diseases and, therefore can be used as diagnosis markers for inflammatory bone diseases (Hu et al., 2021).

Proteomic analysis revealed that in contrast with the young control, aged osteocytes released exosomes with high levels of proinflammatory proteins that regulated immunity, angiogenesis, and wound healing and eliminated oxidative stress. This infers that the exosomes released by the aged osteocyte will act as a shuttle to transfer factors that are responsible for promoting a proinflammatory state, a crucial hallmark of bone aging. Thus, utilizing the knowledge of the exosomal protein composition, they can also be used as criteria for indicating the 'bone wellness', and may be used as tool in the treatment monitoring and the personalized medicine (Al-Sowayan et al., 2020). In cases of bone loss due to radiation, exogenous MSC-derived exosomes restored the balance of osteogenic and adipogenic function of host MSCs, alleviating bone loss by activating Wnt/beta catenin signaling (Zuo et al., 2019).

16.3.4 Osteoporosis

OP can be triggered by factors such as low estrogen levels, inflammation, or negative drug side effects leading to bone resorption (Li et al., 2022b). The diagnosis of OP often involves a radiological scan, or it is not detected until the patient suffers a fracture; the ability to detect OP early is an unmet need (Huang et al., 2022). In OP monitoring, the differences in plasma exosomal transfer RNA (tRF-25, tRF-38, and tRF-18) expression of an osteoporotic patient compared to a healthy individual can be used as a potential biomarker (Li et al., 2022a).

Some studies report differences in the expression of circRNA (hsa_circ_0009127, hsa_circ_0090759, hsa_circ_0058392, hsa_circ_0090247, and hsa_circ_0049484) in the bone marrow exosomes from postmenopausal women and control osteoporotic patients through microarray analysis and were found to play an important role in the osteogenic differentiation through different pathways (Fu et al., 2022). These were implicated as potential postmenopausal osteoporosis biomarkers and as therapeutic targets for OP treatment (Fu et al., 2022). Proteins found in exosomes such as proteasome subunit beta type-9, poly(rc) binding protein 2, V-set immunoregulatory receptor, and aminoacyl t-RNA synthetase are closely related to OP, and therefore, understanding them will help us better understand bone diseases in general (Chen et al., 2020).

In one study, when small RNA sequencing was performed on the exosomes of normal and osteoporotic patients, Chen et al. (2020) detected the upregulation of 11 tRFs (small t RNA-derived fragments) and the downregulation of another 18 tRFs. The main tRFs identified were tRF 25, -38, and -18 and thus can be used as the diagnostic biomarker for OP (Chen et al., 2020). Chen et al. also reported that increased serum miR-214–3p correlated positively with reduced bone formation in elderly women with fracture and in ovariectomized mice, indicating the possible usage of the reported miRNA in osteoporosis diagnosis.

Detecting OP in postmenopausal women is often challenging, but in one report, exosomal miR-642a-3p (analyzed by small RNA sequencing) in the plasma of early postmenopausal women was an effective tool for the early diagnosis of postmenopausal OP (Kong et al., 2021). Has_circ_0006859 was also identified as the most upregulated circRNA in a microarray analysis of the serum exosomes of osteoporotic patients (Zhi et al., 2021). Several new markers are also being identified for OP diagnosis, such as plasma-derived long noncoding RNAs and serum-derived exosomal has_circ_0006859 (Teng et al., 2020; Meng et al., 2022).

16.3.5 Osteoarthritis

The hallmark of OA is the loss of ECM, cartilage breakdown, and synovial inflammation (McCulloch et al., 2017). Zhang et al. (2018) analyzed plasma-derived and synovial-fluid-derived exosomal lncRNAs, and found differences in their expression, specifically in lncRNA prostate-specific transcript 1 (PCGEM1) in the synovial-fluid-derived exosomes in early and late OA, compared with levels in healthy subjects, although the plasma-derived exosomes showed no differences. Therefore, Zhang et al. suggested using lncRNA as a biomarker for the progression of OA and exosomal PCGEM1 as a potential marker to discriminate early from late OA.

Skriner et al. (2006) described the presence of citrullinated proteins that consisted of fibrinogen D fragment, Sp alpha (like CD5 antigen protein) receptor, fibrinogen beta-chain precursor, fibrin beta chain, and fibrin alpha chain fragments in RA that were absent in the case of OA; based on these findings, peptide differences represent distinctions between unique joint diseases. In a very interesting report, Kolhe et al. (2017) described differences in synovial fluid exosomal miRNA in male and female OA patients that indicated the potential use of these differentially expressed proteins as novel diagnostic markers. They ascribed this difference in females to the estrogen response and the signals of toll-like receptors. They also reported that haptoglobin, orosomucoid, and ceruloplasmin expression were enhanced in the exosomes of the synovial fluid of female OA patients, while the apolipoprotein was found to be downregulated.

However, in the case of male OA patients, beta-2-glycoprotein and the complement component five proteins were upregulated, whereas Spt-Ada-Gcn5 acetyltransferase-related factor 29 was downregulated (Kolhe et al., 2017). Exosomes also play a key role in the pathological progression of diseases. Domenis et al. (2017) found that the synovial-fluid-derived exosomes from gonarthrotic patients increased the production of pro-inflammatory factors from macrophages, suggesting their possible role in the pathological events of joint diseases.

Exosome concentrations also vary across different stages of disease progression. For instance, the exosome concentrations in synovial fluid samples from late-stage OA patients were higher than those in early-stage OA patients, and in both conditions, they were significantly higher than those in the control sample (Ni et al., 2020). Additionally, the exosomes from end-stage OAK patients had elevated levels of chemokines that recruited inflammatory cells and thereby inhibited the cartilage degradation, ultimately promoting joint degradation, highlighting the relevance of exosomal diagnosis in OA pathology (Ni et al., 2020).

Researchers also reported higher expression of miR-92A-3p in the exosomes of MSCs in OA patients that interfered with WNT5A expression. These exosomes reduced the expression of COL10A1, MMP-13, and Runx2, thereby inhibiting the rapid development of OA (Mao et al., 2018). Zhang et al. (2021d) characterized the exosomes from RA and OA patients and detected membrane-bound TNF-alpha on the RA patient exosomes but not on the OA patient exosomes. Zhao and Xu (2018) detected higher expression of exosomal lncRNA PCGEM1 in the synovial fluid samples of late-stage OA patients than in the early-stage patients. When compared with the healthy control, lncRNA PCGEM1 expression was also higher in early-stage OA patients, indicating its versatility as a biomarker for the disease (Zhao & Xu, 2018).

CONCLUSION

Despite the great potential of exosomes for treating bone disease and their roles as biomarkers for prognosis and diagnosis, there is a long way to go to achieve clinical efficacy due to the problems we've discussed here. There is still no standardized technique for the production, purification, storage, and isolation of the exosomes, for instance. There is also the problem of low yield in isolation, leading to their failure in clinical treatment with prospective aggregation and protein contamination. Also, many exosomal targets are yet to be discovered, and the potential targets for miRNA require detailed analysis before their clinical usage. Exosomes offer prospective researchers promising avenues for exploring their clinical usage.

ACKNOWLEDGEMENTS

The authors would like to acknowledge the funding received from Ministry of Human Resource Development (MHRD), India and Indian Council of Medical Research, India projects (IMPRINT-6714; UAY/MHRD_IITK_006), MHRD, India project (SPARC/2018–2019/P612/S), Science and Engineering Research Board (SERB), India projects (IPA/2020/000026; CRG/2021/002179), Department of Science and Technology (DST), Govt. of India project (DST/NM/NT-2018/48), Department of Biotechnology (DBT), Govt. of India projects (DBT/IN/SWEDEN/08/AK/2017–18; BT/PR46254/AAQ/1/861/2022), Gangwal School of Medical Sciences and Technology initiation grant, Indian Institute of Technology, Kanpur. Sneha Gupta would like to acknowledge IIT Kanpur for her Ph.D. fellowship. Prerna Singh would like to thank DBT for her research associate fellowship at IIT Kanpur.

LIST OF ABBREVIATIONS

BMP	Bone morphogenetic proteins
CD	Cluster of differentiation
COL	Collagen
COL2A1	Collagen type II alpha 1
DACT1	Dishevelled binding antagonist of beta catenin 1
DANCR	Differentiation antagonizing non-protein coding RNA
Dkk3	Dickkopf-related protein 3
DMM	Destabilization of the medial meniscus
hBMSC	Human bone marrow-derived MSC
HDAC	Histone deacetylase
IL	Interleukin
IPFP	Infrapatellar fat pad
lncRNA	Long noncoding RNA
miR	Micro RNA
MMP	Matrix metalloproteinases
MSCs	Mesenchymal stromal cells
mTOR	Mammalian target of rapamycin
NTA	Nanoparticle tracking analysis
PCGEM	Prostate cancer gene expression marker
PDLSCs	Periodontal ligament stem cells
PHC	Primary human chondrocytes
PTGS2	Prostaglandin-endoperoxide synthase 2
qRT-PCR	Quantitative real time polymerase chain reaction
RalA	Ras-related protein
SEM	Scanning electron microscope

SMSC	Synovium-derived MSC
SOX9	SRY-box transcription factor 9
TEM	Transmission electron microscope
TGF	Transforming growth factor
TNF-alpha	Tumor necrosis factor alpha
VEGF	Vascular endothelial growth factor
Wnt	Wingless-related integration

REFERENCES

Abello, J., Nguyen, T. D. T., Marasini, R., Aryal, S., & Weiss, M. L. (2019). Biodistribution of gadolinium-and near infrared-labeled human umbilical cord mesenchymal stromal cell-derived exosomes in tumor bearing mice. *Theranostics*. 9: 2325.

Al-Sowayan, B., Alammari, F., & Alshareeda, A. (2020). Preparing the bone tissue regeneration ground by exosomes: From diagnosis to therapy. *Molecules*. 25: 4205.

Birt, M. C., Anderson, D. W., Toby, E. B., & Wang, J. (2017). Osteomyelitis: Recent advances in pathophysiology and therapeutic strategies. *J. Orthop*. 14: 45–52.

Boyan, B. D., Asmussen, N. C., Lin, Z., & Schwartz, Z. (2022). The role of matrix-bound extracellular vesicles in the regulation of endochondral bone formation. *Cells*. 11: 1619.

Canalis, E., Bilezikian, J. P., Angeli, A., & Giustina, A. (2004). Perspectives on glucocorticoid-induced osteoporosis. *Bone*. 34: 593–598.

Cao, Z., Wu, Y., Yu, L., Zou, L., Yang, L., Lin, S., Wang, J., Youn, Z., & Dai, J. (2021). Exosomal miR-335 derived from mature dendritic cells enhanced mesenchymal stem cell-mediated bone regeneration of bone defects in athymic rats. *Mol. Med*. 27: 1–13.

Chen, M., Li, Y., Lv, H., Yin, P., Zhang, L., & Tang, P. (2020). Quantitative proteomics and reverse engineer analysis identified plasma exosome derived protein markers related to osteoporosis. *J. Proteomics*. 228: 103940.

Chen, Z., Wang, H., Xia, Y., Yan, F., & Lu, Y. (2018). Therapeutic potential of mesenchymal cell—derived miRNA-150–5p—expressing exosomes in rheumatoid arthritis mediated by the modulation of MMP14 and VEGF. *J. Immunol*. 201: 2472–2482.

Chew, J. R. J., Chuah, S. J., Teo, K. Y. W., Zhang, S., Lai, R. C., Fu, J. H., Lim, L. P., Lim, S. K., & Toh, W. S. (2019). Mesenchymal stem cell exosomes enhance periodontal ligament cell functions and promote periodontal regeneration. *Acta Biomater*. 89: 252–264.

Cui, Y., Luan, J., Li, H., Zhou, X., & Han, J. (2016). Exosomes derived from mineralizing osteoblasts promote ST2 cell osteogenic differentiation by alteration of microRNA expression. *FEBS Letters*. 590: 185–192.

Cui, Y., Fu, S., Sun, D., Xing, J., Hou, T., & Wu, X. (2019). EPC-derived exosomes promote osteoclastogenesis through Lnc RNA-MALAT 1. *J. Cell. Mol. Med*. 23: 3843–3854.

Domenis, R., Zanutel, R., Caponnetto, F., Toffoletto, B., Cifù, A., Pistis, C., Di Benedetto, P., Causero, A., Pozzi, M., Bassini, F., & Fabris, M. (2017). Characterization of the proinflammatory profile of synovial fluid-derived exosomes of patients with osteoarthritis. *Mediators Inflamm*. 2017: 4814987.

Eichholz, K. F., Woods, I., Riffault, M., Johnson, G. P., Corrigan, M., Lowry, M. C., Shen, N., Labour, M. N., Wynne, K., & O'Driscoll, L. (2020). Human bone marrow stem/stromal cell osteogenesis is regulated via mechanically activated osteocyte-derived extracellular vesicles. *Stem Cells Transl Med*. 9: 1431–1447.

Einhorn, T. A., & Gerstenfeld, L. C. (2015). Fracture healing: Mechanisms and interventions. *Nat. Rev. Rheumatol*. 11: 45–54.

Ekström, K., Omar, O., Graneli, C., Wang, X., Vazirisani, F., & Thomsen, P. (2013). Monocyte exosomes stimulate the osteogenic gene expression of mesenchymal stem cells. *PLoS One*. 8: e75227.

Elashiry, M., Elashiry, M. M., Elsayed, R., Rajendran, M., Auersvald, C., Zeitoun, R., Rashid, M. H., Ara, R., Meghil, M. M., Liu, Y., & Arbab, A. S. (2020). Dendritic cell derived exosomes loaded with immunoregulatory cargo reprogram local immune responses and inhibit degenerative bone disease *in vivo*. *JEV*. 9: 1795362.

Ell, B., Mercatali, L., Ibrahim, T., Campbell, N., Schwarzenbach, H., Pantel, K., Amadori, D., & Kang, Y. (2013). Tumor-induced osteoclast miRNA changes as regulators and biomarkers of osteolytic bone metastasis. *Cancer Cell*. 24: 542–556.

Fang, S., He, T., Jiang, J., Li, Y., & Chen, P. (2020). Osteogenic effect of tsRNA-10277-loaded exosome derived from bone mesenchymal stem cells on steroid-induced osteonecrosis of the femoral head. *Drug Des. Devel. and Ther.* 4579–4591.

Fu, M., Fang, L., Xiang, X., Fan, X., Wu, J., & Wang, J. (2022). Microarray analysis of circRNAs sequencing profile in exosomes derived from bone marrow mesenchymal stem cells in postmenopausal osteoporosis patients. *J. Clin. Lab. Anal.* 36: e23916.

Fujiwara, T., Uotani, K., Yoshida, A., Morita, T., Nezu, Y., Kobayashi, E., Yoshida, A., Uehara, T., Omori, T., Sugiu, K., & Komatsubara, T. (2017). Clinical significance of circulating miR-25–3p as a novel diagnostic and prognostic biomarker in osteosarcoma. *Oncotarget.* 8: 33375.

Furuta, T., Miyaki, S., Ishitobi, H., Ogura, T., Kato, Y., Kamei, N., Miyado, K., Higashi, Y., & Ochi, M. (2016). Mesenchymal stem cell-derived exosomes promote fracture healing in a mouse model. *Stem Cells Transl. Med.* 5: 1620–1630.

Garimella, R., Washington, L., Isaacson, J., Vallejo, J., Spence, M., Tawfik, O., Rowe, P., Brotto, M., & Perez, R. (2014). Extracellular membrane vesicles derived from 143B osteosarcoma cells contain pro-osteoclastogenic cargo: A novel communication mechanism in osteosarcoma bone microenvironment. *Transl. Oncol.* 7: 331–340.

Ge, X., Liu, W., Zhao, W., Feng, S., Duan, A., Ji, C., Shen, K., Liu, W., Zhou, J., Jiang, D., & Rong, Y. (2020a). Exosomal transfer of LCP1 promotes osteosarcoma cell tumorigenesis and metastasis by activating the JAK2/STAT3 signaling pathway. *Mol. Ther. Nucleic Acids.* 21: 900–915.

Ge, Y., & Wang, X. (2020). The role and mechanism of exosomes from umbilical cord mesenchymal stem cells in inducing osteogenesis and preventing osteoporosis. *Cell Transplantation.* 30: 09636897211057465.

Guo, S. C., Tao, S. C., Yin, W. J., Qi, X., Sheng, J. G., & Zhang, C. Q. (2016). Exosomes from human synovial-derived mesenchymal stem cells prevent glucocorticoid-induced osteonecrosis of the femoral head in the rat. *Int. J. of Biol. Sci.* 12: 1262.

Gupta, S., Qayoom, I., Gupta, P., Gupta, A., Singh, P., Singh, S., & Kumar, A. (2023). Exosome-functionalized, drug-laden bone substitute along with an antioxidant herbal membrane for bone and periosteum regeneration in bone sarcoma. *ACS Appl. Mater. Interfaces.* 15: 8824–8839.

Hu, G., Drescher, K. M., & Chen, X. M. (2012). Exosomal miRNAs: Biological properties and therapeutic potential. *Front. in Genet.* 3: 56.

Hu, Y., Wang, Y., Chen, T., Hao, Z., Cai, L., & Li, J. (2021). Exosome: Function and application in inflammatory bone diseases. *Oxid. Med. Cell. Longev.* 2021: 6324912.

Huang, G., Zhao, Q., Li, W., Jiao, J., Zhao, X., Feng, D., & Tang, W. (2022). Exosomes: A new option for osteoporosis treatment. *Medicine.* 101: e32402.

Huber, J., Griffin, M. F., Longaker, M. T., & Quarto, N. (2022). Exosomes: A tool for bone tissue engineering. *Tissue Eng. B: Rev.* 28: 101–113.

Huda, M. N., Nafiujjaman, M., Deaguero, I. G., Okonkwo, J., Hill, M. L., Kim, T., & Nurunnabi, M. (2021). Potential use of exosomes as diagnostic biomarkers and in targeted drug delivery: Progress in clinical and preclinical applications. *ACS Biomater.* 7: 2106–2149.

Huynh, N., VonMoss, L., Smith, D., Rahman, I., Felemban, M. F., Zuo, J., Rody Jr, W. J., McHugh, K. P., & Holliday, L. S. (2016). Characterization of regulatory extracellular vesicles from osteoclasts. *J. Dent. Res.* 95: 673–679.

Hwang, J. H., Park, Y. S., Kim, H. S., Kim, D., Lee, S. H., Lee, C. H., Lee, S. H., Kim, J. E., Lee, S., Kim, H. M., & Kim, H. W. (2023). Yam-derived exosome-like nanovesicles stimulate osteoblast formation and prevent osteoporosis in mice. *J. Control. Release.* 355: 184–198.

Jia, Y., Zhu, Y., Qiu, S., Xu, J., & Chai, Y. (2019). Exosomes secreted by endothelial progenitor cells accelerate bone regeneration during distraction osteogenesis by stimulating angiogenesis. *Stem Cell Res. Ther.* 10: 1–13.

Khan, A. A., Sandor, G. K. B., Dore, E., Morrison, A. D., Alsahli, M., Amin, F., Peters, E., Hanley, D. A., Chaudry, S. R., Lentle, B., & Dempster, D. W. (2009). Bisphosphonate associated osteonecrosis of the jaw. *J. Rheumat.* 36: 478–490.

Kim, S. H., Lechman, E. R., Bianco, N., Menon, R., Keravala, A., Nash, J., Mi, Z., Watkins, S. C., Gambotto, A., & Robbins, P. D. (2005). Exosomes derived from IL-10-treated dendritic cells can suppress inflammation and collagen-induced arthritis. *J. Immunol.* 174: 6440–6448.

Kolhe, R., Hunter, M., Liu, S., Jadeja, R. N., Pundkar, C., Mondal, A. K., Mendhe, B., Drewry, M., Rojiani, M. V., Liu, Y., & Isales, C. M. (2017). Gender-specific differential expression of exosomal miRNA in synovial fluid of patients with osteoarthritis. *Sci. Rep.* 7: 2029.

Kong, D., Chen, T., Zheng, X., Yang, T., Zhang, Y., & Shao, J. (2021). Comparative profile of exosomal microRNAs in postmenopausal women with various bone mineral densities by small RNA sequencing. *Genomics*. 113: 1514–1521.

Kuang, M., Huang, Y., Zhao, X. G., Zhang, R., Ma, J., Wang, D., & Ma, X. (2019). Exosomes derived from Wharton's jelly of human umbilical cord mesenchymal stem cells reduce osteocyte apoptosis in glucocorticoid-induced osteonecrosis of the femoral head in rats via the miR-21-PTEN-AKT signalling pathway. *Int. J. of Biol. Sci.* 15: 1861.

Li, Q. C., Li, C., Zhang, W., Pi, W., & Han, N. (2022a). Potential effects of exosomes and their MicroRNA carrier on osteoporosis. *Curr. Pharm. Des.* 28: 899–909.

Li, R., Lin, Q. X., Liang, X. Z., Liu, G. B., Tang, H., Wang, Y., Lu, S. B., & Peng, J. (2018b). Stem cell therapy for treating osteonecrosis of the femoral head: From clinical applications to related basic research. *Stem Cell Res. Ther.* 9: 1–11.

Li, X., Liu, L., Meng, D., Wang, D., Zhang, J., Shi, D., Liu, H., Xu, H., Lu, L., & Sun, L. (2012). Enhanced apoptosis and senescence of bone-marrow-derived mesenchymal stem cells in patients with systemic lupus erythematosus. *Stem Cells Dev.* 21: 2387–2394.

Li, Y., Huang, P., Nasser, M. I., Wu, W., Yao, J., & Sun, Y. (2022b). Role of exosomes in bone and joint disease metabolism, diagnosis, and therapy. *Eur. J. Pharm. Sci.* 176: 106262.

Li, Z., Wang, Y., Xiao, K., Xiang, S., Li, Z., & Weng, X. (2018a). Emerging role of exosomes in the joint diseases. *Cell. Physiol. Biochem.* 47: 2008–2017.

Liang, M., Yin, X., Zhang, S., Ai, H., Luo, F., Xu, J., Dou, C., Dong, S., & Ma, Q. (2021a). Osteoclast-derived small extracellular vesicles induce osteogenic differentiation via inhibiting ARHGAP1. *Mol. Ther.-Nucleic Acids*. 23: 1191–1203.

Liang, Y., Duan, L., Lu, J., & Xia, J. (2021b). Engineering exosomes for targeted drug delivery. *Theranostics*. 11: 3183.

Liu, A., Lin, D., Zhao, H., Chen, L., Cai, B., Lin, K., & Shen, S. G. F. (2021). Optimized BMSC-derived osteoinductive exosomes immobilized in hierarchical scaffold via lyophilization for bone repair through Bmpr2/Acvr2b competitive receptor-activated Smad pathway. *Biomaterials*. 272: 120718.

Liu, J., Li, D., Wu, X., Dang, L., Lu, A., & Zhang, G. (2017a). Bone-derived exosomes. *Curr. Opin. Pharmacol.* 34: 64–69.

Liu, J., Liang, C., Guo, B., Wu, X., Li, D., Zhang, Z., Zheng, K., Dang, L., He, X., Lu, C., & Peng, S. (2017b). Increased PLEKHO1 within osteoblasts suppresses Smad-dependent BMP signaling to inhibit bone formation during aging. *Aging Cell*. 16: 360–376.

Liu, W., Li, L., Rong, Y., Qian, D., Chen, J., Zhou, Z., Luo, Y., Jiang, D., Cheng, L., Zhao, S., & Kong, F. (2020). Hypoxic mesenchymal stem cell-derived exosomes promote bone fracture healing by the transfer of miR-126. *Acta Biomater.* 103: 96–212.

Liu, W., Wu, Y. H., Zhang, L., Xue, B., Wang, Y., Liu, B., Liu, X. Y., Zuo, F., Yang, X. Y., Chen, F. Y., & Duan, R. (2018). MicroRNA-146a suppresses rheumatoid arthritis fibroblast-like synoviocytes proliferation and inflammatory responses by inhibiting the TLR4/NF-kB signaling. *Oncotarget*. 9: 23944.

Liu, W., Zhou, Z., Zhang, Q., Rong, Y., Li, L., Luo, Y., Wang, J., Yin, G., Lv, C., & Cai, W. (2019). Overexpression of miR-1258 inhibits cell proliferation by targeting AKT3 in osteosarcoma. *Biochem. Bioph. Res. Co.* 510: 479–486.

Liu, Y., Zeng, Y., Si, H. B., Tang, L., Xie, H. Q., & Shen, B. (2022). Exosomes derived from human urine—derived stem cells overexpressing miR-140–5p alleviate knee osteoarthritis through downregulation of VEGFA in a rat model. *Am. J. Sports Med.* 50: 1088–1105.

Luo, Z. W., Liu, Y. W., Rao, S. S., Yin, H., Huang, J., Chen, C. Y., Hu, Y., Zhang, Y., Tan, Y. J., Yuan, L. Q., & Chen, T. H. (2019). Aptamer-functionalized exosomes from bone marrow stromal cells target bone to promote bone regeneration. *Nanoscale*. 11: 20884–20892.

Lv, P., Gao, P., Tian, G., Yang, Y., Mo, F., Wang, Z., Sun, L., Kuang, M. J., & Wang, Y. (2020). Osteocyte-derived exosomes induced by mechanical strain promote human periodontal ligament stem cell proliferation and osteogenic differentiation via the miR-181b-5p/PTEN/AKT signaling pathway. *Stem Cell Res. Ther.* 11: 1–15.

Maehara, M., Toyoda, E., Takahashi, T., Watanabe, M., & Sato, M. (2021). Potential of exosomes for diagnosis and treatment of joint disease: Towards a point-of-care therapy for osteoarthritis of the knee. *Int. J. Mol. Sci.* 22: 2666.

Mao, G., Zhang, Z., Hu, S., Zhang, Z., Chang, Z., Huang, Z., Liao, W., & Kang, Y. (2018). Exosomes derived from miR-92a-3p-overexpressing human mesenchymal stem cells enhance chondrogenesis and suppress cartilage degradation via targeting WNT5A. *Stem Cell Res. Ther.* 9: 1–13.

Marsell, R., & Einhorn, T. A. (2011). The biology of fracture healing. *Injury*. 42: 551–555.
Masaoutis, C., & Theocharis, S. (2019). The role of exosomes in bone remodeling: Implications for bone physiology and disease. *Dis. Markers*. 2019: 9417914.
McCulloch, K., Litherland, G. J., & Rai, T. S. (2017). Cellular senescence in osteoarthritis pathology. *Aging Cell*. 16: 210–218.
Meng, F., Xue, X., Yin, Z., Gao, F., Wang, X., & Geng, Z. (2022). Research progress of exosomes in bone diseases: Mechanism, diagnosis and therapy. *Front. Bioeng. Biotech*. 10: 866627.
Miyaki, S., & Asahara, H. (2012). Macro view of microRNA function in osteoarthritis. *Nat. Rev. Rheumatol*. 8: 543–552.
Mohammed, E., Khalil, E., & Sabry, D. (2018). Effect of adipose-derived stem cells and their exo as adjunctive therapy to nonsurgical periodontal treatment: A histologic and histomorphometric study in rats. *Biomolecules*. 8: 167.
Morrell, A. E., Brown, G. N., Robinson, S. T., Sattler, R. L., Baik, A. D., Zhen, G., Cao, X., Bonewald, L. F., Jin, W., Kam, L. C., & Guo, X. E. (2018). Mechanically induced Ca2+ oscillations in osteocytes release extracellular vesicles and enhance bone formation. *Bone Res*. 6: 6.
Muntion, S., Ramos, T. L., Diez-Campelo, M., Rosón, B., Sánchez-Abarca, L. I., Misiewicz-Krzeminska, I., Preciado, S., Sarasquete, M. E., De Las Rivas, J., Gonzalez, M., & Sanchez-Guijo, F. (2016). Microvesicles from mesenchymal stromal cells are involved in HPC-microenvironment crosstalk in myelodysplastic patients. *PloS One*. 11: e0146722.
Ni, Z., Zhou, S., Li, S., Kuang, L., Chen, H., Luo, X., Ouyang, J., He, M., Du, X., & Chen, L. (2020). Exosomes: Roles and therapeutic potential in osteoarthritis. *Bone Res*. 8: 25.
Olszta, M. J., Cheng, X., Jee, S. S., Kumar, R., Kim, Y. Y., Kaufman, M. J., Douglas, E. P., & Gower, L. B. (2007). Bone structure and formation: A new perspective. *Mater. Sci. Eng. R Rep*. 58: 77–116.
Otoukesh, B., Boddouhi, B., Moghtadaei, M., Kaghazian, P., & Kaghazian, M. (2018). Novel molecular insights and new therapeutic strategies in osteosarcoma 11 Medical and health sciences 1112 oncology and carcinogenesis. *Cancer Cell Int*. 18: 1–23.
Plotkin, L. I., & Wallace, J. M. (2021). MicroRNAs and osteocytes. *Bone*. 150: 115994.
Qayoom, I., Teotia, A. K., & Kumar, A. (2019). Nanohydroxyapatite based ceramic carrier promotes bone formation in a femoral neck canal defect in osteoporotic rats. *Biomacromolecules*. 21: 328–337.
Qi, X., Zhang, J., Yuan, H., Xu, Z., Li, Q., Niu, X., Hu, B., Wang, Y., & Li, X. (2016). Exosomes secreted by human-induced pluripotent stem cell-derived mesenchymal stem cells repair critical-sized bone defects through enhanced angiogenesis and osteogenesis in osteoporotic rats. *Int. J. Biol. Sci*. 12: 836.
Ren, L., Song, Z., Cai, Q., Chen, R., Zou, Y., Fu, Q., & Ma, Y. (2019). Adipose mesenchymal stem cell-derived exosomes ameliorate hypoxia/serum deprivation-induced osteocyte apoptosis and osteocyte-mediated osteoclastogenesis *in vitro*. *Biochem. Biophys. Res. Commun*. 508: 138–144.
Rudiansyah, M., El-Sehrawy, A. A., Ahmad, I., Terefe, E. M., Abdelbasset, W. K., Bokov, D. O., Salazar, A., Rizaev, J. A., Muthanna, F. M. S., & Shalaby, M. N. (2022). Osteoporosis treatment by mesenchymal stromal/stem cells and their exosomes: Emphasis on signaling pathways and mechanisms. *Life Sci*. 306: 120717.
Sadat-Ali, M., Al-Dakheel, D. A., Al-Turki, H. A., & Acharya, S. (2021). Efficacy of autologous bone marrow derived Mesenchymal stem cells (MSCs), osteoblasts and osteoblasts derived exosome in the reversal of ovariectomy (OVX) induced osteoporosis in rabbit model. *Am. J. Transl. Res*. 13: 6175.
Schioppo, T., Ubiali, T., Ingegnoli, F., Bollati, V., & Caporali, R. (2021). The role of extracellular vesicles in rheumatoid arthritis: A systematic review. *Clin. Rheumatol*. 40: 3481–3497.
Shimbo, K., Miyaki, S., Ishitobi, H., Kato, Y., Kubo, T., Shimose, S., & Ochi, M. (2014). Exosome-formed synthetic microRNA-143 is transferred to osteosarcoma cells and inhibits their migration. *Biochem. Biophys. Res. Commun*. 445: 381–387.
Skriner, K., Adolph, K., Jungblut, P. R., & Burmester, G. R. (2006). Association of citrullinated proteins with synovial exosomes. *Arthritis Rheumatol*. 54: 3809–3814.
Song, H., Li, X., Zhao, Z., Qian, J., Wang, Y., Cui, J., Weng, W., Cao, L., Chen, X., Hu, Y., & Su, J. (2019). Reversal of osteoporotic activity by endothelial cell-secreted bone targeting and biocompatible exosomes. *Nano Lett*. 19: 3040–3048.
Song, J., Kim, D., Han, J., Kim, Y., Lee, M., & Jin, E. J. (2015). PBMC and exosome-derived Hotair is a critical regulator and potent marker for rheumatoid arthritis. *Clin. Exp. Med*. 15: 121–126.
Sun, W., Zhao, C., Li, Y., Wang, L., Nie, G., Peng, J., Wang, A., Zhang, P., Tian, W., Li, Q., & Song, J. (2016). Osteoclast-derived microRNA-containing exosomes selectively inhibit osteoblast activity. *Cell Discov*. 2: 1–23.

Tavasolian, F., Moghaddam, A. S., Rohani, F., Abdollahi, E., Janzamin, E., Momtazi-Borojeni, A. A., Moallem, S. A., Jamialahmadi, T., & Sahebkar, A. (2020). Exosomes: Effectual players in rheumatoid arthritis. *Autoimmun. Rev*. 19: 102511.

Teng, Z., Zhu, Y., Zhang, X., Teng, Y., & Lu, S. (2020). Osteoporosis is characterized by altered expression of exosomal long non-coding RNAs. *Front. Genet*. 11: 566959.

Tominaga, N., Yoshioka, Y., & Ochiya, T. (2015). A novel platform for cancer therapy using extracellular vesicles. *Adv. Drug Deliv*. 95: 50–55.

Ukai, T., Sato, M., Akutsu, H., Umezawa, A., & Mochida, J. (2012). MicroRNA-199a-3p, microRNA-193b, and microRNA-320c are correlated to aging and regulate human cartilage metabolism. *J. Orthop. Res*. 30: 1915–1922.

Vig, S., & Fernandes, M. H. (2022). Bone cell exosomes and emerging strategies in bone engineering. *Biomed*. 10: 767.

Wang, J. W., Wu, X. F., Gu, X. J., & Jiang, X. H. (2019). Exosomal miR-1228 from cancer-associated fibroblasts promotes cell migration and invasion of osteosarcoma by directly targeting SCAI. *Oncol. Res*. 27: 979.

Wang, M., Li, J., Ye, Y., He, S., & Song, J. (2020a). SHED-derived conditioned exosomes enhance the osteogenic differentiation of PDLSCs via Wnt and BMP signaling *in vitro*. *Differentiation*. 111: 1–11.

Wang, N., Liu, X., Tang, Z., Wei, X., Dong, H., Liu, Y., Wu, H., Wu, Z., Li, X., Ma, X., & Guo, Z. (2022a). Increased BMSC exosomal miR-140–3p alleviates bone degradation and promotes bone restoration by targeting Plxnb1 in diabetic rats. *J. Nanobiotechnology*. 20: 1–20.

Wang, S., Jia, J., & Chen, C. (2021). lncRNA-KCNQ1OT1: A potential target in exosomes derived from adipose-derived stem cells for the treatment of osteoporosis. *Stem Cells Int*. 2021: 7690006.

Wang, Y., Kong, B., Chen, X., Liu, R., Zhao, Y., Gu, Z., & Jiang, Q. (2022b). BMSC exosome-enriched acellular fish scale scaffolds promote bone regeneration. *J. Nanobiotechnology*. 20: 1–11.

Wei, H., Chen, J., Wang, S., Fu, F., Zhu, X., Wu, C., Liu, Z., Zhong, G., & Lin, J. (2019). A nanodrug consisting of doxorubicin and exosome derived from mesenchymal stem cells for osteosarcoma treatment *in vitro*. *Int. J. of Nanomed*. 14: 8603–8610.

Xia, Y., He, X. T., Xu, X. Y., Tian, B. M., An, Y., & Chen, F. M. (2020). Exosomes derived from M0, M1 and M2 macrophages exert distinct influences on the proliferation and differentiation of mesenchymal stem cells. *PeerJ*. 8: e8970.

Xie, X., Xiong, Y., Panayi, A. C., Hu, L., Zhou, W., Xue, H., Lin, Z., Chen, L., Yan, C., Mi, B., & Liu, G. (2020). Exosomes as a novel approach to reverse osteoporosis: A review of the literature. *Front. Bioeng. Biotech*. 8: 594247.

Xing, X., Han, S., Li, Z., & Li, Z. (2020). Emerging role of exosomes in craniofacial and dental applications. *Theranostics*. 10: 8648.

Xiong, Y., Chen, L., Yan, C., Zhou, W., Yu, T., Sun, Y., Cao, F., Xue, H., Hu, Y., Chen, D., & Mi, B. (2020). M2 Macrophagy-derived exosomal miRNA-5106 induces bone mesenchymal stem cells towards osteoblastic fate by targeting salt-inducible kinase 2 and 3. *J. Nanobiotechnology*. 18: 1–16.

Xu, J. F., Wang, Y. P., Zhang, S. J., Chen, Y., Gu, H. F., Dou, X. F., Xia, B., Bi, Q., & Fan, S. W. (2017). Exosomes containing differential expression of microRNA and mRNA in osteosarcoma that can predict response to chemotherapy. *Oncotarget*. 8: 75968.

Xu, R., Shen, X., Si, Y., Fu, Y. U., Zhu, W., Xiao, T., Fu, Z., Zhang, P., Cheng, J., & Jiang, H. (2018). Micro RNA-31a-5p from aging BMSC s links bone formation and resorption in the aged bone marrow microenvironment. *Aging Cell*. 17: e12794.

Xu, T., Luo, Y., Wang, J., Zhang, N., Gu, C., Li, L., Qian, D., Cai, W., Fan, J., & Yin, G. (2020). Exosomal miRNA-128–3p from mesenchymal stem cells of aged rats regulates osteogenesis and bone fracture healing by targeting Smad5. *J. Nanobiotechnology*. 18: 1–18.

Yang, L., Huang, X., Guo, H., Wang, L., Yang, W., Wu, W., Jing, D., & Shao, Z. (2021a). Exosomes as efficient nanocarriers in osteosarcoma: Biological functions and potential clinical applications. *Front. Cell Dev. Biol*. 9: 737314.

Yang, R., Xu, W., Zheng, H., Zheng, X., Li, B., Jiang, L., & Jiang, S. (2021b). Exosomes derived from vascular endothelial cells antagonize glucocorticoid-induced osteoporosis by inhibiting ferritinophagy with resultant limited ferroptosis of osteoblasts. *J. Cell. Physiol*. 236: 6691–6705.

Yang, X., Shi, G., Guo, J., Wang, C., & He, Y. (2018). Exosome-encapsulated antibiotic against intracellular infections of methicillin-resistant Staphylococcus aureus. *Int. J. Nanomed*. 13: 8095.

Ye, Z., Zheng, Z., & Peng, L. (2020). MicroRNA profiling of serum exosomes in patients with osteosarcoma by high-throughput sequencing. *J. Invest. Med.* 68: 893–901.
Yoshida, A., Fujiwara, T., Uotani, K., Morita, T., Kiyono, M., Yokoo, S., Hasei, J., Nakata, E., Kunisada, T., & Ozaki, T. (2018). Clinical and functional significance of intracellular and extracellular microRNA-25–3p in osteosarcoma. *Acta Med. Okayama.* 72: 165–174.
Yu, B., Zhang, X., & Li, X. (2014). Exosomes derived from mesenchymal stem cells. *Int. J. Mol. Sci.* 15: 4142.
Yun, B., Maburutse, B. E., Kang, M., Park, M. R., Park, D. J., Kim, Y., & Oh, S. (2020). Dietary bovine milk—derived exosomes improve bone health in an osteoporosis-induced mouse model. *J. Dairy Sci.* 103: 7752–7760.
Zakeri, Z., Salmaninejad, A., Hosseini, N., Shahbakhsh, Y., Fadaee, E., Shahrzad, M. K., & Fadaei, S. (2019). MicroRNA and exosome: Key players in rheumatoid arthritis. *J. Cell. Biochem.* 120: 10930–10944.
Zhai, M., Zhu, Y., Yang, M., & Mao, C. (2020). Human mesenchymal stem cell derived exosomes enhance cell-free bone regeneration by altering their miRNAs profiles. *Adv. Sci.* 7: 2001334.
Zhang, H., Wang, J., Ren, T., Huang, Y., Liang, X., Yu, Y., Wang, W., Niu, J., & Guo, W. (2020a). Bone marrow mesenchymal stem cell-derived exosomal miR-206 inhibits osteosarcoma progression by targeting TRA2B. *Cancer Letters.* 490: 54–65.
Zhang, K., Dong, C., Chen, M., Yang, T., Wang, X., Gao, Y., Wang, L., Wen, Y., Chen, G., Wang, X., & Yu, X. (2020b). Extracellular vesicle-mediated delivery of miR-101 inhibits lung metastasis in osteosarcoma. *Theranostics.* 10: 411.
Zhang, L., Wang, Q., Su, H., & Cheng, J. (2021b). Exosomes from adipose derived mesenchymal stem cells alleviate diabetic osteoporosis in rats through suppressing NLRP3 inflammasome activation in osteoclasts. *J. Biosci. Bioeng.* 131: 671–678.
Zhang, L., Zhang, P., Sun, X., Zhou, L., & Zhao, J. (2018). Long non-coding RNA DANCR regulates proliferation and apoptosis of chondrocytes in osteoarthritis via miR-216a-5p-JAK2-STAT3 axis. *Biosci. Rep.* 38: BSR20181228.
Zhang, X. B., Hsueh, M. F., Huebner, J. L., & Kraus, V. B. (2021d). TNF-α carried by plasma extracellular vesicles predicts knee osteoarthritis progression. *Front. Immunol.* 12: 758386.
Zhang, X. B., Zhang, R. H., Su, X., Qi, J., Hu, Y. C., Shi, J. T., Zhang, K., Wang, K. P., & Zhou, H. Y. (2021c). Exosomes in osteosarcoma research and preclinical practice. *Am. J. Transl. Res.* 13: 882.
Zhang, Y., Cao, X., Li, P., Fan, Y., Zhang, L., Ma, X., Sun, R., Liu, Y., & Li, W. (2021a). microRNA-935-modified bone marrow mesenchymal stem cells-derived exosomes enhance osteoblast proliferation and differentiation in osteoporotic rats. *Life Sci.* 272: 119204.
Zhang, Z., Shuai, Y., Zhou, F., Yin, J., Hu, J., Guo, S., Wang, Y., & Liu, W. (2020c). PDLSCs regulate angiogenesis of periodontal ligaments via VEGF transferred by exosomes in periodontitis. *Int. J. Med. Sci.* 17: 558.
Zhao, Y., & Xu, J. (2018). Synovial fluid-derived exosomal lncRNA PCGEM1 as biomarker for the different stages of osteoarthritis. *Int. Orthop.* 42: 2865–2872.
Zheng, J., Zhu, L., In, I. I., Chen, Y., Jia, N., & Zhu, W. (2020). Bone marrow-derived mesenchymal stem cells-secreted exosomal microRNA-192–5p delays inflammatory response in rheumatoid arthritis. *Int. Immunopharmacol.* 78: 105985.
Zhi, F., Ding, Y., Wang, R., Yang, Y., Luo, K., & Hua, F. (2021). Exosomal hsa_circ_0006859 is a potential biomarker for postmenopausal osteoporosis and enhances adipogenic versus osteogenic differentiation in human bone marrow mesenchymal stem cells by sponging miR-431–5p. *Stem Cell Res. Ther.* 12: 1–15.
Zhou, J., Dai, Y., Lin, Y., & Chen, K. (2022). Association between serum amyloid A and rheumatoid arthritis: A systematic review and meta-analysis. *Semin. Arthritis Rheumatol.* 52: 151943.
Zhu, M., Liu, Y., Qin, H., Tong, S., Sun, Q., Wang, T., Zhang, H., Cui, M., & Guo, S. (2021). Osteogenically-induced exosomes stimulate osteogenesis of human adipose-derived stem cells. *Cell Tissue Bank.* 22: 77–91.
Zhu, W., Guo, M., Yang, W., Tang, M., Chen, T., Gan, D., Zhang, D., Ding, X., Zhao, A., Zhao, P., & Yan, W. (2020). CD41-deficient exosomes from non-traumatic femoral head necrosis tissues impair osteogenic differentiation and migration of mesenchymal stem cells. *Cell Death Dis.* 11: 293.
Zuo, R., Liu, M., Wang, Y., Li, J., Wang, W., Wu, J., Sun, C., Li, B., Wang, Z., Lan, W., Zhang, C., & Lan, W. (2019). BM-MSC-derived exosomes alleviate radiation-induced bone loss by restoring the function of recipient BM-MSCs and activating Wnt/β-catenin signaling. *Stem Cell Res. Ther.* 10: 1–13.

17 Clinically Relevant Bone Diseases and Bone Fracture Animal Models

Irfan Qayoom, Ekta Srivastava, and Ashok Kumar

17.1 INTRODUCTION

Bone diseases and bone fractures are a significant health concern, affecting millions of people worldwide. There are many different types of bone diseases and fractures, each with their own unique causes, symptoms, and treatment options. Some of the most clinically relevant bone diseases include osteoporosis, osteoarthritis, and rheumatoid arthritis. These conditions can result in decreased bone strength and increased risk of fractures.

Animal models are widely used to study bone diseases and fractures. These models can help researchers understand the underlying mechanisms of these conditions and develop new treatment options. Some of the most commonly used animal models include rodents, such as mice and rats, and larger animals, such as pigs and nonhuman primates (Table 17.1) (Anesi et al., 2020).

Considering the central role of animal models in the study of bone healing, the European Commission devised three Rs rules as fundamental when using animals for experimental purposes:

- Reduction: lowest number possible to achieve scientific evidence
- Refinement: minimal animal suffering
- Replacement: prefer non-animal-based studies

Moreover, in designing animal studies, the specific animal model needs to be selected considering the requirements like the anatomical bone location (femur, tibia, cranium, vertebrae, etc.), size, biomechanical features, densities, and turnover and the specific conditions for bone healing (bone infections, bone cancer, or fractures). Apart from the type of animal models used to study the efficacy of new therapeutic molecules, implants, or tissue-engineered constructs, another challenge is the identical replication of diseases and fractures. An array of different models across the species have been developed to generate clinically relevant bone disease and fracture models. This chapter provides a brief overview of different bone disease models that are commonly used to study the therapeutic potential of new molecules, materials, and implants in bone pathologies.

17.2 CRITICAL-SIZED BONE DEFECT MODELS

Critical-size defects are defects that lack the capacity to regenerate spontaneously. In one experiment, they showed not more than 10% regeneration at the defect sites (Lindsey et al., 2006). Any standard definition is further complicated due to variability in experimental species selected, target bone due to intrinsic regenerative variations, age of experimental species, and technical variations like residual periosteum at defect site (Liebschner, 2004). The four major defect types targeted are calvarial, long bone or segmental, partial cortical, and cancellous bone (Figure 17.1).

DOI: 10.1201/9781003307310-20

TABLE 17.1
Most Common Animal Models for Studying Bone Diseases

Animal	Bone Microscopic and Macroscopic Features	Bone Composition and Remodelling	Animal Management	Best Type of Study
Rodents	Mainly primary bone in long bone cortices and minimal cancellous bone. Cortices are thin and fragile.	Limited cortical remodeling and non-Haversian remodelling. Limited secondary osteon formation. Higher bone healing capacity in craniofacial bones.	Cheap and easily manageable. Rats are more docile and social than mice, although the latter are cheaper to house and maintain.	Osteoinduction. Cartilage regeneration potential. Bone infection. Extraoral surgical approaches.
Rabbit	Cortices are fragile, and there is less cancellous bone than in humans. Quick achievement of skeletal maturity. Small size. Lack of biomechanical data. Dense Haversian bone.	Similar bone density to human. Bone metabolism is similar to human, with Haversian-type remodelling, although at a higher rate than humans.	Availability, housing, and handling are easy. Cage confinement might worsen their bone healing capability.	Musculoskeletal research. Bone implants. Modelling of vertebral fracture repair. Extraoral surgical approaches.
Sheep	High trabecular bone density. Good body weight. Different bone microstructure than humans. Big difference between young and mature sheep due to age-dependent changes in bone structure.	Similar bone healing capacity to humans. Different remodelling processes.	Although docile, their size requires a lot of space.	Orthopaedic research. Bone filler materials in cranial osteotomies. Extraoral surgical approaches.
Goats	Good size. Presence of Haversian systems in the tibia, except for the caudal part.	Similar bone healing potential. Similar bone composition.	Docile and tolerant to environmental conditions. A lot of space is needed.	Bone filler materials in cranial osteotomies. Extraoral surgical approaches. Cartilage, ligaments and menisci regeneration.
Pig	Plexiform bone that shifts to dense secondary osteonal bone. Good development of the Haversian system, with medium canals. Similar to humans.	Similar bone density and bone mineral concentration to humans. Similar bone remodelling.	High body weight and aggressive nature.	Extra- and intraoral approaches. Osteonecrosis surgery. Osteogenic regeneration materials in craniofacial bones. Dental implants.
Dog	Similar cancellous bone to humans. Presence of secondary osteons with small canals. Thinner articular cartilage.	Variability of trabecular bone remodelling depending on site, age and species.	Docile, easy handling. Good size.	Dental implants and peri-implantitis.
Nonhuman primates	Close to humans.	Comparable with humans.	Difficult to handle, and highly trained staff are needed.	Bone implant.

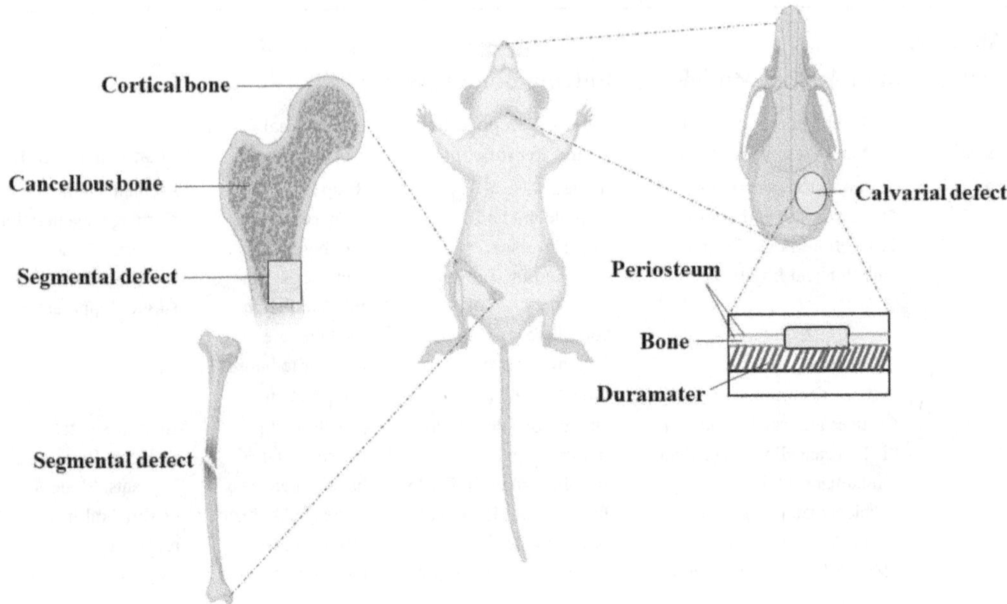

FIGURE 17.1 Major anatomical sites including long bones (femur and tibia) or flat bones (cranium) where critical-sized bone defects are created in animal models to evaluate the efficacy of new therapeutics, biomaterials, and implants to promote bone regeneration.

The defect type must rationalize the objective of the study, possess physiological and pathological analogies to humans, and simulate clinical conditions. Different species are utilized ranging from rodents to large animals like sheep and goat depending upon facilities like easy acquisition, care, and management. The number of implants and duration of experiment should be taken into consideration while selecting appropriate animal models.

17.2.1 Calvarial Defect

The procedure initiates with sagittal incision across the scalp, followed with exposure of calvarial bone. A circular bone defect is created covering the depth of bone entirely, covered with periosteum keeping the dura mater intact (Nakamura et al., 2017). Researchers prefer the model due to standardized reproducibility and lack of any stabilization. The major limitation of the model is lack of physiological mechanical loading at the defect site (Gomes & Fernandes, 2011). Kumar and coworkers demonstrated enhanced bone mineralization and new bone formation in critical-sized calvarial defects in rats and rabbits using functionalized nanohydroxyapatite bioactive ceramic carriers (Teotia et al., 2017, 2019, 2020). Various different studies have been carried out to demonstrate the efficacy of new biomaterials in augmenting bone regeneration using critical-sized calvarial bone defect models across the species (Ji et al., 2017).

17.2.2 Long Bone or Segmental Defect

This type of defect is created by osteotomy, involving the use of a saw or drill to remove the desired segment in long bones. The size of the defect is an important factor to consider. Although standardization of critical-size defect is still warranted and awaited, segmental defect 2–2.5 times the diameter of the long bone's shaft is considered critical size (Lindsey et al., 2006). These defects depend not only on size but also on bone structure, defect location, mechanical loading at defect site, fixation hardware used to stabilize the bone, etc. (Galtt & Mattys, 2014).

The most common sites for creating long bone defects are proximal tibia, femoral neck, and metatarsus (Christou et al., 2014.). Distal femur becomes an important site for implantation after total knee replacement. One such model developed in rabbits is steroid-associated osteonecrosis. Several studies report rabbit as an appropriate animal model, reporting its similar bone mineral density and toughness to that in humans, in addition to its easy handling and housing, although its small size limits their application (Wang et al., 1998). Our group has been working in orthopaedics extensively, and we have generated metaphyseal tibia critical-sized bone defect models in rodents to evaluate the efficacy of different functionalized biomaterials in enhancing bone regeneration and bone healing (Gupta et al., 2021; Raina et al., 2019; Teotia et al., 2016; Teotia et al., 2018). The major limitation of critical-size defect models is the lack of consensus on what constitutes a critical size, making comparison among different studies less calculated. To create a nonunion osteotomy model of critical-sized bone defect in long bones, attempts have been made to maximize fracture healing with the least traumatic side effects.

Typical osteotomy includes a diaphyseal fracture model involving drilling a hole using a small-diameter drill bit or transverse or oblique transections of bone, followed by removal of bone segment. The stabilization of bone is assured with Kirschner wire (K-wire), which is inserted into the medullary canal of the femur in an anterograde fashion, which functions as intramedullary nailing subsequent to creation of segmental defect. Each procedure had limitations like faster healing due to small defect size or difficulty in stabilization with intramedullary K-wire fixation (Russell et al., 2009).

At times, the in-stabilization at the defect site led to pseudoarthrosis formation. Another technique overcoming these limitations is plate fixation, leading to more rigid stabilization preventing micromotion at the osteotomy site. The surgical procedure involves longitudinal incision over lateral femur, followed by careful removal of muscles. The plate is applied to the lateral femoral shaft and secured with stainless steel screws. Reciprocating saw is used to remove a segment of bone, followed by muscles and skin closure (Stewart, 2019). Several modifications have been made to these osteotomy animal models to recapitulate fracture-related infection, osteomyelitis, or osteosarcoma, leading to debridement of a chunk of bone and stabilization (Helbig et al., 2020).

17.3 OSTEOPOROSIS AND OSTEOPOROTIC FRAGILITY FRACTURE MODELS

Osteoporosis is an old-age disease characterized by continuous loss of bone mass and deterioration of bone microarchitecture that weakens the bone and makes them susceptible to fractures. At the cellular level, it is mostly the imbalance in the bone remodelling where there is increased bone resorption; however, the detailed mechanism leading to such cellular events is not fully understood. Moreover, the fractures associated with osteoporosis are so complicated that even after surgical interventions using implants, it is difficult to achieve full success; implants usually fail owing to weak bone structure, leading to secondary osteoporotic fractures.

The research has primarily focussed on understanding bone behaviour in osteoporosis, assessing the efficacy of potent new therapies in osteoporosis and related fractures, and developing new approaches and therapies to augment osteoporotic fragility fractures and at the same time enhance the biomechanical strength of nascent bone at fracture sites. Different animal models have been used to study the pathogenesis of osteoporosis and the efficiency of new therapies in osteoporotic fracture repair. Here we discuss some of the most common surgical procedures for generating osteoporosis and osteoporotic fragility fractures.

17.3.1 OVARIECTOMY

Ovariectomy is one of the safe and simple methods to generate osteoporosis and is most commonly performed in rats (Van Der Jagt et al., 2014). In ovariectomy-induced osteoporosis models, it is the trabecular bone of lumbar vertebrae which show early signs of osteoporosis as measured by reduction in bone mineral density (BMD), T-score, and Z-score. In long bones like the metaphysis of the tibia and the proximal femur, it usually takes six to nine months to show the signs of osteoporosis. In cortical bones, the remodelling and onset of osteoporosis start three months later than in trabecular bones; ovariectomy accompanied with low calcium diet doesn't show marked differences in the time of onset of osteoporosis (Kubo et al., 1999).

17.3.2 Aged Animals

Type 2 osteoporosis is the most common model developed in aged animals which usually after one year in rats and nine years in sheep (Savaridas et al., 2015). The most common animals used to generate osteoporosis by aging are mice due to their short lifespans. However, the cost of maintenance and housing of large animals for longer periods is very high along with variability in ageing between the animals (Perkins et al., 1994).

17.3.3 Accelerated Ageing Strains

Accelerated aging strains are a specialized mice strain called as senescence accelerated mouse (SAM) which have a short lifespan of six to eight months (Okamoto et al., 1995). The SAM prone-6 strains have osteoporotic conditions similar to senile osteoporosis in humans like low adult BMD, insufficient osteoblasts, and developing of spontaneous fractures in old age (D'Ippolito et al., 1999; Melton et al., 2005). The impaired bone formation in these strains is attributed to the downregulation/suppression of the Wnt signalling pathway (Syed & Hoey, 2010). However, the value of SAM-based osteoporotic models remains controversial owing to their complex genetic background.

17.3.4 Osteoporotic Fragility Fracture Models

Osteoporotic fragility fractures occur without any severe trauma, such as from falls from a standing height or less due to the fragile bones. There are no satisfactory treatment strategies for osteoporotic fragility fractures, and around 20% mortality has been observed in the first years after fracture due to long-term hospitalizations (Lane, 2006). The conventional use of prosthetic implants in osteoporotic fracture fixation shows failures due to the limited osteointegration and implant failures (Barrios et al., 1993). This makes it necessary to develop human replicas of osteoporotic fragility fracture models to evaluate the efficacy of new treatment approaches.

Hip fractures are the most common osteoporotic fragility fractures which occur due to fall from a height and are a common site of implant failures. An osteoporotic hip fracture model has been generated in hips of osteoporotic rats that mimics hip fracture in humans (Qayoom et al., 2020a; Raina et al., 2020; Širka et al., 2018). The model was generated by creating a defect 1 mm diameter and 8 mm long in the femoral neck canal of osteoporotic rats from the greater trochanter towards the femur head. The defect was further impacted with functionalized bone substitutes (bone morphogenetic protein and zoledronic acid), and after four months, there was enhanced defect filling and trabecular bone formation with optimum trabecular parameters at the defect site. However, no differences across the groups were observed in the biomechanical strength of the bones after two (Širka et al., 2018), four (Qayoom et al., 2020a), and six (Raina et al., 2020) months. This shows that the time for the osteoporosis to develop in models needs to be optimized such that the cortical bone is also affected, which has been shown to contribute maximally towards the mechanical strength of the long bones (Figure 17.2).

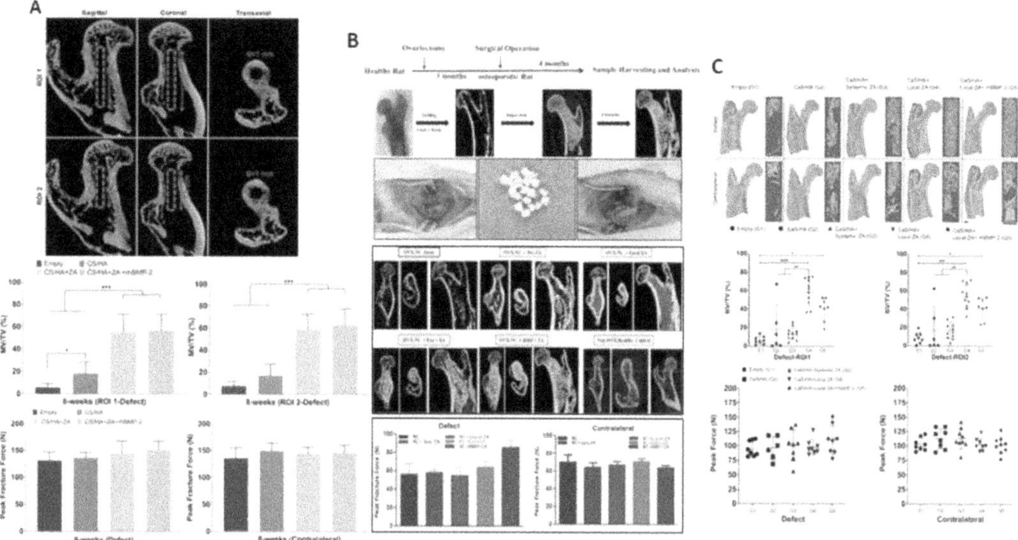

FIGURE 17.2 Evaluation of trabecular bone regeneration and mechanical strength in rat osteoporotic hip fracture model at (A) two months (reproduced under the terms of CC-BY 4.0 (https://creativecommons.org/licenses/by/4.0/) International License from Širka, A., Raina, D. B., Isaksson, H., Tanner, K. E., Smailys, E., Kumar, A., Tarasevičius, S., Tägil, M., & Lidgren, L.: Calcium Sulphate/Hydroxyapatite Carrier for Bone Formation in the Femoral Neck of Osteoporotic Rats. Tissue Eng. Part A. 2018. 24. 23–24. Copyright 2018 Širka et al., published by Mary Ann Liebert, Inc.); (B) four months (reproduced with permission from Qayoom, I., Teotia, A., K., & Kumar, A.: Nanohydroxyapatite Based Ceramic Carrier Promotes Bone Formation in a Femoral Neck Canal Defect in Osteoporotic Rats. ACS Biomacromolecules. 2020a. 2. 328–337. Copyright 2020 American Chemical Society); and (C) six months (reproduced under the terms of CC-BY 4.0 (https://creativecommons.org/licenses/by/4.0/) International License from Raina, D. B., Širka, A., Qayoom, I., Teotia, A. K., Liu, Y., Tarasevicius, S., Tanner, K. E., Isaksson, H., Kumar, A., Tägil, M., & Lidgren, L.: Long-Term Response to a Bioactive Biphasic Biomaterial in the Femoral Neck of Osteoporotic Rats. Tissue Eng., Part A. 2020. 26. 19–20. Copyright 2020 Raina et al., published by Mary Ann Liebert, Inc.).

17.4 INFECTION TREATMENT-INDUCED FRACTURE MODELS

Bone infections, also known as osteomyelitis, are characterized by progressive inflammation caused by infectious microorganism, often bacteria and most commonly Gram-positive *Staphylococcus aureus* (Kavanagh et al., 2018). The infection spreads to other bones via one of three routes: hematogenous, contiguous, and direct inoculation due to peripheral vascular insufficiency. There are also three main aetiologies of osteomyelitis: hematogenous, traumatic, and vascular disease associated as in diabetic foot ulcers (Fritz & McDonald, 2008).

The current treatment approaches involve antimicrobial therapy with antibiotics and/or surgical intervention (Hatzenbuehler & Pulling, 2011). These procedures pose specific risks such as systemic toxicity, antimicrobial drug resistance with prolonged use of antibiotics, and morbidity of target tissue due to surgical debridement. The past decade has witnessed a surge in osteomyelitis cases due to increase in trauma, diabetes, reconstructive surgeries involving prosthetics, and improvement in diagnostic methods (Tran et al., 2013). One of the major hallmarks of osteomyelitis is necrotic bone complemented with conundrum biofilm niche. Biofilms are characterized with a protective slime layer acting as a barrier between immune cells and bacteria, leading to the creation of metabolically or phenotypically resistant bacterial "persisters" (Urish & Cassat, 2020).

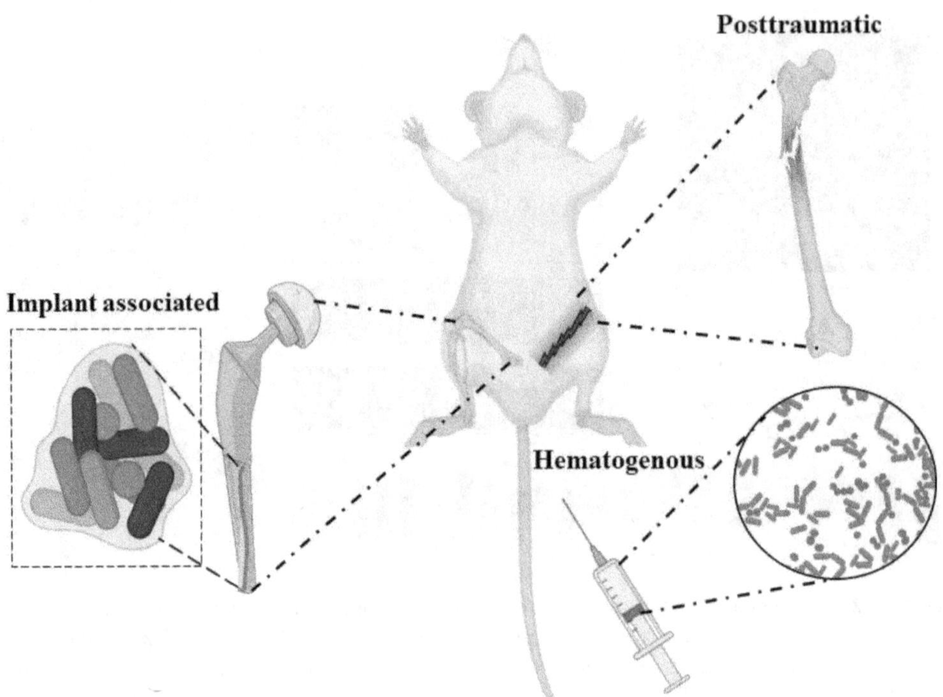

FIGURE 17.3 Commonly used approaches to develop osteomyelitis models in animals including implant-associated osteomyelitis, hematogenous osteomyelitis, and post-traumatic osteomyelitis. Implant-associated infection model is developed by inoculation bacteria along with the implantation of prosthesis. In hematogenous infection models, the bacterial inoculum is injected in the tail vein of the animal model so that it mimics the spread of infection to the bone through blood stream. Trauma-based infection models mimic the inoculation of bacteria in the bone during trauma and fractures.

These outcomes have prompted the usage of various animals like rats, mice, rabbits, avians, dogs, sheep, goats, and pigs to model osteomyelitis to develop improved diagnostic methods and novel therapeutic approaches and refine current treatment approaches (Moreau, 2017). The major steps towards generating a successful model involve inducing mechanical trauma leading to bone injury followed by bacterial colonization through direct inoculation or medical device. There are different routes to administer bacteria at the injured site: directly via bacterial inoculation, foreign hardware with bacterial suspension or biofilm, and/or direct intravenous injection (hematogenous seeding) (Figure 17.3) (Wang et al., 2017). The three major steps towards creation of a successful model are histopathological evidence of osteomyelitis, clinical manifestation of disease, and positive bone cultures (Chadha et al., 1999).

17.4.1 Small Animal Model System

One of the common surgical methods for developing osteomyelitis in small animals involves medial parapatellar arthrotomy to gain access to the femur followed by insertion of K-wire in the medullary cavity and bacterial inoculation into the cavity and closing of wounds (Bernthal et al., 2010). Another widely described model does not involve a longitudinal defect in the medullary canal; the medulla is accessed by drilling a small hole in the bone, followed by direct inoculation and sealing of surgical site (Funao et al., 2012). Long bone models mostly utilize mechanical trauma, placement of foreign bodies, or creation of fractures with sealing to localise infection and prevent soft tissue infection.

Several studies also report the development of acute and chronic hematogenous osteomyelitis by lateral tail vein injection of a single dose of *S. aureus* without any surgical intervention (Horst et al., 2012). These models also provide insight into the pathogenesis of *S. aureus* with utilization of advanced microscopy like transmission electron microscopy to detect the microorganisms residing inside the osteocyte lacuno-canalicular network (de Mesy Bentley et al., 2017). These models have led to the development of different virulence factors associated with biofilm and to deciphering the role of bacteria as intracellular pathogens.

Another interesting study provides insight into implant microstructure as an evasion method for bacteria as bacteria were present within allograft cortical Haversian canal and canaliculi of mouse femur. Such models are being utilized to examine different combinations of antibiotics effective against osteomyelitis (Zoller et al., 2020). In our study, we utilized macroporous gelatin cryogel as a carrier of bacteria to develop an osteomyelitis model in rat tibia (Qayoom et al., 2022).

The defined colony-forming units of *S. aureus* were loaded onto the gelatine cryogel, which was then semi-dried in the laminar hood followed by implantation in a 1 mm hole created in the metaphyseal part of the tibia. The infection was allowed to develop for three weeks with continuous monitoring of systemic inflammation. After the bone lesions and soft tissue inflammation was observed, the infected site was debrided, and soft/hard necrotic tissues were removed followed by implantation. The model was used to evaluate the efficacy of the adjuvant therapy of antibiotic-loaded nanocement to clear the infection and at the same time augment bone regeneration at the debrided site (Figure 17.4) (Qayoom et al., 2020b, 2020c).

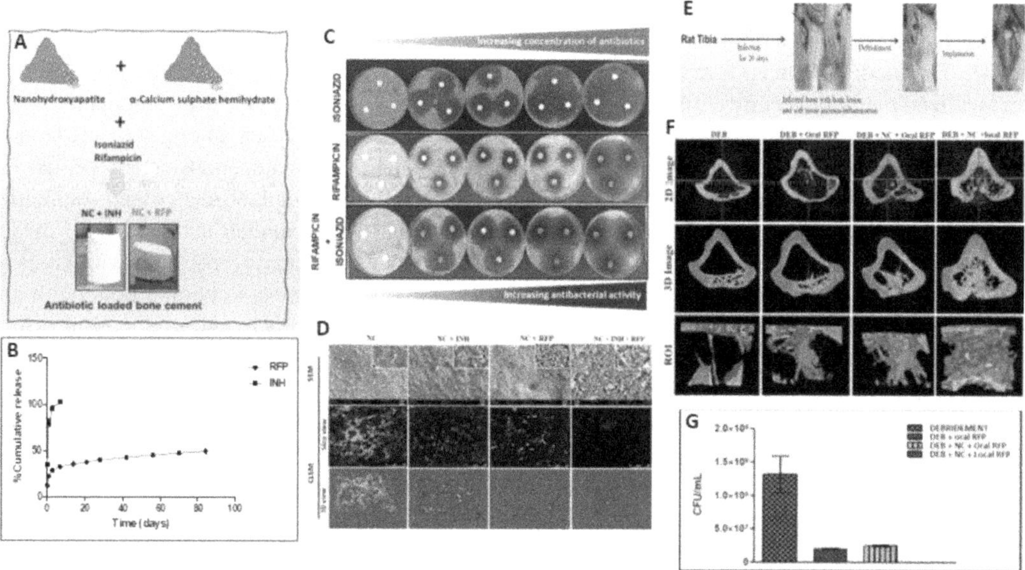

FIGURE 17.4 (A) Fabrication of antibiotic-loaded nanocement using isoniazid (INH) and rifampicin (RFP). (B) In vitro release kinetics of RFP and INH from nanocement showing sustained release of RFP and burst release of INH. (C) & (D) In vitro antibacterial activity and antibiofilm activity of antibiotic-loaded nanocement with mycobacterium smegmatis. (E) Development of osteomyelitis in rat tibia using staphylococcus aureus and implantation of RFP-loaded nanocement at the debrided site (reproduced under the terms of CC-BY 4.0 (https://creativecommons.org/licenses/by/4.0/) International License from Qayoom, I., Verma, R., Murugan, P. A., Raina, D. B., Teotia, A. K., Matheshwaran, S., Nair, N. N., Tägil, M., Lidgren, L., & Kumar, A.: A biphasic nanohydroxyapatite/calcium sulphate carrier containing Rifampicin and Isoniazid for local delivery gives sustained and effective antibiotic release and prevents biofilm formation. Sci. Rep. 2020c. 10. 1–14. Copyright 2020 Qayoom et al., published by Nature Publishing Group). (F) Micro-CT analysis of the debrided site post-sacrifice showing enhanced bone mineralization in local delivery groups when compared with other groups. (G) Complete eradiation of bacterial burden in soft tissues at the infected site after implantation of RFP-loaded nanocement (reproduced with permission from Qayoom, I., Teotia, A. K., Panjla, A., Verma, S., & Kumar, A.: Local and sustained delivery of rifampicin from a bioactive ceramic carrier treats bone infection in rat tibia. ACS Infect. Dis. 2020b. 6. 2938–2949. Copyright 2020 American Chemical Society).

We also developed an osteomyelitis model in distal femur of rats as this part of femur has the highest vasculature and is prone to hematogenous dissemination-based infections (Qayoom et al., 2022). We used this model to evaluate the efficacy of antibiotic-loaded composite cryogel synthesized from nanohydroxyapatite and collagen to prevent the development of infection and also promote bone healing at the fracture site. This model describes a new treatment approach that could be utilized to preclude the development of infection and simultaneously promote bone healing at the fracture site.

The major attractions to using a rat model are small size and ease of genetic and molecular tailoring, facilitating a wide array of investigations, but lacunae arise with multistage surgical procedures owing to their different bone structure, size, and remodelling procedures than with humans. These limitations can be addressed in animals like rabbits as revision surgeries and chronic osteomyelitis can be well established, and full segmental defects in radius can be achieved without stabilization. A few limitations with rabbit include respiratory depression complicating surgical procedures and hindgut fermentation impacting oral antibiotic therapies. Most of these surgeries must be performed in mature rabbits to maximize therapeutic efficacy for clinical translation.

17.4.2 Large Animal Models System

Pigs, sheep, goats, and dogs are utilized to develop animal models for osteomyelitis. The most widely utilized porcine model is hematogenous osteomyelitis, developed with intravenous administration of inoculum of *S. aureus* into lateral ear vein of pigs without additional trauma (Jensen et al., 2010). The model has been further modified by injecting the inoculum into femoral artery leading to localized femoral osteomyelitis (Nielsen et al., 2015). The technique is at times complicated with soft tissue infection, injection site abscess with variable degree of diseases among subjects (Jødal et al., 2019). However, this still is a strong technique for modelling hematogenous osteomyelitis.

Other alternative models are mandibular osteomyelitis and tibial implant-related and traumatic tibial osteomyelitis (Hill & Watkins, 2001). Studies based on porcine models successfully provide insights into the pharmacokinetics of drugs, diagnostic work, and bone regeneration with combinatorial antibiotic therapy. Porcine bone possesses similar fracture stress to human bone with an optimal gastrointestinal tract for oral antibiotic administration, conferring many benefits (Bue et al., 2018). Still, extensive usage is limited by their rapid growth, excessive mature body weight, greater expense, and shorter long bones (Jensen et al., 2017).

Initial surgery procedures to develop an ovine osteomyelitis model involved creating a tibial or femur defect and subsequent bacterial inoculum injection in the medullary cavity of adult sheep or through hardware infected with biofilm or planktonic bacteria (Moriarty et al., 2017). The defects can be unicortical followed with medullary canal inoculation or osteotomies stabilized with infected hardware. Most of these models are utilized to perform multistage revision surgeries as witnessed in clinical settings, administer local antibiotic therapies via injectable hydrogels or titanium plates, and/or implanting orthopaedic hardware; human and ovine bone possess similar torsional stiffness and osteogenesis (Boot et al., 2021). The drawbacks are the risk of sepsis during modelling requiring perioperative antibiotics and the housing and maintenance requirements associated with large animals (Roux et al., 2021).

Caprine models mostly utilize unicortical tibial defects with or without perioperative dose of IV antibiotics, without any report of sepsis (Salgado et al., 2005). Another model includes tibial osteotomy with internal fixation or percutaneous pin placement through tibia. Some interesting studies have used tobramycin-loaded calcium sulphate pellets or applied electrical stimulation to treat osteomyelitis (Tran et al., 2013). Another widely used model is goat, with major advantage of similar composition and size of long bones ideal for multistage surgeries with no record of sepsis, in contrast with sheep (Billings & Anderson, 2022). These models require more exploration in terms of pathogenesis and diagnostic investigations; most researchers utilize them to either develop models or examine treatment options.

Another interesting model was developed using canine to examine the role of VEGF as a rate-limiting step in wound healing. Tibial fracture model of canine osteomyelitis was developed and covered with rotational muscular flap to assess the role of vascularized tissue at defect site. VEGF mRNA levels were higher in animals with flap; the authors concluded that the surgical closure has significant impact on specific signalling (Khodaparast et al., 2003). Using canine as an animal model raises ethical considerations as these are companion models and osteomyelitis is terminal research (Billings & Anderson, 2022).

17.5 DIABETIC BONE INFECTIONS

Diabetes is a metabolic disorder affecting 463 million people worldwide, with an expected rise in adult prevalence to 10.2% by 2030. It can result from increased insulin resistance in target tissue or decreased insulin secretion, resulting in elevated blood glucose levels. Chronic hyperglycaemia further deteriorates the functioning of vital organs like cardiovascular system, kidneys, and blood vessels. Increasing evidence demonstrates the detrimental effect of diabetes on the skeletal system, leading to impaired bone healing, increased risk of fracture, and loss of bone strength, significantly affecting bone quality (Marin et al., 2018).

Different events like inflammation and oxidative stress impede the distribution of oxygen, nutrients, and osteoprogenitor cells to damage sites. Several researchers have identified altered differentiation fates for osteoprogenitor cells to adipose lineage, leading to more fat deposits at the fractured callus. Chronic hyperglycaemia further increases advanced glycation end products, which upon interaction with cell surface receptors leads to increase in nonenzymatic crosslinking in collagen, resulting in decreased stiffness in bone matrix.

Another serious complication associated with diabetes is postoperative orthopaedic infections (Chen et al., 2022). The difficulty fighting infections in a diabetic patient mainly comes from increased adherence of microorganisms to cells, defective innate immune response, and underlying diabetic complications like neuropathy and vasculopathy. Researchers developed an implant-related *S. aureus* infection model in nonobese diabetic mouse and compared the host response with identically infected CD 1 mice; the group found differences in susceptibility to infections due to diabetes based on bacterial load, biofilm formation, and body weight as measured with clinical, microbiological, and histological techniques (Lovati et al., 2013).

Several studies report the adverse effect of diabetes on fracture healing, reporting three- to four-fold higher risk of complications including delayed union, nonunion, redislocation, or pseudoarthrosis. In a study including spontaneously diabetic animals, defective healing of fracture with lowered bone apposition and mineralization was reported. Insulin imbalance leads to reduced osteoblast differentiation, increased osteoclast activity, and altered apoptosis of chondrocytes, disturbing the remodelling of osseous callus. This ultimately results in prolonged healing of fracture by 87% (Jiao et al., 2015).

17.6 CANCER TREATMENT-INDUCED BONE FRACTURE MODELS

Bone is a common site for cancer metastasis, with markedly high mortality rates; it causes insidious pain, pathological fractures, and reduced quality of life (Simmons et al., 2015). The steps involved in the pathogenesis of bone metastasis includes a) primary neoplasm proliferation, b) local tissue invasion, c) intravasation into blood, d) extravasation in bone marrow, e) tumour cell dormancy, f) proliferation in bone tissue, and finally g) modification of local bone microenvironment (Fidler, 2003). Bone tumours have been classified as primary bone tumours (sarcomas), which are uncommon contributing only 0.2% of total bone tumours and secondary bone tumours (metastatic) (Jiang et al., 2020).

Understanding molecular mechanisms to develop new therapeutic molecules/drugs to preclude the growth of bone metastasis makes it necessary to develop animal models which are replicas of bone metastatic cancer in humans (Rosol, 2000). Preclinical animal models are important for devising new treatment strategies which can be used to manage the dead space after debridement of bone cancers, for instance, local delivery of anticancer drugs using bioactive carriers' post-debridement as bone fillers in order to augment bone healing in the dead space and kill dormant cells, simultaneously (Dewhurst et al., 2020).

Researchers have developed an array of bone metastasis animal models including cancer models after chemical or genetic induction, xenograft human models, and clinical trials in companion animals with spontaneous cancers. Each of these ways has its own advantages and limitations, and no single bone metastasis model is considered the ideal. It is important to consider the model based on the question under investigation.

Surgical resection of tumours accompanied with radiotherapy and chemotherapy is one of the conventional therapies to treat bone tumours. However, this procedure is usually unsuccessful in eradicating micrometastasis, eventually resulting in recurrence of tumours (Chen & Yao, 2022). Moreover, during surgical resection, a dead space is created at the debrided site which is prone to fractures and is usually filled with autografts or allografts, which have their own associated limitations.

The bone loss during surgical debridement is the main cause of physical disabilities and postoperative fractures. Different types of preclinical animal models have been developed to mimic the clinically used surgical procedure of debridement in bone tumours so as to design biomaterial fillers as carriers for local delivery of anticancer drugs to eradicate the micrometastasis and augment bone healing, simultaneously. Owing to the urgent need to develop new biomaterials for the treatment of osteosarcoma and associated bone loss, an array of different biomaterials has been designed at different times of history as given in Figure 17.5 (Zhang et al., 2022).

Significant literature shows that the xenograft model is successful in developing osteosarcoma in immunocompromised mice due to quick onset, affordable cost, and ease of handling. The cells injected in the immunocompromised animals, like U2-OS, Saos2, HOS, 143B, UMR 106–01, and K7M2, accumulate and form a solid tumour at the local site within days or weeks (Ek et al., 2006). The xenograft model has been used in screening potent drugs owing to the high rate of incidence, reproducibility, and easily quantifiable tumorigenic potential of injected cells with accurate titration.

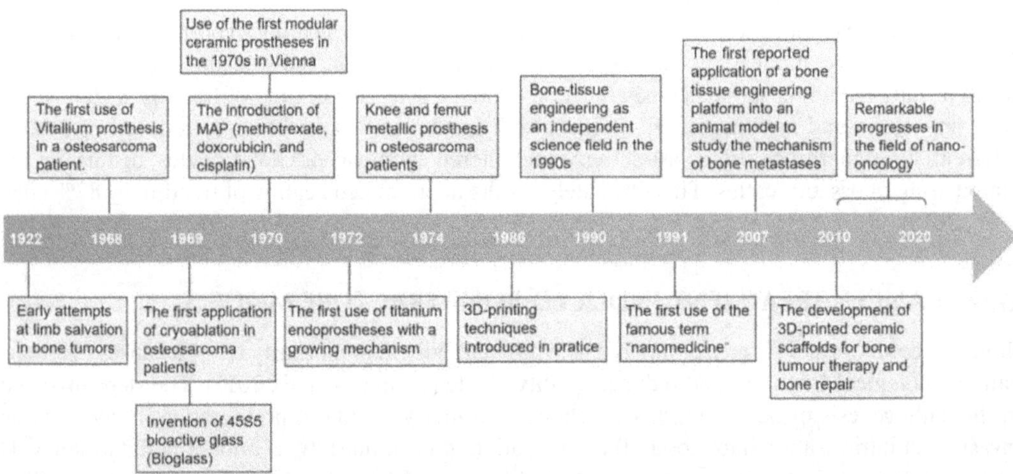

FIGURE 17.5 Timeline of major milestones in the development of materials for bone repair and osteosarcoma treatment (reproduced under the terms of CC-BY 4.0 (https://creativecommons.org/licenses/by/4.0/) International License from Zhang, Y., Wu, Y., Qiao, X., Lin, T., Wang, Y., & Wang, M.: Biomaterial-based strategy for bone tumor therapy and bone defect regeneration: An innovative application option. Front. Mater. 2022. 9. 554. Copyright 2022 Zhang et al., published by Frontiers).

However, xenograft models use fully developed osteosarcoma cell lines and cannot address the contribution of the tumour microenvironment to the tumour behaviours, thus this model is not fit for analyzing the initiation and aetiology of the tumours (Becher & Holland, 2006). Surgical orthotropic implantation was also used to develop a spontaneously metastasizing model of osteosarcoma by transplanting osteosarcoma tissue from a five-year-old girl in nude mice till 32nd passage followed by implantation of intact tumour tissue from xenograft in mice tibia (Crnalic et al., 1997). The surgical orthotropic model is clinically relevant; however, it has several associated limitations like lack of reproducibility, the need for highly technical skills, and the lack of scope for in vitro studies.

17.7 OSTEOCHONDRAL DEFECT MODELS

Osteochondral defects (OCDs) are the leading causes of joint pain, deformity, and dysfunction induced by severe trauma, sports injuries, or physical diseases (Deng et al., 2019). OCDs are also one of the main causes of osteoarthritis (OA). It has been estimated that around 33.6% of women and 24.3% of men with age above 60 years suffer from OA globally (Pereira et al., 2011). Owing to the avascularity, lack of lymphatic vessels, and limited proliferation capacity of chondrocytes, cartilage regeneration poses a major challenge. Moreover, the different healing capacity of cartilage and the subchondral bones, the regeneration of OCDs further increase the complexity of developing novel treatment approaches. This reinforces the significance of optimal animal models for use in studying the healing of critical-sized OCDs. An array of animal models from rats to goats and non-human primates have been used so far to evaluate the efficacy of new drugs and other treatment approaches for the treatment of critical sized OCDs.

17.7.1 Small Animal Models

Small animals provide the flexibility of evaluating proof of concept with ease and using large numbers of animals to induce multiple variations. However, small knee size and thin cartilage limit the use of small animals in replicating human OCD conditions. In case of rodents, rats are clinically more relevant than mice owing to their skeletal maturity around seven months.

The critical size of rat OCD has been defined as 1.4 mm (Katagiri et al., 2017), and the most common OCD in rats is the one with the dimensions of 2 mm diameter and 2 mm depth on the trochlear groove of the femur. The large joints in rabbits with skeletal maturity at nine months provide a suitable model for evaluating the potential of different drugs, biomaterials, or approaches to repairing OCDs (Wang et al., 1998). Rabbit cartilage is relatively thin, with average thicknesses of 0.44 ± 0.08 mm for the trochlear groove and 0.3 ± 0.007 mm for the medial femoral condyle (Rasanen & Messner, 1996). However, the subchondral bone in rabbit trochlea with thickness of 386 ± 160 μm is similar to the human medial femoral condyle with its thickness of 213 ± 116 μm. Both also possess relatively thin bone plates with high porosity and low density in the subchondral bone (Chevrier et al., 2015). In comparison with other species, rabbits have faster skeletal changes and bone turnover (Castañeda et al., 2006). Defects of 3–5 mm diameter and 2–5 mm depth have been developed in rabbit femoral trochlea, medial femoral condyle, and lateral femoral condyle to study the potential of biomaterial in OCD regeneration.

17.7.2 Large Animal Models

The large animal models like goat, sheep, horse, dog and pig provide optimal joint size and clinically relevant joint lesions (Schneider-Wald et al., 2013); however, large animals have more complicated logistics and financial and ethical deliberations. The clinically relevant large animals still have the disadvantages of smaller cartilage volume and thickness than in humans (Frisbie et al., 2006). Dogs could be the most suitable model for studying OA as dogs lack the capacity of intrinsic cartilage regeneration, but the ethical issues with the use of dogs as animal models for preclinical and translational studies limit their use.

Dogs reach skeletal maturity at 12–24 months, and dog models are specific for sports and rehabilitation protocols. The cartilage thickness on medial condyle of dogs is 0.95 mm, and defects of 2 to 10 mm diameter and 4 mm depth have been the most commonly generated (McCarty et al., 2016; Salkeld et al., 2016). Goats have thicker cartilage than canine and softer subchondral bone, rendering them susceptible to OCDs. The defect size of diameter 6 mm has been shown to be critical in goats, and defects of this size don't heal spontaneously. Overcoming the major drawbacks of utilizing large animal models—higher costs and optimal facilities—will make goats a viable large animal model for cartilage and osteochondral lesions, although lesion sizes are still not comparable with those in humans.

Pigs are the most relevant clinical large animal models used in an array of biomedical research. The cartilage thickness in pigs is reported to be around 1.5 mm at the medial femoral condyle, and the defect size of diameter 6.3 mm was found to be critical with limited healing capacity, mimicking articular cartilage lesions (Gotterbarm et al., 2008). The most common model in pigs is the one with defect dimensions of 6 mm to 8 mm diameter or larger with postoperative follow-up period of 3 to 24 months.

Amongst large animals, sheep is the most commonly used in orthopaedic research; the knee of sheep is anatomically similar to humans. However, the thinner cartilage limits their use in osteochondral defects as almost all of the defects are located in the subchondral bone. The cartilage thickness in medial femoral condyle of sheep is reported to be approximately 0.45 mm, and osteochondral defects with dimensions of 6–8 mm diameter and 5–13 mm depth have been developed to study biomaterials for osteochondral defect regeneration.

Horses being robust and long-lived animals are more suitable for studying superficial cartilage and subchondral bone regeneration. The upright knee joint in horses with large joint size, thick articular cartilage, and fully straightened gait process makes them highly relevant clinical animal models. The thickness of articular cartilage in horses is around 1.75 mm (close to humans' 2.35 mm), and the OCD of size 15 mm to 20 mm have been developed in horses for different studies (Meng et al., 2020). However, high cost, inconvenient management, long-term postoperative care, high joint loads, and highly specialized conditions limit the use of horse models, in addition to ethics considerations.

17.8 SPINAL DEFECT MODELS

The animal models used in spinal fusion studies are distinctive: Their main purpose is not to recapitulate the native bone anatomy but to create a mechanically optimal arrangement at the site. Most of the common spine defect models involve stabilizing mechanically disturbed sites caused spondylosis, scoliosis, bone tuberculosis infections, or posttraumatic fractures. Different models have been developed to evaluate fusion efficacy, including anterolateral (anterior cervical and lumbar) and posterolateral (Khan & Lane, 2004) spinal fusion models.

For anterolateral fusion, the sheep cervical spinal fusion model has been used consistently to assess the effects of different biologics to augment the fusion. Kandziora et al. (2002) developed this model utilizing C3-C4 discectomy and a series of growth factors loaded on poly-(D,L-lactide)-coated interbody cage to evaluate the efficient fusion. Zdeblick et al. used a goat model of anterior cervical discectomy and fusion to evaluate the efficacy of coral hydroxyapatite bone substitute in anterior cervical decompression and fusion in presence and absence of anterior cervical plate (Khan & Lane, 2004). The model showed successful outcomes in terms of fusion, but the coral hydroxyapatite bone substitute for anterior cervical fusions caused impactful significant implant failures at 12 weeks; however, the compatibility improved with optimum early creeping substitution by the native bone (Khan & Lane, 2004). Apart from anterolateral cervical spine fusion models, different species are also being utilized to evaluate the efficacy of bone graft substitutes, scaffolds, and engineered constructs.

Posterolateral spine fusion models have been extensively used to evaluate the efficacy of tissue-engineered constructs in promoting fusion including rats, rabbits, canines, sheep, and primates. The rat model of posterolateral intertransverse fusion was used as a proof of concept to examine the efficacy of spinal fusion with gene therapy using a gene for novel osteoinductive protein LIM mineralization protein-1 (Boden et al., 1998). The most feasible model of intertransverse process fusion is the rabbit model because of its similar union rate to humans', and this model has been commonly used for various biomaterials like demineralized bone matrix (DBM), recombinant growth factors, and tissue engineered bone-polymer constructs (Boden et al., 1999; Martin et al., 1999; Poynton et al., 2002).

Sandhu et al. (1996) investigated the optimum dose of recombinant factors for spinal fusion in pivotal studies of canine posterolateral spinal fusion models by testing doses of 58, 230, and 920 μg recombinant human bone morphogenetic protein-2 (rhBMP2). The authors observed that irrespective of decortication in the spines, the animals showed clinical spinal fusion after three months except for one with a low dosage of rhBMP2. They used a posterolateral sheep spinal fusion model to assess the efficacies of composite materials of type I bovine dermal collagen, 65% hydroxyapatite and 35% tricalcium phosphate bone graft substitutes. They also used nonhuman primate models of posterolateral spinal fusion for end-stage efficacy closest to human conditions. The results of autogenous bone grafts, cortical and cancellous allografts, and DBM used in nonhuman primate models has shown outcomes similar to human clinical experiences thereby legitimizing the use of this model (Sandhu & Khan, 2002).

CONCLUSION

Animal models continue to be an indispensable tool in research to develop new therapeutic molecules, biomaterials, bone substitutes/fillers, and treatment strategies for pathological conditions associated with bones like bone fractures, osteoporosis, infections, and cancer. The choice of model and the type of species used in developing the model depend on the question under investigation. However, appropriate in vitro investigation is imperative that should support in vivo evaluation in animal models.

ACKNOWLEDGEMENTS

The authors would like to acknowledge the funding received from Ministry of Human Resource Development (MHRD), India and Indian Council of Medical Research (ICMR), India projects (IMPRINT-6714; UAY/MHRD_IITK_006), MHRD, India project (SPARC/2018–2019/P612/S), Science and Engineering Research Board, India projects (IPA/2020/000026; CRG/2021/002179), Department of Science and Technology, Govt. of India project (DST/NM/NT-2018/48), Department of Biotechnology, Govt. of India projects (DBT/IN/SWEDEN/08/AK/2017–18; BT/PR46254/AAQ/1/861/2022), Gangwal School of Medical Sciences and Technology Initiation Grant, Indian Institute of Technology, Kanpur.

LIST OF ABBREVIATIONS

143B	Human Osteosarcoma Cell Line
BMP	Bone Morphogenetic Protein
HOS	Human Osteosarcoma Cell Line
K7M2	Murine Osteosarcoma Cell Line
K-wire	Kirschner Wire
OA	Osteoarthritis
OCD	Osteochondral Defect
RFP	Rifampicin

UMR 106–01 Rat Osteogenic Cell Line
VEGF Vascular Endothelial Growth Factor
B-TCP Beta-Tricalcium Phosphate

REFERENCES

Anesi, A., di Bartolomeo, M., Pellacani, A., Ferretti, M., Cavani, F., Salvatori, R., Nocini, R., Palumbo, C., & Chiarini, L. (2020). Bone healing evaluation following different osteotomic techniques in animal models: A suitable method for clinical insights. *Appl. Sci.* 10: 7165.

Barrios, C., Broström, L. Å., Stark, A., & Walheim, G. (1993). Healing complications after internal fixation of trochanteric hip fractures: The prognostic value of osteoporosis. *J. Orthop. Trauma.* 7: 438–442.

Becher, O. J., & Holland, E. C. (2006). Genetically engineered models have advantages over xenografts for preclinical studies. *Cancer Res.* 66: 3355–3358.

Bernthal, N. M., Stavrakis, A. I., Billi, F., Cho, J. S., Kremen, T. J., Simon, S. I., Cheung, A. L., Finerman, G. A., Lieberman, J. R., Adams, J. S., & Miller, L. S. (2010). A mouse model of post-arthroplasty staphylococcus aureus joint infection to evaluate in vivo the efficacy of antimicrobial implant coatings. *PLoS One.* 5: e12580.

Billings, C., & Anderson, D. E. (2022). Role of animal models to advance research of bacterial osteomyelitis. *Front. Vet. Sci.* 9: 538.

Boden, S. D., Martin, G. J., Morone, M., Ugbo, J. L., Titus, L., & Hutton, W. C. (1999). The use of coralline hydroxyapatite with bone marrow, autogenous bone graft, or osteoinductive bone protein extract for posterolateral lumbar spine fusion. *Spine.* 24: 320–327.

Boden, S. D., Titus, L., Hair, G., Liu, Y., Viggeswarapu, M., Nanes, M. S., & Baranowski, C. (1998). Lumbar spine fusion by local gene therapy with a cDNA encoding a novel osteoinductive protein (LMP-1). *Spine.* 23: 2486–2492.

Boot, W., Schmid, T., D'Este, M., Guillaume, O., Foster, A., Decosterd, L., Richards, R. G., Eglin, D., Zeiter, S., & Moriarty, T. F. (2021). A hyaluronic acid hydrogel loaded with gentamicin and vancomycin successfully eradicates chronic methicillin-resistant staphylococcus aureus orthopedic infection in a sheep model. *Antimicrob. Agents Chemother.* 65(4): e01840–20.

Bue, M., Hanberg, P., Koch, J., Jensen, L. K., Lundorff, M., Aalbæk, B., Jensen, H. E., Søballe, K., & Tøttrup, M. (2018). Single-dose bone pharmacokinetics of vancomycin in a porcine implant-associated osteomyelitis model. *J. Orthop. Res.* 36: 1093–1098.

Castañeda, S., Largo, R., Calvo, E., Rodríguez-Salvanés, F., Marcos, M. E., Díaz-Curiel, M., & Herrero-Beaumont, G. (2006). Bone mineral measurements of subchondral and trabecular bone in healthy and osteoporotic rabbits. *Skelet. Radiol.* 35: 34–41.

Chadha, H. S., Fitzgerald, J., Wiater, P., Sud, S., Nasser, S., & Wooley, P. H. (1999). Experimental acute hematogenous osteomyelitis in mice. I: Histopathological and immunological findings. *J. Orthop. Res.* 17: 376–381.

Chen, H., & Yao, Y. (2022). Progress of biomaterials for bone tumor therapy. *J. Biomater. Appl.* 36: 945–955.

Chen, Y., Zhou, Y., Lin, J., & Zhang, S. (2022). Challenges to improve bone healing under diabetic conditions. *Front. Endocrinol.* 13: 495.

Chevrier, A., Kouao, A. S. M., Picard, G., Hurtig, M. B., & Buschmann, M. D. (2015). Interspecies comparison of subchondral bone properties important for cartilage repair. *J. Orthop. Res.* 33: 63–70.

Christou, C., Oliver, R. A., Pelletier, M. H., & Walsh, W. R. (2014). Ovine model for critical-size tibial segmental defects. *Comp. Med.* 64: 377–385.

Crnalic, S., Håkansson, I., Boquist, L., Löfvenberg, R., & Broström, L. Å. (1997). A novel spontaneous metastasis model of human osteosarcoma developed using orthotopic transplantation of intact tumor tissue into tibia of nude mice. *Clin. Exp. Metastasis.* 15: 164–172.

de Mesy Bentley, K. L., Trombetta, R., Nishitani, K., Bello-Irizarry, S. N., Ninomiya, M., Zhang, L., Chung, H. L., McGrath, J. L., Daiss, J. L., Awad, H. A., Kates, S. L., & Schwarz, E. M. (2017). Evidence of staphylococcus aureus deformation, proliferation, and migration in canaliculi of live cortical bone in murine models of osteomyelitis. *J. Bone. Miner. Res.* 32: 985–990.

Deng, C., Chang, J., & Wu, C. (2019). Bioactive scaffolds for osteochondral regeneration. *J. Orthop. Translat.* 17: 15–25.

Dewhurst, R. M., Scalzone, A., Buckley, J., Mattu, C., Rankin, K. S., Gentile, P., & Ferreira, A. M. (2020). Development of natural-based bone cement for a controlled doxorubicin-drug release. *Front. Bioeng. Biotech.* 8: 754.

D'Ippolito, G., Schiller, P. C., Ricordi, C., Roos, B. A., & Howard, G. A. (1999). Age-related osteogenic potential of mesenchymal stromal stem cells from human vertebral bone marrow. *J. Bone Miner. Res.* 14: 1115–1122.

Ek, E. T. H., Dass, C. R., & Choong, P. F. M. (2006). Commonly used mouse models of osteosarcoma. *Crit. Rev. Oncol. Hematol.* 60: 1–8.

Fidler, I. J. (2003). The pathogenesis of cancer metastasis: The "seed and soil" hypothesis revisited. *Nat. Rev. Cancer.* 3: 453–458.

Frisbie, D. D., Cross, M. W., & McIlwraith, C. W. (2006). A comparative study of articular cartilage thickness in the stifle of animal species used in human pre-clinical studies compared to articular cartilage thickness in the human knee. *Vet. Comp. Orthop. Traumatol.* 19: 142–146.

Fritz, J. M., & McDonald, J. R. (2008). Osteomyelitis: Approach to diagnosis and treatment. *Phys. Sportsmed.* 36: 50–54.

Funao, H., Ishii, K., Nagai, S., Sasaki, A., Hoshikawa, T., Aizawa, M., Okada, Y., Chiba, K., Koyasu, S., Toyama, Y., & Matsumoto, M. (2012). Establishment of a real-time, quantitative, and reproducible mouse model of staphylococcus osteomyelitis using bioluminescence imaging. *Infect. Immun.* 80: 733.

Galtt, V., & Mattys, R. (2014). Adjustable stiffness, external fixator for the rat femur osteotomy and segmental bone defect models. *J. Vis. Exp.* 92: e51558.

Gomes, P. S., & Fernandes, M. H. (2011). Rodent models in bone-related research: The relevance of calvarial defects in the assessment of bone regeneration strategies. *Lab. Anim.* 45: 14–24.

Gotterbarm, T., Breusch, S. J., Schneider, U., & Jung, M. (2008). The minipig model for experimental chondral and osteochondral defect repair in tissue engineering: Retrospective analysis of 180 defects. *Lab. Anim.* 42: 71–82.

Gupta, S., Teotia, A. K., Qayoom, I., Shiekh, P. A., Andrabi, S. M., & Kumar, A. (2021). Periosteum-mimicking tissue-engineered composite for treating periosteum damage in critical-sized bone defects. *Biomacromolecules.* 22: 3237–3250.

Hatzenbuehler, J., & Pulling, T. J. (2011). Diagnosis and management of osteomyelitis. *Am. Fam. Physician.* 84: 1027–1033.

Helbig, L., Guehring, T., Titze, N., Nurjadi, D., Sonntag, R., Armbruster, J., Wildemann, B., Schmidmaier, G., Gruetzner, A. P., & Freischmidt, H. (2020). A new sequential animal model for infection-related non-unions with segmental bone defect. *BMC Musculoskelet. Disord.* 21: 1–11.

Hill, P. F., & Watkins, P. E. (2001). The prevention of experimental osteomyelitis in a model of gunshot fracture in the pig. *Eur. J. Orthop. Surg. Traumatol.* 11: 237–241.

Horst, S. A., Hoerr, V., Beineke, A., Kreis, C., Tuchscherr, L., Kalinka, J., Lehne, S., Schleicher, I., Köhler, G., Fuchs, T., Raschke, M. J., Rohde, M., Peters, G., Faber, C., Löffler, B., & Medina, E. (2012). A novel mouse model of staphylococcus aureus chronic osteomyelitis that closely mimics the human infection: An integrated view of disease pathogenesis. *Am. J. Pathol.* 181: 1206–1214.

Jensen, H. E., Nielsen, O. L., Agerholm, J. S., Iburg, T., Johansen, L. K., Johannesson, E., Møller, M., Jahn, L., Munk, L., Aalbaek, B., & Leifsson, P. S. (2010). A non-traumatic staphylococcus aureus osteomyelitis model in pigs. *In Vivo.* 24: 257–264.

Jensen, L. K., Koch, J., Dich-Jorgensen, K., Aalbæk, B., Petersen, A., Fuursted, K., Bjarnsholt, T., Kragh, K. N., Tøtterup, M., Bue, M., Hanberg, P., Søballe, K., Heegaard, P. M. H., & Jensen, H. E. (2017). Novel porcine model of implant-associated osteomyelitis: A comprehensive analysis of local, regional, and systemic response. *J. Orthop. Res.* 35: 2211–2221.

Ji, W., Bolander, J., Chai, Y. C., Katagiri, H., Marechal, M., & Luyten, F. P. (2017). Toward advanced therapy medicinal products (ATMPs) combining bone morphogenetic proteins (BMP) and cells for bone regeneration. In *Bone Morphogenetic Proteins: Systems Biology Regulators.* S. Vukicevic, and K. T. Sampath, Eds. Cham: Springer, pp. 127–169.

Jiang, W., Rixiati, Y., Zhao, B., Li, Y., Tang, C., & Liu, J. (2020). Incidence, prevalence, and outcomes of systemic malignancy with bone metastases. *J. Orthop. Surg. (Hong Kong).* 28: 2309499020915989.

Jiao, H., Xiao, E., & Graves, D. T. (2015). Diabetes and its effect on bone and fracture healing. *Curr. Osteoporos. Rep.* 13: 327–335.

Jødal, L., Roivainen, A., Oikonen, V., Jalkanen, S., Hansen, S. B., Afzelius, P., Alstrup, A. K. O., Nielsen, O. L., & Jensen, S. B. (2019). Kinetic modelling of [68Ga]Ga-DOTA-Siglec-9 in porcine osteomyelitis and soft tissue infections. *Molecules.* 24: 4094.

Kandziora, F., Schmidmaier, G., Schollmeier, G., Bail, H., Pflugmacher, R., Görke, T., Wagner, M., Raschke, M., Mittlmeier, T., & Haas, N. P. (2002). IGF-I and TGF-beta1 application by a poly-(D,L-lactide)-coated cage promotes intervertebral bone matrix formation in the sheep cervical spine. *Spine*. 27: 1710–1722.

Katagiri, H., Mendes, L. F., & Luyten, F. P. (2017). Definition of a critical size osteochondral knee defect and its negative effect on the surrounding articular cartilage in the rat. *Osteoarthr. Cartil.* 25: 1531–1540.

Kavanagh, N., Ryan, E. J., Widaa, A., Sexton, G., Fennell, J., O'Rourke, S., Cahill, K. C., Kearney, C. J., O'Brien, F. J., & Kerrigan, S. W. (2018). Staphylococcal osteomyelitis: Disease progression, treatment challenges, and future directions. *Clin. Microbiol. Rev*. 31(2): e00084–17.

Khan, S. N., & Lane, J. M. (2004). Spinal fusion surgery: Animal models for tissue-engineered bone constructs. *Biomaterials*. 25: 1475–1485.

Khodaparast, O., Coberly, D. M., Mathey, J., Rohrich, R. J., Levin, L. S., & Brown, S. A. (2003). Effect of a transpositional muscle flap on VEGF mRNA expression in a canine fracture model. *Plast. Reconstr. Surg*. 112: 171–176.

Kubo, T., Shiga, T., Hashimoto, J., Yoshioka, M., Honjo, H., Urabe, M., Kitajima, I., Semba, I., & Hirasawa, Y. (1999). Osteoporosis influences the late period of fracture healing in a rat model prepared by ovariectomy and low calcium diet. *J. Steroid Biochem. Mol. Biol*. 68: 197–202.

Lane, N. E. (2006). Epidemiology, etiology, and diagnosis of osteoporosis. *Am. J. Obstet. Gynecol*. 194: S3–S11.

Liebschner, M. A. K. (2004). Biomechanical considerations of animal models used in tissue engineering of bone. *Biomaterials*. 25: 1697–1714.

Lindsey, R. W., Gugala, Z., Milne, E., Sun, M., Gannon, F. H., & Latta, L. L. (2006). The efficacy of cylindrical titanium mesh cage for the reconstruction of a critical-size canine segmental femoral diaphyseal defect. *J. Orthop. Res*. 24: 1438–1453.

Lovati, A. B., Drago, L., Monti, L., De Vecchi, E., Previdi, S., Banfi, G., & Romanò, C. L. (2013). Diabetic mouse model of orthopaedic implant-related staphylococcus aureus infection. *PLoS One*. 8: e67628.

Marin, C., Luyten, F. P., Van der Schueren, B., Kerckhofs, G., & Vandamme, K. (2018). The impact of type 2 diabetes on bone fracture healing. *Front. Endocrinol. (Lausanne)*. 9: 6.

Martin, G. J. J., Boden, S. D., Titus, L., & Scarborough, N. L. (1999). New formulations of demineralized bone matrix as a more effective graft alternative in experimental posterolateral lumbar spine arthrodesis. *Spine*. 24: 637–645.

McCarty, E. C., Fader, R. R., Mitchell, J. J., Glenn, R. E., Potter, H. G., & Spindler, K. P. (2016). Fresh osteochondral allograft versus autograft: Twelve-month results in isolated canine knee defects. *Am. J. Sports Med*. 44: 2354–2365.

Melton, L. J., Beck, T. J., Amin, S., Khosla, S., Achenbach, S. J., Oberg, A. L., & Riggs, B. L. (2005). Contributions of bone density and structure to fracture risk assessment in men and women. *Osteoporosis Int*. 16: 460–467.

Meng, X., Ziadlou, R., Grad, S., Alini, M., Wen, C., Lai, Y., Qin, L., Zhao, Y., & Wang, X. (2020). Animal models of osteochondral defect for testing biomaterials. *Biochem. Res. Int*. 2020: 9659412.

Moreau, A. (2017). The next personalized medicine evolution in orthopedics: How diagnosing and treating scoliosis are about to change. *Per. Med*. 14: 89–92.

Moriarty, T. F., Schmid, T., Post, V., Samara, E., Kates, S., Schwarz, E. M., Zeiter, S., & Richards, R. G. (2017). A large animal model for a failed two-stage revision of intramedullary nail-related infection by methicillin-resistant staphylococcus aureus. *Eur. Cells Mater*. 34: 83–98.

Nakamura, T., Shirakata, Y., Shinohara, Y., Miron, R. J., Hasegawa-Nakamura, K., Fujioka-Kobayashi, M., & Noguchi, K. (2017). Comparison of the effects of recombinant human bone morphogenetic protein-2 and -9 on bone formation in rat calvarial critical-size defects. *Clin. Oral Investig*. 21: 2671–2679.

Nielsen, O. L., Afzelius, P., Bender, D., Schønheyder, H. C., Leifsson, P. S., Nielsen, K. M., Larsen, J. O., Jensen, S. B., & Alstrup, A. K. (2015). Comparison of autologous 111In-leukocytes, 18F-FDG, 11C-methionine, 11C-PK11195 and 68Ga-citrate for diagnostic nuclear imaging in a juvenile porcine haematogenous staphylococcus aureus osteomyelitis model. *Am. J. Nucl. Med. Mol. Imaging*. 5: 169–182.

Okamoto, Y., Takahashi, K., Toriyama, K., Takeda, N., Kitagawa, K., Hosokawa, M., & Takeda, T. (1995). Femoral peak bone mass and osteoclast number in an animal model of age-related spontaneous osteopenia. *Anat. Rec*. 242: 21–28.

Pereira, D., Peleteiro, B., Araújo, J., Branco, J., Santos, R. A., & Ramos, E. (2011). The effect of osteoarthritis definition on prevalence and incidence estimates: A systematic review. *Osteoarthr. Cartil.* 19: 1270–1285.

Perkins, S. L., Gibbons, R., Kling, S., & Kahn, A. J. (1994). Age-related bone loss in mice is associated with an increased osteoclast progenitor pool. *Bone.* 15: 65–72.

Poynton, A. R., Zheng, F., Tomin, E., Lane, J. M., & Cornwall, G. B. (2002). Resorbable posterolateral graft containment in a rabbit spinal fusion model. *J. Neurosurg.* 97: 460–463.

Qayoom, I., Srivastava, E., & Kumar, A. (2022). Anti-infective composite cryogel scaffold treats osteomyelitis and augments bone healing in rat femoral condyle. *Biomater. Adv.* 142: 213133.

Qayoom, I., Teotia, A. K., & Kumar, A. (2020a). Nanohydroxyapatite based ceramic carrier promotes bone formation in a femoral neck canal defect in osteoporotic rats. *Biomacromolecules.* 21: 328–337.

Qayoom, I., Teotia, A. K., Panjla, A., Verma, S., & Kumar, A. (2020b). Local and sustained delivery of rifampicin from a bioactive ceramic carrier treats bone infection in rat tibia. *ACS Infect. Dis.* 6: 2938–2949.

Qayoom, I., Verma, R., Murugan, P. A., Raina, D. B., Teotia, A. K., Matheshwaran, S., Nair, N. N., Tägil, M., Lidgren, L., & Kumar, A. (2020c). A biphasic nanohydroxyapatite/calcium sulphate carrier containing rifampicin and isoniazid for local delivery gives sustained and effective antibiotic release and prevents biofilm formation. *Sci. Rep.* 10: 1–14.

Raina, D. B., Qayoom, I., Larsson, D., Zheng, M. H., Kumar, A., Isaksson, H., Lidgren, L., & Tägil, M. (2019). Guided tissue engineering for healing of cancellous and cortical bone using a combination of biomaterial based scaffolding and local bone active molecule delivery. *Biomaterials.* 188: 38–49.

Raina, D. B., Širka, A., Qayoom, I., Teotia, A. K., Liu, Y., Tarasevicius, S., Tanner, K. E., Isaksson, H., Kumar, A., Tägil, M., & Lidgren, L. (2020). Long-term response to a bioactive biphasic biomaterial in the femoral neck of osteoporotic rats. *Tissue Eng., Part A.* 26: 1042–1051.

Rasanen, T., & Messner, K. (1996). Regional variations of indentation stiffness and thickness of normal rabbit knee articular cartilage. *J. Biomed. Mater. Res.* 31: 519–524.

Rosol, T. J. (2000). Pathogenesis of bone metastases: Role of tumor-related proteins. *J. Bone Miner. Res.* 15: 844–850.

Roux, K. M., Cobb, L. H., Seitz, M. A., & Priddy, L. B. (2021). Innovations in osteomyelitis research: A review of animal models. *Animal Model Exp. Med.* 4: 59–70.

Russell, G., Tucci, M., Conflitti, J., Graves, M., Wingerter, S., Woodall, J., Ragab, A., & Benghuzzi, H. (2009). Characterization of a femoral segmental nonunion model in laboratory rats: Report of a novel surgical technique. *J. Invest. Surg.* 20: 249–255.

Salgado, C. J., Jamali, A. A., Mardini, S., Buchanan, K., & Veit, B. (2005). A model for chronic osteomyelitis using staphylococcus aureus in goats. *Clin. Orthop. Relat. Res.* 436: 246–250.

Salkeld, S. L., Patron, L. P., Lien, J. C., Cook, S. D., & Jones, D. G. (2016). Biological and functional evaluation of a novel pyrolytic carbon implant for the treatment of focal osteochondral defects in the medial femoral condyle: Assessment in a canine model. *J. Orthop. Surg. Res.* 11: 155.

Sandhu, H. S., Kanim, L. E. A., Kabo, J. M., Toth, J. M., Zeegen, E. N., Liu, D., Delamarter, R. B., & Dawson, E. G. (1996). Effective doses of recombinant human bone morphogenetic protein-2 in experimental spinal fusion. *Spine.* 21: 2115–2122.

Sandhu, H. S., & Khan, S. N. (2002). Animal models for preclinical assessment of bone morphogenetic proteins in the spine. *Spine.* 27: S32–S38.

Savaridas, T., Wallace, R. J., Dawson, S., & Simpson, A. H. R. W. (2015). Effect of ibandronate on bending strength and toughness of rodent cortical bone: Possible implications for fracture prevention. *Bone Joint Res.* 4: 99–104.

Schneider-Wald, B., Von Thaden, A. K., & Schwarz, M. L. R. (2013). Defect models for the regeneration of articular cartilage in large animals. *Der. Orthopade.* 42: 242–253.

Simmons, J. K., Hildreth, B. E., Supsavhad, W., Elshafae, S. M., Hassan, B. B., Dirksen, W. P., Toribio, R. E., & Rosol, T. J. (2015). Animal models of bone metastasis. *Vet. Pathol.* 52: 827–841.

Širka, A., Raina, D. B., Isaksson, H., Tanner, K. E., Smailys, A., Kumar, A., Tarasevičius, Š., Tägil, M., & Lidgren, L. (2018). Calcium sulphate/hydroxyapatite carrier for bone formation in the femoral neck of osteoporotic rats. *Tissue Eng., Part A.* 24: 1753–1764.

Stewart, S. K. (2019). Fracture non-union: A review of clinical challenges and future research needs. *Malays. Orthop. J.* 13: 1–10.

Syed, F. A., & Hoey, K. A. (2010). Integrative physiology of the aging bone: Insights from animal and cellular models. *Ann. N. Y. Acad. Sci.* 1211: 95–106.

Teotia, A. K., Dienel, K., Qayoom, I., van Bochove, B., Gupta, S., Partanen, J., Seppälä, J., & Kumar, A. (2020). Improved bone regeneration in rabbit bone defects using 3D printed composite scaffolds functionalized with osteoinductive factors. *ACS Appl. Mater. Interfaces.* 12: 48340–48356.

Teotia, A. K., Gupta, A., Raina, D. B., Lidgren, L., & Kumar, A. (2016). Gelatin-modified bone substitute with bioactive molecules enhance cellular interactions and bone regeneration. *ACS Appl. Mater. Interfaces.* 8: 10775–10787.

Teotia, A. K., Qayoom, I., & Kumar, A. (2018). Endogenous platelet-rich plasma supplements/augments growth factors delivered via porous collagen-nanohydroxyapatite bone substitute for enhanced bone formation. *ACS Biomater. Sci. Eng.* 5: 56–69.

Teotia, A. K., Raina, D. B., Isaksson, H., Tägil, M., Lidgren, L., Seppälä, J., & Kumar, A. (2019). Composite bilayered scaffolds with bio-functionalized ceramics for cranial bone defects: An in vivo evaluation. *Multifunct. Mater.* 2: 014002.

Teotia, A. K., Raina, D. B., Singh, C., Sinha, N., Isaksson, H., Tägil, M., Lidgren, L., & Kumar, A. (2017). Nano-hydroxyapatite bone substitute functionalized with bone active molecules for enhanced cranial bone regeneration. *ACS Appl. Mater. Interfaces.* 9: 6816–6828.

Tran, N., Tran, P. A., Jarrell, J. D., Engiles, J. B., Thomas, N. P., Young, M. D., Hayda, R. A., & Born, C. T. (2013). In vivo caprine model for osteomyelitis and evaluation of biofilm-resistant intramedullary nails. *Biomed. Res. Int.* 2013: 674378.

Urish, K. L., & Cassat, J. E. (2020). Staphylococcus aureus osteomyelitis: Bone, bugs, and surgery. *Infect. Immun.* 88: e00932–19.

Van der Jagt, O. P., van der Linden, J. C., Waarsing, J. H., Verhaar, J. A. N., & Weinans, H. (2014). Electromagnetic fields do not affect bone micro-architecture in osteoporotic rats. *Bone Joint Res.* 3: 230–235.

Wang, X., Mabrey, J. D., & Agrawal, C. M. (1998). An interspecies comparison of bone fracture properties. *Biomed. Mater. Eng.* 8: 1–9.

Wang, Y., Cheng, L. I., Helfer, D. R., Ashbaugh, A. G., Miller, R. J., Tzomides, A. J., Thompson, J. M., Ortines, R. v., Tsai, A. S., Liu, H., Dillen, C. A., Archer, N. K., Cohen, T. S., Tkaczyk, C., Stover, C. K., Sellman, B. R., & Miller, L. S. (2017). Mouse model of hematogenous implant-related staphylococcus aureus biofilm infection reveals therapeutic targets. *Proc. Natl. Acad. Sci.* 114: E5094–E5102.

Zhang, Y., Wu, Y., Qiao, X., Lin, T., Wang, Y., & Wang, M. (2022). Biomaterial-based strategy for bone tumor therapy and bone defect regeneration: An innovative application option. *Front. Mater.* 9: 554.

Zoller, S. D., Hegde, V., Burke, Z. D. C., Park, H. Y., Ishmael, C. R., Blumstein, G. W., Sheppard, W., Hamad, C., Loftin, A. H., Johansen, D. O., Smith, R. A., Sprague, M. M., Hori, K. R., Clarkson, S. J., Borthwell, R., Simon, S. I., Miller, J. F., Nelson, S. D., & Bernthal, N. M. (2020). Evading the host response: Staphylococcus “hiding” in cortical bone canalicular system causes increased bacterial burden. *Bone Res.* 8: 1–11.

18 Advanced Biomaterial-Based Strategies for Intervertebral Disc Repair and Regeneration

Akash Yadav, Raghavendra Dhanenawar, and Akshay Srivastava

18.1 INTRODUCTION

Intervertebral disc degeneration (IVDD) is a root cause of lower back pain. Several risk variables, including environment, daily activities, and genetics, are necessary for comprehending the pathophysiology of IVD. Mutations in collagen, aggrecan, vitamin D receptor, and extracellular matrix (ECM)-producing genes that alter metabolic pathways contribute to this disorder (Ravalli & Musumeci, 2021).

According to MRI findings in epidemiological research, IVDD probably begins in adolescence and progresses with age (Mesregah et al., 2022). Research indicates that 77% of the population under 50 years old has severe discomfort in the lumbar area, and 90% of the population over 50 experiences the progressive disc degeneration that leads to the complete loss of IVD functionality. In IVDD, there are three crucial phenomena: (a) increased catabolic cascades, (b) recurrent cell loss, and (c) reduction of cellular activities and anabolic events (Dou et al., 2021).

Mainstream therapeutic approaches both surgical and nonsurgical are centered on symptomatic relief. Surgical therapies emphasize physically alleviating illness at the tissue level, for instance nerve root decompression (discectomy) and removal of the deteriorated disc. Nonsurgical treatments elicit limited effects on the milieu. Traditional treatment approaches do not stimulate disc regeneration and, hence, perhaps cannot reverse the progression of disc degradation.

Some patients relapse following therapy, and the degeneration of adjoining regions may be expedited by disc degradation (Harmon et al., 2020; Harper & Klineberg, 2019). The long-term vision of the biomaterial-based paradigm in tissue engineering rests in establishing techniques that are customized to the extremity levels of disc degeneration in a bid to potentiate the treatment's relevance. The therapeutic feasibility of a treatment is ascertained by reduced IVD pain and dysfunction, and biomaterial-based tissue engineering endeavors to address the pathophysiology behind IVD in its earliest, mildest, and most severe manifestations.

The current need also involves patient-centered biomaterials and tissue engineering frameworks to arrest disease prognosis, induce tissue restoration, and alleviate the underlying cause, namely, discogenic low back pain. The pertinent features for evaluating tissue-engineered intervertebral discs are the biocompatibility, biodegradability, and biomechanical qualities of the material and a structural design that permits the passage of substrates, micronutrients, and prudential substances within and between cells. The ability of biomaterials to adapt to the microenvironment of the host conserves disc structure, sustains tissue homeostasis, and intensifies ECM deposition for morphological tissue healing, thereby generating cohesive mechanical stability. Here, we discuss the biomaterial-based approaches established for offsetting the limitations of the traditional treatment approaches.

DOI: 10.1201/9781003307310-21

18.2 BIOMATERIALS FOR ANNULUS FIBROSUS AND NUCLEUS PULPOSUS REPAIR AND REGENERATION

Several strategies are currently being investigated for the repair and regeneration of IVD (Figure 18.1). They usually involve cell-based biomolecule delivery and bioactive materials either alone or in combination. The biomaterial-based approaches have shown tremendous progress in repairing IVDD by repopulating the disc's native cells, replacing the degraded disc matrix, controlling the inflammation, and even reinstating the whole disc.

The primary goals of biomaterials to restore IVD biomechanical functions are to (a) assist the viability of resident cells, (b) accelerate the production and deposition of discal ECM, (c) reduce pathogenic fibrosis, (d) alleviate inflammation, and (e) enhance the spinal stability. Myriad of polymeric materials of synthetic and natural origin have been explored and utilized for IVD regeneration (Table S18.1). The choice of ideal biomaterial is the foremost important consideration for designing scaffolds. So far both natural and synthetic biomaterials have been explored in IVD tissue engineering. These biomaterials are discussed in the following sections.

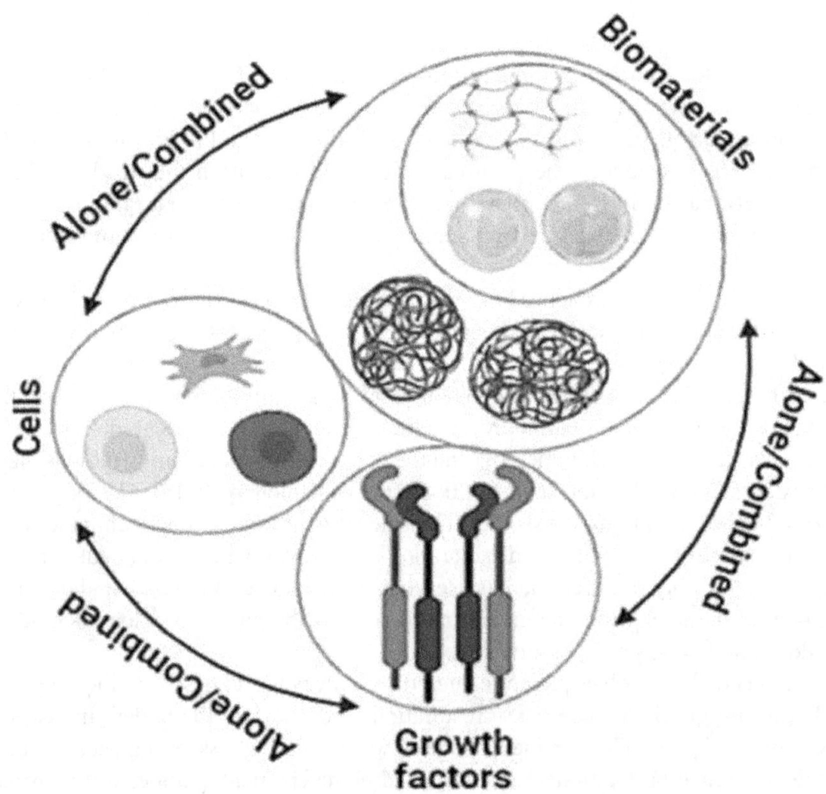

FIGURE 18.1 Strategies for intervertebral disc repair and regeneration (reproduced with permission from Malli, S. E., Kumbhkarn, P., Dewle, A., & Srivastava, A.: Evaluation of Tissue Engineering Approaches for Intervertebral Disc Regeneration in Relevant Animal Models. ACS Appl. Bio Mater.: 2021. 4. 7721–7737. Copyright 2021 American Chemical Society).

18.2.1 Natural Biomaterials

18.2.1.1 Chitosan

Chitosan (CS), a biopolymer composed of polysaccharide of glucosamine and N-acetyl glucosamine units, is produced when chitin is partially deacetylated. Since CS dissolves at low pH, the resultant solution must be neutralized before use. This is difficult because of the crosslinking of CS chains after neutralizing an acidic chitosan solution. Through lysozyme activity, CS is broken down in living organisms. The degradation period is extended while cellular adhesion is improved by increasing the level of de-acetylation (Doench et al., 2019). CS's cationic properties also enable it to bind with anionic glycosaminoglycans, and it promote the interaction of growth factors and other cytokines. CS is a versatile polymer, but it works best when blended with another material to enhance biomechanical characteristics. It has also shown to stimulate chondrogenic differentiation (Garcia et al., 2021). CS-based strategies have been used for IVDD repair, in an example, CS hydrogel augmented with gelatin and Link N have shown to increase the mechanical properties of the hydrogel and demonstrated the cellular adhesion leading to enhanced production of glycosaminoglycans (GAGs) (Adoungotchodo et al., 2021).

Another study reports the development of a thermosensitive, minimally invasive IVDD treatment. Researchers developed a thermosensitive CS hydrogel that could imitate the nucleus pulposus (NP), the central portion of the IVD, by demonstrating indistinguishable mechanistic properties along with cellular adhesion and restorative and regenerative capabilities (Alinejad et al., 2019). Tissue-engineered biomimetic CS-based scaffolds have also been investigated as restorative and regenerative approaches for IVDD.

A study reports the designing and development of a CS-based tissue-engineered biomimetic scaffold processed from poly(lactic-co-glycolic acid) (PLGA) by electrospinning. The developed scaffold showed enhanced mechanical properties with chondro-inductive properties (Garakani et al., 2020; Shen et al., 2021). Recently, researchers developed a minimally invasive treatment that significantly reduced IVD degeneration, namely, intradiscal injection-based delivery of CS hydrogels loaded with transforming growth factor, bone morphogenetic protein, tissue inhibitors of metalloproteinases, and matrix metalloproteinase inhibitors (Gandhi et al., 2020). Researchers studied combined therapy to counter degenerative manifestations by developing gentamicin-loaded CS microsphere–β-tricalcium phosphate reinforced polymer scaffolds that optimally released gentamicin locally to the afflicted defect regions and bolstered bone and tissue regeneration (Liu et al., 2022a).

18.2.1.2 Alginate

Alginate is a highly adaptable substance that has promising potential as a biomaterial for tissue engineering and regeneration, particularly for the NP. Natural biopolymer alginate (alginic acid) is extracted from brown seaweed and is typically made up of β-(1–4)-linked D-mannuronic acid (M) and α-(1–4)-linked L-guluronic acid (G) moieties (Sahoo & Biswal, 2021). Calibrating the weight-to-volume (w/v) proportion of the alginate controls the stiffness of the nanofibers. In terms of stiffness, 2% (w/v) alginate scaffolds are found to be similar to the native NP in certain reports.

Materials made of alginate are intermittently mixed with synthetic polymers like poly(ε-caprolactone) (PCL) and polyglycolic acid (PGA) to improve their mechanical properties (Farokhi et al., 2020). Photo-crosslinking is another method used to enhance the mechanical functionalities of alginate composites; it also enhances ECM synthesis in vivo and promotes cell proliferation. The in vivo degradation is believed to occur by removing the links within the chains. The key disadvantage of employing this material is that the in vivo degradation process is poorly understood (Araiza-Verduzco et al., 2020; Wang et al., 2021).

A preclinical study showed the safety and effectiveness of alginate gel. Ultra-purified alginate gel (UPAL) was implanted into sheep and rabbit IVD demonstrated pronounced biomechanical properties and enhanced GAG production (Tsujimoto et al., 2018). Authors of another recent study investigated the ability of UPAL to alleviate lower back pain. They found that UPAL downregulated the expression of the inflammatory cytokines tumor necrosis factor (TNF-α), interleukin 6, and tyrosine kinase A, leading to reduced nociception and inhibition of IVDD (Ura et al., 2021). A 3D-printed flexible polylactic acid scaffold was investigated for its biocompatibility and biomimetic property; the authors prepared a hydrogel composite of alginate and NP cells along with MSCs (Marshall et al., 2021).

18.2.1.3 Hyaluronic Acid

Hyaluronan or hyaluronic acid (HA) is a heteropolysaccharide derived from connective tissue and is diligently researched for the goal of tissue regeneration. It is made up of repeated units of d-glucuronic acid and *N*-acetyl-d-glucosamine. Clinical uses for HA derivatives include surgical operations and medication administration.

HA is enzymatically degraded by hyaluronidases. Hyaluronidases break down HA by cleaving the glucosaminyl linkages, and the degree of degradation is controlled by introducing methacrylate groups, which are also utilized for photo-crosslinking the HA-based constructs (Fallacara et al., 2018). Optimizing the w/v ratio of HA improves the firmness to the extent that it is comparable with annulus fibrosus (AF) and NP structures. Since HA is a crucial component of the IVD, researchers have used various nanofiber- and hydrogel-based scaffolds (Ji & Kim, 2021; Liu et al., 2018; Varela-Aramburu et al., 2021).

In a recent in vitro study, the inflammatory properties of HA were assessed in human disc cells, and the expression of inflammatory mediators like TNF-α and cyclooxegenase-2 was lower after HA treatment. The authors also reported that HA can substantially alleviate IVDD by attuning the p38 and Erk1/2 pathways (Yamamoto et al., 2021). Another study reports the application of cell-loaded 3D hydrogel in an in vitro inflammatory model and also in vivo into a rat-tail model. The HA hydrogel mimics the ECM components of the disc and the therapeutic impact was demonstrated by the alleviation of neurotrophins and marginalization of hyper-innervation (Srivastava et al., 2016).

A phase-II clinical study (registered under ChiCTR2200058291) recently reported the use of the HA hydrogel loaded with autologous adipose-derived mesenchymal stem cells (ASCs) to counter discogenic back pain (Zhang et al., 2022). The study included 100 suitable patients who were placed randomly into three groups with subsequent dose escalation and one placebo as the control group. The patients were tracked for up to 24 months after the successful transplantation of the HA hydrogel. All the eligible evaluation parameters for the assessment of the phase II clinical study were assessed (Zhang et al., 2022). Interestingly, HA hydrogel has been shown to alleviate pain, reduce nociceptive behavior, and inhibit hyperinnervation. An implanted HA hydrogel altered glycosylation and modulated key inflammatory and regulatory signaling pathways, making HA hydrogel a promising candidate for the regeneration of IVD (Isa et al., 2018).

The core NP comprises chondrocytes, and peripheral AF comprises fibroblasts (Johnson & Roberts, 2003). Autologous NP cells were isolated from healthy lumbar discs and mounted with HA-pNIPAM hydrogel for seeding and distribution, and the hydrogel significantly fostered IVD repair and regeneration (Rosenzweig et al., 2018). In a pilot study, HA hydrogel mixed with platelet-rich plasma was used as a carrier material for the delivery of human mesenchymal stem cells (hMSCs) (Russo et al., 2021). In another example, a combination strategy was also developed where with photocrosslinkable collagen gel patch used for AF repair, while the injectable modified HA hydrogel represents the NP component (Sloan et al., 2017, 2020). This combined approach showed tissue repair and mechanically stabilized the IVD.

18.2.1.4 Collagen

Collagen (Col) is notably the most prevalent protein, accounts for almost one-third of the overall protein weight of the body. The majority of collagens are composed of three distinct amino acids: glycine (33%), which particularly imparts the molecule's stability; proline (15%); and hydroxyproline (15%) (Dong & Lv, 2016). Col fibrils are formed by covalent interactions between Col molecules. In vivo Col crosslinking occurs via enzyme lysyl oxidase using an aldehydic reaction to crosslink Col through the lysine side chains. The extent of crosslinking impacts the mechanical stability, degree of degradation, and interactions between cells and fibers.

Col fibrils are arrays of Col fragments that vary in thickness from 50 nm to just several hundred nm and that are amalgamated to create multiscale and hierarchical structures with a variety of mechanical properties. By limiting the hydrostatic potential of the tightly packed proteoglycans, a robust fibrous network is produced with compressive and tensile strength (Andriotis et al., 2018; Lin et al., 2020); this phenotypic hierarchy produced unique nonlinear, hyperelastic, anisotropic stress–strain behavior.

A self-assembled nanofibrous scaffold developed from Col peptide was reported in a study on IVD restoration. Pro-Hyp-Gly peptide sequences were used to create a Col peptide that exhibited nanofibrous scaffolds, and implanting the Col–peptide scaffolds into degraded rabbit IVD elevated GAG and Col levels. The degeneration index score was used to assess tissue functional recovery, and the biologically active scaffold was proven to rehabilitate IVD degeneration (Uysal et al., 2019). A thiolated-Col hydrogel was used in one study to overcome the challenges with injectable hydrogels and demonstrated excellent cell delivery in tissue regeneration (Pupkaite et al., 2019).

In another study, researchers used a template to create knitted-PGLA-mesh Col scaffolds of different mesh sizes (Xie et al., 2022). First, the authors developed a braided, composite PLGA mesh by producing network-fashioned Col micro-sponges inside the PLGA mesh holes or by covering a thin Col sheet alongside the framework of the PLGA mesh; the mesh was then solvated using an alkaline solution, and eliminating the PLGA matrix template generated Col meshes. The Col meshes enhanced the cellular adhesive and proliferative functionalities of dermal fibroblast cells in the regeneration of dermal tissue (Xie et al., 2022).

Col II are a typical and well-understood biomaterial for NP tissue regeneration as similar Col is present in natural NP tissue; however, lack of crosslinking limits its regeneration applications. Carbodiimide-crosslinked 3D Col II hydrogel demonstrated good outcomes in NP tissue repair and regeneration (Zhou et al., 2016), as did genipin-crosslinked Col hydrogels for NP tissue regeneration (Zhou et al., 2018). Adipose-derived stem cells loaded with Col hydrogel scaffolds were tested in sheep models to evaluate the therapeutic efficacy in IVD regeneration, and the micro-CT analysis revealed the stabilization of the disc height in the ASC-loaded Col hydrogel scaffold treatment group. However, complete regeneration of IVD could not be achieved (Friedmann et al., 2021).

Similarly, human umbilical cord mesenchymal stem cells in combination with type I Col demonstrated restoration of disc height and better regenerative properties (Yi et al., 2016). Moreover, uniquely crosslinked Col gels are also used to repair ring structure of AF in the IVD (Borde et al., 2014). Aligned Col scaffolds also promoted AF tissue regeneration, and aligning Col in a composite material with alginate regenerated NP (Bowles et al., 2010). Because the aligned Col scaffolds lack sufficient mechanical strength, researchers recently fabricated a polycaprolactone-supported electro-compacted type I Col patch that demonstrated high tensile properties; it demonstrated suitability for AF tissue tissue (Dewle et al., 2021).

18.2.1.5 Gelatin

Gelatin is the hydrolytic degradation product of collagen; it is often developed by processing trash, such as the bones and skin of filleted fish. Depending on its source, gelatin exhibits a variety of physical and chemical characteristics as a natural substance that make it intriguing for a variety of applications (Bello et al., 2020). Due to the excellent water solubility of gelatin, crosslinking is necessary after creating the scaffolds; there are a variety of physical crosslinking techniques, such as UV exposure and dehydrothermal treatment.

Chemical crosslinking includes using glutaraldehyde in the form of a liquid or vapor, ethylcarbodiimide-hydrochloride, coupled with *N*-hydroxysuccinimide, and enzymatic techniques including genipin or transglutaminase treatment. The crosslinking significantly affects the chemical and physical characteristics of the final scaffold. Gelatin nanofibers are most commonly made by electrospinning, and crosslinking modifies the ultrathin fibers' structure, affecting their porosity, mechanical characteristics, and capacity to support cell development (Campiglio et al., 2019; Rebers et al., 2021).

In a recent study, multiply layered aligned gelatin scaffolds with biomechanical and anatomical qualities similar to those typical of indigenous AF lamellae were produced, and they showed enhanced cell proliferation and invasion. The scaffolds provided a critical milieu for inducing collagen fibrous tissue formation inside a native AF defect in a porcine model. Scaffold composed of natural polymer enhanced AF healing and prevented IVD herniation and both neural and vascular ingrowth after discectomy (Hu et al., 2022).

A photo-crosslinkable gelatin-*co*-HA-methacrylate (GelHA) hydrogel was designed to foster the NP alike transformation of encapsulated ASCs for IVD repair. In a rat-tail IVDD model, the ASC-encapsulated GelHA hydrogel differentiated ASCs into NP cells; the combinatorial effect of GelHA hydrogel and ASCs encouraged optimum IVD repair in rats, as shown by a much larger percentage of the NP matrix and substantially greater disc height. In conclusion, coupling the GelHA hydrogel with the ASCs induced NP-like transformation and increased the effectiveness of ASCs for disc repair (Chen et al., 2019). Recently, gelatin-poly (γ-glutamic acid) hydrogel showed potential as an adhesive for repairing annular defects in lumbar discectomy. The developed material acted as sealant to fill the AF tears in a minimally invasive way to restore the mechanical properties of IVD (Yang et al., 2021).

18.2.1.6 Fibrin

Fibrin is a common tissue adhesive consisting of fibrinogen and thrombin; it is a nonimmunogenic and biocompatible biomaterial. It modulates the Ca^{2+}, fibrinogen, and thrombin concentrations that alter the physical properties and the binding capacity of the fibrin. Fibrin may be prepared with 2D or 3D scaffolds or phasic properties to facilitate biological and biochemical interactions for minimizing wound manifestations and enhanced functional repair process.

Numerous therapeutic strategies have been devised to enhance the biomechanical, physical, chemical, and physiological attributes of target tissues in response to impairments in those tissues or to altered physiological conditions (Park & Woo, 2018). A fibrin glue showed tremendous potential for the repair of fibrous lesions in a sheep AF model. It significantly enhanced the sealing action of the surgical sutures for the AF defects under continuous axial loading (Du & Zhu, 2019).

MRI scans of the lower back showed that the discs treated with fibrin glue had more of their NP and physiological hydration intact than did those treated with a placebo. The histomorphological analysis also elicited that the fibrin glue slowed or halted the disc degeneration in the damaged vertebrae. Collectively, fibrin glue and surgical suture on the AF increased sealing and thereby healing and reduced disc deterioration (Du & Zhu, 2019).

A clinical study registered under ClinicalTrials.gov identifier: NCT04621799 in phase 2 and 3 aims to effectively establish intra-annular fibrin infusions as a therapy for chronic multilevel discogenic low back pain. The subjects were injected with nonautologous injections of fibrin, and the authors investigated the variables that could contribute to improving pain. Another pilot study reported on intradiscal injections of fibrin as a sealant for lumbar disc distortion. Patients suffering from persistent discogenic low back pain showed promising, safe, and effective results in this pilot research of intradiscal injections of fibrin sealant (Yin et al., 2014). In another study, genipin-crosslinked fibrin hydrogel showed promise as sealant for AF injury. It has shown the restoration of disc height and regeneration of the AF (Scheibler et al., 2018).

18.2.2 Synthetic Biomaterials

18.2.2.1 Polyethylene Glycol

Polyethylene glycol (PEG) is a chemically synthesized polyether that is biodegradable and water-soluble (Kong et al., 2017). PEG refers to macromolecules with molar mass under 20,000 g/mol, whereas polyethylene oxide (PEO) refers to those with mass more than 20,000 g/mol. PEG macromolecules are available in many formations such as branching, star, and comb-like configurations. PEGylation, where PEG is covalently attached to another polymeric material, is a potential therapeutic approach employed to develop various constructs for IVD repair and regeneration (Zarrintaj et al., 2019).

In prior research, saline and PEG mixtures are helpful in regulating hydration levels. Researchers investigated best solution buffers for stabilizing AF specimen hydration in vitro. This was performed by examining a broad range of concentrations of phosphate-buffered saline and PEG buffer.

Researchers examined the link between alterations in tissue hydration and mechanical response by measuring post-failure mechanics. Finite element analysis (FEA) showed the efficacy of PEG in simulating tissue swelling and biomechanical response in the outer environment (Werbner et al., 2022). Authors of another study applied a PEG adhesive featuring trimethylene carbonate (TMC) with hexamethylene diisocyanate functionalization as a promising option for the repair and restoration of biomechanical function attributed to its injectability, adhesive property, and suitability for annular repair. The PEG–TMC adhesives demonstrated strong adhesive strength, delayed degradation, excellent cytocompatibility, and biomechanical effectiveness for the repair of AF (Long et al., 2018).

Earlier literature has also shown that interactions between NP cells and laminin boost cell adhesion and biogenesis, suggesting that an ideal biomaterial will be effective for fostering or sustaining the NP cell phenotype. Therefore, a hydrogel composed of photo-crosslinkable PEG laminin-111 was constructed. NP cellular metabolism and expression of putative phenotypic biomarkers were found to be influenced by hydrogel formulation, notably upregulation of N-cadherin and cytokeratin-8 seen for cells incubated in the hydrogel were reported (Francisco et al., 2014).

In a different study, applying GRAS (generally recognized as safe) plasticizers at very low saturation concentrations improved the compressive strength of PEG gels (20%). For forming tougher gels, photochemical gelation was revealed to be superior to chemical gelation; however, chemical gelation gave more control and product homogeneity. The gelling temperature of 37 °C developed a 30% glycerol PEG scaffold with the optimum yield strength. Introducing alginate and laponite to gels produced at ambient pressure increased their mechanical performance (Golshan et al., 2019).

18.2.2.2 Poly-E-Caprolactone

PCL is a chemically synthesized bio-degradable polyester authorized for application within the body by the US FDA and European Commission. Due to the considerably slower rate of degradation, the biodegradation of PCL can be controlled via blending with polymers like polyvinyl alcohol (PVA)/PGA. As a biopolymer, PCL is mechanically adaptable and chemically versatile, and it has great elasticity.

Although PCL-based scaffolds are often inserted in a solid state, they may be employed as hydrogels by integrating them with other polymers, allowing them to work effectively for a longer period of time. PCL can associate with natural or manufactured monomers including PEG, poly(acrylic) acid, and poly(N-iso-propyl-acrylamide) to generate di- or triblock amphipathic copolymers (Choi et al., 2019).

Recently, 3D-printed PCL scaffolds to repair AF were developed that resembled the natural tissue's architectural and biomechanical properties. By placing PCL struts in contrast to angular alignments, the angle ply configuration of natural AF tissue was replicated in multilayer scaffolds. Morphological and biomechanical properties of constructed AF cellular metabolic activity, cellular alignment, conformation, and protein expressions were investigated in vitro (Christiani et al., 2019).

Using micro-CT and 3D modeling, the IVD architecture was reverse-engineered, culminating via the application of computer-aided design (CAD) that resembles the native rabbit IVD (Van Uden et al., 2015). Later, a 3D-printed PCL scaffold was prepared with a 100% in-fill density with diverse geometries based on the computer-aided design. Scanning electron microscopy analysis of the microstructure of PCL scaffolds confirmed the appropriate fusion adhesion among layers needed for IVD total disc replacements (Van Uden et al., 2015).

Authors of one recent work aimed to simulate the architectural and biomechanical microenvironment of surrounding AF tissue utilizing scaffolds fabricated from a PCL and PLA synthetic biopolymer composite (PLLA). These frameworks promoted cell survival and alignment, optimal tensile strengths, and the secretion of Col type I (Col-1), the primary constituent of AF tissue (Shamsah et al., 2020). The PCL-based IVD prostheses were fabricated with cell-laden collagen–hyaluronic acid material, demonstrated appropriate mechanical strength, and maintained cell viability (Gloria et al., 2020). Furthermore, growth-factor-releasing 3D-printed PCL and a gelatin–hyaluronic acid–sodium alginate scaffold showed anatomically correct mechanical support for reconstructing (Sun et al., 2021).

18.2.2.3 Polyurethane

Polyurethane (PU) is the oldest, yet most desirable, polymer in the modern period due to the diversity of its characteristics and processing. PU is a synthetically developed polymer composed of urethane groups with biological functionalities and excellent mechanical and physical capabilities, including elastic, tensile, and compressive behavior. Owing to its simple manufacturing, broad formulation control from delicate to stiff, and array of shapes. In the clinical setting, these are employed in designing implants and biodegradable membranes for tissues (Reghunadhan & Thomas, 2017).

Utilizing in situ polymerization and freeze drying, a new polyurethane 3D scaffold with high permeability was constructed for a research study. The scaffolds were characterized in terms of their chemical structure, macrostructure, morphology, and mechanical strength. The findings showed that integrating different development techniques achieved high porosity and interconnecting pores, resulting in PU scaffolds with porosity greater than 70% and pore sizes that ranged from 100 to 800 m (Luo et al., 2020).

A cytocompatible NP substitute material based on PU is also reported that is ideal for noninvasive administration, has a modifiable design and permits the quick biomechanical rehabilitation of IVD. A double-phasic PU scaffold composed of material with spontaneous swelling efficiency and a pliable envelope exhibited cytocompatibility with inherent disc cells. Integrating the scaffolds into an incompletely nucleotomized IVD decreased genetic expression, enhanced proteoglycans and Col-II, and reduced Col-1 density in residual NP tissue, indicating the scaffold's capacity to retard degradation and re-establish the IVD cell phenotype (Li et al., 2016).

Agnol et al. (2019) developed a PU adhesive with minimally invasive properties and in situ polymerizing attributes for AF repair and regeneration. The adhesive was moisture resistant for 18 days and needed 10 h of preparation at 60 °C prior to use. The molecules linked irreversibly to gelatin (without a catalyst or an initiator) had a prominent impact on cell proliferation following polymerization, each of which is crucial for clinical translation. These results verified the PU adhesive's efficacy as an AF sealant (Agnol et al., 2019). Notochord cells are observed in neonates at early development of vertebrae and last up to eleven years of age (Cramer & Bakkum, 2013). These notochordal cells differentiate into IVD cells, which were employed for 3D culture on polyurethane film. The developed polyurethane fibrin composite showed proliferation within the 3D culture of autologous IVD cells (Bono et al., 2010).

18.2.2.4 Polylactide-Co-Glycolic Acid

PLGA is a basic and linear aliphatic polyester. It is a stiff, crystalline substance that is immiscible in the majority of organic solvents. The fibers of this biodegradable polymer demonstrate exceptional strength and modulus. Similar to most polyesters, PLGA may be prepared through extrusion, injections, or compression molding, but they are vulnerable to hydrolytic breakdown; their processing methodologies determine the features and degradation rates of PLGA scaffolds. If taken in high quantities, the breakdown product, glycolic acid—a natural substrate—can lead to the buildup of local acid concentrations that can injure tissue (Shetye et al., 2017).

In a relatively new approach, researchers restored IVD biomechanics, including stabilizing the implants and imparting shock absorption in the form of a 4D-printed disc spacer. This innovative method leverages 4D printing to construct components that may change form over time when subjected to diverse environmental stimuli, such as heat. The thermal expansion and allocation of a 4D-printed PLA framework was explored in a bid to achieve the appropriate shape transformation. (Alief et al., 2019).

An FEA study was also conducted to construct an interbody cage that could be embedded into the spinal column and prevent postoperative repercussions (Salleh et al., 2021). The PLA cage was embedded within the lumbar region (L4 and L5) and was employed to build a 3D model of the spine using 3D Slicer software. The developed 3D model was laden with flexion and extensions, axial rotation, lateral flexion, and compression. The developed cage with 50% infill density was found to be the most suitable design with respect to the permissible extent of stresses created, the predicted printability time (Salleh et al., 2021).

18.3 BIOMATERIALS FOR CARTILAGE END PLATE REPAIR

The cartilage end plate (CEP) includes a bony external plate and a cartilaginous interior plate. It helps in providing the nourishment to the avascular IVD required to stimulate biomechanistic function. Percutaneous vertebroplasty is a clinical technique to repair CEP by injecting PMMA (polymethylmethacrylate) and calcium phosphate cement into the vertebrae (Ikeuchi et al., 2001). Gels are being made from natural polymers such as alginate, hyaluronic acid, Col, elastin, and fibrin and synthetic polymers such as polyurethane, CS, silk–elastin copolymer, Col crosslinked with PEG, and photo-curated PEG and being explored for CEP repair (Tang et al., 2020). Among these, a silk–elastin-derived recombinant protein copolymer as an injectable biomaterial for NP replenishment was developed and commercialized as "Nucore an injectable nucleus" by Spine Wave of USA (Boyd & Carter, 2006).

Scaffold-free tissue-engineered structures provide a cutting-edge approach to cell therapy. The development of scaffold-free structures relies on cell sheet engineering, spheroid cell aggregates, tissue strands, and 3D bioprinting (Table S18.2). Scaffolding entails integrating aggregates into large constructs that are suitable for complex tissues and organs. The primary drawbacks are poor mechanical stability, which can damage the cells, and the initial time required for expansion and ECM production (Ovsianikov et al., 2018).

Cell sheet engineering is a more recent approach to scaffold-free tissue engineering. This method involves embedding a single layer of cells, ion channels, extracellular matrix, growth factor receptors, and other cell surface proteins on thermo-responsive surfaces. The thermo-responsive polymer that is most often adopted is Poly (N-isopropyl acrylamide). This cell sheet engineering was used to reconstruct annulus fibrosus by integrating bone-marrow-derived stem cells (BMSCs). In this, multilayered BMSC sheets were developed on a PDMS surface. Later, the sheets were wrapped in opposite directions, rolled, and chopped to form a multilamellar angle ply tissue representing native annulus fibrosus (Chong et al., 2020).

18.4 SCAFFOLD FABRICATION TECHNIQUES FOR IVD REPAIR AND REGENERATION

Hydrogels and nanofibers are the most common formats of biomaterials utilized for IVD repair and regeneration, largely hydrogels for NP repair and nanofibers for AF repair. The most common techniques for hydrogel fabrication are based on chemical and physical crosslinking at various temperatures and pH. Most of the widely explored hydrogels for augmenting the NP region are injectable; similarly, nanofibrous scaffolds with mimicking architecture and tensile properties of AF tissue have been the benchmark. The major focus of scaffold fabrication for IVD treatment is on reducing the complexity associated with the treatment procedures, which involve injectable and defect-filling materials, in situ fixation, and minimally invasive implantation. These procedures and scaffold formats are discussed in greater detail by Bowles and Setton (2017). Recently, advanced fabrication techniques such as 3D printing have gained much attention for repairing a part of IVD or replacing entire IVD.

18.4.1 3D-Printed Biomaterials for IVD Repair and Regeneration

Additive manufacturing, or 3D bioprinting, is a technique of printing a predefined structure by the successive deposition of layers; the concept is understood in contrast with to the concept of sculpturing, or subtractive manufacturing, where the unwanted part is removed. It is a unique strategy that uses micro-CT or X-ray images of the body to build 3D-structured scaffolds. The scaffolds are prepared with readily available polymers like PLA, PCL, and PEG using techniques like fused deposition model, extrusion, inkjet printing, stereolithography, and selective laser sintering (SLS) (Harmon et al., 2020). In further advancement of the technique, digital light processing is used with UV radiation as a light source (Liang et al., 2021).

Another study reported a combined PLA and a double-network of hydrogel of PEG diacrylate and gellan gum to counter IVDD and restore disc biomechanical function. (Schol & Sakai, 2019). The authors used a 3D-bioprinted biomimetic artificial IVD scaffold that combined various biomaterials, poly(l-lactide)/octa-armed polyhedral oligomeric silsesquioxane fibers produced through electrospinning as the AF material, and gellan gum with PEG diacrylate hydrogel along with BMSCs represented NP material (Zhu et al., 2021). A viscoelastic scaffold was 3D printed with configurable biomimetic mechanics for complete spine motion segment operations using PLA (Figure 18.2).

The mechanical characteristics of the 3D-printed scaffolds were tuned by modulating the porosity of the scaffold. The flexible 3D-printed PLA scaffolds had a slower rate of deterioration and, as a result, greater mechanical stability than conventional PLA scaffolds. The NP cell-seeded 3D-printed flexible PLA scaffolds encouraged matrix formation and physiological mechanical properties. MSCs that were grown on the flexible PLA also anchored to the scaffold showed evidence of fibrocartilaginous differentiation (Marshall et al., 2021).

A native porous interbody fusion device was constructed using 3D printing and selective laser melting. The developed device demonstrated less rigidity, which lessened the stress-shielding effect and offered enough flexibility for tissue development, aiding in the progression of device development for degenerated discs (Tsuang et al., 2023). Thermoplastic polyurethane (TPU) was also used to create a 3D-printed IVD implant with a modified "Bucklicrystal" structure. The implant has a distinctive auxetic architecture with blocks affixed face to face. Its remarkable load-bearing capacity and resilience under compression are attained by ensuring a negative Poisson's ratio (Figure 18.3) (Jiang et al., 2023).

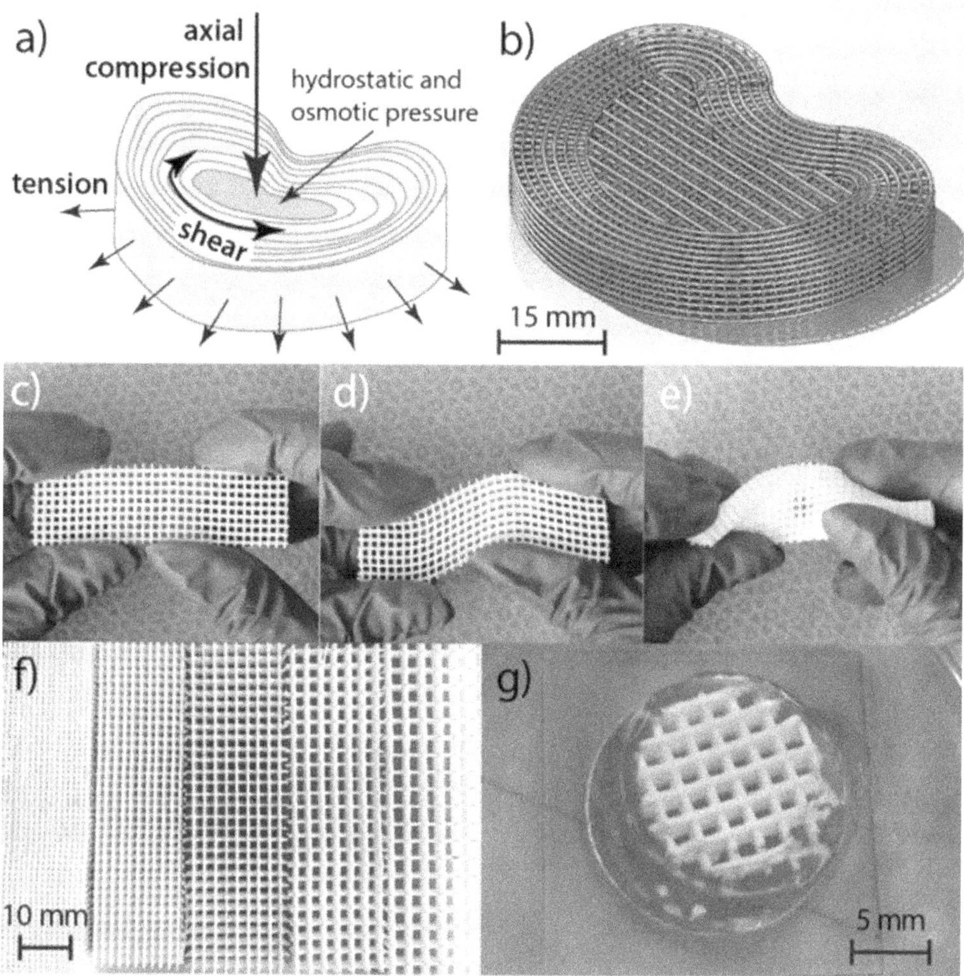

FIGURE 18.2 (a) Schematic showing loading of the intervertebral disc. (b) CAD rendering of a flexible PLA IVD shape. (c–e) Still images extracted from a video showing (c) flexible PLA sheet, (d) bent flexible PLA sheet, and (e) twisted flexible PLA sheet. (f) Flexible PLA scaffolds with different fiber spacing (1, 1.5, 2, 2.5, and 3 mm). (g) Printed 1.5 mm flexible PLA scaffold filled with 1.2% alginate and bovine NP cells (reproduced with permission from Marshall L. S., Jacobsen D. T., Emsbo E., Murali A., Anton K, Liu Z. J., Lu H. H., & Chahine O. N.: Three-Dimensional-Printed Flexible Scaffolds Have Tunable Biomimetic Mechanical Properties for Intervertebral Disc Tissue Engineering. ACS Biomater. Sci. Eng.: 2021. 7. 5836–5849. Copyright 2021 American Chemical Society).

In a recent technique, electrohydrodynamic 3D printing was adopted to produce PCL scaffolds. The structural benefits of the developed scaffolds were validated using FEA. The scaffolds were put together into an AF-like construct to resemble the angle-ply design of the AF lamella. The 3D-printed PCL scaffolds demonstrated good biocompatibility and permitted cellular adhesion and proliferation. In another example, 3D-printed GelMA hydrogel mimicked the NP, contributed to the preservation of disc height, decreased the deficit of NP content, and substantially reinstated the biomechanical functionality of degenerated IVDs after implantation (Liu et al., 2022b).

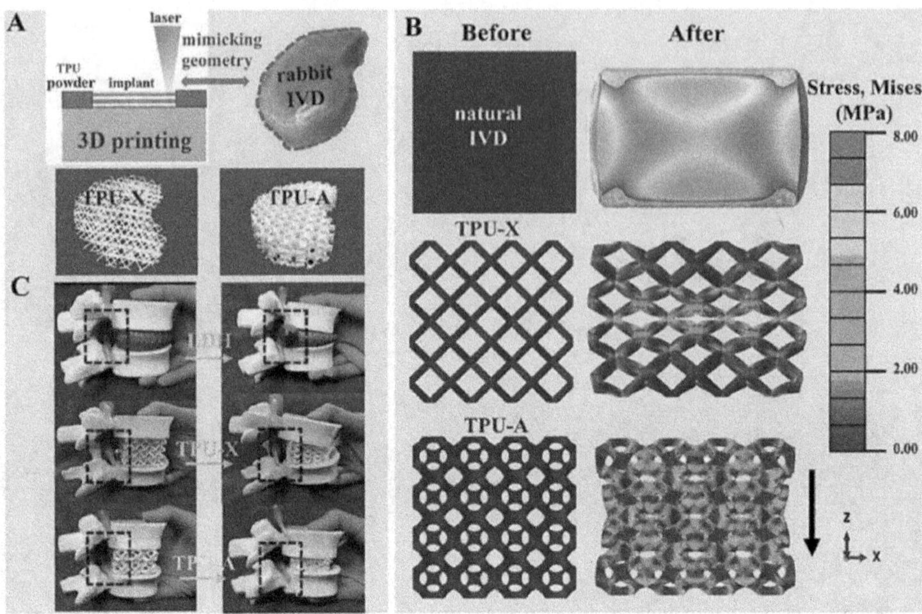

FIGURE 18.3 (A) Schematic illustrating the SLS fabrication process and printed implants with geometry mimicking the rabbit IVD. (B) The stress and deformation distribution within natural IVD, TPU-X, and TPU-A under compression (the mid-sagittal plane of 3D analyses). (C) The behavior of TPU-X and TPU-A under compression using a commercial lumbar disc herniation model (reproduced under the terms of CC-BY 4.0 (https://creativecommons.org/licenses/by/4.0/) International License from Jiang, Y., Shi, K., Zhou, L., He, M., Zhu, C., Wang, J., Li, J., Li, Y., Liu, L., Sun, D., Feng, G., Yi, Y., & Zhang L.: 3D-printed auxetic-structured intervertebral disc implant for potential treatment of lumbar herniated disc, Bioact. Mater.: 2023. 20. 528–538. Copyright 2023 Jiang et al., published by Elsevier).

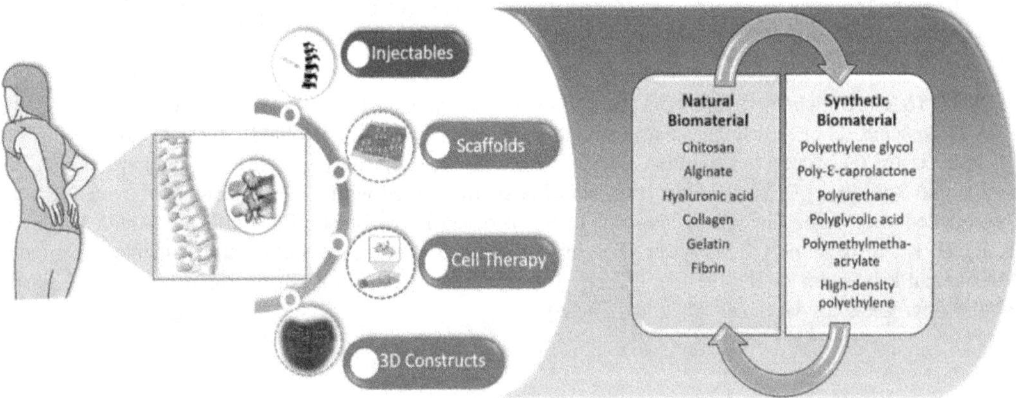

FIGURE 18.4 Biomaterial-based strategies for repairing the nucleus pulposus, annulus fibrosus, and cartilaginous end plate.

CONCLUSION

This chapter summarizes the potential use of biomaterials for the repair and regeneration of IVD. The early success of intervertebral disc repair was modest because early research concentrated only on restoring the degenerated disc structure and disregarded the interaction between cells. Natural polymers such as collagen, hyaluronic acid, gelatin, fibrin and chitosan are the most widely employed, and of these, collagen and hyaluronic acid-based scaffolds hold promise due to their bioactive nature in modulating ECM production and possessing anti-inflammatory properties.

Synthetic biomaterials such as PCL, PEG, PLA, and PLGA have also been utilized for IVD repair, primarily because of their excellent mechanical properties. These materials are easier to process and can mimic the mechanical features of IVD. Several composite materials utilizing synthetic and natural biomaterials are being used to mimic both the mechanical and biological properties of IVD. These materials have been developed in the form of hydrogels, nanofibers, and 3D-printed scaffolds. These scaffolds allow for adding native IVD cells or stem cells and have shown success. Overall, the biomaterial discussed in this chapter can be used in various forms by using specialized fabrication techniques to mimic the mechanical properties while retaining their bioactivity for IVD repair and regeneration.

ACKNOWLEDGEMENTS

I would like to express my deep sense of gratitude toward National Institute of Pharmaceutical Education and Research, Ahmedabad, for its fellowship, infrastructure, and library facilities.

LIST OF ABBREVIATIONS

μ-CT	Micro-Computed Tomography
ADMSC	Adipose Derived Mesenchymal Stem Cells
AF	Annulus Fibrosus
CAD	Computer Aided Design
CEP	Cartilaginous End Plate
COL	Collagen
CS	Chitosan
ECM	Extracellular Matrix
FEA	Finite Element Analysis
GAG	Glycosaminoglycan
GelMA	Gelatin Methacrylate
GF	Growth Factor
HA	Hyaluronic Acid
HA-pNIPAM	Hyaluronic Acid-Poly N-Isopropyl Acrylamide
hMSCs	Human Mesenchymal Stem Cells
IVD	Intervertebral disc
IVDD	Intervertebral Disc Degeneration
MRI	Magnetic Resonance Imaging
MSC	Mesenchymal Stem Cell
NP	Nucleus Pulposus
PCL	Polycaprolactone
PEG	Polyethylene Glycol
PGA	Phospho-Glyceric Acid
PLGA	Poly Lactic-co-Glycolic Acid
PLLA	Poly-L-Lactic Acid
PU	Polyurethane
PVA	Polyvinyl Alcohol
TPU	Thermoplastic Urethane
UPAL	Ultra Purified Alginate
VEGF	Vascular Endothelial Growth Factor
β-TCP	Beta Tricalcium Phosphate

REFERENCES

Adoungotchodo, A., Epure, L. M., Mwale, F., & Lerouge, S. (2021). Chitosan-based hydrogels supplemented with gelatine and link n enhance extracellular matrix deposition by encapsulated cells in a degenerative intervertebral disc environment. *Eur. Cells Mater.* 41: 471–484.

Agnol, L. D., Dias, F. T. G., Nicoletti, N. F., Marinowic, D., Moura e Silva, S., Marcos-Fernandez, A., Falavigna, A., & Bianchi, O. (2019). Polyurethane tissue adhesives for annulus fibrosus repair: Mechanical restoration and cytotoxicity. *J. Biomater. Appl.* 34: 673–686.

Alief, N. A., Supriadi, S., & Whulanza, Y. (2019). Modelling the shape memory properties of 4D printed polylactic acid (PLA) for application of disk spacer in minimally invasive spinal fusion. *AIP Conf. Proc.* 2092.

Alinejad, Y., Adoungotchodo, A., Grant, M. P., Epure, L. M., Antoniou, J., Mwale, F., & Lerouge, S. (2019). Injectable chitosan hydrogels with enhanced mechanical properties for nucleus pulposus regeneration. *Tissue Eng., Part A.* 25: 303–313.

Andriotis, O. G., Desissaire, S., & Thurner, P. J. (2018). Collagen fibrils: Nature's highly tunable nonlinear springs. *ACS Nano.* 12: 3671–3680.

Araiza-Verduzco, F., Rodríguez-Velázquez, E., Cruz, H., Rivero, I. A., Acosta-Martínez, D. R., Pina-Luis, G., & Alatorre-Meda, M. (2020). Photocrosslinked alginate-methacrylate hydrogels with modulable mechanical properties: Effect of the molecular conformation and electron density of the methacrylate reactive group. *Materials.* 13: 2–6.

Bello, A. B., Kim, D., Kim, D., Park, H., & Lee, S. H. (2020). Engineering and functionalization of gelatin biomaterials: From cell culture to medical applications. *Tissue Eng. Part B Rev.* 26: 164–180.

Bono, E., Mathes, S. H., Franscini, N., & Graf-Hausner, U. (2010). Tissue engineering—the gateway to regenerative medicine. *Chimia.* 64: 808–812.

Borde, B., Grunert, P., Hartl, R., & Bonassar, L. (2014). *Method for Repairing Annulus and Collagen Gel Composition* (United States Patent Application Publication).

Bowles, R. D., & Setton, L. A. (2017). Biomaterials for intervertebral disc regeneration and repair. *Biomaterials.* 129: 54–67.

Bowles, R. D., Williams, R. M., Zipfel, W. R., & Bonassar, L. J. (2010). Self-assembly of aligned tissue-engineered annulus fibrosus and intervertebral disc composite via collagen gel contraction. *Tissue Eng., Part A.* 16: 1339–1348.

Boyd, L. M., & Carter, A. J. (2006). Injectable biomaterials and vertebral endplate treatment for repair and regeneration of the intervertebral disc. *Eur. Spine J.* 15: 414–421.

Campiglio, C. E., Negrini, N. C., Farè, S., & Draghi, L. (2019). Cross-linking strategies for electrospun gelatin scaffolds. *Materials.* 12: 2476.

Chen, P., Ning, L., Qiu, P., Mo, J., Mei, S., Xia, C., Zhang, J., Lin, X., & Fan, S. (2019). Photo-crosslinked gelatin-hyaluronic acid methacrylate hydrogel-committed nucleus pulposus-like differentiation of adipose stromal cells for intervertebral disc repair. *J. Tissue Eng. Regen. Med.* 13: 682–693.

Choi, Y., Park, M. H., & Lee, K. (2019). Tissue engineering strategies for intervertebral disc treatment using functional polymers. *Polymers.* 11: 1–25.

Chong, J. E., Santerre, J. P., & Kandel, R. A. (2020). Generation of an in vitro model of the outer annulus fibrosus-cartilage interface. *JOR Spine.* 3: 1–11.

Christiani, T. R., Baroncini, E., Stanzione, J., & Vernengo, A. J. (2019). In vitro evaluation of 3D printed polycaprolactone scaffolds with angle-ply architecture for annulus fibrosus tissue engineering. *Regen. Biomater.* 6: 175–184.

Cramer, G. D., & Bakkum, B. W. (2013). Microscopic anatomy of the zygapophysial joints, intervertebral discs, and other major tissues of the back. In *Clinical Anatomy of the Spine, Spinal Cord, and ANS* (Third Edit). G. D. Cramer, and S. A. Darby, Eds. St. Louis: Elsevier, pp. 586–637.

Dewle, A., Rakshasmare, P., & Srivastava, A. (2021). A polycaprolactone (PCL)-supported electrocompacted aligned collagen type-I patch for annulus fibrosus repair and regeneration. *ACS Appl. Bio. Mater.* 4: 1238–1251.

Doench, I., Tran, T. A., David, L., Montembault, A., Viguier, E., Gorzelanny, C., Sudre, G., Cachon, T., Louback-Mohamed, M., Horbelt, N., Peniche-Covas, C., & Osorio-Madrazo, A. (2019). Cellulose nanofiber-reinforced chitosan hydrogel composites for intervertebral disc tissue repair. *Biomimetics.* 4: 1–17.

Dong, C., & Lv, Y. (2016). Application of collagen scaffold in tissue engineering: Recent advances and new perspectives. *Polymers*. 8: 1–20.

Dou, Y., Sun, X., Ma, X., Zhao, X., & Yang, Q. (2021). Intervertebral disk degeneration: The microenvironment and tissue engineering strategies. *Front. Bioeng. Biotech*. 9: 1–18.

Du, Z. C., & Zhu, L. X. (2019). A heterologous fibrin glue enhances the closure effect of surgical suture on the repair of annulus fibrous defect in a sheep model. *Curr. Med. Sci*. 39: 597–603.

Fallacara, A., Baldini, E., Manfredini, S., & Vertuani, S. (2018). Hyaluronic acid in the third millennium. *Polymers*. 10: 701.

Farokhi, M., Jonidi Shariatzadeh, F., Solouk, A., & Mirzadeh, H. (2020). Alginate based scaffolds for cartilage tissue engineering: A review. *Int. J. Polym. Mater*. 69: 230–247.

Francisco, A. T., Hwang, P. Y., Jeong, C. G., Jing, L., Chen, J., & Setton, L. A. (2014). Photocrosslinkable laminin-functionalized polyethylene glycol hydrogel for intervertebral disc regeneration. *Acta Biomatr*. 10: 1102–1111.

Friedmann, A., Baertel, A., Schmitt, C., Ludtka, C., Milosevic, J., Meisel, H. J., Goehre, F., & Schwan, S. (2021). Intervertebral disc regeneration injection of a cell-loaded collagen hydrogel in a sheep model. *Int. J. Mol. Sci*. 22: 4248.

Gandhi, S. D., Maerz, T., Mitchell, S., Bachison, C., Park, D. K., Fischgrund, J. S., & Baker, K. C. (2020). Intradiscal delivery of anabolic growth factors and a metalloproteinase inhibitor in a rabbit acute lumbar disc injury model. *Int. J. Spine Surg*. 14: 585–593.

Garakani, S. S., Khanmohammadi, M., Atoufi, Z., Kamrava, S. K., Setayeshmehr, M., Alizadeh, R., Faghihi, F., Bagher, Z., Davachi, S. M., & Abbaspourrad, A. (2020). Fabrication of chitosan/agarose scaffolds containing extracellular matrix for tissue engineering applications. *Int. J. Biol. Macromol*. 143: 533–545.

Garcia, C. E. G., Lardy, B., Bossard, F., Martínez, F. A. S., & Rinaudo, M. (2021). Chitosan based biomaterials for cartilage tissue engineering: Chondrocyte adhesion and proliferation. *Food Hydrocoll. Health*. 1: 100018.

Gloria, A., Russo, T., D'Amora, U., Santin, M., De Santis, R., & Ambrosio, L. (2020). Customised multiphasic nucleus/annulus scaffold for intervertebral disc repair/regeneration. *Connect. Tissue Res*. 61: 152–162.

Golshan, A., Curtis, J. A., Lianos, V., Rabbany, S. Y., & De Guzman, R. C. (2019). Compressive strengths of PEG gels with glycerol and bioglass particles. *J. Mater. Res*. 34: 1341–1352.

Harmon, M. D., Ramos, D. M., Nithyadevi, D., Bordett, R., Rudraiah, S., Nukavarapu, S. P., Moss, I. L., & Kumbar, S. G. (2020). Growing a backbone—functional biomaterials and structures for intervertebral disc (IVD) repair and regeneration: Challenges, innovations, and future directions. *Biomater. Sci*. 8: 1216–1239.

Harper, R., & Klineberg, E. (2019). The evidence-based approach for surgical complications in the treatment of lumbar disc herniation. *Int. Orthop*. 43: 975–980.

Hu, M. H., Yang, K. C., Chen, C. W., Chu, P. H., Chang, Y. L., Sun, Y. H., Lin, F. H., & Yang, S. H. (2022). Multilayer electrospun-aligned fibroin/gelatin implant for annulus ibrosus repair: An in vitro and in vivo evaluation. *Biomedicines*. 10: 2107.

Ikeuchi, M., Yamamoto, H., Shibata, T., & Otani, M. (2001). Mechanical augmentation of the vertebral body by calcium phosphate cement injection. *J. Orthop. Sci*. 6: 39–45.

Isa, I. L. M., Abbah, S. A., Kilcoyne, M., Sakai, D., Dockery, P., Finn, D. P., & Pandit, A. (2018). Implantation of hyaluronic acid hydrogel prevents the pain phenotype in a rat model of intervertebral disc injury. *Sci. Adv*. 4: 1–20.

Ji, D., & Kim, J. (2021). Recent strategies for strengthening and stiffening tough hydrogels. *Adv. Nanobiomed. Res*. 1: 2100026.

Jiang, Y., Shi, K., Zhou, L., He, M., Zhu, C., Wang, J., Li, J., Li, Y., Liu, L., Sun, D., Feng, G., Yi, Y., & Zhang, L. (2023). 3D-printed auxetic-structured intervertebral disc implant for potential treatment of lumbar herniated disc. *Bioact. Mater*. 20: 528–538.

Johnson, W. E. B., & Roberts, S. (2003). Human intervertebral disc cell morphology and cytoskeletal composition: A preliminary study of regional variations in health and disease. *J. Anat*. 203: 605–612.

Kong, X. B., Tang, Q. Y., Chen, X. Y., Tu, Y., Sun, S. Z., & Sun, Z. L. (2017). Polyethylene glycol as a promising synthetic material for repair of spinal cord injury. *Neural Regen. Res*. 12: 1003–1008.

Li, Z., Lang, G., Chen, X., Sacks, H., Mantzur, C., Tropp, U., Mader, K. T., Smallwood, T. C., Sammon, C., Richards, R. G., Alini, M., & Grad, S. (2016). Polyurethane scaffold with in situ swelling capacity for nucleus pulposus replacement. *Biomaterials*. 84: 196–209.

Liang, R., Gu, Y., Wu, Y., Bunpetch, V., & Zhang, S. (2021). Lithography-based 3D bioprinting and bioinks for bone repair and regeneration. *ACS Biomater. Sci. Eng*. 7: 806–816.

Lin, J., Shi, Y., Men, Y., Wang, X., Ye, J., & Zhang, C. (2020). Mechanical roles in formation of oriented collagen fibers. *Tissue Eng. Part B Rev*. 26: 116–128.

Liu, Y., He, W., Zhang, Z., & Lee, B. P. (2018). Recent developments in tough hydrogels for biomedical applications. *Gels*. 4: 46.

Liu, Y., Zhao, Q., Chen, C., Wu, C., & Ma, Y. (2022a). B-tricalcium phosphate/gelatin composite scaffolds incorporated with gentamycin-loaded chitosan microspheres for infected bone defect treatment. *PLoS One*. 17: e0277522.

Liu, Z., Wang, H., Yuan, Z., Wei, Q., Han, F., Chen, S., Xu, H., Li, J., Wang, J., Li, Z., Chen, Q., Fuh, J., Ding, L., Wang, H., & Li, B. (2022b). High-resolution 3D printing of angle-ply annulus fibrosus scaffolds for intervertebral disc regeneration. *Biofabrication*. 15: 15015.

Long, R. G., Rotman, S. G., Hom, W. W., Assael, D. J., Illien-Jünger, S., Grijpma, D. W., & Iatridis, J. C. (2018). In vitro and biomechanical screening of polyethylene glycol and poly(trimethylene carbonate) block copolymers for annulus fibrosus repair. *J. Tissue Eng. Regen. Med*. 12: e727–e736.

Luo, K., Wang, L., Chen, X., Zeng, X., Zhou, S., Zhang, P., & Li, J. (2020). Biomimetic polyurethane 3D scaffolds based on polytetrahydrofuran glycol and polyethylene glycol for soft tissue engineering. *Polymers*. 12: 1–12.

Malli, S. E., Kumbhkarn, P., Dewle, A., & Srivastava, A. (2021). Evaluation of tissue engineering approaches for intervertebral disc regeneration in relevant animal models. *ACS Appl. Bio. Mater*. 4: 7721–7737.

Marshall, S. L., Jacobsen, T. D., Emsbo, E., Murali, A., Anton, K., Liu, J. Z., Lu, H. H., & Chahine, N. O. (2021). Three-dimensional-printed flexible scaffolds have tunable biomimetic mechanical properties for intervertebral disc tissue engineering. *ACS Biomater. Sci. Eng*. 7: 5836–5849.

Mesregah, M. K., Repajic, M., Mgbam, P., Fresquez, Z., Wang, J. C., & Buser, Z. (2022). Trends and patterns of cervical degenerative disc disease: An analysis of magnetic resonance imaging of 1300 symptomatic patients. *Eur. Spine J*. 31: 2675–2683.

Ovsianikov, A., Khademhosseini, A., & Mironov, V. (2018). The synergy of scaffold-based and scaffold-free tissue engineering strategies. *Trends Biotechnol*. 36: 348–357.

Park, C. H., & Woo, K. M. (2018). Fibrin-based biomaterial applications in tissue engineering and regenerative medicine. *Adv. Exp. Med. Biol*. 1064: 253–261.

Pupkaite, J., Rosenquist, J., Hilborn, J., & Samanta, A. (2019). Injectable shape-holding collagen hydrogel for cell encapsulation and delivery cross-linked using thiol-Michael addition click reaction. *Biomacromolecules*. 20: 3475–3484.

Ravalli, S., & Musumeci, G. (2021). New horizons of knowledge in intervertebral disc disease. *J. Invest. Surg*. 34: 912–913.

Rebers, L., Reichsöllner, R., Regett, S., Tovar, G. E. M., Borchers, K., Baudis, S., & Southan, A. (2021). Differentiation of physical and chemical cross-linking in gelatin methacryloyl hydrogels. *Sci. Rep*. 11: 1–12.

Reghunadhan, A., & Thomas, S. (2017). Polyurethanes: Structure, properties, synthesis, characterization, and applications. In *Polyurethane Polymers: Blends and Interpenetrating Polymer Networks*. S. Thomas, J. Datta, J. T. Haponiuk, and A. Reghunadhan, Eds. Cambridge: Elsevier, pp. 1–16.

Rosenzweig, D. H., Fairag, R., Mathieu, A. P., Li, L., Eglin, D., Steffen, T., Weber, M. H., Ouellet, J. A., & Haglund, L. (2018). Thermoreversible hyaluronan-hydrogel and autologous nucleus pulposus cell delivery regenerates human intervertebral discs in an ex vivo, physiological. *Eur. Cells Mater*. 36: 200–217.

Russo, F., Ambrosio, L., Peroglio, M., Guo, W., Wangler, S., Gewiess, J., Grad, S., Alini, M., Papalia, R., Vadalà, G., & Denaro, V. (2021). A hyaluronan and platelet-rich plasma hydrogel for mesenchymal stem cell delivery in the intervertebral disc: An organ culture study. *Int. J. Mol. Sci*. 22: 1–14.

Sahoo, D. R., & Biswal, T. (2021). Alginate and its application to tissue engineering. *SN Appl. Sci*. 3: 1–19.

Salleh, N. S. M., Mazlan, M. H., Abdullah, N. S., Ahmad, I. L., Abdullah, A. H., Jalil, M. H. A., Takano, H., & Nordin, N. D. D. (2021). Design and analysis of infill density effects on interbody fusion cage construct based on finite element analysis. *2021 IEEE National Biomedical Engineering Conference (NBEC)*. Kuala Lumpur, Malaysia, pp. 25–29.

Scheibler, A. G., Götschi, T., Widmer, J., Holenstein, C., Steffen, T., Camenzind, R. S., Snedeker, J. G., & Farshad, M. (2018). Feasibility of the annulus fibrosus repair with in situ gelating hydrogels—A biomechanical study. *PLoS One*. 13: 1–15.

Schol, J., & Sakai, D. (2019). Cell therapy for intervertebral disc herniation and degenerative disc disease: Clinical trials. *Int. Orthop*. 43: 1011–1025.

Shamsah, A. H., Cartmell, S. H., Richardson, S. M., & Bosworth, L. A. (2020). Tissue engineering the annulus fibrosus using 3D rings of electrospun PCL: PLLA angle-ply nanofiber sheets. *Front. Bioeng. Biotech*. 7: 1–17.

Shen, Y., Xu, Y., Yi, B., Wang, X., Tang, H., Chen, C., & Zhang, Y. (2021). Engineering a highly biomimetic chitosan-based cartilage scaffold by using short fibers and a cartilage-decellularized matrix. *Biomacromolecules*. 22: 2284–2297.

Shetye, S. S., Miller, K. S., Hsu, J. E., & Soslowsky, L. J. (2017). 7.18 Materials in tendon and ligament repair. *Compr. Biomater. II*. 7: 314–340.

Sloan, S. R., Galesso, D., Secchieri, C., Berlin, C., Hartl, R., & Bonassar, L. J. (2017). Initial investigation of individual and combined annulus fibrosus and nucleus pulposus repair ex vivo. *Acta Biomatr*. 59: 192–199.

Sloan, S. R., Wipplinger, C., Kirnaz, S., Navarro-Ramirez, R., Schmidt, F., McCloskey, D., Pannellini, T., Schiavinato, A., Härtl, R., & Bonassar, L. J. (2020). Combined nucleus pulposus augmentation and annulus fibrosus repair prevents acute intervertebral disc degeneration after discectomy. *Sci. Transl. Med*. 12: eaay2380.

Srivastava, A., Abbah, S. A., Carroll, O., Tiernan, D., Owens, P., Dockery, P., Finn, D., Pandit, A., & Isa, I. L. M. (2016). Modulation of extracellular matrix activity, neurotropic factors and sensory innervation associated pain in intervertebral disc degeneration using a hyaluronic acid hydrogel. *Glob. Spine J*. 6: s-0036–1582591.

Sun, B., Lian, M., Han, Y., Mo, X., Jiang, W., Qiao, Z., & Dai, K. (2021). A 3D-bioprinted dual growth factor-releasing intervertebral disc scaffold induces nucleus pulposus and annulus fibrosus reconstruction. *Bioact. Mater*. 6: 179–190.

Tang, G., Zhou, B., Li, F., Wang, W., Liu, Y., Wang, X., Liu, C., & Ye, X. (2020). Advances of naturally derived and synthetic hydrogels for intervertebral disk regeneration. *Front. Bioeng. Biotech*. 8: 745.

Tsuang, F. Y., Li, M. J., Chu, P. H., Tsou, N. T., & Sun, J. S. (2023). Mechanical performance of porous biomimetic intervertebral body fusion devices: An in vitro biomechanical study. *J. Orthop. Surg. Res*. 18: 1–17.

Tsujimoto, T., Sudo, H., Todoh, M., Yamada, K., Iwasaki, K., Ohnishi, T., Hirohama, N., Nonoyama, T., Ukeba, D., Ura, K., Ito, Y. M., & Iwasaki, N. (2018). An acellular bioresorbable ultra-purified alginate gel promotes intervertebral disc repair: A preclinical proof-of-concept study. *EBioMedicine*. 37: 521–534.

Ura, K., Yamada, K., Tsujimoto, T., Ukeba, D., Iwasaki, N., & Sudo, H. (2021). Ultra-purified alginate gel implantation decreases inflammatory cytokine levels, prevents intervertebral disc degeneration, and reduces acute pain after discectomy. *Sci. Rep*. 11: 1–12.

Uysal, O., Arslan, E., Gulseren, G., Kilinc, M. C., Dogan, I., Ozalp, H., Caglar, Y. S., Guler, M. O., & Tekinay, A. B. (2019). Collagen peptide presenting nanofibrous scaffold for intervertebral disc regeneration. *ACS Appl. Bio. Mater*. 2: 1686–1695.

Van Uden, S., Silva-Correia, J., Correlo, V. M., Oliveira, J. M., & Reis, R. L. (2015). Custom-tailored tissue engineered polycaprolactone scaffolds for total disc replacement. *Biofabrication*. 7: 15008.

Varela-Aramburu, S., Su, L., Mosquera, J., Morgese, G., Schoenmakers, S. M. C., Cardinaels, R., Palmans, A. R. A., & Meijer, E. W. (2021). Introducing hyaluronic acid into supramolecular polymers and hydrogels. *Biomacromolecules*. 22: 4633–4641.

Wang, L., Zhang, H. J., Liu, X., Liu, Y., Zhu, X., Liu, X., & You, X. (2021). A physically cross-linked sodium alginate—Gelatin hydrogel with high mechanical strength. *ACS Appl. Polym. Mater*. 3: 3197–3205.

Werbner, B., Zhou, M., McMindes, N., Lee, A., Lee, M., & O'Connell, G. D. (2022). Saline-polyethylene glycol blends preserve in vitro annulus fibrosus hydration and mechanics: An experimental and finite-element analysis. *J. Mech. Behav. Biomed. Mater*. 125: 104951.

Xie, Y., Kawazoe, N., Yang, Y., & Chen, G. (2022). Preparation of mesh-like collagen scaffolds for tissue engineering. *Mater. Adv*. 3: 1556–1564.

Yamamoto, T., Suzuki, S., Fujii, T., Mima, Y., Watanabe, K., Matsumoto, M., Nakamura, M., & Fujita, N. (2021). Efficacy of hyaluronic acid on intervertebral disc inflammation: An in vitro study using notochordal cell lines and human disc cells. *J. Orthop. Res*. 39: 2197–2208.

Yang, J. J., Lin, Y. Y., Chao, K. H., & Wang, J. L. (2021). Gelatin-poly (γ-glutamic acid) hydrogel as a potential adhesive for repair of intervertebral disc annulus fibrosus: Evaluation of cytocompatibility and degradability. *Spine*. 46: E243–E249.

Yi, W., Yang, D., Cao, H., Li, C., Han, J., Cui, J., Hu, J. F., & Li, T. (2016). Repair of degenerative intervertebral discs in rabbits by human umbilical cord mesenchymal stem cells embedded in type I collagen hydrogel. *Stem Cell Res. Ther*. 1: 53–63.

Yin, W., Pauza, K., Olan, W. J., Doerzbacher, J. F., & Thorne, K. J. (2014). Intradiscal injection of fibrin sealant for the treatment of symptomatic lumbar internal disc disruption: Results of a prospective multicenter pilot study with 24-month follow-up. *Pain Med. (US)*. 15: 16–31.

Zarrintaj, P., Saeb, M. R., Jafari, S. H., & Mozafari, M. (2019). Application of compatibilized polymer blends in biomedical fields. In *Compatibilization of Polymer Blends: Micro and Nano Scale Phase Morphologies, Interphase Characterization, and Properties*. A. R. Ajitha, and S. Thomas, Eds. Cambridge: Elsevier, pp. 511–537.

Zhang, J., Sun, T., Zhang, W., Yang, M., & Li, Z. (2022). Autologous cultured adipose derived mesenchymal stem cells combined with hyaluronic acid hydrogel in the treatment of discogenic low back pain: A study protocol for a phase II randomised controlled trial. *BMJ Open*. 12: e063925.

Zhou, X., Tao, Y., Chen, E., Wang, J., Fang, W., Zhao, T., Liang, C., Li, F., & Chen, Q. (2018). Genipin-cross-linked type II collagen scaffold promotes the differentiation of adipose-derived stem cells into nucleus pulposus-like cells. *J. Biomed. Mater. Res. A*. 106: 1258–1268.

Zhou, X., Tao, Y., Wang, J., Liu, D., Liang, C., Li, H., & Chen, Q. (2016). Three-dimensional scaffold of type II collagen promote the differentiation of adipose-derived stem cells into a nucleus pulposus-like phenotype. *J. Biomed. Mater. Res. A*. 104: 1687–1693.

Zhu, M., Tan, J., Liu, L., Tian, J., Li, L., Luo, B., Zhou, C., & Lu, L. (2021). Construction of biomimetic artificial intervertebral disc scaffold via 3D printing and electrospinning. *Mater. Sci. Eng. C*. 128: 112310.

19 Osteoarthritis Pain and Current Therapeutic Strategies

Erick Orozco Morato and Lakshmi S. Nair

19.1 INTRODUCTION

Osteoarthritis (OA) is a chronic progressive disease that attacks and degrades joints in the body. Obesity and age are two highly associated factors that affect the severity and progression of the disease (Cui et al., 2020). Among all the clinically different arthritis, OA is the most frequently seen, affecting around 300 million people worldwide (Kolasinski et al., 2020). This number is expected to rise as the population continues to age (Barbour et al., 2017; Alliance, 2023). Therefore, continued research to understand the progression, diagnosis and treatment of the disease and associated pain symptoms are of great importance for improving the quality of life of people suffering from OA.

OA typically features different pathologies including but not limited to degeneration of the hyaline cartilage surrounding the joint, bone-on-bone grinding and bone remodeling. This further leads to a decrease in the intra-articular (IA) space, inflammation of the synovium and the new formation of abnormal bone cysts and bone marrow lesions (Haviv et al., 2013; O'Neill & Felson, 2018). Diagnosis of OA is typically based on a combination of clinical, pathological and radiographic evidence (Zhang & Jordan, 2010). However, the primary reason for patients seeking medical aid is pain, and by the time a patient has begun to experience the joint pain, the disease has progressed to a more advanced stage (Glyn-Jones et al., 2015).

While OA might appear as the direct degradation of joint cartilage driven by mechanical forces applied to the affected joints, its pathogenicity is induced by a complex network of mechanical and biological changes, as well as associated risk factors such as age, sex, obesity, injury and genetics (Zhang & Jordan, 2010; Vincent, 2020). The avascular articular cartilage that provides lubrication and proper mobility is made up by chondrocytes and the extracellular matrix (ECM) they produce. The components of the ECM include proteoglycans, collagen and glycosaminoglycans.

Proper mechanical loading of the joints is a key factor in maintaining cartilage homeostasis, as both overloading (obese patient) and deloading (immobilization of a limb) of a joint can lead to decreased or damaged cartilage (Primorac et al., 2020). Dysregulation of the joint can lead to enhanced expression of catabolic enzymes at the joint, such as aggrecanases and matrix metalloproteinases (MMPs). These families of catabolic enzymes target two of the primary components of articular cartilage: aggrecan and type 2 collagen. Loss of these components leads to the early stages of cartilage degeneration and secretion of inflammatory cytokines.

Increased presence of inflammatory cytokines in the synovial fluid leads to the activation and recruitment of macrophages and lymphocytes into the synovium. The breakdown of articular cartilage releases MMPs, activating infiltrating macrophages; this creates a positive feedback loop of cartilage degradation and inflammation at the joint space. As the superficial cartilage layer continues to degenerate from abnormal loading of the joint and the presence of catabolic enzymes and proinflammatory cytokines accumulates, the underlying subchondral bone begins to change. Osteoblast and osteoclast activity is dysregulated, leading to formation of common radiographic middle to late-stage OA pathologies such as cysts, osteophytes and fissures in the subchondral bone.

While this noxious cycle of inflammation and cartilage degeneration are usually the primary painful events that lead patients to seek medical help, that is not always the case (Baker et al., 2010;

DOI: 10.1201/9781003307310-22

Ene et al., 2015; Pearson et al., 2017). There is a discordance between symptomatic and radiographic changes in patients with knee OA. Patients with early OA knee pain may not necessarily present visible radiographic changes such as joint space narrowing or developing osteophytes, or patients who do not present painful symptoms display radiographic changes. This makes the accurate diagnosis and grading of progressive OA somewhat challenging. Therefore, positive diagnosis of OA is based on a combination of pain, swelling, or stiffness with radiographically detected changes to joint morphology (Zhang & Jordan, 2010).

While the damaged articular cartilage in an OA joint lacks nerves and therefore cannot propagate signals of sensitivity or pain, the rest of the tissues surrounding the joint, such as the synovium, ligaments, and subchondral bone, are all highly innervated by nociceptors and therefore are potential sources of the sensitization experienced by patients who suffer from OA. These peripheral nociceptors include nonspecific ion channel receptors such as TRPV1 and voltage-gated sodium channels such as Nav1.7. Activation of these receptors propagates noxious stimuli along the peripheral nervous system, upward to the dorsal root ganglion and then further up to the central nervous system, where the stimuli are interpreted as noxious pain. These peripheral nociceptors also have surface receptors for pro-inflammatory markers, including but not limited to NGF, TNFA, IL6, Substance P and CGRP. Therefore, the inflammatory milieu of the OA joint is not only responsible for cartilage degeneration and remodeling of the joint space, it also leads to inflammation in these peripheral nociceptors that a patient experiences as elevated pain and sensitivity (O'Neill & Felson, 2018; Yu et al., 2022). This chapter will focus on the efficacy and limitations of the current clinical interventions available to manage OA pain.

19.2 OPIOIDS

Opioids have been used as an effective method of inducing analgesia since morphine was first purified in 1803 (Rosenblum et al., 2008). Since then, their use has greatly expanded to treat moderate to severe surgical and chronic pain conditions. Their use has become so widespread that in 2017, over 191 million opioid prescriptions were dispensed in the United States. Opioids work by binding to opioid receptors that are endogenously expressed throughout the peripheral and central nervous system.

Currently, four different opioid receptors (all G-coupled) have been identified: mu (μ), delta (δ), kappa (κ) and opioid receptor like-1. Out of these four opioid receptors, most clinically used opioids induce their analgesic effects by binding to the μ receptor. Once the opioid receptors are activated, they interact downstream with calcium and potassium ion channels, hyperpolarizing the associated nerve and inhibiting neural activity (Al-Hasani & Bruchas, 2011). Common side effects of opioid use include euphoria, sedation, nausea, vomiting, and constipation. However, the most concerning are addiction and respiratory suppression, as most overdose deaths of morphine-like drugs are caused by respiratory arrest (Jamison & Mao, 2015; Inturrisi, 2002).

Gwam et al. (2021) performed a large study that used data from the National Medical Care Survey (NAMCS) to identify and analyze trends in opioid-prescribing practices for patients who suffer from knee OA. The NAMCS data set included all patients (41,389,332) in the United States who visited an outpatient clinic for knee OA treatment between 2007 and 2016. The authors identified that between 2007 and 2016, out of the 41 million patients who visited outpatient clinics, 5.3 million of them (12.8%) were prescribed opioids. There were the most prescriptions in 2013 and 2014, with 23% of patients being prescribed opioids.

Hydrocodone-based opioids are the most commonly prescribed (70.4%), followed by tramadol-based opioids (25.9%), and the remainder comprise formulations including pentazocine, oxycodone, morphine and other codeine-based formulations. The authors noted that this is of particular concern, as there is recent evidence that tramadol has a higher risk of dependency than other opioids. Tramadol also has the side effect of interacting with serotonin and norepinephrine. This places patients who suffer from depression and take selective serotonin reuptake inhibitors at increased risk of seizures induced by tramadol. Overall, this large study by Gwam et al. (2021) emphasize the need for further studies on the safety of opioid prescriptions.

Opioids are typically prescribed to patients who undergo total knee arthroplasty (TKA) for managing postoperative pain; TKA is currently used as a final treatment option for advanced knee OA. Due to the significant side effects of opioids, such as addiction and overdose, there is significant interest in developing alternative therapies that reduce and limit opioid use as a primary method of pain management related to OA.

In a clinical trial, Eckhard et al. (2019) evaluated the viability of reducing post-op opioid use by modifying and optimizing adjuvant treatment of dexamethasone and gabapentin. 160 patients were recruited for the study, with 80 receiving the "old protocol" of 4 mg of dexamethasone daily for two days, 600 mg gabapentin daily for one week, and 80 receiving the "new protocol" of 10 mg dexamethasone daily for two days, 300 mg gabapentin every 8 h for one week. All patients who underwent postsurgical treatment under the "new protocol" had significantly reduced opioid consumption vs the "old protocol" group at 48 h and 78 h post-surgery, but not at 24 h post-surgery. Overall, while this was a small trial, the results show a positive trend in overall reducing opioid consumption by co-administration of other analgesic adjuvants.

19.3 VISCOSUPPLEMENTATION

Hyaluronic acid (HA) is an endogenously secreted polysaccharide found in many tissues such as articular cartilage, synovial fluid, skin and vitreous fluid (Pereira et al., 2018). It is composed of repeating units of glucuronic acid and N-acetyl-d-glucosamine (Schanté et al., 2011). Its molecular weight is variable but can reach between 4000 to 7000 kDa in healthy articular joints (Balazs et al., 1967; Webner et al., 2021). Due to its high solubility in water and high molecular weight, it is also capable of forming highly viscous and injectable hydrogels.

It is this lubricity and viscosity of HA that are thought to provide the necessary lubrication and cushioning for the maintenance of healthy synovial joints (Altman et al., 2015). In osteoarthritic knees, enhanced reactive oxygen species and inflammatory cytokines accumulate at the joint. These inflammatory markers reduce HA concentrations and molecular weights to almost half of the healthy levels, therefore reducing its lubricating capabilities (Balazs et al., 1967; Band et al., 2015; Legre-Boyer, 2015). This decrease in the functional capabilities of HA has been correlated with OA joint pain and disease progression (Sudha & Rose, 2014). This has therefore, become a key target for treating the pain associated with the OA (Band et al., 2015). By injecting supplemental HA into the affected joint, the goal is to directly address the diminished lubricity and enhanced inflammation and pain experienced at the arthritic joint (Nicholls et al., 2018).

Nicholls et al. (2018) recently evaluated the rheological characteristics of clinically approved HA preparations and human synovial fluid to determine which formulation is more representative of healthy human synovial fluid. Of the selected products, Hyalgan®, Supratz®, Orthovisc® and Euflexxa® are all linear HA formulations with molecular weights (mw) ranging from 500 to 3600 kDa. The HA preparations Monovisc®, Gel-One®, Synvisc® and Synvisc-One® are all crosslinked HA formulations with generally larger molecular weights (1000–6000 kDa). In healthy knee joints, HA has a linear chained structure, with mw between 5000–6000 kDa. Of the linear chained formulations, Euflexxa® (2400–3600 kDa) comes closest to the mw of HA in healthy synovial fluid, while of the crosslinked options, Synvisc® and Synvisc-One® (6000 kDa) are most similar to healthy HA (Table 19.1).

TABLE 19.1
Rheological Properties of Clinically Used Intra-Articular Hyaluronic Acid Formulations

Product	Mw (kDa)	Crosslinking	Zero Shear Rate Viscosity ($\eta_{0.1}$ (Pa sec))	Shear Thinning Ratio ($\eta_{0.1}/\eta_{250}$)	Crossover Frequency (Hz)
Hyalgan®	500–730	No	0.27	2.33	>10[e]
Supartz®	620–1170	No	3.07	10.9	3.98
Monovisc®	1000–2900[a]	Yes	56.4	51.5	2.51
Orthovisc®	1000–2900	No	120.8	170.4	0.16
Euflexxa®	2400–3600	No	91.2	237.2	0.10
Gel-One®	N/A[c]	Yes	190.2	243.0	[b]
Synvisc®	6000[d]	Yes	191.7	740.7	<0.01[e]
Synvisc-One®	6000[d]	Yes	184.4	651.2	<0.01[e]

[a] Molecular weight of the monomer used, not the crosslinked product; [b] not observed; [c] not reported as formulation is highly crosslinked; [d] only reflective of the soluble portion; [e] extrapolated.

To evaluate the formulations' capacity to resist deformation under long-term load, Nicholls et al. (2018) analyzed the zero shear rate viscosity of the above-mentioned formulations. Only Supratz®, Monovisc®, Orthovisc® and Euflexxa® fell within the range of HA in healthy joints (from 1 to 175 Pa sec). The authors also measured the shear thinning ratio, which indicates how the viscosity of the product changes under strain. Euflexxa®, Gel-One®, and Orthovisc® were most similar to the values reported for healthy knee synovial fluid based on their shear thinning ratio. Synvisc® and Synvisc-One® had shear thinning ratios much higher than that of healthy synovial fluid.

The authors also studied the crossover frequency of these HA formulations; this parameter represents the changes in the viscoelastic properties of synovial fluid as a person shifts from walking to running motions. The results indicated that the crosslinked formulations only exhibit elastic properties, therefore functioning unlike endogenous HA. Overall, Nicholls et al. concluded that Euflexxa® and Orthovisc®, linear HA formulations, were the clinically available formulations that most accurately recapitulated the viscoelastic properties and molecular weights of healthy synovial fluid (Nicholls et al., 2018).

While IA injections of hyaluronic acid (IAHA) are a very commonly used technique to treat OA joint pain, the overall efficacy remains controversial (Pereira et al., 2022). In fact, there is no clear consensus between the major clinical academies. For example, the American Academy of Orthopaedic Surgeons and the American College of Rheumatology currently do not recommend or recommend against the use of IAHA injections (Kolasinski et al., 2020; American Academy of Orthopaedic Surgeons, 2021). On the other hand, the Osteoarthritis Research Society International and the European Society for Clinical and Economic Aspects of Osteoporosis, Osteoarthritis and Musculoskeletal Diseases (ESCEO), respectively, conditionally and weakly recommend the use of IAHA injections in their most recent clinical guidelines (Bannuru et al., 2019; Bruyère et al., 2019). ESCEO, in its most recent guidelines, states that while IAHA has shown efficacy in several meta-analyses, there is a wide range of heterogeneity in the clinical trial evidence. This discrepancy in clinical evidence might be due to differences in HA products used, which vary in molecular weight and crosslinking (Bruyère et al., 2019).

In 2020, Hummer et al. (2020) conducted a network meta-analysis to directly evaluate the efficacy of high- vs low-molecular-weight IAHA in reducing knee OA pain. The authors selected 14 RCTs encompassing 2796 patients and evaluated high- (at least 6000 kDa) vs low-molecular-weight (less than 750 kDa) IA knee HA injections. To analyze these RCTS, the authors employed a Bayesian network meta-analysis of indirect treatment comparisons in order to evaluate the effectiveness of the following treatments: high- and low-molecular-weight IAHA, IA corticosteroids, conventional therapy and IA placebo.

The selected primary endpoint was the effect size on reported pain scores. When compared against placebo, the low-molecular-weight IAHA injections improved pain scores but not to a statistically significant degree vs placebo. Conversely, high-molecular-weight IAHA did show statistical significance against placebo, with possible clinical significance as well. High molecular weight IAHA also provided enhanced pain relief when compared to low molecular weight IAHA; however, the results were not statistically or clinically significant. Overall, the authors conclude that OA knee pain is reduced by the high molecular weight IAHA and that the negative recommendations of IAHA might be caused by the combination of low and high molecular weight IAHA injection in previous clinical trials (Hummer et al., 2020).

More recently, Pereira et al. (2022) conducted a larger meta-analysis of 24 clinical trials that included 8997 patients. The primary goal of the study was to evaluate the efficacy of IAHA injections to reduce OA knee pain and improve joint function and the safety of each intervention. The authors used a DerSimonian–Laird random-effects model to analyze the clinical data using standard mean differences (SMD) with 95% confidence intervals and selected SMD of −0.37 to indicate minimal clinical significance.

The clinical trials included in this meta-analysis used both low and high molecular weights, as well as linear and crosslinked IAHA preparations. The primary outcome of pain intensity was that the patients who received IAHA injections experienced only a small, non-clinically relevant reduction in pain intensity (SMD −0.08). A similar, nonsignificant improvement was seen in functional improvements in the patients who received IAHA (SMD −0.11). Lastly, the authors identified statistically significant increases in adverse effects (e.g., hospital admission, prolonged hospital stay) in patients receiving IAHA injections vs placebo. These study findings do not support the broad use of IAHA injections to treat knee OA (Pereira et al., 2022).

Like HA, IA corticosteroids are clinically used to treat OA joint pain. Maia et al. (2019) performed a small clinical trial (44 patients) to evaluate the effectiveness of IA injections of hyaluronic acid, dexamethasone (Dex) or a combined treatment of HA and Dex to mitigate OA pain and improve knee proprioception. The patients screened for this study were all 50 years and older, with diagnosed stage 2+ OA based on Kellgren–Lawrence radiographic evidence, and were subdivided into one of three treatment groups: HA (Orthovisc®, three doses in a single shot), HA & Dex (three Orthovisc® doses in a single shot & 4 mg Dex) and Dex (Dex 4 mg).

Patients were evaluated for proprioception and WOMAC score at six weeks, three months and six months post injection. The HA group demonstrated improved knee pain, stiffness and function based on the WOMAC scale, as well as enhanced knee flexion and extension strength for up to six months post-injection. Neither Dex nor HA & Dex showed significant improvement in these parameters. None of the parameters reflected improved knee proprioception throughout the study. The authors postulated that the improved knee strength might have been because patients could properly perform physical therapy due to their decreased joint pain. While this paper presents some interesting direct comparisons at up to six months post-injection of HA and Dex, it is limited based on the small sample size (Maia et al., 2019).

Overall, while the efficacy of joint viscosupplementation remains controversial, it is evident that further investigation and clinical trials are needed that specifically focus on understanding the effects that molecular weight and crosslinking of HA can have on pain and functional outcomes.

19.4 INTRA-ARTICULAR CORTICOSTEROIDS

As with IA HA injections, the primary goal of IA corticosteroid (IACS) injections is to reduce the pain caused by the cartilage degradation and inflammation experienced at the affected joint. In fact, IACS injections are the most commonly prescribed first treatment intervention, with around 25% of all patients who suffer from OA pain receiving IACS (Dysart et al., 2021; Bedard et al., 2018).

Even though IACS injections are frequently used, there remains some debate regarding their ability to modulate joint pain effectively.

Clinical studies have shown varied efficacy of pain reduction from IACS injections. Common factors that appear to indicate enhanced efficacy include (healthy) body weight, early/less severe disease progression and reduced inflammation at the joint (Guermazi et al., 2020). Some of the most prescribed CS for IA injections are methylprednisolone acetate, triamcinolone hexacetonide and triamcinolone acetonide (TA).

Typically, the dosage used for knee IA injections ranges from 20 to 80 mg, and they tend to provide pain relief for a period varying between 4 and 24 weeks, regardless of the CS used (Martin & Browne, 2019; da Costa et al., 2016), possibly for some of the reasons we have already discussed. However, IACS injections also carry counter-indications that attending physicians must account for when considering CS for their patients, such as increased rate of OA progression, reduced healing of subchondral fractures, enhanced osteonecrosis and bone loss (Kompel et al., 2019).

Charnwichai et al. (2023) evaluated potential side effects on articular cartilage in OA patients who received knee IA injections of TA or HA. Articular cartilage samples were collected from patients who had previously received one of three treatments six months before TKA: TA, HA or no injection. These patients were all diagnosed with Kellgren–Lawrence grade 3 or 4 OA. Cartilage samples were fixed and stained with hematoxylin and eosin. Sections were also subjected to alcian blue to evaluate proteoglycan levels in the cartilage, while TUNEL assay staining was performed to evaluate the degree of chondrocyte apoptosis. Histological analysis of the cartilage sections revealed no significant differences in cartilage thickness, proteoglycan or degree of apoptosis between TA and HA joints. These studies may aid medical practitioners in selecting the most appropriate IA injection depending on the patients' specific symptoms of knee OA (Charnwichai et al., 2023).

As mentioned previously, while IACS can reduce knee OA pain, patient response is inconsistent. To improve patient outcomes, Wu et al. (2023) investigated what potential factors could be used as predictors of positive response to IACS injections in patients suffering from knee OA. The authors utilized publicly available data from 4796 patients from the Osteoarthritis Initiative database. Patients included in this study had received at least one IACS injection in one or both of their knees within the first five years of follow-up after the IACS injection; this left a total of 385 patients included in the analysis.

The authors studied the following six variables for analysis as predictors of positive IACS response: BMI, baseline WOMAC pain score, stiffness, disability score and previous use of analgesics. Out of all of the investigated parameters, baseline WOMAC pain score had the most significant association with a positive response to IACS treatments, specifically scores of 5 and higher. However, the authors caution that in order to develop a more accurate predictive model, larger-scale RCTs are still required (Wu et al., 2023).

To reduce the local adverse reactions of multiple IACS injections and prolong the pain relief efficacy of a single injection, extended-release (ER) formulations of these CS are currently being developed and used in the clinic. Zilretta® is a current clinically approved ER formulation for the localized delivery of encapsulated triamcinolone acetonide in a biodegradable PLGA microsphere carrier. Clinical trials of the microsphere ER-TA formulation provided encouraging results for the localized and controlled delivery of corticosteroids. When comparing single injections of ER-TA to free crystalline (CS) TA, Zilretta® showed enhanced residency time in knee synovial fluid (12 weeks vs 6 weeks), indicating the capability of controlled and sustained release of TA at the intra-articular space (Kraus et al., 2018).

A phase 3 trial was conducted to evaluate the efficacy of Zilretta® in modulating OA knee pain compared with placebo and TA. Conaghan et al. (2018) reported that a single injection of Zilretta® provided significant relief from daily pain intensity vs placebo for up to 12 weeks. While no significant differences were identified when comparing Zilretta® vs CS-TA in daily pain intensity, when looking at the WOMAC scores for pain and physical function, Zilretta® showed significant improvement vs CS-TA. Patients who received Zilretta® also reported significant improvements in

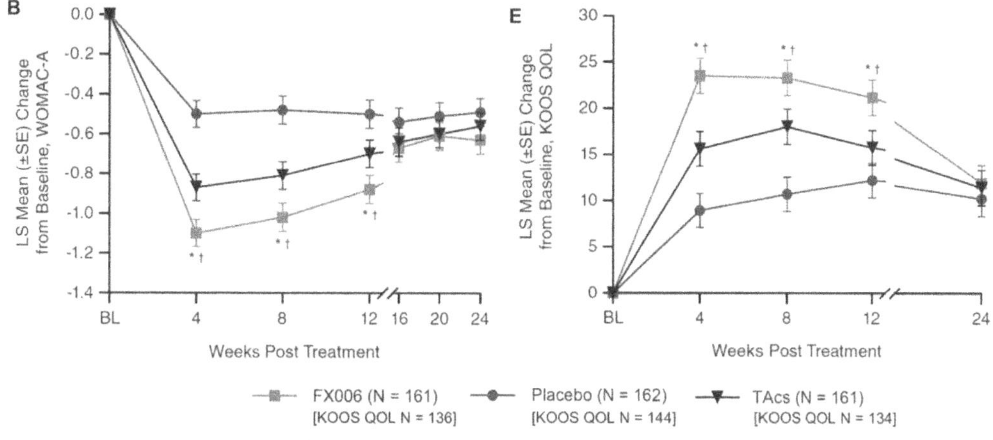

FIGURE 19.1 WOMAC-A (pain) scores for patients receiving Zilretta® (FX006), Placebo, or CS-TA (TAcs) injections (B). KOOS Quality Of Life scores for patients receiving Zilretta® (FX006), Placebo, or CS-TA (TAcs) injections (E). (Reproduced with permission from Conaghan, P. G., Hunter, D. J., Cohen, S. B., Kraus, V. B., Berenbaum, F., Lieberman, J. R., Jones, D.G., Spitzer, A.I., Jevsevar, D.S., Katz, N.P., Burgess, D.J., Lufkin, J., Johnson, J. R., & Bodick, N.: Effects of a single intra-articular injection of a microsphere formulation of triamcinolone acetonide on knee osteoarthritis pain: a double-blinded, randomized, placebo-controlled, multinational study. J. Bone Joint Surg. Am. 2018. 100. 666–677. Copyright 2018 Wolters Kluwer Health, Inc.)

quality of life based on KOOS scale vs CS-TA at the 12-week timepoint (Figure 19.1) (Conaghan et al., 2018).

The safety and efficacy of multiple injections of Zilretta® was also evaluated (Spitzer et al., 2019). In this clinical study, the authors observed that the majority of patients requested a second injection of Zilretta® four months after the first injection, with no adverse effects such as inflammation, infection or radiographic degeneration of the joint detected at the one-year evaluation (Spitzer et al., 2019). This time point is of key importance, as current clinical practice indicates that patients should not receive more than three or four CS injections every 12 months (Martin & Browne, 2019). Current CS-TA provides pain relief for as little as two as four weeks, meaning a patient receiving traditional CS-TA might not be able to receive enough injections per year to manage their pain based on current guidelines. This makes extended-release CS formulations a more clinically favorable therapeutic approach for patients who suffer from arthritic joint pain.

TLC599 is a novel liposomal formulation for the extended release of dexamethasone sodium phosphate to treat OA pain. This formulation is still under development, and phase 2a clinical trial data was recently published (Hunter et al., 2022). The authors evaluated the effects of 12 mg and 18 mg doses of TLC599 over 24 weeks vs placebo. The 72 patients enrolled in this study were all diagnosed with Kellgren–Lawrence grade 2 or 3 OA and self-reported pain scores of 5–9 out of 10.

Patients received a single IA injection of the low-dose (12 mg) TLC, high-dose (18 mg) TLC or placebo (saline) injection into the selected arthritic knee joint. The high-dose TLC formulation did not display a statistically significant pain-relieving effect compared to placebo. However, the low-dose TLC showed significant analgesic efficacy over a placebo for up to 24 weeks (Hunter et al., 2022). The lack of analgesic effect of the higher dose was presumably due to the significant reduction in the rate of Dex release, although the mechanism is still not fully understood. Overall, this indicates that TLC599 is a promising new single-dose analgesic formulation to treat OA pain. Currently, a phase 3 clinical trial for TLC599 has been completed, but the researchers have not yet published any data (https://clinicaltrials.gov/study/NCT04123561).

19.5 LOCAL ANESTHETICS

Local anesthetics (LAs) are incredibly potent pain-modulating drugs that trace their origins back thousands of years to the coca leaf of Peru (Biondich & Joslin, 2016). After the successful isolation of cocaine in 1859, it quickly became widely used in dental and ophthalmological surgery due to its potent anesthetic effects. However, by the 1890s, its negative side effects on the cardiovascular system and the effect of addiction paved the way for the development and discovery of synthetic alternatives (Bhimana & Bhimana, 2018).

The LA molecular structure is based on three small components: an aromatic ring, an intermediate link and a tertiary amine end. LAs are then classified based on what type of intermediate link they possess, amide or ester. Cocaine, the first isolated local anesthetic, as well as procaine and benzocaine are all part of the ester family of LAs; this class is quickly metabolized in the bloodstream by pseudocholinesterase, which also produces the byproduct of para-aminobenzoic acid, the main causative agent of allergic reactions to local anesthetics. Lidocaine, ropivacaine and bupivacaine among others are all amide LAs that, unlike the ester LAs, are metabolized in the liver. This localized degradation of amide LAs increases their duration of action and reduces the possibility of allergic reactions (Wadlund, 2017).

LAs provide anesthetic and analgesic effects by preventing the activation of peripheral nociceptors, which occurs because the LA binds to voltage-gated sodium channels. This in turn inhibits the activation of the channel, and the generation of an action potential in response to a painful stimulus. While these small molecules are incredibly useful in preventing and reducing peripheral pain sensation, they suffer from short duration of relief; for example, lidocaine and bupivacaine can induce anesthesia for a period lasting between 2 h and 8 h.

To prolong this anesthetic effect, LAs are commonly injected with minute amounts of vasoconstrictors such as epinephrine in order to reduce diffusion of the drug away from the area of interest (Butterworth, 2009; Butterworth et al., 2018). An important consideration that has been extensively studied preclinically is LA-induced chondrotoxicity. Kreuz et al. (2018) conducted a systematic analysis of in vitro and ex vivo studies that included both animal and human chondrocytes exposed to various local anesthetics, including but not limited to lidocaine, ropivacaine and bupivacaine. The authors concluded that all local anesthetics present with both time, and dose dependent chondrotoxicity.

Jayaram et al. (2019) identified the same results as Kreuz did, in which chondrotoxicity was induced in a time- and dose-dependent manner. This systematic review, however, focused solely on studies that evaluated LA chondrotoxicity on human knee articular cartilage. The authors of both the studies concluded that while the results linked LA to chondrotoxicity, the studies involved are in vitro work, so the in vivo mechanism is still not completely understood (Kreuz et al., 2018; Chen et al., 2013).

A retrospective study was conducted by Buchko et al. (2015) to evaluate the postoperative chondrotoxic effects of local anesthesia in humans. Patients ($n = 105$) undergoing ACL reconstructive surgery aged 25.5 ± 8.6 years old, with no reported history of previous knee injury, articular damage or surgical repair were selected. One group of patients received a 48 h continuous infusion of bupivacaine via pain pump (IAPP), and the second group were without pain pump (control). Both groups received a single IA injection of bupivacaine or lidocaine at the end of the surgery.

While the control groups did not show chondrolysis, 28% (13/46) of patients in the IAPP group developed chondrolysis. In addition, LAs showed dose-dependent effects on the extent of chondrolysis. For instance, 0.5% bupivacaine via IAPP showed significantly higher incidence of chondrolysis than 0.25% bupivacaine. Even though the authors did not examine the effects of single versus multiple injections of LA on chondrolysis, the findings showed the dose-dependent chondrotoxicity of LAs. In conclusion, the authors recommended continuous intra-articular LA infusions (Buchko et al., 2015).

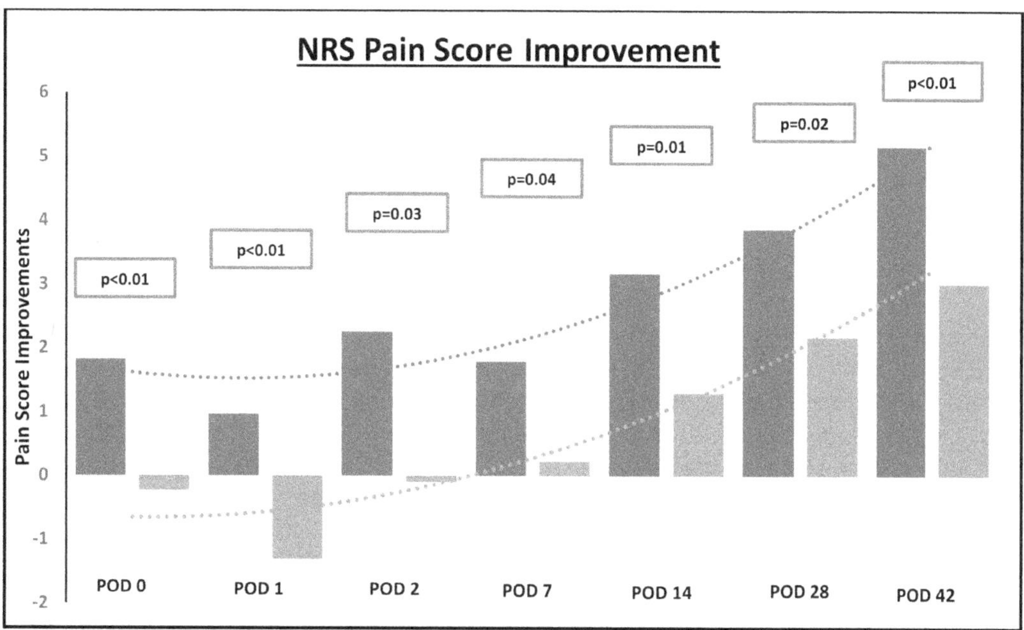

FIGURE 19.2 Patient reported pain scores using a numerical rating scale. Scores were recorded from post-op day (POD) 0 to 42. Exparel® (blue bars) provides significant improvement in pain outcomes from POD0 to POD42 compared with control (green bars) (reproduced with permission from Malige, A., Pellegrino, A. N., Kunkle, K., Konopitski, A. K., Brogle, P. J., & Nwachuku, C. O.: Liposomal bupivacaine in adductor canal blocks before total knee arthroplasty leads to improved postoperative outcomes: a randomized controlled trial. J. Arthroplasty. 2022. 37. 1549–1556. Copyright 2022 Elsevier).

Similar to Zilretta®, Exparel® is a clinically approved biomaterial-based extended-release formulation composed of multivesicular liposomal bupivacaine. In preclinical animal studies, Exparel® showed reduced chondrotoxicity in vitro and in vivo when compared with free bupivacaine solution, directly addressing one of the drawbacks of LA therapy (Shaw et al., 2018; Farmer et al., 2020). The focus of clinical data on the pain relief efficacy of Exparel® appears to be its value as a pre- or post-operative TKA anesthetic. For example, Malige et al. (2022) published RCT results in which patients received Exparel® or ropivacaine adductor canal block as a presurgical injection before TKA. The results were highly encouraging, as patients who received the Exparel® injection reported decreased hospital stay postsurgery, decreased opioid use and overall decrease in postsurgical pain (Figure 19.2).

A different clinical study conducted by Lonza et al. (2023) corroborates the advantages of liposomal bupivacaine for pain management. The authors evaluated the reported pain scores of patients who received liposomal bupivacaine vs continuous nerve block with pain pump delivering bupivacaine solution and reported no significant differences in pain scores for up to 72 h postsurgery, in morphine use, or in length of stay post-surgery. The liposomal bupivacaine showed significant improvements: ease of administration, reduced catheter-associated complications and significant cost savings to the patient and hospital (Lonza et al., 2023).

While studies provide encouraging support for the use of liposomal bupivacaine, there is still some controversy regarding its enhanced efficacy compared with that of more traditional anesthetic injections. In a recent meta-analysis, Chen et al. (2023) compared the effectiveness of liposomal bupivacaine vs bupivacaine periarticular injections in patients undergoing TKA. The authors identified a significant decrease in morphine use in patients who received liposomal bupivacaine vs traditional anesthetic injections within the first 48 h postsurgery. However, when the authors looked at other important factors such as post-op pain score, nausea and length of hospital stay, no significant differences were detected between the patients who received liposomal bupivacaine and traditional anesthetic injections.

To evaluate the clinical efficacy of Exparel® for postsurgical TKA, Feng et al. (2021) compared Exparel® to traditional bupivacaine injections. Patients were divided into two treatment groups, given either periarticular Exparel® or periarticular 0.25% bupivacaine injections following the surgery. A total of 1,677 patients around 65 years old were enrolled in this study.

The authors evaluated the efficacy of the treatments based on patients' self-reported verbal rating scale (VRS) pain scores, quantity of morphine milligram equivalents and postoperative function (AM-PAC). When comparing Exparel® vs traditional bupivacaine treatment, Feng et al. (2021) detected no significant differences in VRS pain scores, opioid use or AM-PAC functional assessment were identified measured at 72 h, 96 h and 24 h postsurgery. the authors concluded that the increased clinical cost of using Exparel® over traditional bupivacaine injections was not justified. The evidence is clearly still conflicting regarding the efficacy and benefits of using sustained-release local anesthetic formulations to treat OA and postoperative pain. However, due to the high chondrotoxicity, and short window of efficacy, of LAs, their the continued development and optimization of sustained release formulations is of great value to the clinical setting.

An alternative therapeutic strategy to address the short anesthetic window, and chondrotoxicity of local anesthetic is the use of a genicular nerve block. This approach utilizes ultrasound guidance to precisely administer targeted local anesthetic injections to the main nerve branches that innervate the knee. The primary nerve is the genicular nerve, which branches off to the superolateral genicular nerve (SLGN), the superomedial genicular nerve (SMGN) and the inferomedial genicular nerve (IMGN). These nerve branches are the most commonly targeted locations for GNB (Yasar et al., 2015).

Recently, Shanahan et al. (2023) reported the results of a small clinical trial where they compared the effect of GNB using 0.5% bupivacaine injections vs placebo saline over 12 weeks. In their study, patients received three US-guided perineural injections at the SLGN, SMGN and IMGN branches of the genicular nerve and were followed up for pain assessment for 12 weeks. Physical function and pain score as measured by VAS and WOMAC scores improved significantly for the entire 12 weeks of the study; scores improved two weeks post injection with a diminishing (yet significant) effect for the remaining period of the study (Shanahan et al., 2023).

19.6 PLATELET-RICH PLASMA

Platelet-rich plasma (PRP) injections have been an area of great interest for treating OA over the past 20 years. PRP is a blood product that through its autologous nature has reduced risk of inducing allergic reactions. The preparation of PRP is relatively simple: Whole blood is centrifuged for a short period of time to pellet down red blood cells. This allows for reconstituting platelets in the plasma at higher concentrations than those found endogenously in blood (Jayaram et al., 2023).

PRP is rich in bioactive molecules such as insulin-like growth factor, vascular endothelial growth factor, and platelet-derived growth factor among many others; it also secretes potent anti-inflammatory modulators such as IL1, TNF-R and IL10. These signaling molecules make PRP a target of great interest as a treatment for OA as they are involved in a multitude of signaling pathways with anti-inflammatory, chondroprotective and chondrogenic effects (Xie et al., 2014).

The efficacy of IA PRP injections vs saline injections was evaluated in a randomized clinical trial by Bennell et al. (2021). The trial encompassed 288 patients with Kellgren-Lawrence grade 2 or 3 symptomatic OA. These patients received three weekly IA PRP injections of leukocyte-poor PRP, or saline, and were evaluated over a 12 month period. Injected PRP was prepared using a commercial product by Regen Lab.

The primary outcomes of this study were changes in knee pain and medial tibial cartilage volume. At the 12 month evaluation, patients who received PRP injections had no statistically significant improvement in reported knee pain or measured medial tibial cartilage volume loss when compared with saline injections. Potentially influencing factors such as body mass index, presence of knee effusion at time of injection or degree of OA severity were accounted for and did not affect the outcome measurements. The authors concluded that based on the evidence of this clinical trial, the use of IA PRP injections for knee OA is not supported. However, they also mentioned that these results were inconsistent with other reported clinical trials that have identified significant benefits when PRP injections compared to placebo. The authors postulated that these differences might be caused by injection regiment, outcome measurements or preparation technique of the PRP itself (Bennell et al., 2021).

Typically, PRP is subcategorized based on the degree of leukocytes present in plasma. Leukocyte-poor plasma (LP-PRP) contains equal or lower levels of leukocytes than whole blood, whereas leukocyte-rich plasma (LR-PRP) contains higher levels of leukocytes than whole blood. Currently, there is no consensus or specific formulation of PRP that provides optimal results for knee OA treatment; therefore, further investigation and optimization are required.

To address this question, Jayaram et al. (2023) recently conducted a study that focused on identifying and characterizing differences in mediators of pain and inflammation within LP-PRP and LR-PRP human samples. The authors collected blood samples and isolated LP and RP PRP from six male and six female patients suffering from Kellgren-Lawrence OA grade 2. These samples were then subjected through a Luminex panel to evaluate changes in inflammatory mediators such as TNFA, IL1B, MMP9, IL1Ra, IL4, IL6 IL8 and IL10.

To evaluate changes in modulators of nociceptive pain, the authors also measured changes in nerve growth factor (NGF) and tartrate resistant acid phosphatase 5 (TRAP5). Their results revealed that LR-PRP expressed more IL1Ra, IL4, IL8 and MMP9 than did LP-PRP. The authors detected no significant differences between TNFA, IL1B, IL6, IL10, NGF or TRAP5 expression between LR-PRP and LP-PRP. The authors conclude that the strong presence of anti-inflammatory mediators in LR-PRP makes it a potential beneficial therapy for knee OA (Jayaram et al., 2023). However, further studies need to be conducted to evaluate the long-term effect of OA progression due to the detected enhanced expression of MMP9.

Belk et al. (2023) published a meta-analysis of published clinical studies to compare the safety and efficacy of HA, PRP or blood marrow aspirate concentrate (BMAC) to treat knee OA. They selected 27 clinical studies encompassing a total of 2396 patients and analyzed the data using network and non-network meta-analysis statistics as required. The results indicated that both BMAC and PRP were significantly more effective in improving WOMAC, VAS and IKDC scores than IAHA injections; however, there were no significant differences in outcome scores between PRP and BMAC.

The authors postulated that this effect, particularly for PRP, may be due to the growth factors within PRP modulating and suppressing the inflammatory and catabolic environment of the OA joint. They also reported significant post-injection improvements in patients who received LR-PRP compared with IAHA as assessed by outcome scores. The authors attributed the improved outcome identified in patients receiving BMAC vs IAHA to the presence of growth factors and bone marrow mesenchymal stem cells within BMAC, in a similar manner to PRP (Belk et al., 2023).

Filardo et al. (2021) also conducted a meta-analysis of RCT to evaluate the efficacy of IA PRP treatments for OA knee pain. While Belk et al. (2023) only included comparisons with IAHA injections, Filardo et al. (2021) also evaluated potential treatment differences in PRP vs placebo, PRP vs HA and PRP vs steroids using a total of 34 clinical trials encompassing 3277 patients. The authors used changes in WOMAC score as their primary outcome at 6 and 12 months post intervention, as well as AS and KOOS pain scores as the secondary outcomes. They conducted statistical analysis using a z test on pooled mean differences and pooled risk ratio.

PRP provided a clinically significant difference vs placebo at the 12 month followup based on WOMAC score but not at the earlier 6 month time point. When evaluating PRP vs IAHA, the authors saw a clinically significant difference favoring PRP injections at both the 6 and 12 months. Finally, the authors reported that a meta-analysis of PRP vs steroid could not be carried out because there were only two studies, but both studies did report significant benefit of PRP (Filardo et al., 2021).

Individually, PRP and HA show varied efficacy in treatin OA pain. To understand the clinical efficacy and safety of combined treatment of HA and PRP, Zhao et al. (2020) conducted a meta-analysis composed of 940 patients across five RCTs and two cohort studies. The patients were between 40 and 60 years old, with varied severity of OA ranging from Kellgren-Lawrence grade 1 to grade 4. Pain scores and adverse effects were evaluated for 6–12 months post-intervention.

Dual HA-PRP treatment significantly improved VAS score vs HA alone six months post-intervention, and WOMAC score was significantly higher at 12 months post-treatment than with PRP alone. While significant improvements were detected at 6 and 12 months post-treatment, no significant differences were observed at 1 month or 3 months post-treatment. The authors therefore proposed that this dual therapy was of particular benefit for patients predicted to have long-term knee OA pain. When adverse effects were evaluated, the combined HA-PRP therapy showed no significant differences compared with single injections of HA or PRP, further supporting the safety of this treatment (Zhao et al., (2020). These studies provide strong evidence for the improved clinical outcome of PRP as a treatment of OA pain. However, further work is needed to standardize the preparation parameters and leukocyte composition of PRP injections.

Overall, several therapeutic strategies are currently used to manage OA. However, optimal strategies to manage pain associated with a progressive disease such as OA are currently not available. There is a critical need to develop novel therapeutic strategies and sustained release formulations to address the issue of long-term pain associated with OA.

ACKNOWLEDGEMENTS

We acknowledge funding from the National Institute of Arthritis and Musculoskeletal and Skin Diseases (RO1 AR075143 and RO1 AR075143-S1).

LIST OF ABBREVIATIONS

BMAC	Blood Marrow Aspirate Concentrate
CS	Corticosteroids
ER	Extended-release
HA	Hyaluronic acid
IAHA	Intra-articular injections of hyaluronic acid
LA	Local anesthetic
OA	Osteoarthritis
PRP	Platelet-rich plasma
PLGA	Poly-lactic-co-glycolic-acid
SMD	Standard mean differences
TKA	Total knee arthroplasty
TA	Triamcinolone acetonide
VRS	Verbal rating scale

REFERENCES

Al-Hasani, R., & Bruchas, M. R. (2011). Molecular mechanisms of opioid receptor-dependent signaling and behavior. *Anesthesiology*. 115: 1363–1381.

Alliance, O. A. (2023). *OA Prevalence and Burden*. https://oaaction.unc.edu/oa-module/oa-prevalence-and-burden/

Altman, R. D., Manjoo, A., Fierlinger, A., Niazi, F., & Nicholls, M. (2015). The mechanism of action for hyaluronic acid treatment in the osteoarthritic knee: A systematic review. *BMC Musculoskelet. Disord.* 16: 1–10.

American Academy of Orthopaedic Surgeons. (2021). *Management of Osteoarthritis of the Knee (NonArthroplasty) Evidence-Based Clinical Practice Guideline.* www.aaos.org/oak3cpg

Baker, K., Grainger, A., Niu, J., Clancy, M., Guermazi, A., Crema, M., Hughes, L., Buckwalter, J., Wooley, A., Nevitt, M., & Felson, D. T. (2010). Relation of synovitis to knee pain using contrast-enhanced MRIs. *Ann. Rheum. Dis.* 69: 1779–1783.

Balazs, E. A., Watson, D., Duff, I. F., & Roseman, S. (1967). Hyaluronic acid in synovial fluid. I. Molecular parameters of hyaluronic acid in normal and arthritic human fluids. *Arthritis Rheumatol.* 10: 357–376.

Band, P. A., Heeter, J., Wisniewski, H. G., Liublinska, V., Pattanayak, C. W., Karia, R. J., Stabler, T., Balazs, E. A., & Kraus, V. B. (2015). Hyaluronan molecular weight distribution is associated with the risk of knee osteoarthritis progression. *Osteoarthr. Cartil.* 23: 70–76.

Bannuru, R. R., Osani, M. C., Vaysbrot, E. E., Arden, N. K., Bennell, K., Bierma-Zeinstra, S. M. A., Kraus, V. B., Lohmander, L. S., Abbott, J. H., Bhandari, M., & Blanco, F. J. (2019). OARSI guidelines for the non-surgical management of knee, hip, and polyarticular osteoarthritis. *Osteoarthr. Cartil.* 27: 1578–1589.

Barbour, K. E., Helmick, C. G., Boring, M., & Brady, T. J. (2017). Vital signs: Prevalence of doctor-diagnosed arthritis and arthritis-attributable activity limitation—United States, 2013–2015. *Morb. Mortal. Wkly. Rep.* 66: 246–253.

Bedard, N. A., DeMik, D. E., Glass, N. A., Burnett, R. A., Bozic, K. J., & Callaghan, J. J. (2018). Impact of clinical practice guidelines on use of intra-articular hyaluronic acid and corticosteroid injections for knee osteoarthritis. *J. Bone Joint Surg.* 100: 827–834.

Belk, J. W., Lim, J. J., Keeter, C., McCulloch, P. C., Houck, D. A., McCarty, E. C., Frank, R. M., & Kraeutler, M. J. (2023). Patients with knee osteoarthritis who receive platelet-rich plasma or bone-marrow aspirate concentrate injections have better outcomes than patients who receive hyaluronic acid: Systematic review and meta-analysis. *Arthroscopy.* 39: 1714–1734.

Bennell, K. L., Paterson, K. L., Metcalf, B. R., Duong, V., Eyles, J., Kasza, J., Wang, Y., Cicuttini, F., Buchbinder, R., Forbes, A., & Harris, A. (2021). Effect of intra-articular platelet-rich plasma vs placebo injection on pain and medial tibial cartilage volume in patients with knee osteoarthritis: The RESTORE randomized clinical trial. *JAMA.* 326: 2021–2030.

Bhimana, D., & Bhimana, V. (2018). The historical perspective of local anesthetics. *Dev. Anaesth. Pain Manag.* 1: 1–8.

Biondich, A. S., & Joslin, J. D. (2016). Coca: The history and medical significance of an ancient Andean tradition. *Emerg. Med. Int.* 2016: 4048764.

Bruyère, O., Honvo, G., Veronese, N., Arden, N. K., Branco, J., Curtis, E. M., Al-Daghri, N. M., Herrero-Beaumont, G., Martel-Pelletier, J., Pelletier, J. P., & Rannou, F. (2019). An updated algorithm recommendation for the management of knee osteoarthritis from the European Society for Clinical and Economic Aspects of Osteoporosis, Osteoarthritis and Musculoskeletal Diseases (ESCEO). *Semin. Arthritis Rheumatol.* 49: 337–350.

Buchko, J. Z., Gurney-Dunlop, T., & Shin, J. J. (2015). Knee chondrolysis by infusion of bupivacaine with epinephrine through an intra-articular pain pump catheter after arthroscopic ACL reconstruction. *Am. J. Sports Med.* 43: 337–344.

Butterworth, J. F. (2009). Clinical pharmacology of local anesthetics. In *Hadzic's Textbook of Regional Anesthesia and Acute Pain Management.* A. Hadzic, Ed. New York: McGraw-Hill Education, pp. 96–113.

Butterworth, J. F., Mackey, D. C., & Wasnick, J. D. (2018). Adjuncts to anesthesia. In *Morgan and Mikhail's Clinical Anesthesiology.* J. F. Butterworth, D. C. Mackey, and J. D. Wasnick, Eds. New York: McGraw-Hill Education.

Charnwichai, P., Tammachote, R., Tammachote, N., Chaichana, T., & Kitkumthorn, N. (2023). Histological features of knee osteoarthritis treated with triamcinolone acetonide and hyaluronic acid. *Biomed. Rep.* 18: 1–8.

Chen, J. J., Wu, Y. C., Wang, J. S., & Lee, C. H. (2023). Liposomal bupivacaine administration is not superior to traditional periarticular injection for postoperative pain management following total knee arthroplasty: A meta-analysis of randomized controlled trials. *J. Orthop. Surg. Res.* 18: 206.

Chen, T. W., Wardill, T. J., Sun, Y., Pulver, S. R., Renninger, S. L., Baohan, A., Schreiter, E. R., Kerr, R. A., Orger, M. B., Jayaraman, V., & Looger, L. L. (2013). Ultrasensitive fluorescent proteins for imaging neuronal activity. *Nature.* 499: 295–300.

Conaghan, P. G., Hunter, D. J., Cohen, S. B., Kraus, V. B., Berenbaum, F., Lieberman, J. R., Jones, D. G., Spitzer, A. I., Jevsevar, D. S., Katz, N. P., & Burgess, D. J. (2018). Effects of a single intra-articular injection of a microsphere formulation of triamcinolone acetonide on knee osteoarthritis pain: A double-blinded, randomized, placebo-controlled, multinational study. *J. Bone Joint Surg. Am.* 100: 666–677.

Cui, C., Zheng, L., Fan, Y., Zhang, J., Xu, R., Xie, J., & Zhou, X. (2020). Parathyroid hormone ameliorates temporomandibular joint osteoarthritic-like changes related to age. *Cell Proliferation.* 53: e12755.

da Costa, B. R., Hari, R., & Jüni, P. (2016). Intra-articular corticosteroids for osteoarthritis of the knee. *JAMA.* 316: 2671–2672.

Dysart, S., Utkina, K., Stong, L., Nelson, W., Sacks, N., Healey, B., & Niazi, F. (2021). Insights from real-world analysis of treatment patterns in patients with newly diagnosed knee osteoarthritis. *Am. Health Drug Benefits.* 14: 56–62.

Eckhard, L., Jones, T., Collins, J. E., Shrestha, S., & Fitz, W. (2019). Increased postoperative dexamethasone and gabapentin reduces opioid consumption after total knee arthroplasty. *Knee Surg. Sports Traumatol. Arthrosc.* 27: 2167–2172.

Ene, R., Sinescu, R. D., Ene, P., Cîrstoiu, M. M., & Cîrstoiu, F. C. (2015). Synovial inflammation in patients with different stages of knee osteoarthritis. *Rom. J. Morphol. Embryol.* 56: 169–173.

Farmer, T., Morris, S. C., Quigley, R., Amin, N. H., Wongworawat, M. D., & Syed, H. M. (2020). Chondrotoxicity of local anesthetics: Liposomal bupivacaine is less chondrotoxic than standard bupivacaine. *Adv. Pharmacol. Pharm. Sci.* 2020: 5794187.

Feng, J. E., Ikwuazom, C. P., Mahure, S. A., Waren, D. P., Slover, J. D., Schwarzkopf, R. S., Long, W. J., & Macaulay, W. B. (2021). Discontinuation of the liposomal delivery of bupivacaine has no effect on pain management after primary total knee arthroplasty: No effect on pain scores, opioid consumption, or functional status. *Bone Joint J.* 103: 102–107.

Filardo, G., Previtali, D., Napoli, F., Candrian, C., Zaffagnini, S., & Grassi, A. (2021). PRP injections for the treatment of knee osteoarthritis: A meta-analysis of randomized controlled trials. *Cartilage.* 13: 364S–375S.

Glyn-Jones, S., Palmer, A. J., Agricola, R., Price, A. J., Vincent, T. L., & Weinans, H. (2015). Osteoarthritis. *Lancet.* 386: 376–387.

Guermazi, A., Neogi, T., Katz, J. N., Kwoh, C. K., Conaghan, P. G., Felson, D. T., & Roemer, F. W. (2020). Intra-articular corticosteroid injections for the treatment of hip and knee osteoarthritis-related pain: Considerations and controversies with a focus on imaging—Radiology scientific expert panel. *Radiology.* 297: 503–512.

Gwam, C. U., Emara, A. K., Ogbonnaya, I. A., Zuskov, A., Luo, T. D., & Plate, J. F. (2021). Addressing national opioid prescribing practices for knee osteoarthritis: An analysis of an estimated 41,389,332 patients with knee arthritis. *J. Am. Acad. Orthop. Surg.* 29: e337–e344.

Haviv, B., Bronak, S., & Thein, R. (2013). The complexity of pain around the knee in patients with osteoarthritis. *Isr. Med. Assoc. J.* 15:178–181.

Hummer, C. D., Angst, F., Ngai, W., Whittington, C., Yoon, S. S., Duarte, L., Manitt, C., & Schemitsch, E. (2020). High molecular weight Intraarticular hyaluronic acid for the treatment of knee osteoarthritis: A network meta-analysis. *BMC Musculoskelet. Disord.* 21: 1–10.

Hunter, D. J., Chang, C. C., Wei, J. C. C., Lin, H. Y., Brown, C., Tai, T. T., Wu, C. F., Chuang, W. C. M., & Shih, S. F. (2022). TLC599 in patients with osteoarthritis of the knee: A phase IIa, randomized, placebo-controlled, dose-finding study. *Arthritis Res. Ther.* 24: 1–11.

Inturrisi, C. E. (2002). Clinical pharmacology of opioids for pain. *Clin. J. Pain.* 18: S3–S13.

Jamison, R. N., & Mao, J. (2015). Opioid analgesics. *Mayo Clin. Proc.* 90: 957–968.

Jayaram, P., Kennedy, D. J., Yeh, P., & Dragoo, J. (2019). Chondrotoxic effects of local anesthetics on human knee articular cartilage: A systematic review. *PM&R.* 11: 379–400.

Jayaram, P., Mitchell, P. J., Shybut, T. B., Moseley, B. J., & Lee, B. (2023). Leukocyte-rich platelet-rich plasma is predominantly anti-inflammatory compared with leukocyte-poor platelet-rich plasma in patients with mild-moderate knee osteoarthritis: A prospective, descriptive laboratory study. *Am. J. Sports Med.* 51: 2133–2140.

Kolasinski, S. L., Neogi, T., Hochberg, M. C., Oatis, C., Guyatt, G., Block, J., Callahan, L., Copenhaver, C., Dodge, C., Felson, D., & Gellar, K. (2020). 2019 American College of Rheumatology/Arthritis Foundation guideline for the management of osteoarthritis of the hand, hip, and knee. *Arthritis Rheumatol.* 72: 220–233.

Kompel, A. J., Roemer, F. W., Murakami, A. M., Diaz, L. E., Crema, M. D., & Guermazi, A. (2019). Intra-articular corticosteroid injections in the hip and knee: Perhaps not as safe as we thought? *Radiology.* 293: 656–663.

Kraus, V. B., Conaghan, P. G., Aazami, H. A., Mehra, P., Kivitz, A. J., Lufkin, J., Hauben, J., Johnson, J. R., & Bodick, N. (2018). Synovial and systemic pharmacokinetics (PK) of triamcinolone acetonide (TA) following intra-articular (IA) injection of an extended-release microsphere-based formulation (FX006) or standard crystalline suspension in patients with knee osteoarthritis (OA). *Osteoarthr. Cartil.* 26: 34–42.

Kreuz, P. C., Steinwachs, M., & Angele, P. (2018). Single-dose local anesthetics exhibit a type-, dose-, and time-dependent chondrotoxic effect on chondrocytes and cartilage: A systematic review of the current literature. *Knee Surg. Sports Traumatol. Arthrosc.* 26: 819–830.

Legre-Boyer, V. (2015). Viscosupplementation: Techniques, indications, results. *Orthop. Traumatol.- Sur.* 101: S101–S108.

Lonza, G. C., Yuan, F., Pham, F. M., Wright, C. T., Arellano-Kruse, A., & Andrawis, J. (2023). Liposomal bupivacaine versus continuous nerve block: Liposomal bupivacaine may be non-inferior and more cost effective. *J. Arthroplasty.* 38: 831–835.

Maia, P. A. V., Cossich, V. R. A., Salles-Neto, J. I., Aguiar, D. P., & de Sousa, E. B. (2019). Viscosupplementation improves pain, function and muscle strength, but not proprioception, in patients with knee osteoarthritis: A prospective randomized trial. *Clinics.* 74: e1207.

Malige, A., Pellegrino, A. N., Kunkle, K., Konopitski, A. K., Brogle, P. J., & Nwachuku, C. O. (2022). Liposomal bupivacaine in adductor canal blocks before total knee arthroplasty leads to improved postoperative outcomes: A randomized controlled trial. *J. Arthroplasty.* 37: 1549–1556.

Martin, C. L., & Browne, J. A. (2019). Intra-articular corticosteroid injections for symptomatic knee osteoarthritis: What the orthopaedic provider needs to know. *J. Am. Acad. Orthop. Surg.* 27: e758–e766.

Nicholls, M., Manjoo, A., Shaw, P., Niazi, F., & Rosen, J. (2018). A comparison between rheological properties of intra-articular hyaluronic acid preparations and reported human synovial fluid. *Adv. Ther.* 35: 523–530.

O'Neill, T. W., & Felson, D. T. (2018). Mechanisms of osteoarthritis (OA) pain. *Curr. Osteoporos. Rep.* 16: 611–616.

Pearson, M. J., Herndler-Brandstetter, D., Tariq, M. A., Nicholson, T. A., Philp, A. M., Smith, H. L., Davis, E. T., Jones, S. W., & Lord, J. M. (2017). IL-6 secretion in osteoarthritis patients is mediated by chondrocyte-synovial fibroblast cross-talk and is enhanced by obesity. *Sci. Rep.* 7: 3451.

Pereira, H., Sousa, D. A., Cunha, A., Andrade, R., Espregueira-Mendes, J., Oliveira, J. M., & Reis, R. L. (2018). Hyaluronic acid. In *Osteochondral Tissue Engineering: Challenges, Current Strategies, and Technological Advances.* J. M. Oliveira, S. Pina, R. L. Reis, and J. S. Roman, Eds. Cham: Springer, pp. 137–153.

Pereira, T. V., Jüni, P., Saadat, P., Xing, D., Yao, L., Bobos, P., Agarwal, A., Hincapié, C. A., & da Costa, B. R. (2022). Viscosupplementation for knee osteoarthritis: Systematic review and meta-analysis. *BMJ.* 378: e069722.

Primorac, D., Molnar, V., Rod, E., Jeleč, Ž., Čukelj, F., Matišić, V., Vrdoljak, T., Hudetz, D., Hajsok, H., & Borić, I. (2020). Knee osteoarthritis: A review of pathogenesis and state-of-the-art non-operative therapeutic considerations. *Genes.* 11: 854.

Rosenblum, A., Marsch, L. A., Joseph, H., & Portenoy, R. K. (2008). Opioids and the treatment of chronic pain: Controversies, current status, and future directions. *Exp. Clin. Psychopharmacol.* 16: 405–416.

Schanté, C. E., Zuber, G., Herlin, C., & Vandamme, T. F. (2011). Chemical modifications of hyaluronic acid for the synthesis of derivatives for a broad range of biomedical applications. *Carbohydr. Polym.* 85: 469–489.

Shanahan, E. M., Robinson, L., Lyne, S., Woodman, R., Cai, F., Dissanayake, K., Paddick, K., Cheung, G., & Voyvodic, F. (2023). Genicular nerve block for pain management in patients with knee osteoarthritis: A randomized placebo-controlled trial. *Arthritis Rheumatol.* 75: 201–209.

Shaw, K. A., Moreland, C., Jacobs, J., Hire, J. M., Topolski, R., Hoyt, N., Parada, S. A., & Cameron, C. D. (2018). Improved chondrotoxic profile of liposomal bupivacaine compared with standard bupivacaine after intra-articular infiltration in a porcine model. *Am. J. Sports Med.* 46: 66–71.

Spitzer, A. I., Richmond, J. C., Kraus, V. B., Gomoll, A., Jones, D. G., Huffman, K. M., Peterfy, C., Cinar, A., Lufkin, J., & Kelley, S. D. (2019). Safety and efficacy of repeat administration of triamcinolone acetonide extended-release in osteoarthritis of the knee: A phase 3b, open-label study. *Rheumatol. Ther.* 6: 109–124.

Sudha, P. N., & Rose, M. H. (2014). Beneficial effects of hyaluronic acid. *Adv. Food Nutr. Res.* 72: 137–176.

Vincent, T. L. (2020). Of mice and men: Converging on a common molecular understanding of osteoarthritis. *Lancet Rheumatol.* 2: e633–e645.

Wadlund, D. L. (2017). Local anesthetic systemic toxicity. *AORN J.* 106: 367–377.

Webner, D., Huang, Y., & Hummer III, C. D. (2021). Intraarticular hyaluronic acid preparations for knee osteoarthritis: Are some better than others? *Cartilage.* 13: 1619S–1636S.

Wu, R., Ma, Y., Li, M., Li, Q., Deng, Z., Chen, Y., Zheng, Q., & Fu, G. (2023). Baseline knee pain predicts long-term response of intra-articular steroid injection in symptomatic knee osteoarthritis: Data from OAI. *Cartilage.* 14: 144–151.

Xie, X., Zhang, C., & Tuan, R. S. (2014). Biology of platelet-rich plasma and its clinical application in cartilage repair. *Arthritis Res. Ther.* 16: 1–15.

Yasar, E., Kesikburun, S., Kılıç, C., Güzelküçük, Ü., Yazar, F., & Tan, A. K. (2015). Accuracy of ultrasound-guided genicular nerve block: A cadaveric study. *Pain Physician.* 18: E899–E904.

Yu, H., Huang, T., Lu, W. W., Tong, L., & Chen, D. (2022). Osteoarthritis pain. *Int. J. Mol. Sci.* 23: 4642.

Zhang, Y., & Jordan, J. M. (2010). Epidemiology of osteoarthritis. *Clin. Geriatr. Med.* 26: 355–369.

Zhao, J., Huang, H., Liang, G., Zeng, L. F., Yang, W., & Liu, J. (2020). Effects and safety of the combination of platelet-rich plasma (PRP) and hyaluronic acid (HA) in the treatment of knee osteoarthritis: A systematic review and meta-analysis. *BMC Musculoskelet. Disord.* 21: 1–12.f

Index

Note: Page numbers in *italics* indicate a figure and page numbers in **bold** indicate a table on the corresponding page.

D

E

F

G

O

P

Q

R

S

T

U

V

W

X

Z

For Product Safety Concerns and Information please contact our EU representative GPSR@taylorandfrancis.com
Taylor & Francis Verlag GmbH, Kaufingerstraße 24, 80331 München, Germany

www.ingramcontent.com/pod-product-compliance
Lightning Source LLC
LaVergne TN
LVHW081313110826
845149LV00006B/1495

* 9 7 8 1 0 3 2 3 0 9 3 2 3 *